Surgical Techniques in Rectal Cancer

Giovanni Dapri • John H Marks
Editors

Surgical Techniques in Rectal Cancer

Transanal, Laparoscopic and Robotic Approach

Springer

Editors
Giovanni Dapri
Saint-Pierre University Hospital
Department of Gastrointestinal Surgery
European School of Laparoscopic Surgery
Brussels
Belgium

John H Marks
Minimally Invasive Colorectal Surgery
Lankenau Medical Center
Main Line Healthcare
Wynnewood, PA
USA

ISBN 978-4-431-55578-0 ISBN 978-4-431-55579-7 (eBook)
https://doi.org/10.1007/978-4-431-55579-7

Library of Congress Control Number: 2017954362

Printed on acid-free paper

This Springer imprint is published by Springer Nature
The registered company is Springer Japan KK
The registered company address is: Chiyoda First Bldg. East, 3-8-1 Nishi-Kanda, Chiyoda-ku, Tokyo 101-0065, Japan

Foreword 1

Perhaps it is providence that set the stage for the sea change in rectal cancer management that has occurred in the last decade. After nearly a century of relatively sparse production of new and acceptable scientific information regarding rectal cancer, the recent surgical revolution has changed everything. The explosion of interest and performance of minimally invasive surgery with the involvement of an entirely new breed of surgeons, youthful and energetic, has led to new and imaginative ways to accomplish surgical objectives. A small cadre of surgeons who focus their talents upon rectal cancer treatment has developed procedures that are beyond ordinary imagination. These methods are capable of reducing perioperative discomfort, increasing patient safety and curability while maximizing the preservation of normal sphincter function; and as a result these new methods, despite the technical challenge, are gaining traction in the surgical community. Based on a platform of neoadjuvant therapy that the surgical–oncologic world has accepted as beneficial, these new surgical techniques have become transformational.

With this backdrop of dramatic changes in rectal cancer surgery, this book, *Surgical Techniques in Rectal Cancer*, is timely and serves a powerful need. The book is also a celebration of the energy, creativity, courage, and pioneering spirit of the authors. This text is predicted to become a standard reference for contemporary cutting-edge comprehensive rectal cancer management. Rectal cancer's reputation among patients and surgeons alike as one of the most dreaded visceral neoplasms may diminish with the adoption of the surgical techniques and multidisciplinary treatment plans described in this text. Having spent almost seven decades in search of better ways to treat rectal cancer, I have the distinct privilege and honor to offer this commentary and to salute the author heroes who through their talents and new ideas have provided new hope and promise for the rectal cancer patient.

Gerald Marks, MD, F.A.C.S., F.A.S.C.R.S
Lankenau Medical Center
Wynnewood, PA, USA

Founding President
Society of American Gastrointestinal
Endoscopic Surgeons (SAGES)

Foreword 2

There has never been a time in coloproctology when there are so many "known unknowns." This book brilliantly sets out to update us on each of them and to inform us of where each new technology stands in the spectrum of our specialty. In a book so dazzling with new technology for surgery and endoscopy, it is good that the first great "known unknown"—the Complete Response—is given the priority it deserves. I believe that it is now urgent for the profession to recognize that a pathological complete response (pCR) on a histology report after major surgery usually represents one or more errors of judgment or communication by the attending physicians. In their hands a major technological achievement has been reduced for the patient to a truly "hollow victory." That there should be a whole chapter on the management of such cases by surveillance is testament to the balanced editorship of this volume. All the old-fashioned human skills and ability to communicate with the patient are challenged in the face of this new "known unknown."

The year 2016 is indeed a battleground for so many new technologies. Many patients have been led to believe that a robot performing their operation will be superior to a human. Patients need to understand that a bad surgeon with the very best robot is a bad choice when compared with a good surgeon with the instruments of yesteryear—sharp long scissors, the St. Marks retractor, a good light, and the "Patience of Job." Nevertheless, the future will belong to the surgeon who takes those same qualities and applies them with all the advantages of magnification, superior vision, the best diathermy, the ligasure, and all the panoply of aids to modern precision and hemostasis. He will certainly win the everlasting battle for the best outcome.

So many new technologies also threaten the patient with the "hammer and nail" syndrome—if the only tool you have is a hammer the world becomes populated with nails! Throughout medicine the super-specialist with one procedure needs restraint: "because it can be done is not necessarily a reason for doing it!" Another old-fashioned skill required of the attending physician is that of the broker who puts the patient into the right hands.

All the new technologies require patience, skill, and practice, and the specialist colorectal unit of the future will need a wide menu of available alternatives. Laparoscopy, robotics, and endo-luminal tools of the future—all will be needed along with an improved anatomical grasp of the fascial layers of the pelvis, a keen pursuit of the neuro-anatomy of sex and continence—all these will need to be combined with recognition that "practice makes perfect." Sadly, as Sir Edmund Hillary of Mount Everest fame said, "If it is more difficult it will be done worse by some." Teaching, auditing, peer review, and a willingness to accept criticism and improvement—all these mean that the impending struggle between technologies needs to be backed by great skill, hard work, and humility from the surgeons of the next generation. For coloproctology "know-how" they can start by reading this book.

Bill Heald, M.D.
Pelican Cancer Foundation
Basingstoke, UK

Preface

In the last century, the treatment of rectal cancer has been predicated on an abdominoperineal resection (APR). The last decade has seen an explosion of alternatives for rectal cancer specialists to use for the cure of their patients. Widespread use of neoadjuvant chemoradiation, total mesorectal excision (TME), transanal abdominal transanal surgery (TATA), and minimally invasive surgery (MIS) have allowed for the expansion of sphincter preservation and greater cure for the rectal cancer patient. The merger of these approaches has promoted an emphasis on both curing the cancer and maximizing the quality of life.

However, while an impressive multitude of options are now available, the quantity of techniques coupled with the variety of technology and the judgment required to offer an individualized treatment for the rectal cancer patient can leave both the beginning surgeon and the experienced practitioner at a loss as to how best to proceed.

This book has been created to offer the clearest explanation and description of the most cutting-edge options available to treat rectal cancer. Starting with the introductions by Bill Heald, the father of TME surgery, and Gerald Marks, a pioneer in sphincter preservation after radiation therapy and TATA, the 32 chapters have been assigned to an all-star cast of worldwide pioneers in rectal cancer. Each chapter has been written with care and precision to offer to the reader an emphasis on the critical technical points as well as the major take-home messages. The clarity of the text is enhanced immeasurably by the numerous figures and illustrations, permitting complete understanding of each surgical technique from its beginning until the final step.

The two forewords, offered by giants in the field, introduce the reader to the tremendous content of this book. The organization of the book was created to take the reader from presentation of the cancer, through the essential anatomy, neoadjuvant treatment options, and then to the operating room.

This book on rectal cancer has been divided into three main parts: I. History, Anatomy, Evaluation and Medical Treatment; II. Abdominal Laparoscopy and Robot-Assisted; and III. Transanal Laparoscopy and Robot-Assisted.

The book has been written to be useful for everyone involved in rectal cancer management. From internists, gastroenterologists, endoscopists, oncologists, radiotherapists, and radiologists involved in the treatment of rectal cancer during their daily practice, to surgeons specialized in colorectal surgery, to junior faculty, to trainees all interested in new and innovative techniques, this book is for you. We hope you enjoy it!

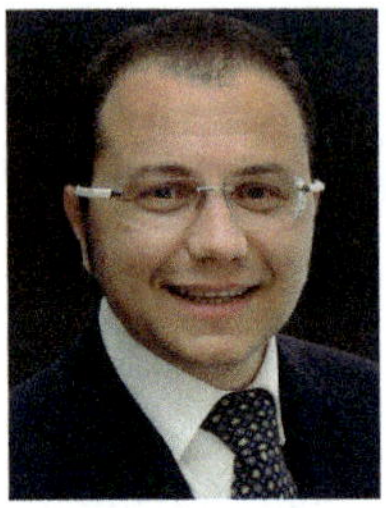

Giovanni Dapri

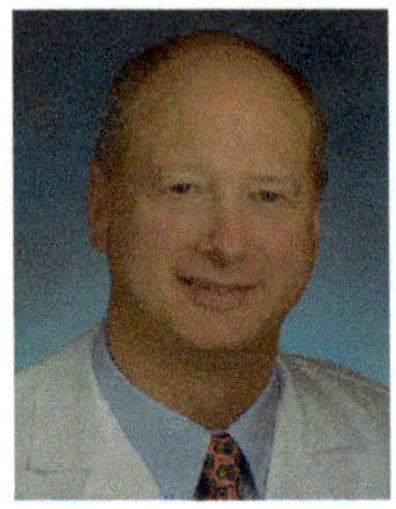

John H Marks

Contents

Part II Abdominal Laparoscopy and Robot-Assisted

Part I

History, Anatomy, Evaluation and Medical Treatment

History of Rectal Cancer Surgery

1

Sharaf Karim Perdawood

Abstract

The surgical treatment of rectal cancer is very challenging and is one of the most rapidly advancing. At this time, different varieties of treatment options exist and new surgical methods are being explored. Thanks to numerous great pioneers in colorectal surgery in the last century, surgery for rectal cancer has changed from being purely palliative to one that made this solid malignancy a curable disease in the vast majority of cases. The evolution path has started few centuries ago, with early efforts to relieve symptoms by limited excisions. With the evolvement of general anesthesia, more extensive resections were made possible and different approaches could be tried. With the accumulation of experience, tumor removal could be combined with conservation of bowel continuity, an option which was not possible earlier. Advances in the understanding of the pathophysiology of rectal cancer, has led to increasing chances of cure through adoption of different surgical principles. However, rectal cancer is still challenging and its treatment options continue to evolve. This chapter focuses on some important landmarks in the surgical treatment of rectal cancer and on some of those pioneers who have contributed to it and to shape the modern rectal cancer surgery.

Keywords

Rectal cancer • History • Surgery

S.K. Perdawood, M.D.
Consultant Colorectal Surgeon, Department of Surgery, Slagelse Hospital, Faelledvej 11, 4200 Slagelse, Denmark
e-mail: sharaf73@hotmail.com

G. Dapri, J.H. Marks (eds.), *Surgical Techniques in Rectal Cancer*,
https://doi.org/10.1007/978-4-431-55579-7_1

1.1 Stomas

Colorectal surgery is inseparable from stomas, thus studying the history of rectal cancer surgery necessitates knowledge of the history of stomas. This is as ancient as history of abdominal trauma, in which "stoma" was an inevitable result of. A clear reference to this is found in the Bibel, describing Eglons belly after being stabbed by Ehud "Even the handle sank in after the blade, and his bowels discharged. Ehud did not pull the sword out, and the fat closed in over it" [1]. For centuries, purposeful stoma formation was advocated to treat abdominal traumas and bowel obstruction. The later often due to incarcerated hernias or tumors, including obstructing rectal cancer. While evidence of stoma creation to relieve bowel obstruction can be found in the writing of the Greek Praxagorus in 400 B.C. "…he (an unknown doctor) seemed to be a very bold practitioner for in this distemper (bowel obstruction) if the remedies did not operate, he ordered an incision to be made into the belly and even into the gut itself and the excrements to be drawn out and the wound sewed up again" [2], the history does not tell us much about purposeful stoma formation until the beginnings of the eighteenth century.

In 1710, Alexis Littré suggested stoma creation for imperforated anus [3]. One of earliest reports of stoma creation to treat obstructing rectal cancer is by Daniel Pring, an English surgeon who performed a lumbar colostomy [3], a procedure which was invented by the Danish surgeon Duret Callisen [4], and later developed by Jean Zulema Amussat [3]. Being regarded as a palliative measure for many decades, the importance of stoma creation increased with the advances in the surgery for rectal cancer.

1.2 Perineal Approach

The first description of signs and symptoms of rectal cancer was made by the English surgeon John Arderne as early as in 1376 [5]. Rectal resection was, however not done until 1793, when Jean Faget performed the first ever mentioned rectal resection. The procedure was done for an extensive ischiorectal abscess, which appeared to be a perforated rectal cancer [6]. The procedure was, thus not planned to treat cancer. In the nineteenth century, the French surgeon Jacques Lisfranc performed the first planned rectal resection for cancer. This was done in 1826 in the pre-anesthetic era. Lisfranc's resection was a very limited one, composed basically of a wide local excision by removing the lower part of the rectum. In his paper which was read before the Academic Royale de Medecine 5 years later, he reported his initial results in nine patients. Six of these patients has survived and albeit surprisingly almost continent [7]. Similar procedures were performed in England by Hubert Mayo of the Middlesex Hospital in 1833, and James Wardrop in 1834 [8]. In Germany, Johann Dieffenbach reported a similar operation in 30 cases, all survived and were probably disease free for a year [9]. At that time, rectal cancer procedures were mostly palliative and with this perineal approach, exposure was very limited, allowed only the lowest part of the rectum and the anal canal to be removed.

1.3 Posterior Approach

With the advent of anesthesia, it became easier to operate and more extensive resections could be performed. Of particular interest is the change in the operative technique for rectal excision, which took the form of removal of the coccyx. This has served as a measure that could allow for more extensive excisions and more effective drainage of the blood which was particularly a problem at that era, due to lack of effective intraoperative hemostatic measures. One of the pioneers, who have contributed to the spread of coccyx removal was Verneuil, who in 1873 and encouraged by the French surgeon Jean Zulema Amussat, excised the coccyx to extend the limits of excision [10]. Theodore Kocher in Germany (Fig. 1.1) also adopted coccyx excision in 1874 [11].

While these advances were adopted by increasing number of surgeons, these excisions could be criticized due to the dangers of bleeding, sepsis, and incontinence. The English surgeon Thomas Curling of the London Hospital and President of the Royal College of Surgeons (Fig. 1.2) wrote in 1876: "Excision of the carcinomatous rectum was practiced formerly by Lisfranc and Dieffenbach and is

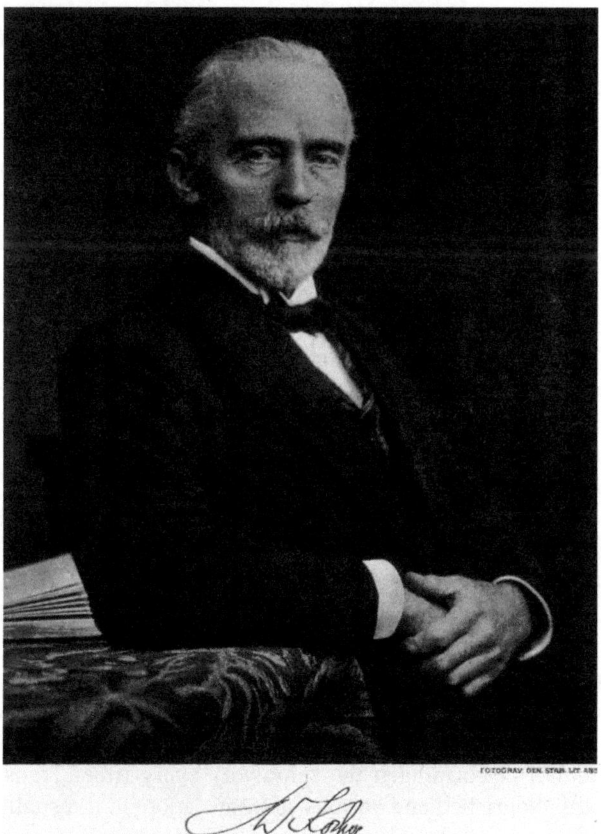

Fig. 1.1 Emil Theodor Kocher (1841-1917)

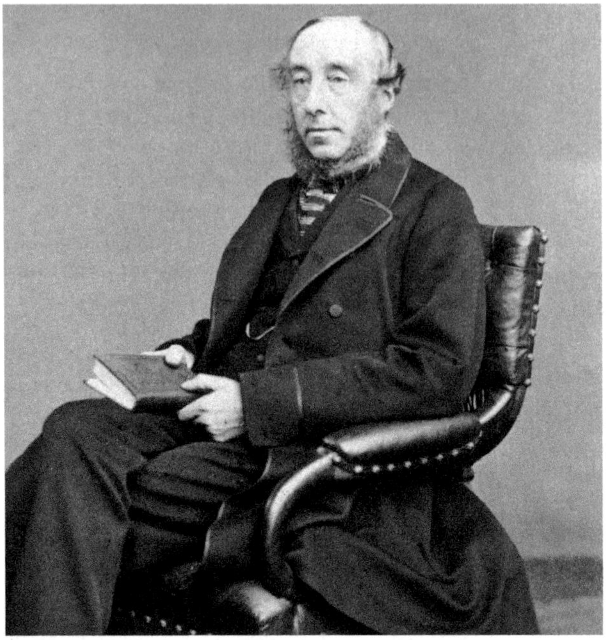

Fig. 1.2 Thomas Blizard Curling (1811–1888)

resorted to in the present day by several German surgeons. I am unwilling to discourage any attempt to relieve so dire a disease as cancer of the rectum, but knowing the danger that must be incurred from haemorhage in the operation, the misery likely to ensue from incontinence of faeces as well as the prospect of early return of the disease, I cannot think that a chance even of a prolongation of life is worth acceptance on the terms offered of such an operation" [12]. Despite critics from Curling and other contemporary surgeons, increasing number of rectal excisions were performed. In 1876, William Harrison Cripps presented 53 cases operated between 1826 and 1875. The mortality rate was 20% and it seemed that survivors had their lives prolonged, the incontinence was not "too high." The main cause of death was peritonitis.

Another landmark in the history of rectal excision is the popularization of transsacral approach by the German surgeon Paul Kraske (Fig. 1.3). He was at a time Director of the Clinic at Freiberg, and after practicing the approach described by Kocher, he wanted to have a better exposure for lesions higher up in the rectum as well as to achieve a better control of hemorrhage [11]. Kraske made a new posterior approach removing the coccyx and part of the sacrum as well. His results in two patients were read to the 14th Congress of the German Society of Surgeons in Berlin 1885. This new approach was probably not standardized and even Kraske himself was not performing it the same way every time. Transsacral approach has afterwards flourished and various surgeons adopted it, usually adding their own modifications, like Julius Hochenegg who brought out the upper cut end of the bowel through the anus (pull through technique).

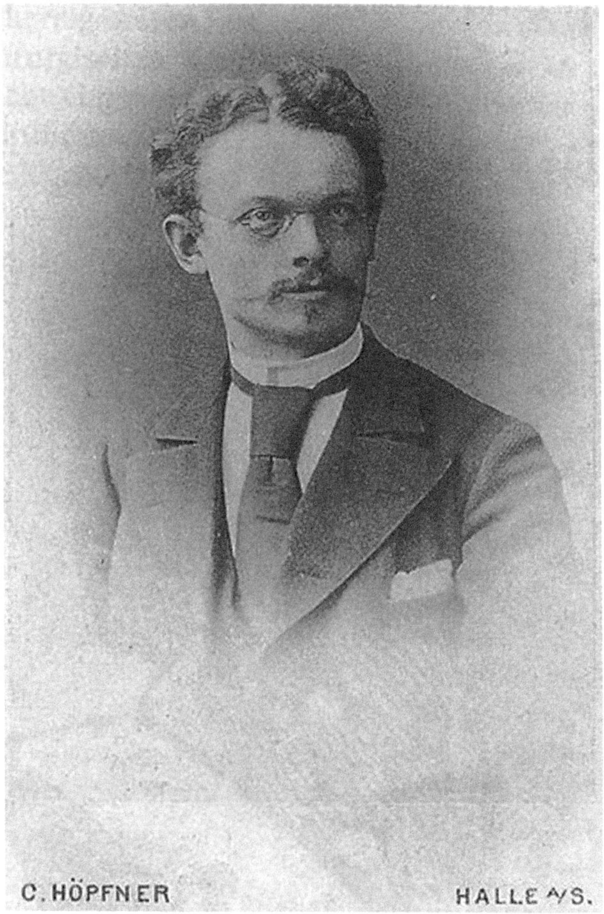

Fig. 1.3 Paul Kraske (1851–1930)

Due to the mutilating nature of these approaches, attempts to find better and less invasive methods continued. One of the controversial approaches is the transvaginal approach. A.T. Norton described in 1889 a transvaginal resection with the reestablishment of continuity and postoperative continence [13]. William Heath Byford (Fig. 1.4) performed a transvaginal resection, combined with excision of the posterior vaginal wall and sutured both ends of the bowel to the vaginal defect. He then closed the vaginal introitus, and has maintained bowel continuity [14]. Another modification of this transvaginal procedure with utilization of the vaginal lumen is the method advocated by L. L. McArthur [15]. He used the vaginal lumen to replace the excised rectum, and claimed that the patient was continent. Byford postulated the following advantages of the transvaginal approach: replacement of the excised rectum by vagina, excision of as high tumors through this method as in transsacral approach with less trauma for the patient, exploration of the peritoneal cavity prior to resection itself and lastly, the procedure could be aborted and could end as a diagnostic procedure without much trauma for the patient.

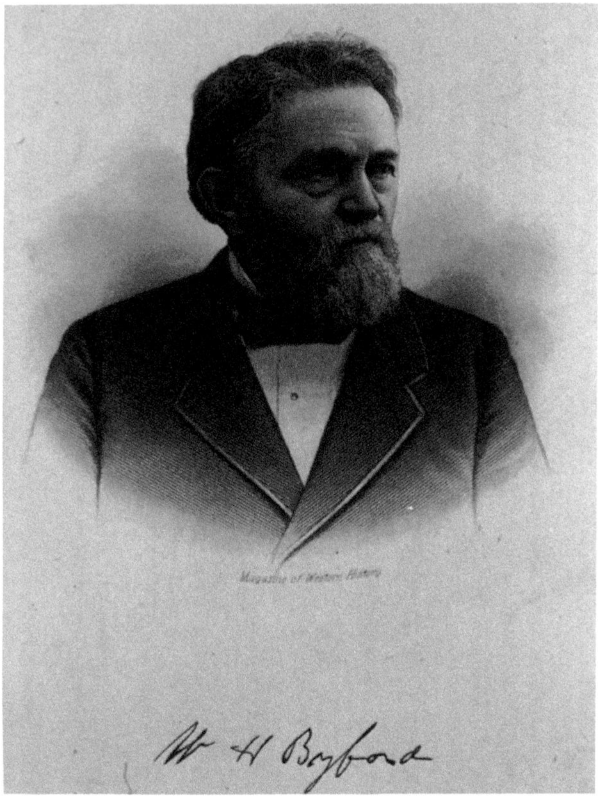

Fig. 1.4 William Heath Byford (1817–1890)

1.4 Abdominoperineal Excision

The first surgeon who performed a combined abdomino (anterior)—perineal (posterior) excision for rectal cancer is the German surgeon Vincent Czerny (Fig. 1.5) in 1883. The procedure was probably done merely by chance, as it was planned as a routine transsacral approach for a high rectal cancer. However, it seems that Czerny was unable to complete the procedure through a transsacral route for some reason. He then simply turned the patient to a supine position and completed the procedure by transabdominal approach. The operation was, however unsuccessful in terms of patient survival [16]. Nonetheless, this accidentally performed procedure marks a new era in the surgical treatment of rectal cancer in terms of being able to do a synchronous abdominoperineal rectal resection.

At the end of the nineteenth century and the beginning of twentieth century, abdominoperineal excision was performed in a way that the rectum was removed as a tube without mesorectum and without removing the lymphatics. At the same time, a growing attention was paid to local disease recurrence. Early results of that kind

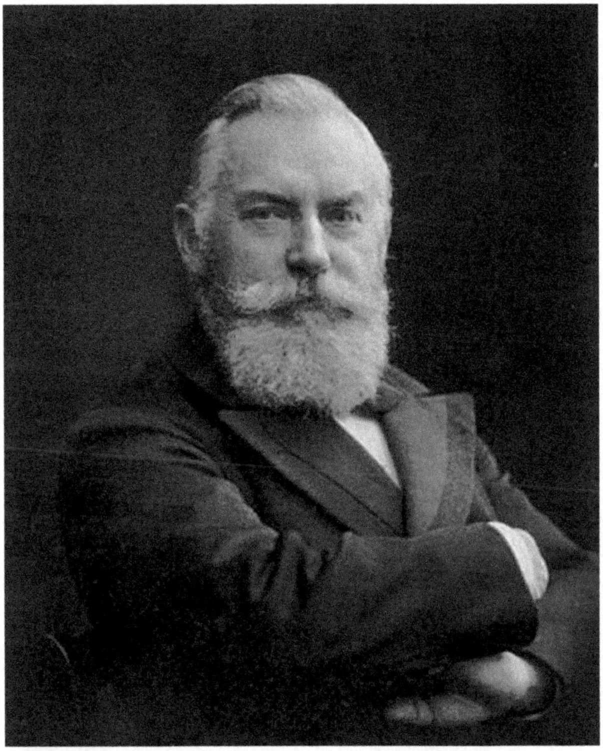

Fig. 1.5 Vincenz Czerny (1842–1916)

of surgery showed very high recurrence rates (Table 1.1). It was during that period where one of great pioneers of rectal cancer surgery appeared on the scene, represented by the English surgeon Ernst Miles, who was appointed assistant surgeon at the Royal Cancer Hospital. Miles had similar high recurrence rates as his contemporary surgeons. After performing autopsy on his own patients who died from recurrence, he invented a new approach. According to Miles, those very high recurrence rates were due to insufficient removal of tissue and thus attention needed to be paid to the lymphatic spread of cancer. He adopted a wide "cylindrical excision" to include lymphatics in the removed rectal specimen. Miles published his first results after performing this extensive excision in 1908 [17]. A similar observation and a similar new method of excision were done by Charles Mayo (Fig. 1.6) [18]. The procedure was associated with high mortality in the early period of adoption although it appeared, on the other hand, that the oncological results were improving dramatically. One of early adopters of Mile's operation was JP Lockert-Mummery, a senior surgeon in St. Mark's Hospital. He had at that time, introduced several modifications of the existing operations. He considered that Mile's operation was associated with high mortality and modified it as well.

While an extended abdominoperineal excision became a reality with obvious benefits in terms of improved oncological quality, concerns began to rise further about the mutilating nature of the procedure and ways to minimize complications, as well as selection of patients for whom a less invasive procedure would be satisfactory.

Table 1.1 Some oncological results of rectal cancer surgery in the beginning of the twentieth century

Surgeon	Number of patients	Recurrence rate (%)
Allingham	18	100
Cripps	85	38
Vogel	1500	80
Miles	57	95

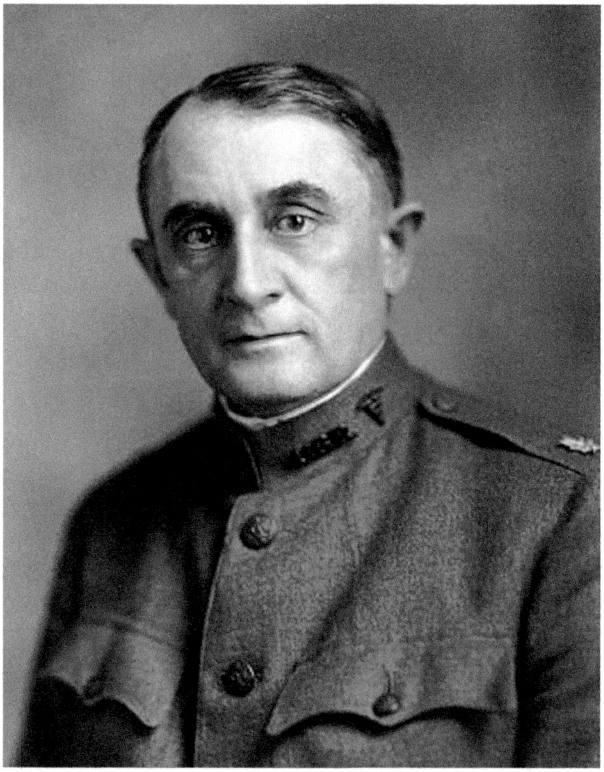

Fig. 1.6 Charles Horace Mayo (1865–1939)

1.5 Hartmann's Operation

Hartmann's operation involves resection of the sigmoid colon and/upper rectum, closure of the remaining rectal stump and fashioning a colostomy. It is performed nowadays mainly for the surgical treatment of diverticulitis. The idea of preserving the distal part of the rectum not involved by cancer came from the need to reduce morbidity and mortality associated with abdominoperineal excision. The first procedure of this art was probably performed by the Austrian surgeon Karl Gussenbauer (Fig. 1.7) in 1879 [19]. The French surgeon Henri Albert Hartmann (Fig. 1.8), who was once professor of surgery at Hotel Dieu in Paris, has later popularized the procedure. This has probably happened between 1909 and 1923 [20], and the procedure ended up bearing Hartmann's name when some unknown surgeon in the 1930s performed a two-staged procedure of sigmoid resection and colostomy with anastomosis at the second stage.

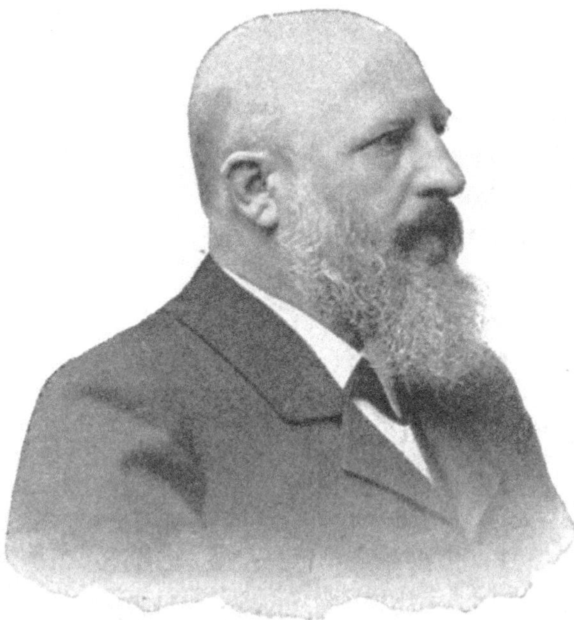
Hofrat Professor Dr. Karl Gussenbauer,
Rector magnificus der Wiener Universität.

Fig. 1.7 Karl Gussenbauer (1842–1903)

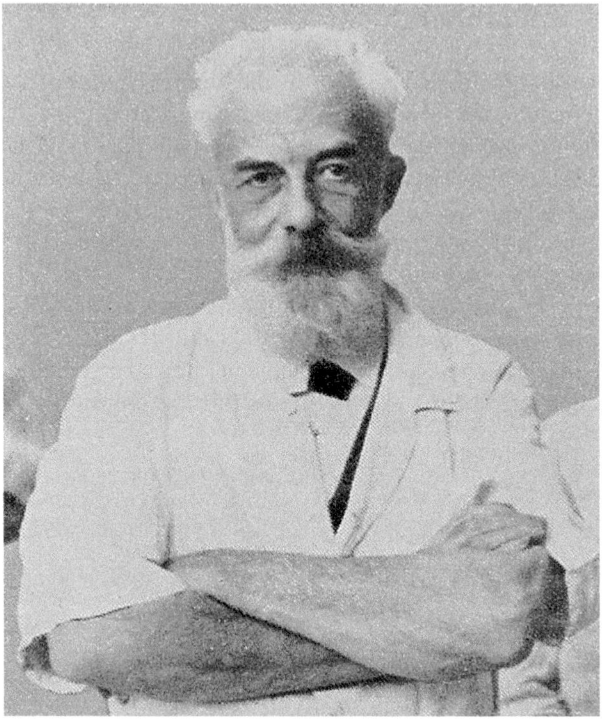

Fig. 1.8 Henri Albert Hartmann (1860–1952)

1.6 Sphincter Preservation

At the beginning of twentieth century, Mile's abdominoperineal excision reached a state of standard surgical procedure for excision of rectal cancer, regardless of tumor height from anal verge. Needless to say, this was mutilating and for patients with high rectal cancers, its necessity was doubtful. The main disadvantage was the need for permanent colostomy. In 1910, the first attempt at performing anastomosis was described by the American surgeon Donald Church Balfour. He performed an abdominal rectal resection and an end-end anastomosis [21]. Balfour's method, which included the use of a tube to support the anastomosis, had a very high anastomotic leak rate and did not gain popularity. Furthermore, at that time where Mile's extensive excision has convinced surgeons due to its oncological benefits, preservation of some distal part of the rectum to perform the anastomosis, was concerning and even not oncologically correct, as formulated by William Mayo (Fig. 1.9) "the operation is probably not radical enough" [22].

However, thanks to the extensive research by Dukes who could demonstrate the safety of sphincter preservation, efforts continued to limit the resections and preserve sphincters. Dukes showed that the lateral and downward spread of cancer was overestimated by Ernst Mile's, as downward lymphatic spread appeared to be the case in only a minority of patients with advanced disease [23]. In 1951 Goligher et al. [24] analyzed 1500 rectal specimens and found that the distal spread of tumor

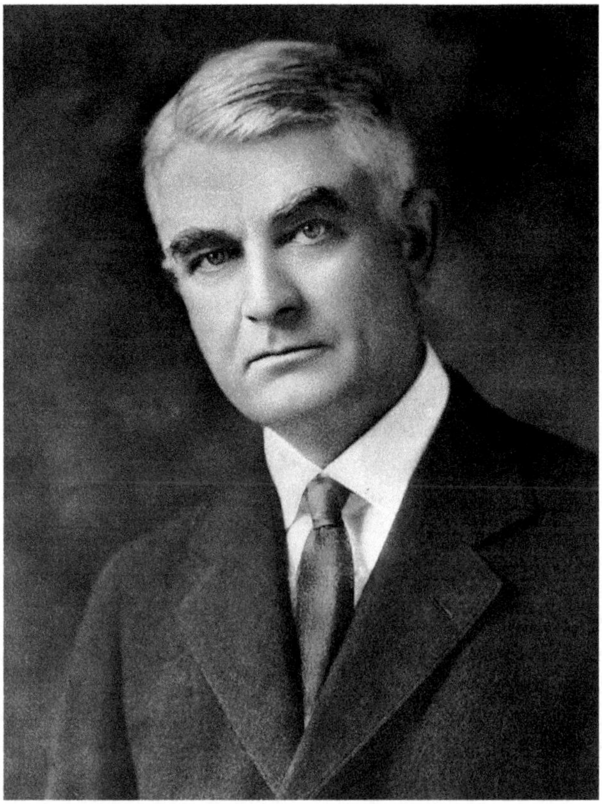

Fig. 1.9 William James Mayo (1861–1939)

cells more than 2 cm did not exceed 2%. A safety margin of only 5 cm could therefore be considered enough to achieve radicality.

Ultimately, the safety of sphincter preservation could be established by Claude Dixon of Mayo Clinic in 1948. He could demonstrate an impressive 5-year survival rate of 64% among 400 patients, results he presented at the meeting of the American Surgical Association in Quebec, Canada [25, 26]. Thus, Mile's theory was rejected and anterior resection became the standard of care for the treatment of mid and upper rectum cancer. Abdominoperineal excision, on the other hand came to stay for many years including present time, in the treatment of lower lesions. While the general believe was that an adequate resection required at least 5 cm distal resection margin, research results showed that lymphatic spread was limited to the level of the tumor or higher up. What encouraged the preservation of the sphincters was the increasing number of papers that showed even a distal margin of 2 cm did not compromise the oncological safety [27]. In the late 1970s, an almost radical shift from abdominoperineal excision to anterior resection is observed.

While preserving the anal sphincter appeared to be safe, another challenge was to actually perform the anastomosis. A positive innovation enabled a shift from the technical difficulty of performing a hand sewn colorectal or coloanal anastomosis, to a smarter way represented by the use of circular stapler devices. The circular devices were developed by Russian surgeons. The breakthrough in the use of staplers happened in 1972 when the American surgeon with a Russian born father, Mark Mitchell Ravitich could be introduced to one of hand-crafted staplers during his visit to Kiev in 1958. He could take one of these devices back to the USA. Several years later, staplers were widely available [28].

1.7 Total Mesorectal Excision

Throughout the first seven decades of the twentieth century, surgery for carcinoma of the rectum has evolved from being a limited transanal or transsacral excision, to a wider excision with unnecessary removal of an extensive amount of tissue of the rectal wall and its surroundings. This has yielded oncologically superior results as expected. However, it seems that with the rejection of Ernst Mile's theory of downward lymphatic spread, the procedure returned almost to the original description with mere removal of the rectal tube. This was the case for surgeries involved anterior resection, which included a blunt dissection in the pelvis, leaving inevitably the mesorectum and endangering the oncological safety. Recurrence rates were high at the end 1970s, when the English pathologist Phil Quirke has renewed the interest for the lateral lymphatic spread in the mid-1980s. He found a correlation between an involved radial resection margin and the development of local recurrence and poor survival [29]. This was a call for action, to improve the quality of rectal cancer surgery.

The English surgeon RJ (Bill) Heald has, since 1982 contributed for the major change in the principles of rectal dissection. He could show improved local recurrence rates through invention of a new resection technique that ensures complete removal of the mesorectal envelope. Surgical planes in Heald's Total Mesorectal Excision are defined embryologically, as the mesorectum has a separate embryological origin than the surrounding tissue. The technique involved a complete removal of the rectum together with the mesorectum down to the levator muscles, through a sharp and precise dissection and a gentle traction avoiding breach in the mesorectal envelope [30–32]. Heald could demonstrate a dramatic improvement in 5-year disease-free survival from around 50% at that time to an impressive 80% and showed local recurrence rate of only 4% [33]. Total Mesorectal Excision has become the gold standard for removal of mid and low rectal cancers in most parts of the world.

The improved oncological outcomes after the introduction of TME were not the only point of focus. Life quality issues, genitourinary function and the importance of nerve preservation have all gained significant amount of attention and research still ongoing to identify ways of improving functional results after rectal cancer surgery.

1.8 Lateral Lymph Node Dissection

In Japan, a more extensive procedure to achieve local tumor control has been advocated for, the so called lateral lymph node dissection [34–36]. The principles of this technique were described in 1950s by Deddish [19] and Bacon [37]. The procedure is not considered a standard of care in the western countries due to several reasons, amongst which the high rates of complications especially nerve damage leading to urogenital dysfunction. Furthermore, more blood loss, longer operation time, and the fact that it may represent a sign of distant tumor spread has discouraged colorectal surgeons to indulge into this practice.

1.9 Laparoscopic and Robotic Surgery

Laparoscopic surgery for rectal cancer was reported for the first time in 1990s [38]. With its obvious advantages like less blood loss, and shorter recovery, laparoscopy has gained its place as a standard method in colorectal surgery. Laparoscopic surgery for colorectal cancer is, at this time widely implemented in the Western world, especially in Europe. The pathological results are more controversial, with several major trials demonstrating contradicting results of laparoscopic rectal cancer surgery compared with open technique [39–41].

Robotics are being increasingly used in the recent years, with promising first experiences [42]. The main arguments for their use in rectal surgery are better visualization with three-dimensional cameras and angulated instruments providing better ergonomics for the surgeon. Thus potential advantages are lower conversion and better preservation of urogenital function. The proof of superiority over laparoscopic surgery is, however lacking. Robotic rectal resection has been otherwise shown to be safe and feasible [43–45]. Robotic rectal resection takes longer time, probably due to longer preparations needed to start the procedure and the subsequent steps not directly related to dissection itself [46]. The real benefits of robotic rectal resection are to be proved through randomized controlled trials, and the results of one such are being awaited to be published [47].

1.10 Transanal Procedures

In the early 1980s, Total Mesorectal Excision was reported and began to gain widespread interest. Simultaneously, in 1983 the German surgeon Gerhard Friedrich Buess introduced a new procedure for the treatment of benign rectal lesions. The method as based on a transanal local tumor excision, thus avoiding major surgery. He called the procedure Transanal Endoscopic Microsurgery (TEM) [48]. The interest for local excision of early rectal cancer has been growing, especially with advances in chemoradiation and the implementation of screening colonoscopies for colorectal cancer and the expected increase in the detection of higher number of early rectal lesions.

In the recent years, transanal endoscopic surgery has gained enormous interest due to its potentials, not only in local excisions, but in rectal resections as well. Through a transanal approach, a potentially better view of the most difficult part of the anatomy could be achieved allowing for a more precise and safe procedure. Transanal or perineal dissection has been shown to be feasible and safe [49–51]. The procedure has evolved from dissection without instruments [52], to the use of transanal endoscopic ports which allowed that Total Mesorectal Excision to be feasible in both cadaveric series [53], as well as human series. The first reported case of transanal TME in a patient using transanal port was reported in 2010 [54]. There are numerous publications in the years followed that, showing that transanal TME is feasible with potentially several benefits.

The future of rectal cancer surgery will definitely follow the same path as its history, with focus on more radical approaches through less invasive methods. One thing is for sure; the job is not done yet, and the history of rectal cancer surgery will not stagnate.

References

1. Bible. Judges. 2:3:22.
2. Le Clerc D. History of Physics. London: D Brown; 1699. p. 406.
3. Dinnick T. The origins and evolution of colostomy. Br J Surg. 1934;22:142–53.
4. Systema Chiruoqoe Hodierne. 1800:688.
5. Shelton A, Goldberg SM. Modern management of cancer of the rectum. Berlin: Springer; 2001. p. 1–5.
6. Meade RH. An introduction to the history of general surgery. Philadelphia: Saunders; 1968. p. 277–314.
7. Rankin FW. How surgery of the colon and rectum developed. Surg Gynecol Obstet. 1937;64:705–10.
8. Allingham W. Diseases of the rectum and anus. 5th ed. London: J. & A. Churchill; 1888.
9. Dieffenbach JF. Die operative Chirurgie. Leipzig: F.A. Brockhaus; 1848.
10. Colcock BP. Surgical progress in the treatment of rectal cancer. Surg Gynecol Obstet. 1965;121:997–1003.
11. Bacon HE. Anus, rectum, sigmoid colon: diagnosis and treatment. Philadelphia: Lippincott; 1949.
12. Curling TD. Observations on disease of the rectum. 4th ed. London: J. & A. Churchill; 1876.
13. Norton AT. A case of epithelioma of the rectum: excision-restoration of function. Trans Clin Soc. 1890;23:222–3.
14. Byford HT. Extirpation of the rectum per vaginum, with utilization of the vagina to replace the lost rectal tissue. Ann Surg. 1896;24:631–3.
15. McArthur LL. Cancer of the rectum. J Obstet. 1891;24:567–73.
16. Morgan CN. Carcinoma of the rectum. Ann R Coll Surg. 1965;36:73–97.
17. Miles WA. Method of performing abdomino-perineal excision for carcinoma of the rectum and of the terminal portion of the pelvic colon (1908). CA Cancer J Clin. 1971;21(6):361–4.
18. Mayo CH. Cancer of the large bowel. Med Sentinel. 1904;12:466–73.
19. Goligher J. Surgery of the anus, rectum and colon. London: Baillíére Tindall; 1984. p. 590–779.
20. Hartmann H. Chirugie du Rectum. Paris: Masson et Cie; 1931.
21. VIII Balfour DC. A method of anastomosis between sigmoid and rectum. Ann Surg. 1910;51(2):239–41.
22. Nicholls RJ. Rectal cancer: anterior resection with per anal colo-anal anastomosis. The results in 76 patients treated by Sir Alan Parks. Bull Cancer. 1983;70(4):304–7.
23. Ravitch MM. The use of stapling instruments in surgery of the gastrointestinal tract, with a note on a new instrument for end-to-end low rectal and oesophagojejunal anastomoses. Aust N Z J Surg. 1978;48(4):444–7.
24. Goligher JC, Dukes CE, Bussey HJ. Local recurrences after sphincter saving excisions for carcinoma of the rectum and rectosigmoid. Br J Surg. 1951;39(155):199–211.
25. Parc R, Tiret E, Frileux P, Moszkowski E, Loygue J. Resection and colo-anal anastomosis with colonic reservoir for rectal carcinoma. Br J Surg. 1986;73(2):139–41.
26. Dixon CF. Anterior resection for malignant lesions of the upper part of the rectum and lower part of the sigmoid. Trans Meet Am Surg Assoc Am Surg Assoc Meet. 1948;66(Trans. 68. meeting):175–92.

27. Da Silva GM, Berho M, Wexner SD, Efron J, Weiss EG, Nogueras JJ, et al. Histologic analysis of the irradiated anal sphincter. Dis Colon Rectum. 2003;46(11):1492–7. https://doi.org/10.1097/01.dcr.0000093642.89267.67.
28. Ravitch MM, Steichen FM, Fishbein RH, Knowles PW, Weil P. Clinical experiences with the Soviet mechanical bronchus stapler (UKB-25). J Thorac Cardiovasc Surg. 1964;47:446–54.
29. Quirke P, Durdey P, Dixon MF, Williams NS. Local recurrence of rectal adenocarcinoma due to inadequate surgical resection. Histopathological study of lateral tumour spread and surgical excision. Lancet. 1986;2(8514):996–9.
30. Heald RJA. New approach to rectal cancer. Br J Hosp Med. 1979;22(3):277–81.
31. Heald RJ, Husband EM, Ryall RD. The mesorectum in rectal cancer surgery – the clue to pelvic recurrence? Br J Surg. 1982;69(10):613–6.
32. Heald RJ, Ryall RD. Recurrence and survival after total mesorectal excision for rectal cancer. Lancet. 1986;1(8496):1479–82.
33. Heald RJ, Moran BJ, Ryall RD, Sexton R, MacFarlane JK. Rectal cancer: the Basingstoke experience of total mesorectal excision, 1978-1997. Arch Surg. 1998;133(8):894–9.
34. Hojo K, Koyama Y, Moriya Y. Lymphatic spread and its prognostic value in patients with rectal cancer. Am J Surg. 1982;144(3):350–4.
35. Moriya Y, Hojo K, Sawada T, Koyama Y. Significance of lateral node dissection for advanced rectal carcinoma at or below the peritoneal reflection. Dis Colon Rectum. 1989;32(4):307–15.
36. Nagawa H, Muto T, Sunouchi K, Higuchi Y, Tsurita G, Watanabe T, et al. Randomized, controlled trial of lateral node dissection vs. nerve-preserving resection in patients with rectal cancer after preoperative radiotherapy. Dis Colon Rectum. 2001;44(9):1274–80.
37. Bacon HE. Abdominoperineal proctosigmoidectomy with sphincter preservation; five-year and ten-year survival after pull-through operation for cancer of rectum. J Am Med Assoc. 1956;160(8):628–34.
38. Plasencia G, Jacobs M, Verdeja JC, Viamonte M III. Laparoscopic-assisted sigmoid colectomy and low anterior resection. Dis Colon Rectum. 1994;37(8):829–33.
39. Bonjer HJ, Deijen CL, Abis GA, Cuesta MA, van der Pas MH, de Lange-de Klerk ES, et al. A randomized trial of laparoscopic versus open surgery for rectal cancer. N Engl J Med. 2015;372(14):1324–32. https://doi.org/10.1056/NEJMoa1414882.
40. Fleshman J, Branda M, Sargent DJ, Boller AM, George V, Abbas M, et al. Effect of laparoscopic-assisted resection vs open resection of stage II or III rectal cancer on pathologic outcomes: the ACOSOG Z6051 randomized clinical trial. JAMA. 2015;314(13):1346–55. https://doi.org/10.1001/jama.2015.10529.
41. Stevenson AR, Solomon MJ, Lumley JW, Hewett P, Clouston AD, Gebski VJ, et al. Effect of laparoscopic-assisted resection vs open resection on pathological outcomes in rectal cancer: the ALaCaRT randomized clinical trial. JAMA. 2015;314(13):1356–63. https://doi.org/10.1001/jama.2015.12009.
42. Hellan M, Anderson C, Ellenhorn JD, Paz B, Pigazzi A. Short-term outcomes after robotic-assisted total mesorectal excision for rectal cancer. Ann Surg Oncol. 2007;14(11):3168–73. https://doi.org/10.1245/s10434-007-9544-z.
43. Mirnezami AH, Mirnezami R, Venkatasubramaniam AK, Chandrakumaran K, Cecil TD, Moran BJ. Robotic colorectal surgery: hype or new hope? A systematic review of robotics in colorectal surgery. Colorectal Dis. 2010;12(11):1084–93. https://doi.org/10.1111/j.1463-1318.2009.01999.x.
44. Scarpinata R, Aly EH. Does robotic rectal cancer surgery offer improved early postoperative outcomes? Dis Colon Rectum. 2013;56(2):253–62. https://doi.org/10.1097/DCR.0b013e3182694595.
45. Mak TW, Lee JF, Futaba K, Hon SS, Ngo DK, Ng SS. Robotic surgery for rectal cancer: a systematic review of current practice. World J Gastrointest Oncol. 2014;6(6):184–93. https://doi.org/10.4251/wjgo.v6.i6.184.
46. Staderini F, Foppa C, Minuzzo A, Badii B, Qirici E, Trallori G, et al. Robotic rectal surgery: state of the art. World J Gastrointest Oncol. 2016;8(11):757–71. https://doi.org/10.4251/wjgo.v8.i11.757.

47. Collinson FJ, Jayne DG, Pigazzi A, Tsang C, Barrie JM, Edlin R, et al. An international, multicentre, prospective, randomised, controlled, unblinded, parallel-group trial of robotic-assisted versus standard laparoscopic surgery for the curative treatment of rectal cancer. Int J Color Dis. 2012;27(2):233–41. https://doi.org/10.1007/s00384-011-1313-6.
48. Buess G, Theiss R, Hutterer F, Pichlmaier H, Pelz C, Holfeld T, et al. Transanal endoscopic surgery of the rectum - testing a new method in animal experiments. Leber Magen Darm. 1983;13(2):73–7.
49. Marks JH, Frenkel JL, D'Andrea AP, Greenleaf CE. Maximizing rectal cancer results: TEM and TATA techniques to expand sphincter preservation. Surg Oncol Clin N Am. 2011;20(3): 501–520., viii-ix. https://doi.org/10.1016/j.soc.2011.01.008.
50. Denost Q, Adam JP, Rullier A, Buscail E, Laurent C, Rullier E. Perineal transanal approach: a new standard for laparoscopic sphincter-saving resection in low rectal cancer, a randomized trial. Ann Surg. 2014;260(6):993–9. https://doi.org/10.1097/sla.0000000000000766.
51. Pontallier A, Denost Q, Van Geluwe B, Adam JP, Celerier B, Rullier E. Potential sexual function improvement by using transanal mesorectal approach for laparoscopic low rectal cancer excision. Surg Endosc. 2016;30(11):4924–33. https://doi.org/10.1007/s00464-016-4833-x.
52. Funahashi K, Koike J, Teramoto T, Saito N, Shiokawa H, Kurihara A, et al. Transanal rectal dissection: a procedure to assist achievement of laparoscopic total mesorectal excision for bulky tumor in the narrow pelvis. Am J Surg. 2009;197(4):e46–50. https://doi.org/10.1016/j.amjsurg.2008.07.060.
53. Telem DA, Han KS, Kim MC, Ajari I, Sohn DK, Woods K, et al. Transanal rectosigmoid resection via natural orifice translumenal endoscopic surgery (NOTES) with total mesorectal excision in a large human cadaver series. Surg Endosc. 2013;27(1):74–80. https://doi.org/10.1007/s00464-012-2409-y.
54. Sylla P, Rattner DW, Delgado S, Lacy AM. NOTES transanal rectal cancer resection using transanal endoscopic microsurgery and laparoscopic assistance. Surg Endosc. 2010;24(5):1205–10. https://doi.org/10.1007/s00464-010-0965-6.

Epidemiology and Carcinogenesis of Rectal Cancer

2

Jai Bikhchandani, Alan G. Thorson, and Henry T. Lynch

Abstract

Cancer of the colon and rectum is extremely common in the Western hemisphere. The etiopathogenesis of colorectal cancer is an intertwined play of several genetic and environmental factors to which an individual is exposed to during the lifetime. The predominance of one factor over another decides the timing of development of this cancer with respect to the individual's age. Familial syndromes like Lynch syndrome and familial adenomatous polyposis predispose an individual to cancer early in their lifespan since they carry the genetic mutation. A sporadic cancer, on the other hand, follows a very interesting and often predictable path from a polyp to carcinoma. There are three such pathways which the colonic epithelium may undertake toward the development of cancer. Each of the pathways has its own unique set of genotypic and phenotypic expression which needs to be understood well to accomplish our ultimate goal for prevention of colorectal cancer.

Keywords

Colorectal cancer • Epidemiology • Lynch syndrome • Carcinogenesis • Polyp-carcinoma sequence

J. Bikhchandani, M.D. • H.T. Lynch, M.D. (✉)
Department of Preventive Medicine, Creighton University,
2500 California Plaza, Hixson-Lied Science Building, Rm 202, Omaha, NE 68178, USA
e-mail: htlynch@creighton.edu

A.G. Thorson, M.D.
Colon and Rectal Surgery Inc., Omaha, NE, USA

G. Dapri, J.H. Marks (eds.), *Surgical Techniques in Rectal Cancer*,
https://doi.org/10.1007/978-4-431-55579-7_2

2.1 Epidemiology

Colorectal cancer (CRC) is the third most common cause of cancer in the United States among both men and women [1]. It is also the second most common cause of cancer-related death among cancers that affect both genders. As per 2009 data, 147,000 new cases were diagnosed with colorectal cancer. Of these, 40,000 patients were diagnosed with new rectal cancers. In the same year, there were 50,000 deaths from cancer of colon and rectum [1]. Worldwide, around 1 million new patients get diagnosed with colorectal cancer every year. These figures seem to be rising which may be multifactorial and associated with improved diagnosis and an aging patient population around the world [2]. Historically, Western countries have a higher incidence of colorectal cancer when compared to Asia and Africa. Interestingly, the variation between countries in rectal cancer incidence is lesser as compared to the incidence of colon cancer [3].

Even though colorectal cancer can occur at any age, increasing age is the most identifiable risk factor for colorectal cancer with over 90% of cases diagnosed in patients over 50 years of age [4]. A recent increase in the incidence of colorectal cancer younger than 40 years of age has been reported [5]. Overall, the incidence of CRC in men is 61 per 100,000 males as compared to 45 per 100,000 females [4]. At birth, the probability of developing colorectal cancer in women is 5.5% and in men 5.9% [6]. Cancer of the rectum appears to be more common in men. The proportion of colorectal cancers developing in colon versus rectum is 2:1 in males and 3:1 in females [4]. Race and ethnicity also affect the risk of colorectal cancer. The incidence of CRC is higher in African-Americans of either sex as compared to white Americans, who are at higher risk than Hispanics or Asian Americans [4]. Ashkenazi Jews appear to be at a slightly increased risk of CRC due to higher prevalence of APC gene mutation. The rates of colorectal cancer in Caucasian Americans have shown a downward trend between 1998 and 2005 with reduced incidence of distal colorectal cancers [1]. Unfortunately, a similar trend has not been seen in African-Americans.

2.2 Etiopathogenesis

Colorectal cancer remains one of the most preventable cancers of all. It almost always arises from benign neoplasms like adenomatous or serrated polyps over a prolonged period of time. There are a large number of factors that play a role, directly or indirectly in driving the polyp to carcinoma sequence. Some of these interactions may be modifiable and help in primary and/or secondary prevention of colorectal cancers. The complex interplay between the various environmental factors and the genetic susceptibility of host from genetic mutations, either acquired or inherited, is important to understand, as that will ultimately play a role in the development of colorectal cancer. Factors that lead to malignant neoplasms of rectum have been studied in common with all colorectal cancers and will be discussed in detail here.

2.3 Polyp to Cancer Transformation

Histologically, colonic polyps may be broadly classified as neoplastic, hyperplastic, hamartomatous, and inflammatory polyps. An adenomatous polyp or an adenoma is a neoplastic polyp with abnormal proliferation of glands in the epithelium. By definition, it is a low-grade dysplastic lesion that has the potential for progression of dysplasia to an invasive cancer. Grossly, these lesions can be pedunculated (mushroom like) or sessile with a broader base. Adenomas may be subclassified as tubular, villous, or tubulovillous. A tubular adenoma is composed of uniform-sized tubules and glands. As the tubules become more elongated with less stroma between glands, they are termed villous in character. A tubular adenoma may have up to 20–25% villous gland-like features and still be considered a "tubular adenoma," while villous adenomas (5–10% of all adenomas) contain more than 50–75% villous features. Hyperplastic polyps are considered metaplastic with well-formed glands and a number of goblet cells that produce a layer of mucous lining them.

Over 90% of colorectal cancers (CRC) are considered to arise in adenomas. The malignant potential of an adenoma is dependent on two main factors—the proportion of villous component in the polyp and the degree of dysplasia [7]. Concurrent existence of adenomas and adenocarcinomas in resected cancer specimens is a circumstantial evidence that an adenoma may lead to cancer [8]. Data from the cancer registry in Norway show that the occurrence of adenomas precedes carcinomas by 5 years [9]. Acceptance of this pathogenic mechanism is the rationale behind worldwide screening measures and surveillance colonoscopy for removal of polyp(s) that may turn into cancer.

In 1951, Jakman and Mayo coined the term "adenoma-carcinoma sequence" [10]. However, the genetic mechanisms behind the process as described later in the text were not well understood until later. Development of invasive cancer in a benign polyp has been observed as a three-step process of initiation, promotion, and progression. All along this sequence, gene mutations, epigenetic alterations, and inflammatory changes are noticed. Some of these mutations may be acquired, in which case the lifestyle and environmental factors have a major role to play, while other patients are born with germline mutations. In these patients, the influence of environmental factors is small compared with the contribution from the underlying genetic mutations and, therefore, manifest with hereditary and familial cancers at a younger age. The classical examples for colorectal cancer in patients with germline mutations are those being associated with familial adenomatous polyposis and Lynch syndrome.

2.4 Genetics and Epigenetics of Colorectal Cancer

There are three major categories of genes that function as policemen for the genome and prevent development of cancer. These are (1) oncogenes, (2) tumor suppressor genes, and (3) mismatch repair genes. Proto-oncogene is a normal human growth-related gene, which when becomes abnormally activated (known as an oncogene) drives the cell through the cell cycle resulting in clonal proliferation. This effect from

Table 2.1 Genes with an integral role in colorectal carcinogenesis

Pathway	Category of gene	Gene	Chromosomal location	Phenotypic effect
APC/LOH	TS gene	APC	5	Early adenoma
		DCC	18	Late adenoma
		P53	17	Invasive cancer
	Oncogene	KRAS	12	Intermediate adenoma
MSI	MMR gene	MLH1	3	Enhanced adenoma carcinoma sequence
		MSH2	2	
		MSH6	2	
		PMS1	2	
		PMS2	7	
Serrated	Heterogeneous	KRAS, MSI	Varied	Hyperplastic-like polyps

oncogenes is in a dominant fashion, and hence alteration of only one allele is necessary. The normal function of tumor suppressor genes is to stop the cell cycle whenever there is abnormal proliferation of the cell as a result of oncogene activation. Tumor suppressor genes act in a recessive manner and promote cancer only when they are inactivated by mutations in both alleles. If cells cannot repair DNA damage, tumor suppressor genes such as p53 drive the cell into a suicide mode called apoptosis. Mismatch repair (MMR) genes act as a watchdog for any errors that may get introduced in the genetic code as a result of replication. Bi-allelic activation of these MMR genes will result in mutations that may lead to cancer. Accumulation of inherited and acquired genetic and epigenetic changes transforms normal glandular epithelial cells into invasive adenocarcinomas. The current understanding of the genetics educates us that colonic epithelium may take one of the three pathways to cancer. The commonly implicated genes in colorectal carcinogenesis can be found in Table 2.1.

2.4.1 APC (or Loss of Heterozygosity) Pathway

The most common pathway is the inactivation of the APC (adenomatous polyposis coli) gene. It is the first event in 70–80% of colorectal carcinomas. The *APC* gene, located on the long arm of chromosome 5 (5q), is considered a gatekeeper gene of colorectal carcinogenesis [11]. APC changes are mostly inactivating mutations that occur very early in the sequence of cancer progression. Inactivation of this gene results in increased cell proliferation predisposing to subsequent mutations. The mechanism involves truncation of the APC protein with altered ability to direct the degradation of β-catenin protein, such that higher levels of β-catenin protein accumulate in the cell cytoplasm and nucleus, leading to deregulation of the Wnt-APC-β-catenin signaling pathway and changes in expression in a range of WNT targets including C-MYC [12]. APC mutation results in a change of normal epithelium to hyperproliferative epithelium. One of these hyperproliferating cells gives rise to a small adenoma in which the genome is hypomethylated. Conventional tubular adenomas are initiated by bi-allelic inactivation of the APC (adenomatous polyposis coli) tumor-suppressor gene [13]. Mutated APC is inherited in familial adenomatous polyposis coli syndrome (FAP) in which hundreds of adenomatous polyps develop and act as precursors for colorectal cancer at a much earlier age.

The next genetic event involves activation of the KRAS oncogene on the chromosome 12p mutation to form the intermediate adenoma. KRAS-activating mutations are found in about 40–45% of both colorectal adenomas and carcinomas, and this is thought mostly to occur during the early stages of adenoma progression [14, 15]. Mutations are usually found in particular positions within the KRAS protein at codons 12, 13, and 61 substituting the original amino acid for a different amino acid that affects the enzymic function of the KRAS protein, reducing or preventing enzymic cleavage of the terminal phosphate group of RAS-bound guanosine triphosphate, which would normally be converted to guanosine diphosphate [14, 15]. This tends to lock the KRAS protein into the active guanosine triphosphate-bound state (unable to convert to the RAS-guanosine diphosphate inactive state) mediating excessive signaling through the RAS-RAF-MEK-ERK pathway that drives cell proliferation. Colorectal cancers can be tested for the presence of mutated KRAS, as such tumors do not benefit from anti-epidermal growth factor receptor therapy. Whereas KRAS wild-type tumors do benefit as their epidermal growth factor receptor-KRAS signaling axis is functioning and can be inhibited by such therapy [16].

The "deleted in colon cancer" (DCC) gene on chromosome 18q is next to be deactivated or lost and results in the development of a late adenoma [17]. The final genetic alteration found consistently in colorectal carcinoma is loss and/or mutation of the p53 tumor suppressor gene on chromosome 17p [17]. The p53 gene is altered in 50% of all human carcinomas and in 70% of colorectal carcinomas. p53 slows the cell cycle, facilitates DNA repair during replication, and, if repair is not feasible, induces apoptosis. This mutation appears to occur late in the carcinogenic sequence. In addition, *p53* expression may be an independent prognostic marker in patients with CRC [18, 19]. Most studies demonstrate a lower survival rate in patients with advanced cancers that are *p53* negative as compared to those whose tumors express *p53* gene product, particularly in those who receive chemotherapy.

2.4.2 Microsatellite Instability Pathway

The second major pathway of adenomagenesis is characterized by the presence of microsatellite instability (MSI) due to defective DNA mismatch repair (MMR) genes [17]. MMR genes are needed for cells to repair DNA replication errors and spontaneous base pair loss. Mismatch repair gene defects initiate a cancer pathway as a consequence of replication errors [18, 19]. This pathway to colorectal carcinoma is found in approximately 20% of cancers [20]. Lynch syndrome patients inherit a single defective allele of a mismatch repair gene and require an additional somatic mutation to inactivate the second allele. Patients who develop spontaneous cancers via this pathway are hit by two somatic events that inactivate the relevant gene. In either case, inactivation leads to a marked increase in replication errors. As

Table 2.2 DNA mismatch repair (MMR) gene mutations in Lynch syndrome

Gene	No. of mutations	No. of polymorphisms
MLH1	164	20
MSH2	121	24
MSH6	31	43
PMS1	1	0
PMS2	5	5

errors accumulate in microsatellite regions of the genome, there is malfunction of genes that contain or are near affected microsatellites. Aaltonen et al. found the RER-positive phenotype in 77% of colorectal carcinomas from HNPCC patients compared with only 13% of patients with sporadic carcinoma [21].

The DNA mismatch repair (MMR) gene mutations found in patients with Lynch syndrome are enlisted in Table 2.2. When both copies of these genes are inactivated, DNA mismatch repair is defective, and the cell exhibits an increased frequency of errors in DNA replication, thereby accelerating the progression to oncogenesis. In sporadic colorectal cancers, this is almost always due to the acquired promoter hypermethylation of the MLH1 gene that silences its expression. In the setting of inherited colorectal cancer susceptibility i.e., Lynch syndrome (LS), the two most commonly inherited mutant genes are MLH1 and MSH2, accounting for around 40% to 45% each of LS families. Studies of DNA methylation in colorectal cancers and their precursors to investigate the role of epigenetic silencing of cancer-related genes in these tumors have identified promoter methylation of the MLH1, MGMT, PTEN, DNMT3B, and other genes involved in the WNT/APC/B-CATENIN signaling pathway [11].

2.4.3 Serrated Pathway

The term "serrated adenoma" was coined by Longacre and Fenoglio-Preiser in 1990 to describe a newly recognized entity of mixed hyperplastic polyp/adenomatous polyp [22]. Premalignant serrated polyps more frequently arise in the proximal colon and are associated with the CIMP, which is a phenotype recognized by having an exceptionally high frequency of aberrantly methylated CpG dinucleotides [23]. The original proposal that only tubular and tubulovillous adenomas had the potential to progress to carcinoma was proven false with the recognition that serrated polyps also have the potential for malignant transformation [13, 24]. Serrated polyps are an alternative pathway to malignancy whereby a subset of hyperplastic polyps, most likely microvesicular hyperplastic polyps, progresses to the serrated pathway [25].

Molecular alterations, such as BRAFV600E mutations, are characteristically found more often in tumors arising via the serrated neoplasia pathway [26]. The serrated adenoma pathway has marked molecular heterogeneity. The various genetic alterations include KRAS mutation, low- or high-level microsatellite instability, 1pLOH, and methylation of HPP1/TPEF (a putative anti-adhesion molecule). Colorectal carcinoma is envisioned to arise from hyperplastic-like polyps (or sessile serrated polyps) in which the earliest events might be BRAF mutation along with a methylated and silenced pro-apoptotic gene. Subsequent methylation of hMLH1 or MGMT then predisposes to mutation, dysplastic change, and finally to malignancy that is frequently characterized by MSI-H or MSI-L status. KRAS mutation may substitute for BRAF in methylator pathways culminating in MSI-L and some MSS (microsatellite stable) colorectal carcinomas [24].

2.5 Genetic Syndromes Predisposing to Colorectal Cancer

A comprehensive list of the various genetic polyposis syndromes is shown in Table 2.3. We will discuss familial adenomatous polyposis (FAP) and Lynch syndrome (LS) in detail below.

Familial adenomatous polyposis—FAP—is an inherited, Mendelian-dominant disease characterized by the progressive development of hundreds or thousands of adenomatous polyps throughout the entire colon [20]. The incidence of FAP is one in 7000 live births [27]. The clinical diagnosis is based on the histologic confirmation of at least 100 adenomas. Although the disease is congenital, there is no available evidence that adenomas have ever been present since birth. A phenotypic alteration of the classical syndrome is seen in affected families with the total number of adenomas being less than 50 [17]. This condition is called attenuated FAP syndrome. The onset of colorectal cancer is at a later average age (approximately 55 years) than that of classic familial adenomatous polyposis (approximately 39 years).

Using genetic-linkage analysis, it has been determined that FAP is caused by a mutation in the tumor suppressor gene APC located on the long arm of chromosome 5q21–22 [17]. The genetic alterations found in the FAP patient's colon and rectal carcinoma are similar to those noted in sporadic carcinoma, except that an APC mutation is already present constitutionally at birth, i.e., a germline mutation. Mutations causing classic FAP are located in the central region, and mutations between codons 1250 and 1464 are associated with particularly severe polyposis.

Table 2.3 Genetics and incidence of polyposis syndromes

Genetic syndrome	Incidence	Gene	Cancer risk
Familial adenomatous polyposis	1/5000	APC	Colorectal, duodenal, thyroid, pancreatic, CNS
Hyperplastic polyposis syndrome	1/100,000	Multiple	Colorectal
MYH-adenomatous polyposis	1/5000	MYH	Colorectal
Juvenile polyposis syndrome	1/100,000	SMAD4	Colorectal, gastric, duodenal, pancreatic
Cowden syndrome	1/200,000	PTEN	Breast, thyroid, uterine, renal cell
Peutz-Jeghers syndrome	1/30,000	STK11	Colorectal, small intestine, stomach, pancreatic, breast
Birt-Hogg-Dube syndrome	1/200,000	BHD	Renal

Bi-allelic inactivation of APC is typically achieved by the combination of an inherited germline mutation in one allele and a chromosomal deletion of the remaining wild-type allele. Thirty-four mutations causing AFAP have been reported to date; these are clustered either at the five prime ends (before codon 436) or at the three prime ends (after codon 1596) of the APC gene. In AFAP (panel B), the mechanism of APC inactivation is different. Germline mutations involved in AFAP may lead to the formation of alternative APC proteins that are initiated from an internal translation site that is located distal to the truncating mutation. This alternative APC protein does have functional activity. Because of this residual gene activity, an additional "hit" is necessary to fully inactivate APC.

2.6 Lynch Syndrome

The key features of Lynch syndrome are elaborated in Table 2.4. There is an earlier average age at the onset of cancer at approximately 45 years as compared to 63 years in general population [28]. A particular pattern of primary cancers is seen within the pedigree, such as colonic and endometrial cancer [28, 29]. The third is better survival that differs from the norm for the specific cancer [30]. The fourth is distinguishing pathological features, and the fifth and sine qua non is the identification of a germline mutation in affected members of the family [31]. Cancers in Lynch syndrome are more often poorly differentiated, with an excess of mucoid and signet-cell features, a Crohn's-like reaction (lymphoid nodules, including germinal centers, located at the periphery of infiltrating colorectal carcinomas), and the presence of infiltrating lymphocytes within the tumor [32–35].

Lynch syndrome or previously called hereditary nonpolyposis colorectal cancer syndrome is caused by a germline mutation in one of the above listed mismatch repair genes. A hallmark of tumors in hereditary nonpolyposis colorectal cancer is microsatellite instability [21, 36, 37]. Microsatellites are genomic regions in which short DNA sequences or a single nucleotide is repeated. There are hundreds of thousands of microsatellites in the human genome. During DNA replication, mutations

Table 2.4 Features of Lynch syndrome

• Autosomal dominant inheritance pattern
• Earlier average age of CRC onset
• Proximal (right-sided) colonic cancer predilection
• Accelerated carcinogenesis
• High risk of metachronous CRCs
• Increased risk for malignancy at certain extra-colonic sites: endometrium, ovary, stomach, small bowel, hepatobiliary tract, pancreas, upper uroepithelial tract (transitional cell carcinoma of the ureter and renal pelvis), prostate, breast
• Pathology—poorly differentiated, with an excess of mucoid and signet-cell features, a Crohn's-like reaction, and a significant excess of infiltrating lymphocytes within the tumor
• Better survival from CRC

occur in some microsatellites owing to the misalignment of their repetitive subunits and result in contraction or elongation ("instability"). These abnormalities are usually repaired by the mismatch repair proteins. However, repair is inefficient in tumors with a deficiency of these proteins. This is a dominantly inherited syndrome. About 70% to 80% of individuals with a predisposing mutation will develop colorectal cancer [38]. The disease is heterogeneous. Adenomas in patients carrying Lynch syndrome gene mutations show microsatellite instability, confirming that mismatch repair defects are important early events in colorectal carcinogenesis. Carcinoma formation requires inactivation of both copies of a given mismatch repair gene, one copy by germline mutation and the other by somatic (acquired) mutation [38].

2.7 Environmental Factors

Geographic variation in the incidence of colorectal cancer across the world supports the hypothesis that there is a defined role of environmental influences on the occurrence of cancer in the colon and rectum. Several factors have been studied and proposed to impact the process of colorectal carcinogenesis (Table 2.5). Burkitt observed that populations in low-risk areas of the third world had greater stool bulk, a faster colonic transit time, and higher dietary fiber intake than populations in high-risk, Westernized regions [39]. It is logical to think that diet should play an important role in colorectal carcinogenesis. Epidemiological and clinical studies show that Western diets contain various mutagens and carcinogens which may be classified as (1) naturally occurring chemicals that include mycotoxins and plant alkaloids, (2) synthetic compounds, i.e., food additives and pesticides, and (3) compounds like polycyclic aromatic hydrocarbons and heterocyclic amines produced by cooking [40]. A number of case control studies have been reported. Jain et al. examined patients with colorectal cancer and compared them with population and hospital controls [41]. An increased risk was found in persons with an increased intake of saturated fat as well as calories, total protein, total fat, oleic acid, and cholesterol. The strongest effect was that of saturated fat. Potter and McMichael found that dietary protein was the strongest predictor of colon carcinoma with a two- to threefold relative risk [42]. A positive association

Table 2.5 Environmental and lifestyle factors that play a role in development of colorectal cancer

• Dietary fat
• Dietary fiber
• Red meat in diet
• Total calories
• Fruits and vegetables
• Bile salts
• Calcium
• Body habitus
• Physical activity
• Alcohol
• Smoking

for the risk of colon carcinoma with egg consumption, coffee intake, and weight greater than 125% of ideal weight has also been reported [43]. No association was noted for use of meat, cheese, milk, or green salad. Garland et al. [44] failed to note any association between dietary fat, animal or vegetable protein, ethanol, or energy intake and subsequent colorectal carcinoma. The authors did note a negative association between vitamin D and calcium intake and subsequent colorectal carcinoma.

2.7.1 Dietary Fiber

Diets with a high roughage content result in the production of soft, bulky, frequent stools. A potential carcinogen in a patient with infrequent stools remains in contact with the colonic and rectal mucosa longer. Experimental work by Fleiszer et al. [45] supported this hypothesis by showing that a high-fiber diet results in a diminished incidence of dimethylhydrazine (DMH)-induced carcinoma of the colon in rats. Nonetheless, the potential protective effect of fiber is controversial. Authors have shown an inverse association between a high-fiber diet and the risk of colon carcinoma [46]. A meta-analysis of 12 case-control studies showed protection with an odds ratio of 0.57 (95% CI, 0.50–0.64) [47]. Asano and McLeod [48] conducted a systematic review and meta-analysis to assess the effect of dietary fiber on the incidence or recurrence of colorectal adenomas. Five studies with 4349 subjects met the inclusion criteria. The interventions were wheat bran fiber, ispaghula husk, or a comprehensive dietary intervention with high-fiber whole food sources alone or in combination. When the data were combined, there was no difference between the intervention and control groups. Fuchs et al. [49] conducted a prospective study of 88,757 women who were 34 to 59 years old and had no history of carcinoma, inflammatory bowel disease, or familial polyposis. During a 16-year follow-up period, 787 cases of colorectal carcinoma were documented. In addition, 1012 patients with adenomas of the distal colon and rectum were found among 27,530 participants who underwent endoscopy during the follow-up period. After adjustment for age, established risk factors, and total energy intake, they found no association between the intake of dietary fiber and the risk of colorectal carcinoma or colorectal adenoma.

2.7.2 Dietary Fat

Populations with diets high in fat and protein are thought to be associated with a high incidence of colorectal carcinoma. The proposed mechanism is a high concentration of fecal bile acids and cholesterol which stimulates cell proliferation and acts as promoters of carcinogenesis. The risk has been observed to be proportionate to the amount as well as type of fat ingested. In a prospective study on a cohort of about 100,000 nurses, a total of 150 nurses developed colon carcinoma with a trend for risk with total fat intake ($p < 0.05$) and animal fat ($p < 0.01$) [50]. Nonetheless, the data currently available are far from being conclusive. In a systematic review by Howe et al. [51], authors cumulatively looked at 5287 cases of colorectal cancer and compared with 10,470 controls. There was a positive association of colorectal cancer with total energy intake.

When the data were controlled for total energy intake, the odds ratio of developing cancer with high-dietary fat intake was 0.90 (95% CI 0.72–1.13). In another randomized controlled trial, 48,835 females were randomized to a modified diet (low dietary fat, high fruits and vegetables) versus no dietary modification. Patients were followed for 8 years [52]. With a 70% of target dietary fat reduction, no significant difference in the incidence of colorectal cancer was observed between the two groups [52].

2.7.3 Red Meat

Larsson et al. [53] prospectively examined the association of red meat consumption with the site of colorectal carcinoma. Diet was assessed at baseline using a self-administered food-frequency questionnaire. Over a mean follow-up of 13.9 years, they observed a significant positive association between red meat consumption and risk of distal colon carcinoma but not of the proximal colon or rectum. Another prospective study followed roughly half a million men and women from Europe for 5 years and identified 1329 colorectal cancers [54]. Colorectal carcinoma risk was positively associated with intake of red and processed meat [highest (>160 g/day) and lowest (<20 g/day) intake, HR 1.35 and of fish (>80 g/day vs. <10 g/day, HR 0.69)] but was not related to poultry intake. In this study population, the absolute risk of development of colorectal carcinoma within 10 years for a study subject aged 50 years was 1.71% for the highest category of red and processed meat intake, 1.28% for the lowest category of intake, 1.86% for subjects in the lowest category of fish intake, and 1.28% for subjects in the highest category of fish intake.

2.8 Lifestyle Factors

Intake of alcohol has been shown to be associated with colorectal cancer with an odds ratio of 2.6 [55]. Daily alcohol drinkers experience a twofold increase in risk of colorectal carcinomas [56]. Sharpe et al. [57] found the daily consumption of alcohol of any type was associated with increased risks of carcinoma of the distal colon and the rectum but not with an increased risk of a carcinoma of the proximal colon. An interesting relationship has been observed between the developments of rectal carcinoma in association with beer consumption [58]. The association of smoking (odds ratio for >40 pack years, 3.31) with adenomas has been reported [59]. Smoking for 20 years has a strong relation to formation of adenomas, but it appears that an induction period of at least 35 years is necessary for colorectal carcinoma [60, 61].

2.9 Obesity

Several authors have reported on a strong association between high body mass index and incidence of colorectal cancer [62–64]. Another indicator of obesity, the waist-to-hip ratio, has been independently related to increasing risk of colon cancer (RR 1.43, 95% CI 1.08–1.33) [65]. The hypothesis is that insulin resistance observed in obese patients is a precursor for hyperinsulinemia and high levels of insulin-like growth factor resulting into cellular proliferation and colonic neoplasia [62].

2.10 Level of Physical Activity

A high level of physical activity offers protective effect against development of colorectal cancer. A large meta-analysis with data pooled from 28 case-control and 19 cohort studies confirm this with a RR of 0.78 in males and 0.71 in females [66]. An estimate of the increased risk seen with a sedentary lifestyle is between 1.6 and 2 times. The effect of physical activity on the risk of development of rectal cancer is weaker compared to colon cancer [66–68]. In the NIH-AARP study, there was a nonsignificant trend toward protection from rectal cancer in men (RR = 0.76, $P = 0.07$) but no protective effect in women (RR = 0.95, $P = 0.23$) [67].The biological mechanisms that explain the relationship between physical activity and CRC risk are unclear.

2.11 Influence of NSAIDs and Aspirin

Data from observational studies show the protective effects of aspirin and other nonsteroidal anti-inflammatory drugs (NSAIDs) by reducing the formation of aberrant crypt foci, adenoma, and carcinoma. The protective mechanisms are not completely understood [69]. A Cochrane meta-analysis [70] reviewed one population-based prevention trial (including 22,071 people) [71], three secondary prevention trials in patients with sporadic polyps (including 2028 patients) [72–74], and four trials in 150 patients with familial adenomatous polyposis [75–78]. The authors conclude that there is some evidence for the effectiveness of intervention strategies using NSAIDs for the prevention of colorectal adenoma. However, the single primary prevention trial reviewed [71] did not demonstrate a decreased incidence of CRC in the intervention group. A recent pooled analysis of two large randomized trials from the UK with over 20 years of follow-up revealed a statistically significant reduction in CRC incidence in aspirin users (RR = 0.63; 95% CI, 0.47–0.85, $P = 0.002$, if allocated to aspirin for 5 years or more), but only after a latency period of 10 years or longer [79]. NSAIDs and aspirin may play an important role in secondary chemoprevention. Logan et al. [80] reported a randomized, double-blind trial of aspirin and folate in the prevention of recurrent colorectal adenomas. Patients randomized to aspirin 300 mg/day had a significantly reduced risk of recurrent adenoma compared to the placebo group (RR = 0.79; 95% CI, 0.63–0.99). It is important to recognize the risks of chemoprophylaxis with aspirin or NSAIDs which may outweigh the benefits. Serious GI complications occur in regular users of aspirin and NSAIDs. A number of authors have evaluated the cost-effectiveness of chemoprevention of CRC with NSAIDs [81] or COX-2 inhibitors [82] and found that chemoprophylaxis with these compounds is not cost-effective.

2.12 Inflammatory Bowel Disease

About 1–2% of all colorectal cancers arise in the setting of ulcerative colitis (UC) or Crohn's disease. Patients with pan-ulcerative colitis for more than 10 years carry a higher risk of dysplasia-carcinoma cascade. The reported risk of long-standing inflammatory bowel disease is variable depending on referral centers versus population-based studies as well as the surveillance practices followed. A meta-analysis of 116 studies evaluating the risk of CRC in ulcerative colitis patients found a prevalence rate of 3.7% (95% CI, 3.2–4.2%) [83]. In 19 of the studies reviewed, there was a cumulative probability of CRC of 2% after 10 years of disease, 8% after 20 years, and 18% after 30 years. The extent of disease also influences the risk of CRC in UC. In a Swedish population-based cohort of 3117 patients with UC, less extensive disease was associated with a lesser risk of CRC [84]. As a ratio of the observed-to-expected incidence, the increased risk of CRC in this cohort was 1.7 for those with ulcerative proctitis (95% CI, 0.8–3.2); 2.8 for those with left-sided colitis (95% CI, 1.6–4.4); and 14.8 for those with pancolitis (95% CI, 11.4–18.9). Coexistence of primary sclerosing cholangitis also modifies the risk of CRC in patients with UC [85]. For patients with long-standing, extensive UC, proctocolectomy is an effective strategy for the prevention of CRC. Other strategies include endoscopic surveillance for dysplasia and/or the use of chemopreventive agents. Although the efficacy of endoscopic surveillance has not been definitively proven in a randomized trial, a recent Cochrane review found that although there was no direct evidence of prolonged survival, patients with UC in surveillance programs tended to have cancers diagnosed earlier with a correspondingly improved prognosis [86]. Despite a lack of definitive evidence, endoscopic surveillance is commonly performed in patients with pancolitis for more than 10 years duration who wish to avoid colectomy. The relationship between Crohn's disease and the development of CRC has been less consistently demonstrated. In a Canadian population-based cohort study, the risk of CRC in 2857 patients with Crohn's disease was compared to a randomly selected group of controls matched 10:1 for age, sex, and geographic location [87]. Patients with Crohn's disease were found to have an elevated risk of colon cancer (incidence rate ratio (IRR) = 2.6; 95% CI, 1.69–4.12) but not rectal cancer (IRR = 1.08; 95% CI, 0.43–2.70).

2.13 Summary

Development of colorectal carcinogenesis is a complex interplay of genetic, environmental, dietary, and lifestyle factors. A thorough understanding of all these factors is essential in formulating an effective prevention strategy for this extremely common cancer.

Acknowledgments This work was supported by revenue from Nebraska cigarette taxes awarded to Creighton University by the Nebraska Department of Health and Human Services. Its contents are solely the responsibility of the authors and do not necessarily represent the official views of the State of Nebraska or the Nebraska Department of Health and Human Services.

References

1. Jemal A, Siegel R, Ward E, Hao Y, Xu J, Thun MJ. Cancer statistics 2009. CA Cancer J Clin. 2009;59:225–49.
2. Boyle P, Langman JS. ABC of colorectal cancer: epidemiology. BMJ. 2000;321:805–8.
3. Wingo PA, Cardinez CJ, Landis SH, Greenlee RT, Ries LA, Anderson RN, et al. Long-term trends in cancer mortality in the United States, 1930–1998. Cancer. 2003;97:3133–275.
4. American Cancer Society Website Cancer Facts and Figures. http://www.cancer.org/downloads/STT/500809web.pdf. Accessed 16 Dec 2009.
5. O'Connell JB, Maggard MA, Liu JH, Etzioni DA, Livingston EH, Ko CY. Rates of colon and rectal cancers are increasing in young adults. Am Surg. 2003;69:866–72.
6. Jemal A, Thomas A, Murray T, Thun M. Cancer statistics, 2002. CA Cancer J Clin. 2002;52:23–47. [Erratum, CA Cancer J Clin 2002;52:119, 181-2]
7. Eide TJ. Natural history of adenomas. World J Surg. 1991;15:3–6.
8. Vogelstein B, Fearon ER, Hamilton SR, Kern SE, Preisinger AC, Leppert M, et al. Genetic alterations during colorectal-tumor development. N Engl J Med. 1988;319:525–32.
9. Kronborg O, Fenger C. Clinical evidence of the adenoma–carcinoma sequence. Eur J Cancer Prev. 1999;8:573–86.
10. Jackman RJ, Mayo CW. The adenoma-carcinoma sequence in cancer of the colon. Surg Gynecol Obstet. 1951;93:327–30.
11. Church JM, Williams BR, Casey G. Molecular genetics and colorectal neo- plasia. In: A primer for the clinician. New York: Igaku-Shoin Medical Publishers; 1996.
12. Arends MJ. Pathways of colorectal carcinogenesis. Appl Immunohistochem Mol Morphol. 2013;21(2):97–102.
13. Goldstein NS. Serrated pathway and APC (conventional)-type colorectal polyps: molecular-morphologic correlations, genetic pathways, and implications for classification. Am J Clin Pathol. 2006;125:146–53.
14. Andreyev HJ, Norman AR, Cunningham D, Oates JR, Clarke PA. Kirsten ras mutations in patients with colorectal cancer: the multicenter "RASCAL" study. J Natl Cancer Inst. 1998;90: 675–84.
15. Naguib A, Wilson CH, Adams DJ, Arends MJ. Activation of K-RAS by co- mutation of codons 19 and 20 is transforming. J Mol Signal. 2011;6:2.
16. Karapetis CS, Khambata-Ford S, Jonker DJ, O'Callaghan CJ, Tu D, Tebbutt NC, et al. K-ras mutations and benefit from cetuximab in advanced colorectal cancer. N Engl J Med. 2008;359: 1757–65.
17. Gordon PH. Malignant neoplasms of the colon. In: Gordon PH, Nivatvongs S, editors. Principles and practice of surgery for the colon, rectum and anus. 3rd ed. New York, London: Informa Healthcare; 2007. p. 489–643.
18. Rosati G, Chiacchio R, Reggiardo G, De Sanctis D, Manzione L. Thymidylate synthase expression, p53, bcl-2, Ki-67 and p27 in colorectal cancer: relationships with tumor recurrence and survival. Tumor Biol. 2004;25:258–63.
19. Resnick MB, Routhier J, Konkin T, Sabo E, Pricolo VE. Epidermal growth factor receptor, c-MET, beta-catenin, and p53 expression as prognostic indicators in stage II colon cancer: a tissue microarray study. Clin Cancer Res. 2004;10:3069–75.
20. Lynch HT, de la Chapelle A. Hereditary colorectal cancer. N Engl J Med. 2003;348:919–32.
21. Aaltonen LA, Peltomaki P, Leach FS, Sistonen P, Pylkkanen L, Mecklin JP, et al. Clues to the pathogenesis of familial colorectal cancer. Science. 1993;260:812–6.
22. Longacre TA, Fenoglio-Preiser CM. Mixed hyperplastic adenomatous polyps serrated adenomas. A distinct form of colorectal neoplasia. Am J Surg Pathol. 1990;14:524–37.

23. Baker K, Zhang Y, Jin C, Jass JR. Proximal versus distal hyper- plastic polyps of the colorectum: different lesions or a biological spectrum? J Clin Pathol. 2004;57:1089–93.
24. Jass JR. Hyperplastic polyps and colorectal cancer: is there a link? Clin Gastroenterol Hepatol. 2004;2:1–8.
25. Bettington M, Walker N, Clouston A, Brown I, Leggett B, Whitehall V. The serrated pathway to colorectal carcinoma: current concepts and challenges. Histopathology. 2013;62:367–86.
26. Grady WM, Markowitz SD. The molecular pathogenesis of colorectal cancer and its potential application to colorectal cancer screening. Dig Dis Sci. 2015;60:762–72.
27. Lynch HT, Smyrk T, McGinn T, Lanspa S, Cavelieri J, Lynch J, et al. Attenuated familial adenomatous polyposis (AFAP). A phenotypically and genotypically distinct variant of FAP. Cancer. 1995;76:2427–33.
28. Bulow S. The Danish polyposis registry. Dis Colon Rectum. 1984;27:351–5.
29. Watson P, Lynch HT. The tumor spectrum in HNPCC. Anticancer Res. 1994;14:1635–9.
30. Gryfe R, Kim H, Hsieh ET, Aronson MD, Holowaty EJ, Bull SB, et al. Tumor microsatellite instability and clinical outcome in young patients with colorectal cancer. N Engl J Med. 2000;342:69–77.
31. Vogelstein B, Kinzler KW, editors. The genetic basis of human cancer. New York: McGraw-Hill; 1998.
32. Smyrk TC, Watson P, Kaul K, Lynch HT. Tumor-infiltrating lymphocytes are a marker for microsatellite instability in colorectal carcinoma. Cancer. 2001;91:2417–22.
33. Alexander J, Watanabe T, Wu T-T, Rashid A, Li S, Hamilton SR. Histopathological identification of colon cancer with microsatellite instability. Am J Pathol. 2001;158:527–351998.
34. Jass JR, Do K-A, Simms LA, Lino H, Wynter C, Pillay SP, et al. Morphology of sporadic colorectal cancer with DNA replication errors. Gut. 1998;42:673–9.
35. Jass JR, Stewart SM. Evolution of hereditary non-polyposis colorectal cancer. Gut. 1992; 33:783–6.
36. Peltomaki P, Lothe RA, Aaltonen LA, Pylkkanen L, Nystrom-Lahti M, Seruca R, et al. Microsatellite instability is associated with tumors that characterize the hereditary non-polyposis colorectal carcinoma syndrome. Cancer Res. 1993;53:5853–5.
37. Boland CR, Thibodeau SN, Hamilton SR, Sidransky D, Eshleman JR, Burt RW, et al. A National Cancer Institute workshop on microsatellite instability for cancer detection and familial predisposition: development of international criteria for the determination of microsatellite instability in colorectal cancer. Cancer Res. 1998;58:5248–57.
38. Cunningham C, Dunlop MG. Molecular genetic basis of colorectal cancer sus- ceptibility. Br J Surg. 1996;83:321–9.
39. Burkitt DP. Related disease–related cause? Lancet. 1969;2:1229–31.
40. Nagao M, Sugimura T. Carcinogenic factors in food with relevance to colon. cancer development. Mutat Res. 1993;290:43–51.
41. Jain M, Cook GM, Davis FG, Grace MG, Howe GR, Miller AB. A case-control study of diet and colorectal cancer. Int J Cancer. 1980;26:757–68.
42. Potter JD, McMichael AJ. Diet and cancer of the colon and rectum: a case- control study. J Natl Cancer Inst. 1986;76:557–69.
43. Phillips RL, Snowdon DA. Dietary relationships with fatal colorectal cancer among seventh-day Adventists. J Natl Cancer Inst. 1985;74:307–17.
44. Garland C, Shekelle RD, Barrett-Connor E, Criqui MH, Rossof AH, Paul O. Dietary vitamin D and calcium and risk of colorectal cancer: a 19 year prospective study in men. Lancet. 1985;1:307–9.
45. Fleiszer D, Murray D, MacFarlane J, Brown RA. Protective effect of dietary fiber against chemically induced bowel tumors in rats. Lancet. 1978;2:552–3.
46. Greenwald P, Lanza E, Eddy GA. Dietary fiber in the reduction of colon cancer. J Am Diet Assoc. 1987;87:1178–88.
47. Trock B, Lanza E, Greenwald P. Dietary fiber, vegetables and colon cancer: critical review and meta-analysis of the epidemiological evidence. J Natl Cancer Inst. 1990;82:650–61.
48. Asano T, McLeod RS. Dietary fiber for the prevention of colorectal adenomas and carcinomas. Cochrane Database Syst Rev. 2002;2:CD003430.
49. Fuchs CS, Giovannucci EL, Colditz GA, Hunter DJ, Stampfer MJ, Rosner B, et al. Dietary fiber and the risk of colorectal cancer and adenoma in women. N Engl J Med. 1999;340:169–76.

50. Willett WC, Stampfer MJ, Colditz GA, Rosner BA, Speizer FE. Relation of meat, food, and fiber intake to the risk of colon cancer in a prospective study amongst women. N Engl J Med. 1990;323:1664–72.
51. Howe GR, Aronson KJ, Benito E, Castelleto R, Cornee J, Duffy S, et al. The relationship between dietary fat intake and risk of colorectal cancer: evidence from the combined analysis of 13 case-control studies. Cancer Causes Control. 1997;8:215–28.
52. Beresford SA, Johnson KC, Ritenbaugh C, Lasser NL, Snetselaar LG, Black HR, et al. Low-fat dietary pattern and risk of colorectal cancer: the Women's health initiative randomized controlled dietary modification trial. JAMA. 2006;295:643–54.
53. Larsson SC, Rafter J, Holmberg L, Bergvist L, Wolk A. Red meat consumption and risk of cancers of the proximal colon, distal colon and rectum: the Swedish mammography cohort. Int J Cancer. 2005;113:829–34.
54. Norat T, Bingham S, Ferrari P, Slimani N, Jenab M, Mazuir M, Overvad K, et al. Meat, fish, and colorectal cancer risk: the European prospective investigation into cancer and nutrition. J Natl Cancer Inst. 2005;97:906–16.
55. Peters U, Sinha R, Chatterjee N, Subar AF, Ziegler RG, Kulldorff M, et al. Dietary fibre and colorectal adenoma in a colorectal cancer early detection program. Lancet. 2003;361:1491–5.
56. Lognecker MP. A case-control study of alcoholic beverage consumption in relation to risk of cancer of the right colon and rectum in men. Cancer Causes Control. 1990;1:5–14.
57. Sharpe CR, Siemiatycki J, Rachet B. Effects of alcohol consumption on the risk of colorectal cancer among men by anatomical subsite (Canada). Cancer Causes Control. 2002;13:483–91.
58. Correa P, Haenszel W. The epidemiology of large bowel cancer. Adv Cancer Res. 1978;26: 1–141.
59. Kikendall JW, Bowen PE, Burgess MB, Magnetti C, Woodward J, Langenberg P, et al. Cigarettes and alcohol as independent risk factors for colonic adenomas. Gastroenterology. 1989;97:660–4.
60. Giovannucci E, Rimm EB, Stampfer MJ, Colditz GA, Ascherio A, Kearney J, et al. A prospective study of cigarette smoking and risk of colorectal adenoma and colorectal cancer in U.S. men. J Natl Cancer Inst. 1994;86:183–91.
61. Giovannucci E, Colditz GA, Stampfer MJ, Hunter D, Rosner BA, Willett WC, et al. A prospective study of cigarette smoking and risk of colorectal adenoma and colorectal cancer in U.S. women. J Natl Cancer Inst. 1994;86:192–9.
62. Lin J, Zhang SM, Cook NR, Rexrode KM, Lee IM, Buring JE. Body mass index and risk of colorectal cancer in women (United States). Cancer Causes Control. 2004;15:581–9.
63. Reeves GK, Pirie K, Beral V, Green J, Spencer E, Bull D. Cancer Incidence and mortality in relation to body mass index in the million women study: cohort study. BMJ. 2007;335:1134.
64. Sturmer T, Buring JE, Lee IM, Gaziano JM, Glynn RJ. Metabolic abnormalities and risk for colorectal cancer in the physicians' health study. Cancer Epidemiol Biomarkers Prev. 2006;15: 2391–7.
65. Larsson SC, Wolk A. Obesity and colon and rectal cancer risk: a meta-analysis of prospective studies. Am J Clin Nutr. 2007;86:556–65.
66. Samad AK, Taylor RS, Marshall T, Chapman MA. A meta-analysis of the association of physical activity with reduced risk of colorectal cancer. Colorectal Dis. 2005;7:204–13.
67. Howard RA, Freedman DM, Park Y, Hollenbeck A, Schatzkin A, Leitzmann MF. Physical activity, sedentary behavior, and the risk of colon and rectal cancer in the NIH-AARP diet and health study. Cancer Causes Control. 2008;19:939–53.
68. Harriss DJ, Atkinson G, Batterham A, George K, Cable NT, Reilly T, et al. Lifestyle factors and colorectal cancer risk (2): a systematic review and meta- analysis of associations with leisure-time physical activity. Colorectal Dis. 2009;11:689–701.
69. Hawk ET, Umar A, Viner JL. Colorectal cancer chemoprevention – an overview of the science. Gastroenterology. 2004;126:1423–47.
70. Asano TK, McLeod RS. Non steroidal anti-inflammatory drugs (NSAID) and Aspirin for preventing colorectal adenomas and carcinomas. Cochrane Database Syst Rev. 2004;(2): CD004079.

71. Gann PH, Manson JE, Glynn RJ, Buring JE, Hennekens CH. Low-dose aspirin and incidence of colorectal tumors in a randomized trial. J Natl Cancer Inst. 1993;85:1220–4.
72. Baron JA, Cole BF, Sandler RS, et al. A randomized trial of aspirin to prevent colorectal adenomas. N Engl J Med. 2003;348:891–9.
73. Sandler RS, Halabi S, Baron JA, Budinger S, Paskett E, Keresztes R, et al. A randomized trial of aspirin to prevent colorectal adenomas in patients with previous colorectal cancer. N Engl J Med. 2003;348:883–90.
74. Benamouzig R, Deyra J, Martin A, Girard B, Jullian E, Piednoir B, et al. Daily soluble aspirin and prevention of colorectal adenoma recurrence: one-year results of the APACC trial. Gastroenterology. 2003;125:328–36.
75. Giardiello FM, Hamilton SR, Krush AJ, Piantadosi S, Hylind LM, Celano P, et al. Treatment of colonic and rectal adenomas with sulindac in familial ade- nomatous polyposis. N Engl J Med. 1993;328:1313–6.
76. Giardiello FM, Yang VW, Hylind LM, Krush AJ, Petersen GM, Trimbath JD, et al. Primary chemo- prevention of familial adenomatous polyposis with sulindac. N Engl J Med. 2002;346:1054–9.
77. Labayle D, Fischer D, Vielh P, Drouhin F, Pariente A, Bories C, et al. Sulindac causes regression of rectal polyps in familial adenomatous polyposis. Gastroenterology. 1991;101:635–9.
78. Steinbach G, Lynch PM, Phillips RK, Wallace MH, Hawk E, Gordon GB, et al. The effect of celecoxib, a cyclooxygenase-2 inhibitor, in familial adenomatous polyposis. N Engl J Med. 2000;342:1946–52.
79. Flossmann E, Rothwell PM. Effect of aspirin on long-term risk of colorectal cancer: consistent evidence from randomized and observational studies. Lancet. 2007;369:1603–13.
80. Logan RF, Grainge MJ, Shepherd VC, Armitage NC, Muir KR. Aspirin and folic acid for the prevention of recurrent colorectal adenomas. Gastroenterology. 2008;134:29–38.
81. Suleiman S, Rex DK, Sonnenberg A. Chemoprevention of colorectal cancer by aspirin: a cost-effectiveness analysis. Gastroenterology. 2002;122:78–84.
82. Hur C, Simon LS, Gazelle GS. The cost-effectiveness of aspirin versus cyclooxygenase-2-selective inhibitors for colorectal carcinoma chemoprevention in healthy individuals. Cancer. 2004;101:189–97.
83. Eaden JA, Abrams KR, Mayberry JF. The risk of colorectal cancer in ulcerative colitis: a meta-analysis. Gut. 2001;48:526–35.
84. Ekbom A, Helmick C, Zack M, Adami HO. Ulcerative colitis and colorectal cancer. A population-based study. N Engl J Med. 1990;323:1228–33.
85. Oetikno RM, Lin OS, Heidenreich PA, Young HS, Blackstone MO. Increased risk of colorectal neoplasia in patients with primary sclerosing cholangitis and ulcerative colitis: a meta-analysis. Gastrointest Endosc. 2002;56:48–54.
86. Collins PD, Mpofu C, Watson AJ, Rhodes JM. Strategies for detecting colon cancer and/or dysplasia in patients with inflammatory bowel disease. Cochrane Database Syst Rev. 2006;(2): CD000279.
87. Gillen CD, Walmsley RS, Prior P, Andrews HA, Allan RN. Ulcerative colitis and Crohns disease: a comparison of the colorectal cancer risk in extensive colitis. Gut. 1994;35:1590–2.

Neoadjuvant Chemoradiotherapy and Neoadjuvant Chemotherapy

3

Mohamed E. Salem and John L. Marshall

Abstract

Rectal cancer is a challenging disease to treat, and its optimal management requires a multidisciplinary approach with involvement of surgical, medical, and radiation oncologists.

The significant advancements in the surgical techniques, preoperative treatment, and medical imaging technology have altered the therapeutic landscape and led to substantial improvements in both local disease control and patient survival. Currently, preoperative (neoadjuvant) chemoradiation (chemoradiotherapy; CRT) is the established standard of care for patients with locally advanced rectal cancer. This treatment paradigm consists of concurrent radiotherapy and infusional-5-FU- or oral capecitabine-based chemotherapy, followed by recovery time, and then total mesorectal excision (TME). Sometimes adjuvant chemotherapy follows surgery. Despite the therapeutic benefits and excellent local control achieved with such a treatment model, CRT remains associated with significant side effects. Therefore, potential practice changing trials are currently ongoing to put forth a new treatment strategy that will enable us to better select patients and deliver the precise therapy for that particular individual, aiming at changing the old concept of "one size fits all" to a new one of "custom-made therapy." A more tailored approach to therapy allows for adaptive therapies based on individual patients and their treatment response, whether this response is to neoadjuvant chemotherapy alone or induction chemotherapy followed by chemoradiation. The results of these ongoing efforts could result in a paradigm shift and an ideal tailored approach to the management of rectal cancer.

M.E. Salem, M.D. (✉) • J.L. Marshall, M.D.
Division of Hematology/Oncology, Georgetown University, 3800 Reservoir Road, N.W., Washington, DC 20007, USA

Lombardi Comprehensive Cancer Center, Georgetown University, 3800 Reservoir Road, N.W., Washington, DC 20007, USA
e-mail: Mohamed.E.Salem@gunet.georgetown.edu

G. Dapri, J.H. Marks (eds.), *Surgical Techniques in Rectal Cancer*,
https://doi.org/10.1007/978-4-431-55579-7_3

The focus of this chapter is to highlight the scientific evidence for managing locally advanced rectal cancer using preoperative CRT, discuss how this treatment has evolved to become the current standard of care, and address the future treatment of this disease.

Keywords
Rectal cancer • Neoadjuvant chemotherapy • Neoadjuvant chemoradiotherapy

3.1 Introduction

Colorectal cancer (CRC) currently presents a significant global health problem: it is one of the leading causes of cancer-related death in the United States and around the world. It is estimated that approximately 1.25 million new cases of CRC are diagnosed annually worldwide, and approximately 600,000 patients are expected to die due to this disease each year [1]. Of these cancers, approximately 30% arise in the rectum.

3.2 Current Standard of Care for Locally Advanced Rectal Cancer

The treatment for rectal cancer has been revolutionized, leading to substantial improvements in disease management over the last 2 decades [2]. Treatment choice for rectal cancer is based on numerous considerations; however, the use of trimodality therapy depends to a great extent upon the stage of tumor and its location in the rectum. In patients with locally advanced rectal cancer, preoperative chemoradiation (chemoradiotherapy; CRT) was established as the standard of care, and this treatment paradigm currently consists of approximately 6 weeks of neoadjuvant CRT (infusional 5-FU- or oral capecitabine-based), followed by 8–12 weeks of recovery prior to surgery—usually involving total mesorectal excision (TME)—possibly followed by adjuvant chemotherapy.

It follows that the decision to carry out preoperative CRT is largely based on the patient's disease stage. Hence, accurate preoperative staging of the rectal cancer is one of the most critical steps in the management of this disease. The basis for a tailored therapeutic approach is the selection of the proper treatment modality for each patient, which is profoundly dependent upon accurate preoperative locoregional staging.

3.3 Staging of Rectal Tumors

Endoscopic ultrasound (EUS) and magnetic resonance imaging (MRI) are the most commonly used modalities in preoperative locoregional staging of rectal cancer; the choice of either one depends mainly on local expertise. Although endoscopic ultrasound allows accurate staging of early rectal cancers (T1 and T2 tumors) with high sensitivity and specificity, its accuracy in predicting mesorectal nodal involvement is about 70%, and it cannot assess the status of circumferential resection margin (CRM).

On the other hand, a thin section (high-resolution) surface pelvic phased-array coil MRI of the pelvis allows excellent soft tissue spatial and contrast resolution.

The MERCURY (Magnetic Resonance Imaging and Rectal Cancer European Equivalence) study group's multicenter trial analysis yielded data on the ability of MRI to predict extramural invasion depth and demonstrated that MRI has an accuracy of 91% in predicting a clear CRM [3]. Thus, MRI is generally preferred over EUS for locoregional staging of rectal cancer due to its greater utility in assessing the CRM.

Once locoregional staging is completed, patients will either undergo surgical resection or neoadjuvant CRT depending on the final TNM stage (treatment algorithm as per Fig. 3.1).

In this chapter, we focus on highlighting the scientific evidence for managing locally advanced rectal cancer using preoperative CRT. We also address how preoperative CRT has evolved to become the current standard of care and discuss future perspectives on such therapies.

3.3.1 Patient Selection

The selection of patients that should undergo preoperative neoadjuvant CRT remains imprecise. Although the only definitive indication for preoperative neoadjuvant CRT is the presence of a T3 or T4 tumor, there may be a convincing argument to use preoperative neoadjuvant CRT in other clinical situations. For example, if a patient has

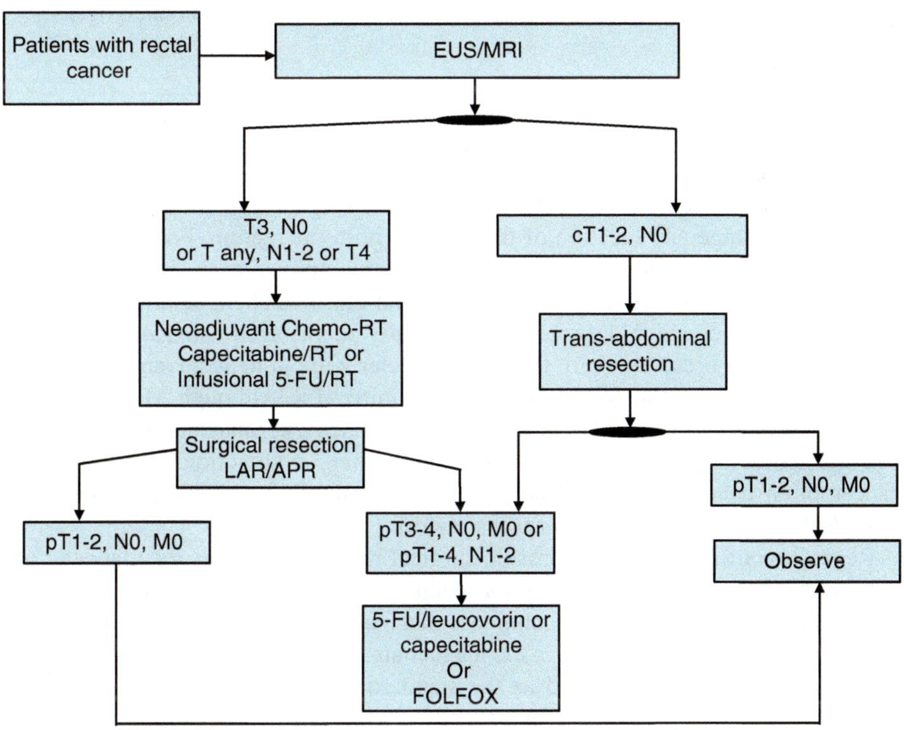

Fig. 3.1 Treatment algorithm for rectal cancer

distal rectal tumors for which an abdominoperineal resection (APR) is believed to be necessary, a major goal is to convert APR to a sphincter-preserving operation—such as low anterior resection (LAR) with coloanal anastomosis—using neoadjuvant CRT.

Furthermore, it is important to note that the accuracy of preoperative EUS and/or MRI for staging of mid to distal T3N0 rectal cancer remains imperfect; approximately 20% of patients may be understaged or overstaged by preoperative MRI and or EUS imaging [3]. Following their review of 188 patients, Guillem et al. (2008) reported that 22% of individuals who were thought, preoperatively, to have stage T3N0 tumors by transrectal ultrasound/MRI received preoperative CRT but were found to have positive lymph nodes on pathological examination of the resected specimen [4]. Thus about 20% of patients were understaged, and, given the anticipated downstaging effect of CRT, one can assume that the percentage with preoperative node-positive disease and incorrect staging was even greater. Conversely, as shown below in the seminal German study, about 18% may be overstaged and therefore overtreated [5, 6]. These observations underscore that the accuracy of preoperative ERUS/MRI for staging mid to distal cT3N0 rectal cancer is limited, and thus, the optimal management strategy for patients with clinical stage T3N0 rectal cancer (based upon preoperative EUS and/or MRI) remains unsatisfactory.

3.4 Multimodality Therapy in Treatment of Rectal Cancer

Rectal cancer is a challenging disease, and, ideally, its treatment should take place in a multidisciplinary setting including surgical, medical, and radiation oncologists.

3.4.1 Surgical Resection

Surgical resection is the keystone treatment for rectal cancer and is the curative modality for this disease. Nonetheless, the required surgical approach varies greatly depending on stage and location of the tumor within the rectum. For instance, for patients with small rectal adenocarcinomas that are confined to the rectal wall (T1 or T2), local excision might be sufficient and can offer excellent results. Similarly, tumors in the upper and middle rectum can usually be managed with LAR, coloanal anastomosis, and preservation of the anal sphincter without neoadjuvant therapy.

On the other hand, low rectal tumors will require APR. Although APR results in excellent local control, the APR procedure necessitates a permanent colostomy and is associated with high incidence of sexual and urinary dysfunction. These circumstances often have a substantial negative impact on quality of life and therefore make APR an unattractive option for the majority of patients.

Regardless of the specific approach, surgical resection remains the mainstay of treatment; it is the curative modality for rectal cancer, and there is no doubt that the remarkable advances in surgical techniques that have evolved over the last 2 decades have resulted in an improvement in the local control of rectal cancer. One technique in particular, TME, has emerged as the standard of care. This procedure entails complete removal of the primary tumor and the associated perirectal lymph nodes, without disruption of the mesorectum.

3.4.2 Radiation Therapy

Advances in surgical resection techniques enable curative potential for rectal cancer; however, local and distant tumor recurrence following surgical resection alone continues to be problematic, and this necessitates further efforts to improve initial local control [7–9]. Additionally, most patients understandably find a permanent colostomy to be of major concern; hence additional treatment options are needed to improve outcome while avoiding the use of colostomy, especially among those with low-lying tumors.

The combination of surgery with other anticancer therapeutic modalities has been explored in the hope of improving outcome. Radiation therapy (radiotherapy; RT) was introduced and then integrated into the treatment paradigm for rectal cancer. This approach was evaluated in several randomized trials, first in the postoperative and then in the preoperative settings [10–19], resulting in reduced local recurrence rates but with little impact on disease-free survival (DFS) and overall survival (OS).

An added local recurrence benefit from combining RT with surgery is evident on data analysis from both pre- and post-TME eras. This was demonstrated in the Dutch neoadjuvant trial of short-course preoperative RT (5 × 5 Gy). This study utilized the modern surgical approach, TME, and demonstrated a consistent benefit of improved local control [2].

3.4.3 Chemoradiotherapy

It became evident that the combination of RT with surgery leads to an improvement in the rate of local control; however, no study to date demonstrates an RT-induced improvement in patient survival. Thus, in continued efforts to improve outcome, the next rational step was to attempt augmentation of RT with chemotherapy. Several phase III trials were conducted to examine whether the addition of fluorouracil-based chemotherapy to RT resulted in a better pathological response and better outcome.

In a landmark study conducted by Krook and colleagues (1991), chemotherapy was combined with RT—postoperatively—in an attempt to reduce recurrences and deaths, as compared with RT alone. A total of 204 patients with high-risk (T3/4 or node-positive) rectal cancer were randomly assigned to receive postoperative RT (4500–5040 cGy) with or without fluorouracil followed by a cycle of systemic therapy with fluorouracil plus semustine (methyl-CCNU). After a median follow-up of 7 years, local recurrence and distant metastases were reduced by 46% ($P = 0.036$) and 37% ($P = 0.011$), respectively. In addition, combined therapy reduced the rate of cancer-related deaths by 36% ($P = 0.0071$) and the overall death rate by 29 % ($P = 0.025$). The authors concluded that the combination of RT and fluorouracil postoperative therapy, followed by continued systemic therapy with a fluorouracil-based regimen, improves disease and survival outcomes for rectal cancer patients, as compared with postoperative RT alone [20].

On the basis of this finding, along with several others, including the GITSG trial [19], it became evident that chemotherapy has benefits when added to RT. Hence, a National Institutes of Health consensus conference recommended postoperative adjuvant CRT as standard treatment for patients with rectal cancer patients who have the adverse prognostic factors of regional nodal metastasis, invasion of perirectal fat or adjacent organs, or both [21]. By the early 1990s, CRT was established as the standard of care in the management of advanced rectal cancer.

3.4.4 Neoadjuvant Chemoradiotherapy

Krook and colleagues [20] examined the benefits of adding chemotherapy to RT in the postoperative setting, but several other prospective randomized trials examined the benefits of adding chemotherapy to RT (compared with RT alone) for the management of locally advanced rectal cancer in the preoperative setting. Subsequently, several other research groups examined both the benefit of preoperative CRT (neoadjuvant CRT) versus preoperative RT alone as well as the contribution of added postoperative chemotherapy in both of these settings.

In 1993, the EORTC Radiotherapy Group initiated the EORTC 22921 trial, using a 2 × 2 factorial design. The aim of the study was to assess the value of adding chemotherapy (5-FU and leucovorin) to preoperative RT (neoadjuvant CRT), as well as the value of added postoperative (adjuvant) chemotherapy (4 cycles of 5-FU and leucovorin), and whether these approaches could improve OS and progression-free survival (PFS) of patients with T3-4 resectable rectal cancer [22].

More than 1000 patients were enrolled onto the trial and then randomly assigned to receive one of the following four treatments: (1) preoperative RT (the control arm), (2) preoperative CRT, (3) preoperative RT and postoperative chemotherapy, or (4) preoperative CRT and postoperative chemotherapy (Fig. 3.2).

Radiotherapy consisted of 45 Gy delivered to the posterior pelvis in 25 fractions of 1.8 Gy over a period of 5 weeks. Preoperative chemotherapy was delivered in 2 × 5-day courses during the first and fifth weeks of RT. Fluorouracil was given at a dose of 350 mg/m^2 per day and leucovorin at a dose of 20 mg/m^2 per day. Surgery was scheduled to take place 8–12 weeks after treatment.

CRT resulted in downsizing and downstaging of tumors and increased local control rates. Local failure rates were significantly lower in all 3 groups receiving chemotherapy compared with the control group, regardless of whether it was given prior to or following surgery.

Patients undergoing preoperative CRT had a significantly higher rate of pathological complete response (pCR, 14% versus 5%). However, the addition of chemotherapy, either concurrently with RT or postoperatively (adjuvant), was not associated with any improvement in PFS or OS.

Updated, long-term results from this study were published in Lancet Oncology in 2014 [23]: the cumulative incidence of local relapse at 10 years was reported as 22.4% with RT alone, compared with 11–15% in the 3 groups receiving chemotherapy. Ten-year DFS was similar in patients receiving preoperative CRT versus RT alone (46% versus 44%), as was OS (51% versus 49%). Additionally, adjuvant fluorouracil-based chemotherapy after preoperative RT (with or without chemotherapy) still did not affect DFS or OS.

Other studies, such as the Fédération Francophone de Cancérologie Digestive (FFCD) trial 9203, revealed similar results and showed that the addition of fluorouracil to RT significantly increased the pCR and local disease control rate [24].

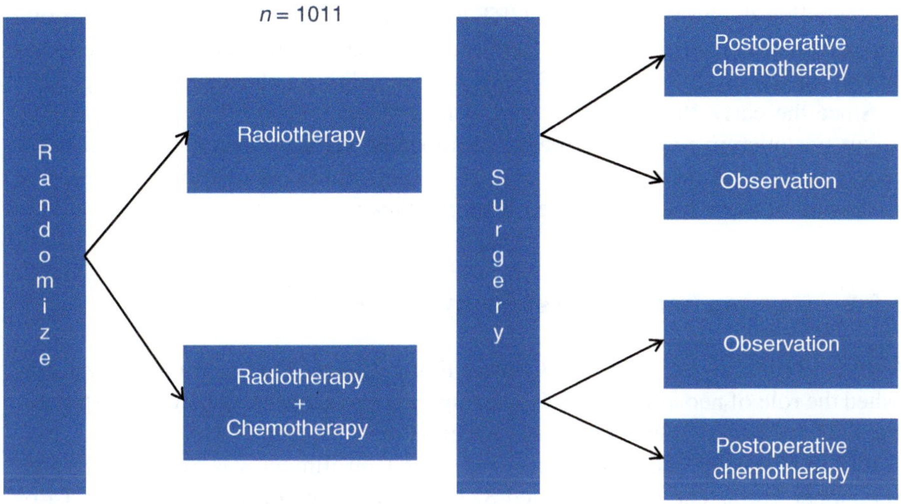

Fig. 3.2 EORTC 22921 trial design

In a meta-analysis that included the EORTC 22921 trial and 5 other studies [24–28], the addition of chemotherapy to preoperative RT in the treatment of locally advanced (T3–4, node-positive) rectal cancer was associated with less local recurrence (odds ratio [OR] for local recurrence 0.56, 95% CI, 0.42 to 0.75) [29].

However, there was no significant difference in OS between RT and CRT. Additionally, there was a higher rate of grade 3 and 4 treatment-related adverse events with CRT (OR 3.96, 95% CI, 3.03 to 5.17).

Despite the lack of improved OS, the addition of chemotherapy to conventional fractionation RT has become a standard approach to neoadjuvant combined modality therapy in the treatment of locally advanced (T3–4, node-positive) rectal cancer, likely because of the reduction in local recurrence and improvement in pathologic complete response (pCR) rates observed with CRT.

3.5 Preoperative Versus Postoperative

At a certain point, adjuvant CRT following resection was considered the standard treatment for stage II–III operable rectal cancer. However, with the growing evidence of the benefits of CRT in the neoadjuvant setting in terms of pCR and local control of disease (in comparison to RT alone), several questions were raised:

(1) What is the best sequence of CRT in relation to surgery?

(2) What is the optimal chemotherapy regimen?

(3) Will delivering more efficient systemic therapy early in the course of treatment result in better outcomes and perhaps have the potential to eradicate subclinical metastatic disease?

(4) How are the compliance issues associated with postoperative chemotherapy to be avoided?

Regarding the best sequence of CRT to use in relation to surgery, there are two major strategies: neoadjuvant CRT followed by surgery, followed by adjuvant chemotherapy, or surgery followed by CRT, followed by adjuvant chemotherapy (Fig. 3.3).

Since the early 1990s, several studies have attempted to compare preoperative versus postoperative CRT in patients with locally advanced rectal cancer to better understand the optimal sequence of CRT administration in relation to surgery. A discussion of these studies and their results follows.

3.5.1 German Rectal Cancer Study Group Trial

A seminal trial carried out by the German Rectal Cancer Study Group firmly established the role of neoadjuvant CRT by comparing preoperative CRT with postoperative CRT for locally advanced rectal cancer patients [5] (Fig. 3.4).

The trial was initiated in February 1995, and enrollment was extended through September 2002. The study enrolled 823 patients with clinical stage T3 or T4 or node-positive disease. Patients were then randomized to receive either preoperative ($N = 421$) or postoperative ($N = 402$) CRT. The preoperative treatment consisted of 5040 cGy delivered in fractions of 180 cGy per day, 5 days per week, concurrently with 5-fluorouracil (5-FU, 1000 mg/m^2 daily for 5 days during the first and fifth weeks of RT). All patients underwent total mesorectal excision 6 weeks after the completion of CRT. One month after this surgery, 4 additional cycles of adjuvant single agent 5-FU (500 mg/m^2 bolus daily for 5 days, every 4 weeks) were administered. With the exception of the delivery of a boost of 540 cGy, CRT administration was identical in the postoperative treatment group. The primary endpoint was OS.

Results from the 46-month median follow-up analysis showed that preoperative CRT was associated with a significantly lower cumulative incidence of local relapse than postoperative CRT (6% versus 13%; P=0.006) [6]. After 11 years of follow-up, the difference was smaller but still persisted (7% versus 10% for pre- versus post-surgical CRT, respectively) [6]. The 5-year DFS rate was 68% versus 65%, and the

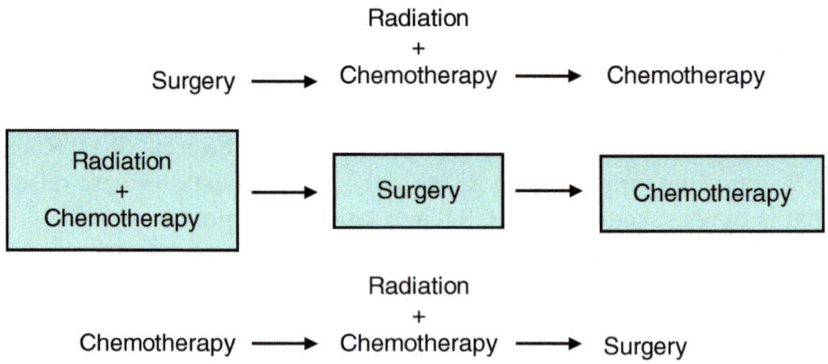

Fig. 3.3 Possible CRT sequences in the treatment of rectal cancer

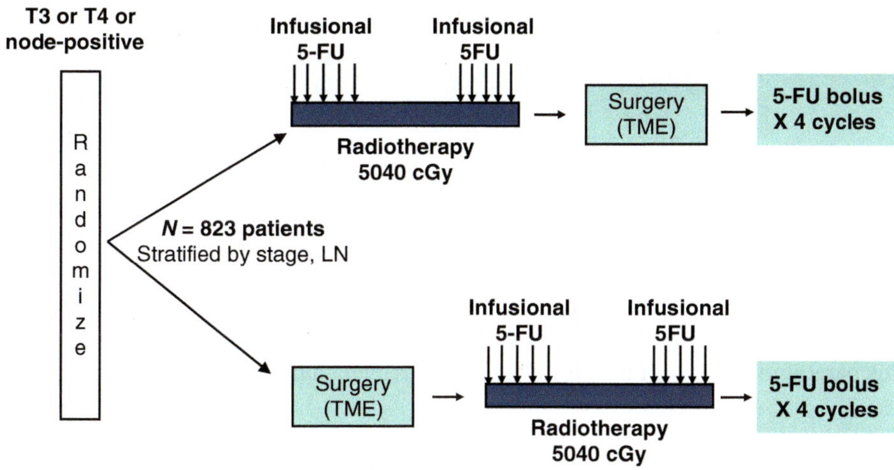

Fig. 3.4 The German Rectal Cancer Study Group trial: preoperative versus postoperative chemoradiotherapy for rectal cancer

5-year OS rates were 76% and 74%, respectively ($P = 0.80$). Ten-year survival rates were similar between pre- and postsurgical CRT (DFS was approximately 68% and OS was approximately 60% [taking the average of both pre- and post- groups]). The long-term toxic effects in the preoperative and postoperative patients were 14% and 24%, respectively ($P = 0.01$).

Following preoperative CRT, there was a significant shift toward earlier TNM staging, suggestive of significant downstaging effects ($P < 0.001$) due to preoperative CRT. Furthermore, 8% of the patients in the preoperative CRT group had a complete response, and only 25% (as compared with 40 % in the postoperative treatment group) had positive lymph nodes [5, 6].

Among patients with tumors that were initially determined to require an abdominoperineal excision, sphincter-preserving surgery was performed pre- and post-chemoradiotherapy in a total of 78 and 116 patients, respectively; however sphincter preservation was actually achieved in 19% of patients undergoing surgery before CRT, compared with 39% undergoing surgery after CRT ($P = 0.004$) [5]. In other words, patients who underwent preoperative CRT were twice as likely to undergo a sphincter-sparing operation.

As a side note, 18% of patients in the postoperative treatment group (no CRT prior to surgery) that were determined preoperatively to have T3 or T4 disease or lymph node metastasis were found to actually have T1 or T2, node-negative tumors on pathological examination of the resected specimen. This important observation clearly highlights the limitations of preoperative staging and perhaps the overtreatment of some patients; it stresses the need for accurate staging to avoid unnecessary treatment of patients with early-stage tumors.

Importantly, some retrospective data suggest that administration of infusional rather than bolus 5-FU during RT increases the likelihood of a pCR in patients with locally advanced rectal cancer [30]. In addition to results from the 1995 German

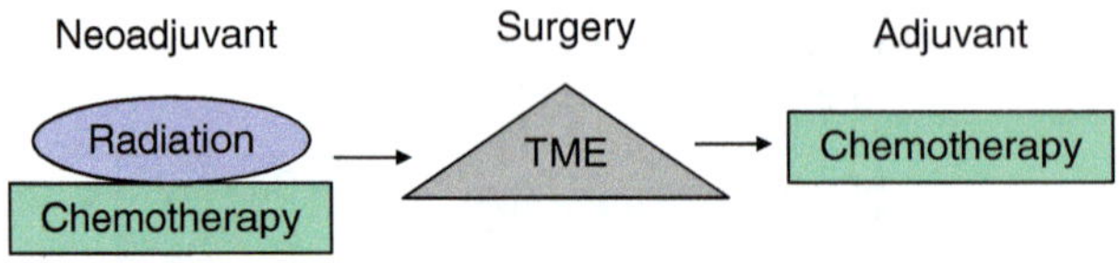

Fig. 3.5 The current standard of care (SOC) for rectal cancer (established in 2004)

national intergroup trial, O'Connell et al. (1994) [31] demonstrated further improvement in outcomes when 5-FU was given continuously during postoperative RT with the use of ambulatory infusion pumps [31].

By 2004, preoperative CRT was established as the standard of care (Fig. 3.5). This paradigm shift was made following the German study results.

3.5.2 Risk Stratification of Rectal Cancer

The German trial not only established a new standard treatment paradigm for the management of rectal cancer, but it also shed light on some very important aspects of rectal cancer treatment: the risk stratification of rectal cancer patients undergoing neoadjuvant CRT and the best way to predict DFS after preoperative therapy.

In a subsequent exploratory analysis of the German Rectal Cancer Study [32], the pathological T stage and the nodal status after CRT were found to be the most important independent prognostic factors for DFS. The 5-year DFS was 85% for ypN0, 65% for ypN1, and 18% for ypN2 (the "y" added to a pathological stage indicate a TNM stage that is given following CRT). The poor outcomes seen in patients with ypN2 disease in this report suggest that positive lymph nodes after neoadjuvant CRT may indicate a more aggressive disease. It is therefore feasible to argue that such patients should undergo prolonged postoperative chemotherapy.

In addition to the nodal status after CRT, prognosis following neoadjuvant CRT was also associated with TRG (tumor regression grading). TRG incorporates the degree of fibrosis as well as the percentage of viable tumor cells [32] and in an updated report of long-term results after a median follow-up of 132 months, the 10-year DFS rates for patients with TRG-4 were 90%, TRG 2 to 3 were 74%, and TRG 0–1 were 63% [33].

Whether the pathological T stage, nodal status, and TRG could or should be used to modify postoperative treatment strategies and whether or not adjuvant chemotherapy should be avoided or augmented in those with a favorable or poor prognosis remain unclear. This is an active area of research and has the potential to offer a unique opportunity to improve the current treatment paradigm and select the optimal therapy.

In addition to the German study, two other prospective randomized trials aimed to compare the efficacy of preoperative CRT with postoperative CRT for rectal cancer. These studies were initiated in the United States by the Radiation Therapy Oncology Group (RTOG; trial 94-01) and the National Surgical Adjuvant Breast and Bowel Project (NSABP; protocol R-03). Unfortunately, both studies were closed prematurely due to poor accrual.

3.5.3 NSABP Trial R-03

Similar to the German study, the NSABP R-03 trial [34] was conceived to determine the best time to administer CRT therapy to patients with stage II and III rectal cancer. The primary intent of this study was to determine whether a difference in DFS is observed following neoadjuvant versus adjuvant CRT for locally advanced rectal cancer. The intended sample size was 900 patients, but after 6 years of slower-than-anticipated accrual, the protocol was closed, having accrued a total of 267 patients. All 267 patients were included in the final analysis.

Between August 1993 and June 1999, 267 patients with clinical T3 or T4 or node-positive rectal cancer were randomized to preoperative CRT ($N = 123$) or postoperative CRT ($N = 131$). Preoperative therapy consisted of one cycle of weekly bolus 5-FU with leucovorin for 6 weeks and 2 courses of 5-FU and leucovorin (daily for 5 days during the first and fifth course of RT) concomitant with pelvic irradiation (50.4 Gy). This was followed by surgery and then 4 cycles of postoperative weekly bolus 5-FU with leucovorin. The postoperative CRT regimen consisted of surgery, followed by one cycle of weekly bolus 5-FU with leucovorin, 2 cycles of 5-FU and leucovorin concomitant with pelvic RT (similar to preoperative CRT), and then 4 cycles of weekly bolus 5-FU and leucovorin.

At the 8.4-year median follow-up, the 5-year DFS for patients in the preoperative group was 64.7% versus 53.4% for the postoperative group ($P = 0.011$). There was only a trend toward better OS (75% versus 66%, $P = 0.065$) and no difference in locoregional control (5-year cumulative incidence of locoregional recurrence was 11% in both arms). The clinical pCR rate after preoperative therapy was 15%. No preoperative patient with a pCR had experienced a recurrence at the time the findings were presented. The authors concluded that preoperative CRT, when compared with postoperative CRT, significantly improved DFS and showed a trend toward improved OS [34]. It is important to reiterate, however, that accrual did not reach planned levels and the protocol was closed early as a result.

3.5.4 Korean Trial

Park and colleagues (2011) reported a single-institution prospective randomized phase III trial comparing preoperative with postoperative CRT (capecitabine (1650 mg/m^2/day administered concurrently with 50 Gy × 25 RT) for patients with locally advanced rectal cancer [35]. Between March 2004 and April 2006, 240 patients with clinical T3 or T4, or node-positive rectal cancer were enrolled then randomly assigned to receive CRT followed by mesorectal excision or mesorectal excision followed by CRT. All patients completed treatment with further adjuvant chemotherapy (4 cycles of oral or IV bolus fluoropyrimidine).

At a median follow-up of 52 months, 3- and 5-year DFS, OS, and cumulative incidence of local recurrence were similar between the two arms. The sphincter-sparing rate was similar in the 2 groups, although among patients with low-lying tumors, the preoperative CRT arm had a higher rate of sphincter preservation (68% versus 42%, $P = 0.008$).

Conceivably, the German Rectal Cancer Study Group study assisted in defining the optimal time to use CRT in relation to surgery; however shortly thereafter, more questions emerged. For example, can orally active fluoropyrimidines replace infusional 5-FU and can oxaliplatin be beneficial as a component of neoadjuvant therapy?

3.6 Can Orally Active Fluoropyrimidines (Capecitabine) Replace Infusional 5-FU?

Several studies in colon cancer have demonstrated non-inferiority and perhaps superiority of the oral fluoropyrimidine, capecitabine, when compared with 5-FU. Whether such findings hold true for rectal cancer and whether capecitabine can replace infusional 5-FU during RT in the neoadjuvant treatment of stage II and III rectal cancer were examined. Two clinical trials studied the effect of capecitabine, in place of infusional 5-FU, combined with RT on pCR, sphincter-sparing surgery, and surgical downstaging.

The first trial, carried out by the German investigators [36], was a neoadjuvant, open-label, multicenter, "non-inferiority," randomized phase 3 study that began in March 2002. The study explored the substitution of infusional with oral fluorouracil [36]. Specifically, the trial directly compared CRT (50.4 Gy) using capecitabine (825 mg/m^2 twice daily, on days 1–38) with CRT (50.4 Gy) using infusional 5-FU (1000 mg/m^2 by continuous infusion on days 1–5 and 29–33).

A total of 401 patients with locally advanced rectal cancer were enrolled and randomized to either the oral or IV fluoropyrimidine group. Five-year OS in the capecitabine group was non-inferior to that in the fluorouracil group (76% versus 67%; $P = 0.0004$), and 3-year DFS was 75% in the capecitabine group and 67% in the fluorouracil group ($P = 0.07$). The local recurrence rate was similar between capecitabine (6%) and IV 5-FU (7%; $P = 0.67$), but fewer patients developed distant metastases in the capecitabine group (19% versus 28% for capecitabine and IV 5-FU, respectively; $P = 0.04$). Patients receiving capecitabine had significantly more hand foot syndrome, fatigue, and proctitis, but less neutropenia.

The second phase III trial, which was conducted by the NSABP group [37], employed a 2 × 2 factorial non-inferiority design to compare 4 preoperative chemotherapy regimens administered concomitantly with RT (45 Gy in 25 fractions over 5 weeks followed by a boost). The trial evaluated the substitution of capecitabine for IV 5-FU as well as the intensification of chemotherapy by adding oxaliplatin.

Between September 2004 and August 2010, a total of 1608 patients with clinical stage II or III rectal cancer were enrolled into the trial and randomized to undergo preoperative CRT consisting of one of the following 4 regimens: RT plus 5-FU as a continuous infusion (225 mg/m^2 daily, 5 days per week) with or without oxaliplatin (50 mg/m^2 weekly) or capecitabine (825 mg/m^2 twice daily 5 days per week) with or without oxaliplatin (50 mg/m^2 weekly). There were no significant differences between capecitabine and infusional 5-FU regimens (regardless of oxaliplatin treatment) for the rates of pCR (21% versus 18% for capecitabine and infusional 5-FU regimens, respectively), sphincter-sparing surgery, or surgical downstaging. Patients receiving capecitabine (regardless of oxaliplatin treatment) had comparable rates of locoregional control (the primary endpoint), with a 3-year incidence of any locoregional events being 12% (capecitabine) versus 11% (IV 5-FU). OS rates were also comparable (81% versus 80%).

Thus, data support the equivalency of daily oral capecitabine and intravenous 5-FU during RT for neoadjuvant therapy; however different toxicity profiles are evident.

3.7 The Optimal Chemotherapy Regimen

Although preoperative CRT combined modality treatment has been established as the standard of care for patients with locally advanced rectal cancer, the optimal chemotherapy regimen administered concurrently with preoperative RT and then postoperatively remains unknown. Indeed, whether intensification of chemotherapy will enhance rectal cancer outcomes is still under investigation.

3.7.1 Oxaliplatin as a Component of Neoadjuvant Therapy

In combination with a fluoropyrimidine, oxaliplatin demonstrated DFS and OS benefits in both adjuvant and palliative treatment of patients with colon cancer [38]. Additionally, preclinical studies showed oxaliplatin to be a potent radiosensitizing agent [39]. Therefore, the addition of oxaliplatin to the standard CRT regimen using 5-FU for the preoperative treatment of patients with rectal cancer appears to be a reasonable step in the quest for improved local control and improved survival.

The efficacy of adding oxaliplatin to both preoperative fluorouracil-based CRT and postoperative chemotherapy of patients with locally advanced rectal cancer was examined in several studies (Table 3.1), most of which demonstrated greater toxicity from an oxaliplatin-containing regimen but with conflicting efficacy data.

3.7.1.1 STAR-01 Trial

In the Italian STAR-01 trial [40], a total of 747 patients with resectable, locally advanced (cT3-4 and/or cN1-2) adenocarcinoma of the mid-low rectum were enrolled and then randomly assigned to receive 5-FU-based CRT (50.4 Gy in 28 daily fractions). 5-FU was infused at a dose of 225 mg/m^2/day, with or without oxaliplatin (60 mg/m^2 weekly × 6 weeks). The primary endpoint was OS.

The addition of weekly oxaliplatin to preoperative 5-FU and RT had no effect on primary tumor response. The rate of pCR was identical in the 2 arms (16%), and sphincter preservation was similar (APR was required in 19% of patients in the oxaliplatin arm compared with 21% in those who did not receive oxaliplatin). However, the addition of oxaliplatin to the CRT regimen significantly increased toxicity (rates of any grade 3 or 4 toxicity during preoperative treatment was 24% with oxaliplatin versus 8% without oxaliplatin). The authors concluded that adding oxaliplatin to fluorouracil-based preoperative CRT significantly increased toxicity without affecting primary tumor response.

3.7.1.2 ACCORD 12/0405 PRODIGE-1 Trial

The ACCORD 12/0405 PRODIGE-1 trial [41] was a multicenter phase III study that randomly assigned 598 patients with T3 or resectable T4N0/1/2 rectal cancer to 5 weeks of treatment with RT (45 Gy/25 fractions) with concurrent capecitabine (800 mg/m^2 twice daily for 5 days per week) or RT (50 Gy/25 fractions) with

Table 3.1 Oxaliplatin as a component of neoadjuvant therapy

Study	No. patients	Chemoradiotherapy		pCR (%)	AEs (Grade 3/4) (%)	Outcomes
		Chemo	RT			
STAR-01 [40]	379	5-FU 225 mg/m²/d	50.4 Gy in 28 daily fractions	16	8	APR 19%
	368	5-FU 225 mg/m²/d + oxaliplatin 60 mg/m²/d	50.4 Gy in 28 daily fractions	16	24	21%
ACCORD [41]	295	Capecitabine 800 mg/m² twice daily 5 days	45 Gy/25 fractions	14	11	OS 88%
	292	Capecitabine 800 mg/m² twice daily + oxaliplatin 50 mg/m²/weekly	50 Gy/25 fractions	19	25	88%
PETACC-6 [42]	544	Capecitabine 825 mg/m² twice daily	45 Gy in 25 fractions	11.3	15.1	3-year DFS 73.9%
	537	Capecitabine 825 mg/m² twice daily + oxaliplatin 50 mg/m² weekly	45 Gy in 25 fractions	13.3	36.7	74.5%
German CAO/ARO/AIO-04 [45]	623	5-FU 1000 mg/m²/day	50.4 Gy in 28 fractions	13	20	3-year DFS 71.2%
	613	FOLFOX	50.4 Gy in 28 fractions	17	24	75.9%
NSABP R-04 [44]	719	5-FU (CI) ± oxaliplatin 50 mg/m²/weekly	50.4 Gy in 28 fractions	18.8		
	707	Capecitabine 825 mg/m² ± oxaliplatin 50 mg/m²	50.4 Gy in 28 fractions	22.2		

No. number, *AEs* adverse events, *5-FU* fluorouracil, *APR* abdominoperineal resection, *chemo* chemotherapy, *DFS* disease-free survival, *FOLFOX* leucovorin + fluorouracil + oxaliplatin, *Gy* Gray, *OS* overall survival, *pCR* pathologic complete response, *RT* radiation therapy, *CI* continuous infusion

capecitabine (800 mg/m² twice daily 5 days per week) *plus* oxaliplatin (50 mg/m² once weekly). The primary endpoint was complete sterilization of the operative specimen (ypCR). Similar to the Italian study, the addition of oxaliplatin increased toxicity (any grade 3–4 toxicity during preoperative therapy occurred at a rate of 25% with oxaliplatin versus 11% without oxaliplatin) and failed to improve pCR rates (19% with oxaliplatin versus 14% without oxaliplatin; $P = 0.09$). The addition of weekly oxaliplatin to preoperative capecitabine and RT had no effect on the likelihood of sphincter-preserving surgery (78% versus 75%), local control rates (4.4% versus 6.1%), or OS (88% in both groups).

3.7.1.3 The PETACC-6 Trial

The PETACC-6 trial [42] investigated whether the addition of oxaliplatin to preoperative oral fluoropyrimidine-based CRT, and postoperative adjuvant fluoropyrimidine-based chemotherapy improves DFS in locally advanced rectal cancer patients.

In total, 1094 patients with T3–T4 and/or node-positive rectal cancer were randomly assigned to receive 5 weeks of preoperative CRT with capecitabine, followed by 6 cycles of adjuvant capecitabine (1000 mg/m^2 twice daily on days 1–15 of every 21 day cycle) with or without the addition of oxaliplatin before (50 mg/m^2 weekly during RT) and after surgery (130 mg/m^2 on day 1, every 21 days). The authors concluded that the addition of oxaliplatin to preoperative fluoropyrimidine-based CRT was not beneficial: it did not improve surgical outcomes and furthermore led to decreased treatment compliance and increased toxicity. In a subsequent analysis presented at the 2014 ASCO annual meeting, after a median follow-up of 31 months, the addition of oxaliplatin to capecitabine plus RT was found to have no impact on DFS (73.9% versus 74.5%) [43].

3.7.1.4 NSABP Trial R-04

The NSABP trial R-04 [44] aimed to compare efficacy of 4 chemotherapy regimens administered concomitantly with preoperative RT (45 Gy in 25 fractions) in a 2 × 2 factorial design in patients with clinical stage II or III rectal cancer undergoing neoadjuvant CRT. In total, 1608 patients were randomly assigned to continuous infusional fluorouracil (225 mg/m^2, 5 days per week), with or without intravenous oxaliplatin (50 mg/m^2 weekly for 5 weeks), or capecitabine (825 mg/m^2 twice per day, 5 days per week), with or without oxaliplatin (50 mg/m^2 weekly for 5 weeks).

The addition of oxaliplatin to either capecitabine or infusional-5-FU during preoperative CRT did not improve outcomes (neither pCR rate nor sphincter-preserving surgery rate were altered). However, oxaliplatin was associated with significantly higher rates of grade 3+ toxicity, including grade 3 or 4 diarrhea ($P < 0.001$). In a preliminary report presented at the 2014 ASCO GI symposium, locoregional control, DFS, and OS were not improved in the oxaliplatin groups.

3.7.1.5 German CAO/ARO/AIO-04 Trial

Contrary to the aforementioned trials, the recently published German CAO/ARO/AIO-04 trial evaluated 2 separate combinations of preoperative CRT, surgery, and adjuvant chemotherapy [45]. This multicenter, open-label, randomized phase 3 study included 1265 patients who had cT3-4 or cN1-2 rectal tumors that were within 12 cm of the anal verge. Patients were randomly assigned to receive preoperative CRT (50.4 Gy with 5-FU [1000 mg/m^2 per day on days 1–5 and 29–33]), followed by surgery, and then adjuvant chemotherapy (IV bolus 5-FU at a dose of 500 mg/m^2 daily for 5 days, every 29 days for 4 courses) or preoperative CRT with infusional 5-FU plus oxaliplatin, followed by surgery and 4 months of adjuvant therapy with modified FOLFOX6. The primary endpoint was DFS.

Disease-free survival at 3 years in the oxaliplatin-treated patients was 75.9%, compared with 71.2% in the non-oxaliplatin-treated group (hazard ratio [HR] 0.79, 95% CI, 0.64–0.98; $P = 0.03$). There was no difference in the rate of complete resection

(R0), but the addition of preoperative oxaliplatin did appear to increase pCR rates (17% [oxaliplatin] versus 13% [no oxaliplatin]: OR 1.40, 95% CI, 1.02–1.92; $P = 0.038$).

In corroboration with other trials, preoperative grade 3–4 adverse events occurred in a greater number of patients who received oxaliplatin along with their preoperative 5-FU-based CRT (24% [oxaliplatin] versus 20% [no-oxaliplatin]. Of the patients who received adjuvant FOLFOX, 36% had grade 3–4 toxicity, which was identical to those who did not receive oxaliplatin in their adjuvant regimen.

The authors concluded that adding oxaliplatin to fluorouracil-based neoadjuvant CRT and adjuvant chemotherapy significantly improved DFS of patients with clinically staged cT3-4 or cN1-2 rectal cancer, compared with oxaliplatin-free regimens. They also concluded that the oxaliplatin-containing regimen could be deemed a new treatment option for patients with locally advanced rectal cancer. However, in his editorial that accompanied the publication entitled "Is the benefit of oxaliplatin in rectal cancer clinically relevant?" Bengt Glimelius argued that adding oxaliplatin to both pre- and postoperative treatment of locally advanced rectal cancer could result in a pronounced overtreatment, thereby risking long-lasting neuropathy in many patients [46]. Glimelius also questioned whether the observed improvement in 3-year DFS was meaningful.

Overall the role of neoadjuvant oxaliplatin in the treatment of locally advanced rectal cancer remains controversial (Table 3.1).

3.7.2 Irinotecan

As was done for oxaliplatin, the benefits of adding irinotecan to the standard 5-FU-based CRT regimen for rectal cancer was examined. In a multi-institutional RTOG trial, a total of 106 patients with locally advanced distal rectal cancer were randomly assigned to receive preoperative CRT with continuous infusional 5-FU concurrent with hyperfractionated RT or continuous infusional 5-FU plus irinotecan concurrent with conventional fractionation RT. The pCR rate was similar in both arms (26% with irinotecan versus 30% without irinotecan), as was the locoregional recurrence rate (17% versus 16%, respectively) [47].

3.8 Future Directions

3.8.1 Neoadjuvant Chemotherapy Alone

As outlined above, the present treatment model uses neoadjuvant CRT followed by surgery, followed by adjuvant chemotherapy for all patients with stage II and III rectal cancer. Although preoperative CRT reduces toxicity compared with postoperative treatment [5], there is still no doubt that CRT is associated with significant side effects. As current surgical techniques achieve very good results and enable excellent local control rates—and the majority of disease recurrence in individuals represents distant metastatic disease—why is trimodality therapy necessary for all patients if the purpose of radiotherapy is to decrease local recurrence rates only? This reasoning led to significant debate as to whether all patients with stage II and III rectal cancer require such an intensive treatment approach, especially if they are surgeon-confirmed TME candidates (a procedure with favorable low rates of local recurrence). Some experts have argued that RT could be eliminated in certain patient populations, particularly those diagnosed as T3N0/T3N1.

Several studies [48–51] have been conducted in an attempt to explore the possibility of excluding radiation from rectal cancer therapy, and although some of the data for neoadjuvant chemotherapy alone followed by resection of the tumor are promising, the small number of patients taking part in these trials significantly limits our ability to make any definitive conclusion (Table 3.2).

The PROSPECT study (NCT01515787) (Fig. 3.6) is a prospective randomized phase II/III trial that was conceived to challenge the existing paradigm for the treatment of patients with rectal cancer (Fig. 3.5). The idea of this trial is to avoid overtreatment by administering the most appropriate therapy to all patients and tailoring treatment based on tolerance and response to induction chemotherapy. Patients with stage II/III (T3N0, T3N1, or T2N1) rectal cancer are initially randomized to preoperative FOLFOX versus standard preoperative CRT. In the preoperative FOLFOX arm, initial chemotherapy is followed by comprehensive restaging using MRI. Those patients experiencing a less than 20% reduction in their rectal tumor following initial FOLFOX will go on to receive preoperative CRT. In all study arms, surgery involves TME, and postoperative chemotherapy will be administered (Fig. 3.6). The primary endpoint of the study is DFS.

In 2016 it was reported that 566 (37%) of the 1531 screened patients thus far met the PROSPECT trial eligibility criteria. Eligible patients were reported to be more

Table 3.2 Studies of neoadjuvant chemotherapy alone in rectal cancer

	Study	No. patients	Inclusion criteria	Chemotherapy	pCR (%)	Outcomes
High risk	Uehara et al. [51]	32	MRI-defined poor risk	Oxaliplatin, capecitabine, and bevacizumab × 12 weeks	13	R0 resection rate = 90% postoperative complication = 43%
	Hasegawa et al. [48]	25	T4 or lymph node-positive	XELOX (4 cycles) plus bevacizumab (3 cycles)	4	R0 resection rate = 92% postoperative complication = 26%
	Ishii et al. [49]	26	T3 or T4 and N0-2	IFL × 2 cycles	3.8	5-year DFS = 74% 5-year OS = 84% LR = 11%
	Schrag et al. [50]	32	Clinical stages II to III	FOLFOX (6 cycles) + bevacizumab (on cycles 1–4)	25	R0 resection rate = 100% 4-year LR = 0% 4-year DFS = 84%

XELOX capecitabine + oxaliplatin, *OS* overall survival, *DFS* disease-free survival, *FOLFOX* leucovorin + fluorouracil + oxaliplatin, *LR* local recurrence, *MRI* magnetic resonance imaging, *No.* number, *IFL* irinotecan + 5-FU + leucovorin, *pCR* pathologic complete response

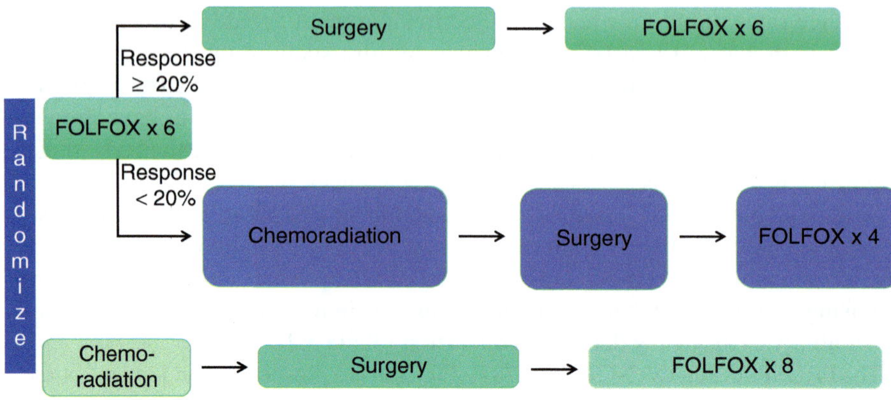

Fig. 3.6 The PROSPECT trial design

likely to have improved performance status ($P = .0003$) and negative circumferential resection margins ($P < .0001$) compared to PROSPECT-ineligible patients. In univariate analyses, these patients had improved DFS (hazard ratio [HR], 0.75; 95% confidence interval [CI], 0.61–0.91), OS (HR, 0.73; 95% CI, 0.57–0.95), and RFS (HR, 0.68; 95% CI, 0.54–0.86), although, only RFS was significantly improved in a multivariate analysis (HR, 0.75; 95% CI, 0.57–1.00, $P = .0499$) [52].

Other studies evaluating a similar approach with preoperative chemotherapy alone are ongoing. The BACCHUS trial (NCT01650428) is a phase II trial aimed at examining the efficacy of 6 cycles of FOLFOX plus bevacizumab versus 6 cycles of FOLFOXIRI plus bevacizumab, with selective use of CRT. The primary endpoint is pCR rate. Additionally, there is a 3-armed randomized phase II trial ongoing in China (NCT01211210) [53]. This study is randomizing patients to one of the following three regimens: (1) 4 cycles of preoperative FOLFOX, (2) FOLFOX followed by FOLFOX-based CRT, and (3) CRT using 5-FU alone. The primary endpoint is 3-year DFS.

These trials will play a key role in the continued quest for the ideal rectal cancer treatment algorithm. However, until study endpoints are reached and results are available, neoadjuvant chemotherapy alone remains only an investigational approach.

3.8.2 Neoadjuvant Chemotherapy (Induction) Followed by Chemoradiation

The current standard treatment timeline consists of 5–6 weeks of combined modality treatment (CRT), followed by 4–6 weeks of recovery time, followed by total mesorectal excision, followed by 4–6 weeks of postoperative recovery time, and followed by initiation of postoperative, adjuvant chemotherapy. Hence, this current treatment paradigm does not allow for the delivery of full systemic chemotherapy until approximately 16 weeks after initiation of neoadjuvant CRT, and such a delay could theoretically allow for metastatic dissemination of disease.

As a result, no systemic therapy is delivered to treat micrometastases for over 4 months after treatment initiation. This delay may create a window of opportunity for the development of metastatic disease. Thus, one could hypothesize that administering chemotherapy at an earlier point might treat the micrometastases, thereby reducing the incidence of distant recurrence.

Such is the rationale for moving full systemic chemotherapy treatment forward to an earlier point in the rectal cancer treatment algorithm. This rationale makes the strategy of induction chemotherapy followed by CRT a very attractive one.

Several trials with various designs and sample sizes have been conducted to examine the strategy of induction chemotherapy followed by CRT (Fig. 3.7). A summary of clinical trials using induction chemotherapy followed by CRT is available in Table 3.3.

3.8.3 The EXPERT Trial

The EXPERT trial [54] was a phase II study that enrolled 105 patients with poor-risk rectal cancer, defined by high-resolution MRI, to receive 12 weeks of neoadjuvant chemotherapy (capecitabine [1000 mg/m^2 twice daily for 14 days every 3 weeks] and oxaliplatin [130 mg/m^2 on day 1 of each 3 week cycle]) followed by CRT (RT, 54 Gy over 6 weeks; capecitabine, 825 mg/m^2 twice daily) prior to TME, which was performed 6 weeks after the completion of CRT. Postoperatively, patients received another 12 weeks of adjuvant capecitabine at a dose of 1250 mg/m^2 twice daily for 14 days every 3 weeks followed by 7 days of rest. Pathological complete response rate (the primary endpoint of the study) was 21% (intention to treat) and 24% (among those who underwent potentially curative surgery). After neoadjuvant capecitabine/oxaliplatin, the tumor response rate was 88%, which was increased to 97% after CRT. The 3-year progression-free and overall survivals were 68% and 83%, respectively. The 3-year relapse-free survival for patients who had complete resection was 74%.

3.8.4 The Spanish GCR-3 Study

The Spanish GCR-3 study [55] was a randomized phase II trial that compared the current conventional treatment paradigm (preoperative CRT, followed by surgery,

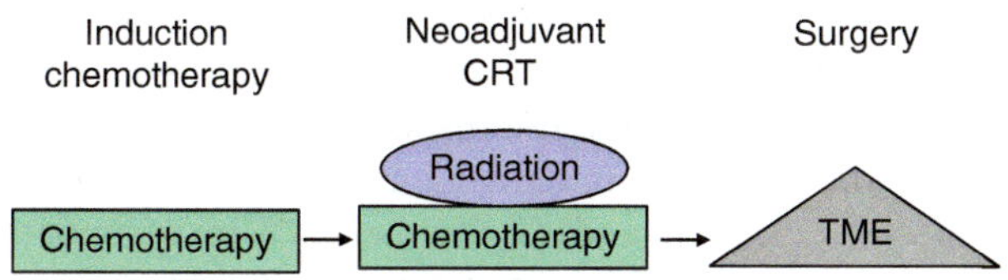

Fig. 3.7 Induction chemotherapy followed by neoadjuvant CRT—an investigative strategy

Table 3.3 Studies of neoadjuvant (induction) chemotherapy followed by chemoradiation in the treatment of rectal cancer

Study	No. patients	Induction chemotherapy	CRT regimen	Adjuvant	pCR (%)	Outcomes
EXPERT [54] (Phase II)	105	CAPOX × 12 weeks	CRT with capecitabine	Capecitabine × 12 weeks	24	R0 resection rate = 99% 3-yrs DFS = 68%; 3-yrs OS = 83%
GCR-3 [55] (Phase II, randomized)	108	–	CRT with CAPOX	CAPOX × 4	13	Distant metastases = 21% 5-y DFS = 62%; 5-yrs OS = 77%
		CAPOX for 4 cycles	CRT with CAPOX	–	14	Distant metastases = 23% 5-yrs DFS = 64%; 5-yrs OS = 74%
CONTRE [56]	39	FOLFOX × 8 cycles	CRT with capecitabine	–	33	R0 resection = 100%
Maréchal et al. [59] (Phase II, randomized)	57	–	CRT with infusional—5-FU	–	34	Closed prematurely for futility
		FOLFOX × 2 cycles	CRT with 5-FU	–	32	
Schou et al. [57]	85	CAPOX × 2 cycles	CRT with capecitabine	–	23	5-yrs DFS = 63% 5-yrs OS = 67%
Koeberle et al. [58]	60	XELOX × 1 cycle	CRT with capecitabine	–	23	R0 resection rate = 98% Sphincter preservation = 84%

5-FU fluorouracil, *XELOX* and *CAPOX* capecitabine + oxaliplatin, *CRT* chemoradiotherapy, *DFS* disease-free survival, *FOLFOX* leucovorin + fluorouracil + oxaliplatin, *No.* number, *OS* overall survival, *pCR* pathologic complete response

followed by postoperative adjuvant therapy) with induction chemotherapy followed by CRT then surgery. The primary endpoint was pCR.

The study enrolled a total of 108 rectal cancer patients with distal or middle third, locally advanced (T3–T4 and/or node-positive) disease, determined using MRI. Patients were then randomly assigned to preoperative CRT followed by surgery and 4 cycles of postoperative adjuvant CAPOX (standard arm, $n = 52$) or 4 cycles of CAPOX followed by CRT and surgery (experimental arm, $n = 56$). The pCR rates were 13% (standard arm) versus 14% (experimental arm). In a recently updated follow-up report published in Annals of Oncology, the median follow-up time was 69.5 months, and the 5-year DFS rates were 64% for the standard arm and 62% for the experimental arm ($P = 0.85$) [55]. The 5-year cumulative incidences of local relapse were 2% and 5%, respectively ($P = 0.61$). No significant difference in either the 5-year cumulative incidence of distant metastases or 5-year OS was detected (21.1% [standard] versus 23.2% [experimental]; $P = 0.80$) and (77.9% [standard] versus 74.7% [experimental]; $P = 0.64$). The authors concluded that both approaches yield similar 5-years outcomes. In this study, the implementation of induction chemotherapy prior to CRT did not improve outcomes.

3.8.5 CONTRE Study

The CONTRE study [56] was a single-arm phase II trial that enrolled 39 patients with clinical stage II to III (T3–T4 and/or N1–N2) rectal cancer. Patients received induction therapy with 8 cycles of modified FOLFOX6 followed by preoperative CRT (50.4 Gy intensity-modulated RT administered concurrently with capecitabine 825 mg/m bid). Surgery was performed 6–10 weeks after CRT. Eighty-nine percent of patients received therapy as planned. Pathological complete response was demonstrated in 33% of patients.

3.8.6 Danish Group

Schou et al. [57] reported results from a single-arm phase II study that included 85 patients with locally advanced rectal cancer (T4 tumors; all T3N+ tumors; and T3 tumors involving, or ≤1 mm from, the mesorectal fascia) who were treated with 2 cycles of CAPOX followed by RT concomitant with capecitabine prior to surgery. TME was carried out 6 weeks after the completion of CRT. R0 resection was seen in 94% of cases, and in the "intention-to-treat" group, pCR was seen in 23% of patients. Five-year DFS and OS were 63% and 67%, respectively.

3.8.7 The Swedish Group

Koeberle et al. [58] reported findings from a Swedish multicenter single-arm phase II study that included 60 patients with locally advanced rectal cancer who received one cycle of XELOX followed by CRT (1.8 Gy fractions 5 days per week for 5 weeks plus XELOX). Surgery was recommended 5 weeks after completion of CRT. The primary endpoint was pCR. In this population, the pCR rate was 23%; R0 resection and sphincter preservation were achieved at rates of 98% and 84%, respectively.

3.8.8 Belgian Group

Maréchal et al. [59] reported results from a randomized phase II study that included 57 patients—with T2–T4 and/or node-positive disease—that were randomly assigned to standard therapy with preoperative CRT (infusional 5-FU combined with RT) followed by surgery or 2 cycles of induction FOLFOX followed by CRT and then surgery. The primary endpoint was the rate of ypT0-1N0 stage achievement.

At the investigators' planned interim analysis, the ypT0-1N0 rates were 34.5% and 32.1%, respectively, and the study was closed prematurely due to futility. It is worth noting that there were no statistically significant differences in any endpoints, including pCR, tumor regression, and sphincter preservation.

Additionally, several studies have evaluated the benefit of adding targeted therapies to induction chemotherapy, such as EXPERT-C [60] and AVACROSS [61] trials (Table 3.4).

3.8.9 Bevacizumab

Early results reported from the AVACROSS study [61] reveal that the incorporation of bevacizumab into both induction chemotherapy and preoperative CRT regimens is feasible, with an impressive pCR rate of 36%. Additionally, 98% of patients were able to undergo an R0 resection. However, in light of a reoperation rate of 24% and an anastomotic leakage rate of 17%, surgical morbidity appears to be a significant problem when intensifying preoperative regimens with antiangiogenic agents.

3.8.10 The COPERNICUS Trial

The COPERNICUS trial [62] is a phase II single-arm study aimed at evaluating the feasibility of administering 4 cycles of neoadjuvant FOLFOX prior to short-course preoperative RT and followed immediately by surgery. The primary endpoint was the proportion of patients completing protocol treatment, including surgery. In a preliminary report presented at the 2015 ASCO Annual meeting, 95% of patients received all 4 cycles of FOLFOX, followed by RT, and underwent surgery [62]. The

Table 3.4 Studies of neoadjuvant (induction) chemotherapy with targeted therapies followed by chemoradiation in the treatment of rectal cancer

Study	No. patients	Induction chemotherapy	CRT regimen	Adjuvant	pCR (%)	Outcomes
EXPERT-C [60]	165 (90)[a]	CAPOX + cetuximab × 4 cycles	CRT with capecitabine + cetuximab	CAPOX × 4 cycles	11[a]	[b]Complete response rate = 15.8% $p = 0.31$
		CAPOX × 4 cycles	CRT with capecitabine	CAPOX × 4 cycles	9[a]	[b]Complete response rate = 7.5%
AVACROSS [61]	47	XELOX + bevacizumab × 12 weeks	CRT with capecitabine + bevacizumab	–	35	Ro resection = 98%

XELOX and *CAPOX* capecitabine + oxaliplatin, *CRT* chemoradiotherapy, *No.* number, *pCR* pathologic complete response

[a]KRAS wild-type patients

[b]Results for analysis of RAS wild-type population

rate of R0 resection was 100%. The median gap between completing neoadjuvant FOLFOX and starting preoperative RT was 10 days, as was the gap between completing radiotherapy and surgery.

Although the results from some trials are promising, it remains difficult to form a firm conclusion on the use of induction chemotherapy given the small sample size, the use of single-arm studies, and the fact that the only randomized study reported showed no difference in the long-term outcome. It is also important to note that multiple trials have examined similar strategies in other tumor types, such as head and neck cancer and nasopharyngeal cancer, and failed to demonstrate an improvement in outcome following or support the routine use of induction chemotherapy over CRT.

Clearly there is a need to test induction chemotherapy strategies in appropriately well-designed controlled randomized studies. Currently there is an ongoing phase III trial evaluating the induction chemotherapy approach with preoperative chemotherapy alone—the French PRODIGE 23 trial (NCT01804790).

The PRODIGE 23 trial investigators' aim is to randomize 460 patients with locally advanced rectal cancer to receive either neoadjuvant chemotherapy with FOLFIRINOX followed by preoperative CRT (arm 1) or standard preoperative CRT alone (arm 2). The results from this trial will hopefully help us to better understand the role of induction therapy in rectal cancer and to shape the treatment paradigm going forward.

It is our opinion that, for now, the use of neoadjuvant (induction) chemotherapy prior to CRT in the patients with rectal cancer should remain investigational and thus be used only in the context of clinical trials.

Acknowledgments We would like to thank Marion L. Hartley, Ph.D., for her editing assistance.

References

1. Jemal A, Bray F, Center MM, Ferlay J, Ward E, Forman D. Global cancer statistics. CA Cancer J Clin. 2011;61(2):69–90.
2. van Gijn W, Marijnen CA, Nagtegaal ID, Kranenbarg EM, Putter H, Wiggers T, et al. Preoperative radiotherapy combined with total mesorectal excision for resectable rectal cancer: 12-year follow-up of the multicentre, randomised controlled TME trial. Lancet Oncol. 2011;12(6):575–82.
3. Group MS. Extramural depth of tumor invasion at thin-section MR in patients with rectal cancer: results of the MERCURY study. Radiology. 2007;243(1):132–9.
4. Guillem JG, Diaz-Gonzalez JA, Minsky BD, Valentini V, Jeong SY, Rodriguez-Bigas MA, et al. cT3N0 rectal cancer: potential overtreatment with preoperative chemoradiotherapy is warranted. J Clin Oncol. 2008;26(3):368–73.
5. Sauer R, Becker H, Hohenberger W, Rodel C, Wittekind C, Fietkau R, et al. Preoperative versus postoperative chemoradiotherapy for rectal cancer. N Engl J Med. 2004;351(17):1731–40.
6. Sauer R, Liersch T, Merkel S, Fietkau R, Hohenberger W, Hess C, et al. Preoperative versus postoperative chemoradiotherapy for locally advanced rectal cancer: results of the German CAO/ARO/AIO-94 randomized phase III trial after a median follow-up of 11 years. J Clin Oncol. 2012;30(16):1926–33.
7. Galandiuk S, Wieand HS, Moertel CG, Cha SS, Fitzgibbons RJ Jr, Pemberton JH, et al. Patterns of recurrence after curative resection of carcinoma of the colon and rectum. Surg Gynecol Obstet. 1992;174(1):27–32.

8. Minsky BD, Mies C, Recht A, Rich TA, Chaffey JT. Resectable adenocarcinoma of the rectosigmoid and rectum. I. Patterns of failure and survival. Cancer. 1988;61(7):1408–16.
9. Phillips RK, Hittinger R, Blesovsky L, Fry JS, Fielding LP. Local recurrence following "curative" surgery for large bowel cancer: I. The overall picture. Br J Surg. 1984;71(1):12–6.
10. Medical Research Council Rectal Cancer Working Party—second report. The evaluation of low dose preoperative X-ray therapy in the management of operable rectal cancer; results of a randomly controlled trial. Br J Surg. 1984;71:21–5.
11. Balslev I, Pedersen M, Teglbjaerg PS, Hanberg-Soerensen F, Bone J, Jacobsen NO, et al. Postoperative radiotherapy in Dukes' B and C carcinoma of the rectum and rectosigmoid. A randomized multicenter study. Cancer. 1986;58(1):22–8.
12. Douglass HO Jr, Moertel CG, Mayer RJ, Thomas PR, Lindblad AS, Mittleman A, et al. Survival after postoperative combination treatment of rectal cancer. N Engl J Med. 1986;315(20):1294–5.
13. Fisher B, Wolmark N, Rockette H, Redmond C, Deutsch M, Wickerham DL, et al. Postoperative adjuvant chemotherapy or radiation therapy for rectal cancer: results from NSABP protocol R-01. J Natl Cancer Inst. 1988;80(1):21–9.
14. Gerard A, Buyse M, Nordlinger B, Loygue J, Pene F, Kempf P, et al. Preoperative radiotherapy as adjuvant treatment in rectal cancer. Final results of a randomized study of the European Organization for Research and Treatment of Cancer (EORTC). Ann Surg. 1988;208(5):606–14.
15. Higgins GA, Humphrey EW, Dwight RW, Roswit B, Lee LE Jr, Keehn RJ. Preoperative radiation and surgery for cancer of the rectum. Veterans Administration Surgical Oncology Group Trial II. Cancer. 1986;58(2):352–9.
16. Rider WD, Palmer JA, Mahoney LJ, Robertson CT. Preoperative irradiation in operable cancer of the rectum: report of the Toronto trial. Can J Surg. 1977;20(4):335–8.
17. Roswit B, Higgins GA, Keehn RJ. Preoperative irradiation for carcinoma of the rectum and rectosigmoid colon: reportof a National Veterans Administration randomized study. Cancer. 1975;35(6):1597–602.
18. Wassif SB, Langenhorst BL, Hop WCJ. The contribution of preoperative radiotherapy in the management of borderline operability rectal cancer Adjuvant therapy of cancer II. Grune & Stratton: New York; 1979. p. 613–20.
19. Gastrointestinal Tumor Study Group. Prolongation of the disease-free interval in surgically rectal carcinoma. N Engl J Med. 1985;312(23):1465–72.
20. Krook JE, Moertel CG, Gunderson LL, Wieand HS, Collins RT, Beart RW, et al. Effective surgical adjuvant therapy for high-risk rectal carcinoma. N Engl J Med. 1991;324(11):709–15.
21. NIH Consensus Conference: adjuvant therapy for patients with colon and rectal cancer. JAMA. 1990;264:1444–50.
22. Bosset JF, Calais G, Mineur L, Maingon P, Radosevic-Jelic L, Daban A, et al. Enhanced tumoricidal effect of chemotherapy with preoperative radiotherapy for rectal cancer: preliminary results—EORTC 22921. J Clin Oncol. 2005;23(24):5620–7.
23. Bosset JF, Calais G, Mineur L, Maingon P, Stojanovic-Rundic S, Bensadoun RJ, et al. Fluorouracil-based adjuvant chemotherapy after preoperative chemoradiotherapy in rectal cancer: long-term results of the EORTC 22921 randomised study. Lancet Oncol. 2014;15(2):184–90.
24. Gerard JP, Conroy T, Bonnetain F, Bouche O, Chapet O, Closon-Dejardin MT, et al. Preoperative radiotherapy with or without concurrent fluorouracil and leucovorin in T3-4 rectal cancers: results of FFCD 9203. J Clin Oncol. 2006;24(28):4620–5.
25. Boulis-Wassif S, Gerard A, Loygue J, Camelot D, Buyse M, Duez N. Final results of a randomized trial on the treatment of rectal cancer with preoperative radiotherapy alone or in combination with 5-fluorouracil, followed by radical surgery. Trial of the European Organization on Research and Treatment of Cancer Gastrointestinal Tract Cancer Cooperative Group. Cancer. 1984;53(9):1811–8.
26. Bujko K, Nowacki MP, Nasierowska-Guttmejer A, Michalski W, Bebenek M, Kryj M. Long-term results of a randomized trial comparing preoperative short-course radiotherapy with preoperative conventionally fractionated chemoradiation for rectal cancer. Br J Surg. 2006;93(10):1215–23.
27. Latkauskas T, Pauzas H, Gineikiene I, Janciauskiene R, Juozaityte E, Saladzinskas Z, et al. Initial results of a randomized controlled trial comparing clinical and pathological downstag-

ing of rectal cancer after preoperative short-course radiotherapy or long-term chemoradiotherapy, both with delayed surgery. Colorectal Dis. 2012;14(3):294–8.
28. Ngan SY, Burmeister B, Fisher RJ, Solomon M, Goldstein D, Joseph D, et al. Randomized trial of short-course radiotherapy versus long-course chemoradiation comparing rates of local recurrence in patients with T3 rectal cancer: Trans-Tasman Radiation Oncology Group trial 01.04. J Clin Oncol. 2012 Nov 1;30(31):3827–33.
29. McCarthy K, Pearson K, Fulton R, Hewitt J. Pre-operative chemoradiation for non-metastatic locally advanced rectal cancer. Cochrane Database Syst Rev. 2012;12:CD008368.
30. Mohiuddin M, Regine WF, John WJ, Hagihara PF, McGrath PC, Kenady DE, et al. Preoperative chemoradiation in fixed distal rectal cancer: dose time factors for pathological complete response. Int J Radiat Oncol Biol Phys. 2000 Mar 1;46(4):883–8.
31. O'Connell MJ, Martenson JA, Wieand HS, Krook JE, Macdonald JS, Haller DG, et al. Improving adjuvant therapy for rectal cancer by combining protracted-infusion fluorouracil with radiation therapy after curative surgery. N Engl J Med. 1994 Aug 25;331(8):502–7.
32. Rodel C, Martus P, Papadoupolos T, Fuzesi L, Klimpfinger M, Fietkau R, et al. Prognostic significance of tumor regression after preoperative chemoradiotherapy for rectal cancer. J Clin Oncol. 2005 Dec 1;23(34):8688–96.
33. Fokas E, Liersch T, Fietkau R, Hohenberger W, Beissbarth T, Hess C, et al. Tumor regression grading after preoperative chemoradiotherapy for locally advanced rectal carcinoma revisited: updated results of the CAO/ARO/AIO-94 trial. J Clin Oncol. 2014 May 20;32(15):1554–62.
34. Roh MS, Colangelo LH, O'Connell MJ, Yothers G, Deutsch M, Allegra CJ, et al. Preoperative multimodality therapy improves disease-free survival in patients with carcinoma of the rectum: NSABP R-03. J Clin Oncol. 2009 Nov 1;27(31):5124–30.
35. Park JH, Yoon SM, CS Y, Kim JH, Kim TW, Kim JC. Randomized phase 3 trial comparing preoperative and postoperative chemoradiotherapy with capecitabine for locally advanced rectal cancer. Cancer. 2011;117(16):3703–12.
36. Hofheinz RD, Wenz F, Post S, Matzdorff A, Laechelt S, Hartmann JT, et al. Chemoradiotherapy with capecitabine versus fluorouracil for locally advanced rectal cancer: a randomised, multicentre, non-inferiority, phase 3 trial. Lancet Oncol. 2012;13(6):579–88.
37. O'Connell MJ, Colangelo LH, Beart RW, Petrelli NJ, Allegra CJ, Sharif S, et al. Capecitabine and oxaliplatin in the preoperative multimodality treatment of rectal cancer: surgical end points from National Surgical Adjuvant Breast and Bowel Project trial R-04. J Clin Oncol. 2014;32(18):1927–34.
38. Andre T, Boni C, Mounedji-Boudiaf L, Navarro M, Tabernero J, Hickish T, et al. Oxaliplatin, fluorouracil, and leucovorin as adjuvant treatment for colon cancer. N Engl J Med. 2004;350(23):2343–51.
39. Blackstock AW, Hess S, Chaney S. Oxaliplatin: In vitro evidence of its radiation sensitizing activity – Pre-clinical observations relevant to clinical trials. Int J Radiat Oncol Biol Phys. 1999;45:253–4.
40. Aschele C, Cionini L, Lonardi S, Pinto C, Cordio S, Rosati G, et al. Primary tumor response to preoperative chemoradiation with or without oxaliplatin in locally advanced rectal cancer: pathologic results of the STAR-01 randomized phase III trial. J Clin Oncol. 2011;29(20):2773–80.
41. Gerard JP, Azria D, Gourgou-Bourgade S, Martel-Laffay I, Hennequin C, Etienne PL, et al. Comparison of two neoadjuvant chemoradiotherapy regimens for locally advanced rectal cancer: results of the phase III trial ACCORD 12/0405-Prodige 2. J Clin Oncol. 2010;28(10):1638–44.
42. Schmoll HJ, Haustermans K, Price TJ. Preoperative chemoradiotherapy and postoperative chemotherapy with capecitabine and oxaliplatin versus capecitabine alone in locally advanced rectal cancer: first results of the PETACC-6 randomized phase III trial. J Clin Oncol. 2013;31 (Suppl; abstr 3531).
43. Schmoll HJ, Haustermans K, Price TJ. Preoperative chemoradiotherapy and postoperative chemotherapy with capecitabine and oxaliplatin versus capecitabine alone in locally advanced rectal cancer: disease-free survival results at interim analysis. J Clin Oncol. 2014;32(5s; abstr 3501).
44. Allegra CJ, Yothers G, O'Connell MJ. Neoadjuvant therapy for rectal cancer: mature results from NSABP protocol R-04. J Clin Oncol. 2014; 32(Suppl 3; abstr 390).

45. Rodel C, Graeven U, Fietkau R, Hohenberger W, Hothorn T, Arnold D, et al. Oxaliplatin added to fluorouracil-based preoperative chemoradiotherapy and postoperative chemotherapy of locally advanced rectal cancer (the German CAO/ARO/AIO-04 study): final results of the multicentre, open-label, randomised, phase 3 trial. Lancet Oncol. 2015;16(8):979–89.
46. Glimelius B. Is the benefit of oxaliplatin in rectal cancer clinically relevant? Lancet Oncol. 2015;16(8):883–5. doi:10.1016/S1470-2045(15)00018-2. Epub 2015 Jul 15
47. Mohiuddin M, Paulus R, Mitchell E, Hanna N, Yuen A, Nichols R, et al. Neoadjuvant chemoradiation for distal rectal cancer: 5-year updated results of a randomized phase 2 study of neoadjuvant combined modality chemoradiation for distal rectal cancer. Int J Radiat Oncol Biol Phys. 2013;86(3):523–8.
48. Hasegawa J, Nishimura J, Mizushima T, Miyake Y, Kim HM, Takemoto H, et al. Neoadjuvant capecitabine and oxaliplatin (XELOX) combined with bevacizumab for high-risk localized rectal cancer. Cancer Chemother Pharmacol. 2014;73(5):1079–87.
49. Ishii Y, Hasegawa H, Endo T, Okabayashi K, Ochiai H, Moritani K, et al. Medium-term results of neoadjuvant systemic chemotherapy using irinotecan, 5-fluorouracil, and leucovorin in patients with locally advanced rectal cancer. Eur J Surg Oncol. 2010;36(11):1061–5.
50. Schrag D, Weiser MR, Goodman KA, Gonen M, Hollywood E, Cercek A, et al. Neoadjuvant chemotherapy without routine use of radiation therapy for patients with locally advanced rectal cancer: a pilot trial. J Clin Oncol. 2014;32(6):513–8.
51. Uehara K, Hiramatsu K, Maeda A, Sakamoto E, Inoue M, Kobayashi S, et al. Neoadjuvant oxaliplatin and capecitabine and bevacizumab without radiotherapy for poor-risk rectal cancer: N-SOG 03 Phase II trial. Jpn J Clin Oncol. 2013;43(10):964–71.
52. Bosse D, Mercer J, Raissouni S, Dennis K, Goodwin R, Jiang D, et al. PROSPECT eligibility and clinical outcomes: results from the Pan-Canadian rectal cancer consortium. Clin Colorectal Cancer. 2016;15(3):243–9. doi:10.1016/jclcc201602003. Epub 2016 Feb 13
53. Glynne-Jones R, Hava N, Goh V, Bosompem S, Bridgewater J, Chau I, et al. Bevacizumab and Combination Chemotherapy in rectal cancer Until Surgery (BACCHUS): a phase II, multicentre, open-label, randomised study of neoadjuvant chemotherapy alone in patients with high-risk cancer of the rectum. BMC Cancer. 2015;15:764. doi:10.1186/s12885-015-1764-1.
54. Chua YJ, Barbachano Y, Cunningham D, Oates JR, Brown G, Wotherspoon A, et al. Neoadjuvant capecitabine and oxaliplatin before chemoradiotherapy and total mesorectal excision in MRI-defined poor-risk rectal cancer: a phase 2 trial. Lancet Oncol. 2010;11(3):241–8.
55. Fernandez-Martos C, Garcia-Albeniz X, Pericay C, Maurel J, Aparicio J, Montagut C, et al. Chemoradiation, surgery and adjuvant chemotherapy versus induction chemotherapy followed by chemoradiation and surgery: long-term results of the Spanish GCR-3 phase II randomized trialdagger. Ann Oncol. 2015;26(8):1722–8.
56. Perez K, Safran H, Sikov W, Vrees M, Klipfel A, Shah N, et al. Complete neoadjuvant treatment for rectal cancer: the Brown University oncology group CONTRE study. Am J Clin Oncol. 2014.
57. Schou JV, Larsen FO, Rasch L, Linnemann D, Langhoff J, Hogdall E, et al. Induction chemotherapy with capecitabine and oxaliplatin followed by chemoradiotherapy before total mesorectal excision in patients with locally advanced rectal cancer. Ann Oncol. 2012;23(10):2627–33.
58. Koeberle D, Burkhard R, von Moos R, Winterhalder R, Hess V, Heitzmann F, et al. Phase II study of capecitabine and oxaliplatin given prior to and concurrently with preoperative pelvic radiotherapy in patients with locally advanced rectal cancer. Br J Cancer. 2008;98(7):1204–9.
59. Marechal R, Vos B, Polus M, Delaunoit T, Peeters M, Demetter P, et al. Short course chemotherapy followed by concomitant chemoradiotherapy and surgery in locally advanced rectal cancer: a randomized multicentric phase II study. Ann Oncol. 2012;23(6):1525–30.
60. Dewdney A, Cunningham D, Tabernero J, Capdevila J, Glimelius B, Cervantes A, et al. Multicenter randomized phase II clinical trial comparing neoadjuvant oxaliplatin, capecitabine, and preoperative radiotherapy with or without cetuximab followed by total mesorectal excision in patients with high-risk rectal cancer (EXPERT-C). J Clin Oncol. 2012;30(14):1620–7.
61. Nogue M, Salud A, Vicente P, Arrivi A, Roca JM, Losa F, et al. Addition of bevacizumab to XELOX induction therapy plus concomitant capecitabine-based chemoradiotherapy in

magnetic resonance imaging-defined poor-prognosis locally advanced rectal cancer: the AVACROSS study. Oncologist. 2011;16(5):614–20.

62. Gollins S, Sebag-Montefiore D, Saunders MP, Grieve R, Scott N, Brown G, et al. A phse II single arm feasibility trial of neoadjuvant chemotherapy (NAC) with oxaliplatin/fluorouracil (OxMdG) then short-course preoperative radiotherapy (SCPRT) then immediate surgery in operable rectal cancer (ORC): COPERNICUS (NCT01263171). J Clin Oncol. 2015;33 (Suppl; abstr 3609).

Neoadjuvant Radiotherapy

4

Te Vuong and Aurelie Garant

Abstract
Over the last two decades, radiation treatment has evolved significantly, not only through its application in serial randomized clinical trials but in many other aspects. One of these key factors is modern imaging, such as computerized tomography and magnetic resonance imaging (MRI), which has become an essential component in determining treatment strategies. In the era of total mesorectal excision surgery (TME), preoperative radiotherapy (RT) reduces local recurrence and can be given either with long-course RT with 5-fluorouracil (5-FU)-based regimen or short-course RT (SCRT). For patients with positive circumferential radial margin (CRM), tumor down-staging is highly desirable, and SCRT is not as effective to prevent local recurrence. Contemporary pattern of recurrence suggests that it is possible to lower the upper limit of the treatment field level. In an effort to reduce radiation-related toxicity, field adjustments along with exploration of new radiation targeted radiation modalities are desirable.

Keywords
Radiation therapy • Local control • Randomized clinical trials • Treatment-related toxicities • Overall survival • Treatment volumes • Radiation modalities

T. Vuong, M.D. (✉) • A. Garant, M.D.
Division of Radiation Oncology, Jewish General Hospital,
3755 Cote Ste. Catherine Road, Montreal, QC, Canada, H3T 1E2
e-mail: tvuong@jgh.mcgill.ca

G. Dapri, J.H. Marks (eds.), *Surgical Techniques in Rectal Cancer*,
https://doi.org/10.1007/978-4-431-55579-7_4

4.1 Introduction

Radiation therapy is a local treatment that was introduced as a mean to improve regional control in conjunction with surgery for patients with locally advanced rectal cancer (RC). Over the last two decades, this treatment modality has evolved significantly, not only through its application in serial randomized clinical trials but also through the advances in technology along with the introduction of computerized imaging techniques that have allowed accurate evaluation of clinical target volumes. Modern imaging, such as computerized scans (CT) and MRI, is now an essential component in determining treatment strategies. Finally, the transition to TME and changes in the pattern of local relapse justify a reexamination of the contemporary radiation practice.

4.2 Rationale for Radiation Therapy

In recent years, the treatment of patients with rectal cancer has seen significant improvements in local control (LC) with the introduction of TME along with new preoperative therapeutic modalities. Locally advanced RC patients include stage II and III cancers with a range of T2–T4 tumors. These patients are currently treated with similar strategies as per NCCN recommendations (http://www.nccn.org/clinical.asp). In the era of modern tumor imaging, pelvic MRI in particular allows for the precise estimation of the circumferential radial margin (CRM) [1, 2], which represents the most important factor for predicting local recurrence (LR) and systemic disease. The Mercury trial [1] reported that for patients with positive CRM on preoperative MRI imaging, the risks of LR and systemic spread were significantly higher than for those with negative CRM.

4.2.1 Radiotherapy Trials

Surgery remains the cornerstone of rectal cancer treatment for locally advanced (T3–4 tumors). To further improve LC in rectal cancer, neoadjuvant (NA) RT has been added to surgery. The benefit of NA SCRT had first been shown by the Swedish Rectal Cancer Group [3] in the pre-TME era. After a median follow-up of 5 years, the LR risk was 11% in the irradiated group and 27% in the non-irradiated group, and the overall survival (OS) rates were 58% and 48%, respectively. In spite of these excellent LC results, the role of RT was questioned after the introduction of TME. In the Dutch TME study [4], the benefit of SCRT followed by immediate TME was demonstrated, with a 10-year LR rate of 11% for patients treated with TME alone vs. 5% for patients treated with SCRT followed by TME S [5]. In the MRC-CR07 study [6], which has a comparable design, patients with respectable rectal cancer were randomized between NA SCRT followed by immediate S vs. S alone. The

S-alone patients received postoperative chemotherapy (CT) long-course (LC) RT when the CRM was involved. The LR rate was 5% in the NA SCRT patients and 12% in patients undergoing S alone ($p < 0.001$), demonstrating that selective postoperative CT-LCRT is not able to provide the same results as preoperative treatment. It has been established that NA RT (either SCRT alone or CT-LCRT) provides significantly better LC than postoperative CT-LCRT, while LR rates are significantly improved in patients receiving NA SCRT. In this study, the benefits of NA SCRT were observed at all tumor levels including the upper third tumor and significant even for patients with specimen obtained within the mesorectal plane. So far no survival benefit has been demonstrated for irradiated patients operated with the TME technique. In the Dutch TME trial [5], NA SCRT had no effect on OS or cancer-specific survival when all randomized patients were included in the analyses. However, in operated patients with a negative CRM, RT significantly improved cancer-specific survival. Unfortunately, this benefit was offset by an increase in other causes of death, resulting in an equal OS rate compared with S-alone group. A subgroup analysis demonstrated that for patients with TNM stage III cancer with a negative CRM, 10-year survival was 50% in the NA SCRT group vs. 40% in the S-alone group ($p = 0.032$). In most studies, the LR rate was reduced from over 10% for patients treated with S only to 5% for patients treated with NA RT and S.

NA RT, in conjunction with TME, improves local control but does not improve OS

4.2.2 Role of CRM

In the Dutch TME trial [4], non-irradiated patients with a positive CRM had a LR risk of 23.3%, whereas those who received radiation showed a drop in LR risk to 15.5% ($p = 0.16$). The MRC-CR07 trial [6] showed a LR rate of 13.8% in patients receiving NA SCRT with 5×5 Gy and a LR rate of 20.7% in patients receiving postoperative CT-LCRT (p nonsignificant). In the EORTC 22921 trial, a similar result was observed in patients treated with chemoradiotherapy (OR = 0.73, 95% CI: 0.39–1.37, $p = 0.33$) when compared to those treated with LCRT alone [7]. However, the polish-randomized trial [8] comparing SCRT to CT-LCRT demonstrated a significant lower CRM-positive rate in the favor of the latter approach.

In patients with positive CRM, CT-LCRT is more effective than SCRT to achieve negative CRM

4.2.3 Multimodality Treatment Approaches

Several Northern European randomized clinical trial (RCT) studies have demonstrated a significant reduction in the LR rate after SCRT. There exists a controversy concerning optimal treatment for the different stages of rectal cancer and prioritization of treatment modalities. In Northern Europe, SCRT is the standard of care for most stage II and III rectal cancer patients. *CT-LCRT is reserved for more advanced cases with positive CRM*. On the other hand, in America and southern Europe, patients are treated with NA LCRT (LCRT, 45–50 Gy) in combination with chemotherapy (CT). Furthermore, as the EORTC 22921 [9] and FFCD 9203 [10] studies demonstrated that the addition of CT to preoperative LCRT is beneficial to LC in locally advanced tumors (T3–4) and this was also recently confirmed by a recent Cochrane review [11], patients are now treated with CT-LCRT, followed by TME.

4.2.4 Randomized Trials Comparing NA SCRT with CT-LCRT

Two published RCT were conducted comparing SCRT to CT-LCRT: the Polish trial with 312 patients [8] and the Australian trial [12] with 326 patients. Both studies had a similar design, and sample size was calculated to demonstrate a difference of 15% in the rate of sphincter preservation (SPS) and 10% in LR, respectively. Both trials showed higher rates of early radiation toxicity in the CT-LCRT arm when compared with the SCRT group; grade III to IV acute toxicity rates were 18% versus 3% ($p = 0.001$) in the Polish trial and 28% versus 1.9% ($p = 0.001$) in the Australian study. In the Polish trial, the SPS rate did not differ between the groups: 61% in the SCRT group and 58% in the CT-LCRT ($p = 0.57$). In this trial, the LR rate was slightly lower in the SCRT group than in the CT-LCRT group 10.6% vs. 15.6% ($p = 0.21$), whereas the opposite tendency was seen in the Australian study at 7.5% versus 4.4% ($p = 0.24$). In this latter trial, a LR rate difference was observed in the group of tumors at 5 cm from the anal verge or below, with 6 out of 48 patients in the SCRT arm vs. 1 out of 31 patients after CT-LCRT although not statistically significant ($p = 0.21$). Additionally, no increase in late toxicity rates was seen in the SCRT irradiation group compared with the CT-LCRT group. In the Polish study, severe late toxicity was observed in 10.1% of patients after SCRT and in 7.1% of patients after CT-LCRT compared to 5.8% of patients after SCRT vs.8.2% of patients after CT-LCRT ($p = 0.53$) in the Australian trial (Table 4.1).

At present, as no consensus has been reached regarding the superiority of one radiation schedule over the other, standard radiation treatment can be defined as either SCRT or CT-LCRT in patients with negative CRM.

There are five contemporary RCT studies testing the oxaliplatin-based chemotherapy regimen published so far: STAR-0145 [14], ACCORD 12/0405-Prodige 246 [15], NSABP R-04 [16], CAO/ARO/AIO-0448 [17], and the PETACC-6 trial [18] which compared standard NA 5-fluorouracil (5-FU)-based CT and LCRT

Table 4.1 5-year local control and overall survival rates results from selected randomized clinical trials using preoperative fluorouracil-based chemotherapy and LCRT/SCRT

RCT	T/stage (S) status	Number of patients	Median age (years)	Local recurrence rate at 5 years %	OS at 5 years %	pCR rate %
German trial: pre op [13]	T1–T4	405	62	6	76	1.9
German trial: post op [13]	T1–T4	394	62	13	74	0 ($p < .001$)
Dutch trial TME S alone [4]	S1–4	908	66	10.9	63.5	0
Dutch trial NA SCRT + TME [4]	S1–4	897	65	5.6	64.2	0
MRC CR07 NA SCRT [6]	S1–4	674	65	4.7	70.3	n/a
MRC CR07 post OP CT-LCRT [6]	S1–4	676	65	11.5	67.9	n/a
Polish trial SCRT [8]	T3–4	155	60	9	67.2 (4y)	0.7
Polish trial CT-LCRT [8]	T3–4	157	59	14.2	66.2 (4y)	16.1 (p n/a)
Trans-Tasman SCRT [12]	T3	162	63	7.5 (3 y)	74	0
Trans-Tasman CT-LCRT [12]	T3	161	64	4.4 (3 y)	70	12.4 (p n/a)
FFCD 9203 NA LCRT [10]	T3–4	367	63	16.5	67.9	3.6
FFCD 9203 NA CT-LCRT [10]	T3–4	375	64	8.1	67.4	11.4 ($p < .0001$)

n/a not available

(CT-RT) to oxaliplatin and 5-FU CT and NA LCRT. Patients with T3 or T4 rectal cancer were recruited sequentially. All but the CAO/ARO/AIO-0448 [17] reported higher morbidity without any improvement in early endpoints such as pathological complete response (pCR) rate (Table 4.2).

Therefore, it can be concluded that the 5-Fu-based chemotherapy regimen remains standard when long-course radiation therapy is used.

Table 4.2 Tumor pCR rate from published randomized clinical trials using preoperative oxaliplatin and 5-fluorouracil-based chemotherapy and LCRT

RCT	T/stage status	Number of patients	Median age (years)	pCR rate %
ACCORD 12: Capecitabine + LCRT [15]	T2–T4	293	63	13.9
ACCORD 12: Capecitabine + oxaliplatin + LCRT [15]	T2–T4	291	61	19.2 ($p = .09$)
STAR-01: 5-FU + LCRT [14]	T1–T4	377	63	16
STAR-01: 5-FU + oxaliplatin + LCRT [14]	T1–T4	362	62	16 ($p = .904$)
NSABP R-04: 5-FU + LCRT [16]	SII–SIII	804	n/a	19.1
NSABP R-04: 5-FU + oxaliplatin + LCRT [16]	SII–SIII	804	n/a	20.9 ($p = .46$)
CAO/ ARO/ AIO-04: 5-FU + LCRT [17]	T1–T4	623	63	13
CAO/ ARO/ AIO-04: 5-FU + oxaliplatin + LCRT [17]	T1–T4	613	64	17 ($p = .038$)
PETACC-6: Capecitabine + LCRT [18]	T3–T4	547	n/a	11.3
PETACC-6: Capecitabine + oxaliplatin + LCRT [18]	T3–T4	547	n/a	13.3 ($p = 0.31$)

n/a not available

4.2.5 Radiation Treatment Volumes

TME now provides optimal tumor bed resection together with the perirectal nodes within the mesorectal fascia, but it is not addressing the pelvic nodes. The Dutch CKVO 95-04 study [4, 5] is unique, having an arm with more than 908 patients treated with TME alone. In this trial, the LR rate was 5% vs. 11% after a median follow-up of 12 years [5]. Most of the recurrences were located below the S2–3 interspace [19] in patients with negative nodes and negative CRM, therefore consistent with the Swedish experience reporting on the level of S1–S2 interspace [20]. The addition of radiation therapy reduced mostly the central recurrence.

In North America, the definition of clinical target volume for the treatment of rectal cancer has been based on consensus by a panel of experts [21] to include coverage of the tumor bed, entire mesorectum and perirectal, and presacral and internal iliac nodes which is supported by the patterns of local recurrence literature. It is imperative to note that the majority of these data were derived before the implementation of quality imaging such as pelvic MRI and the introduction of TME.

4.2.6 Radiation-Related Toxicities

If the value of radiation therapy is now well established, cumulative data on long-term toxicities associated with external beam (EBRT) raise concerns. In a meta-analysis, Camma et al. [22] reported an increased risk of septic complications in irradiated patients compared to non-irradiated patients: 21% vs. 15.2% ($p \leq 0.001$). Moreover, there was an increased risk of overall complications in the irradiated group: 21% vs. 5.2% ($p < 0.003$). Postoperative adverse events were also higher in the radiation treatment group: 57.4% vs. 42.3% ($p < 0.02$). Finally, irradiated patients had a 15% higher risk of death from vascular or infectious causes compared to non-irradiated patients ($p = 0.02$). The Cochrane Database Systematic Review in 2007 by Wong et al. [23], assessing the effect of preoperative RT vs. surgery alone for rectal cancer patients, confirmed the benefits of preoperative RT in reducing LR (HR 0.71, 95% CI 0.64–0.78) with borderline significance with respect to cancer-specific and overall survival (OS) (HR 0.93, 95% CI 0.87–1.0). Late toxicities including pelvic fractures, venothrombosis events, intestinal obstruction, postoperative fistula, cardiovascular death, bowel obstruction, and anal sphincter and sexual dysfunction were all increased.

Thus, if neoadjuvant EBRT has been effective in decreasing local recurrence, the number of patients requiring treatment will need to be weighed against the substantial morbidity risks and long-term side effects related to EBRT. Reducing treatment volumes to the level of S1/S2 might be the most effective and simple means to improve therapeutic index

4.3 Other Perioperative Radiation Treatment Options

4.3.1 Intraoperative Radiation Therapy

The majority of patients with rectal cancer are doing well with current management, but there are less favorable cases with positive CRM or recurrent tumors after previous pelvis radiation therapy that remains a clinical management challenge. There are other radiation modalities, apart from EBRT, that could be considered.

The likelihood of achieving tumor down-staging and/or R0 improves as a function of dose. Wiltshire et al. [24] investigated the value of dose escalation with 5-FU CT in a phase II trial for patients with operable rectal cancer. The three dose levels were 40 Gy in 20 fractions, 46 Gy in 23 fractions, and 50 Gy in 25 fractions and included 46, 52, and 36 patients, respectively. The pCR rates were 15%, 23%, and 33% ($p = 0.07$), respectively, and the 2-year relapse-free survival was 72%, 90%, and 89%, respectively ($p = 0.02$). In Lyon RCT study, R96-0256 [25] NA RT alone using 39 Gy in 13 fractions was compared to the same RT with boost (85 Gy in 3 fractions) using contact X-ray for 88 patients with low rectal cancer. A significant improvement in pCR rate was seen in the contact X-ray boost arm (2% vs. 24%), along with a complete or near complete sterilization of the operative specimen (34% vs. 57%) resulting in a significant increase in SPS in the boost group (44% vs. 76%, $p = 0.04$). At a median follow-up time of 152 months, although there was no difference in OS and LC, however, the rate of colostomy-free survival was 37% vs. 71% ($p = 0.001$) in favor of the boost arm. Using modern preoperative staging imaging, Jakobsen et al. [26] conducted a recent RCT trial on T3–4 tumors with dose escalation, comparing CT-LCRT delivering 50.4 Gy in 28 fractions vs. a dose escalation to 60 Gy with the same regimen (50.4 Gy/28) and high-dose rate endorectal brachytherapy (HDREBT) as boost modality to deliver 10 Gy. For T3 tumors a negative CRM rate of 90% vs. 99%, respectively, was observed ($p = 0.03$) in favor of the boost arm.

Intraoperative radiation therapy (IORT) has been developed in order to further optimize local control especially in this unfavorable tumor group. Most studies have investigated IORT in combination with EBRT. It delivers a higher radiation dose to the CTV at the time of surgical exploration with the advantage of accurate treatment delivery to the area of maximum concern, with adjacent normal structures displaced from the irradiation field. As it is given at the time of surgery, IORT can only be given in a single dose usually varying from 10 to 20 Gy with the peripheral nerve defined as principal dose limiting normal tissue. The benefits of IORT as a means to deliver higher doses and to improve LC have been reported, and some data were quite compelling despite being small retrospectives series [27] due to the limited access of IORT equipment worldwide. The results are most beneficial in patients undergoing complete resection. The IORT literature includes a large spectrum of tumors as the selection criteria varied from one center to another, making the evidence of benefits difficult to ascertain. However, Dubois et al. [28] reported on the unique IORT RCT with 142 patients with T3–4 primary and/or recurrent tumors comparing EBRT using 40 Gy alone to the same EBRT with IORT boost (an additional 18 Gy) and did not confirm any disease-free survival (DFS) benefits ($p = 0.7808$) from the addition of IORT. In this series, the composite population of T3 and T4 tumors did possibly contribute to these negative results.

4.3.2 Intensity-Modulated Radiation Therapy

Radiation therapy was initially based on two-dimensional (2D) planning with standard treatment fields using anatomical bony landmarks. Then, in the early 1990s, three-dimensional imaging radiation-planning system (3D planning) were introduced which allowed for 3D definition of the target and normal tissues by using thin section computed tomography (CT) scan. A decade later, the new generation of linear accelerators were equipped with dynamic multileaf collimators (MLC) capable of following the projection of the target as the accelerator gantry arcs around the patient. As a result, MLC delivery and accurate tumor localization of areas at risk, a safe dose to targets in a variety of areas, have led to an improvement in local tumor control while reducing the dose to normal structures. This technology has significantly contributed to the therapeutic index of radiation therapy of head and neck cancer. Subsequently, IMRT was tested for treatment of pelvic tumors, in particular with anal canal cancer, and showed to be of value in reducing skin and GI toxicities. However, in rectal cancer, there are few preliminary studies, and the benefits of IMRT are lacking. The acute toxicity data from the multi-institutional RTOG study 0822 [29] was not significantly convincing with 51% of ≥ grade 2 GI toxicity versus 58% ($p = 0.31$) in the conventional 3D-based RTOG 0247. Major differences in the clinical target volumes (CTV) contributed to inconsistent results.

In gynecological and anal canal cancer, external iliac and inguinal nodes are routinely included, whereas in rectal cancer, the CTV is posterior. Since radiation is currently given in the context of a NA setting, it is unusual that small bowel loops are closed unlike in the era of adjuvant treatment. Consequently, even with the conventional 3D technique, the incidence of grave GI toxicity is unusual, especially if the CTV superior limit is adjusted to S1–S2 level.

IMRT had interesting virtues and allowed superior dose conformation within the CTV with the ability to limit normal tissue radiation dose. At the Jewish General Hospital (McGill University), in the less favorable T4 tumors, where optimal tumor down-staging is highly desirable, IMRT was explored as a means to dose escalation with 60 Gy in 25 fractions during neoadjuvant treatment for 60 patients selected by pelvic MRI with positive CRM [30]. The R0 rate was 90% and a multivisceral resection rate was 29.5%. The overall acute toxicity profile was acceptable with a distribution of ≥ grade 3 rate of 16.6% for GI, 18% for skin, and 10% for bone marrow.

The role of IMRT requires further demonstration of meaningful clinical benefits in patient outcomes to further substantiate their routine application in the treatment of rectal cancer.

4.3.3 High-Dose Rate Endorectal Brachytherapy (HDREBT)

At the Jewish General Hospital (McGill University), image-guided HDREBT [31, 32] was developed as a highly targeted RT neoadjuvant modality for low T2 with positive CRM and selected T3 rectal cancer. The treatment consists of 26 Gy in 4 consecutive fractions prescribed to the deepest aspect of the tumor bed. It is performed in the ambulatory setting, without CT. Acute proctitis was the only toxicity observed with 1% of grade 3 toxicity. In 678 patients treated [33], at a median follow-up time of 63 months, the LR rate was 4.5%, and the overall 5-year survival was 71%, which compared favorably to NA CT-LCRT. In contrast to EBRT, HDREBT does allow for lower normal tissues exposure to radiation and is given without chemotherapy; thus it is less costly and toxic. An important observation from this institutional experience remains the excellent LC rate despite the absence of attempt to treat pelvic nodes and significant smaller treatment volume when compared to the standard volume used with external beam radiation. There is no randomized study to compare HDREBT to CT-LCRT or SCRT. The main obstacle is presently the lack of brachytherapy expertise in the radiation oncology GI community. However, a matched pair study [34] was conducted between our institution with 141 patients treated with HDREBT, and a national Dutch reference center for rectal cancer with 145 patients treated external beam (EBRT) with either NA CT-LCRT or SCRT, for patients with non-metastatic MRI staged T3 tumor, matched for time period, stage, age, and gender. The objectives were to compare the effect of preoperative treatment strategies on overall survival, cancer-specific deaths, and local recurrence [34]. The 5-year OS was 70.9% (95% CI 62.6%–77.7%) in the EBRT patients compared to 86.9% (80.1%–91.6%) in HDREBT-treated patients, resulting in an adjusted HR of 0.70 (98% CT 0.39–1.26;p = 0.233). Of the 145 patients treated with EBRT, 6.9% (95%

CI 2.8%–11.0%) had local recurrence and 17.9% (95% CI 11.7%–24.2%) patients died of rectal cancer, compared to 4.3% (95%,CI 0.9%–7.5%) local recurrences and 10.6% (95% CI 5.5%–15.7%) rectal cancer deaths of the HDEBT treated patients. This study results suggested the needs of an RCT to evaluate the potential benefits of HDREBT as a NA radiation strategy for rectal cancer.

4.4 Summary

In the era of TME, preoperative RT reduces local recurrence and can be given either with long-course RT with 5-Fu-based regimen or SCRT. For patients with positive CRM, tumor down-staging is highly desirable and SCRT is not as effective to prevent local recurrence. Contemporary pattern of recurrence suggests that it is possible to lower the upper limit of the treatment field level. In an effort to reduce radiation-related toxicity, field adjustment along with exploration of new radiation options is desirable.

References

1. Mercury Study group. Diagnostic accuracy of preoperative magnetic resonance imaging in predicting curative resection of rectal cancer surgery. BMJ. 2006;333(7572):779.
2. Beet-Tan RG, Beets GL, Vliegen RF, et al. Accuracy of magnetic resonance imaging in prediction of tumor free resection margin in rectal cancer surgery. Lancet. 2001;7(9255):497–504.
3. Swedish rectal cancer Trial. Improved survival with pre operative radiotherapy radiotherapy in resectable rectal cancer. N Engl J Med. 1997;336(14):980–7.
4. Kapiteijn E, Marijnen CAM, Nagtegall ID, et al. Preoperative radiotherapy combined with total mesorectal excision for resectable rectal cancer. N Engl J Med. 2001;345:638–46.
5. Gijn WV, Marijnen CAM, Nagtegaal ID, et al. Preoperative radiotherapy combined with total mesorectal excision for resectable rectal cancer: 12-year follow-up of the multicentre, randomised controlled TME trial. Lancet Oncol. 2011;12:575–82.
6. Sebag-Montefiore D, Stephens RJ, Steele R, et al. Preoperative radiotherapy versus selective postoperative chemoradiotherapy in patients with rectal cancer (MRC CR07 and NCIC-CTG C016): a multicentre, randomised trial. Lancet. 2009;373:811–20.
7. Den Dulk M, Collette L, Van de Velde CJM, et al. Quality of surgery in T3-4 rectal cancer: involvement of circumferential resection margin not influenced by preoperative treatment. Results from EORTC trial 22921. Eur J Cancer. 2007;43(12):1821–8.
8. Bujko K, Nowacki MP, Nasierowska-Guttmejer A, et al. Long-term results of a randomized trial comparing preoperative short-course radiotherapy with preoperative conventionally fractionated chemoradiation for rectal cancer. Br J Surg. 2006;93:1215–23.
9. Bosset JF, Collette L, Calais G, et al. Chemotherapy with preoperative radiotherapy in rectal cancer. N Engl J Med. 2006;355:1114–23.
10. Gerard JP, Conroy T, Bonnetain F, et al. Preoperative radiotherapy with or without concurrent fluorouracil and leucovorin in T3-4 rectal cancers: results of FFCD 9203. J Clin Oncol. 2006;24:4620–5.
11. De Caluwe L, Van Nieuwenhove Y, Ceelen WP, et al. Preoperative chemoradiation versus radiation alone for stage II and III resectable rectal cancer. Cochrane Database Syst Rev. 2013;2:CD006041.
12. Ngan SY, Burmaister B, Fisher RJ, et al. Randomized trial of short-course radiotherapy versus long course chemoradiation comparing rates of local recurrence in patients with T3

rectal cancer: trans-tasman radiation oncology group trial 01.04. J Clin Oncol. 2012;30: 3827–33.
13. Sauer R, Becker H, Hohenberger W, et al. Pre operative versus postoperative chemoradiotherapy for rectal cancer. N Engl J Med. 2004;351:1731–40.
14. Aschele C, Cionini L, Lonardi S, et al. Primary tumor response to preoperative chemoradiation with or without oxaliplatin in locally advanced rectal cancer: pathologic results of the STAR-01 randomized phase III trial. J Clin Oncol. 2011;29:2773–80.
15. Gerard JP, Azria D, Gourgou-Bourgade S, et al. Comparison of two neoadjuvant chemoradiotherapy regimens for locally advanced rectal cancer: results of the phase III trial ACCORD 12/0405-Prodige 2. J Clin Oncol. 2010;28:1638–44.
16. O'Connell MJ, Colangelo LH, Beart RW, et al. Capecitabine and oxaliplatin in the preoperative multimodality treatment of rectal cancer: surgical end points from national surgical adjuvant breast and bowel project trial R-04. J Clin Oncol. 2014;32(18):1927–34.
17. Rodel C, Graeven U, Fietkau R, et al. Oxaliplatin added to fluorouracil-based preoperative chemoradiotherapy and postoperative chemotherapy of locally advanced rectal cancer (the German CAO/ARO/AIO-04 study): final results of the multicentre, open-label, randomised, phase 3 trial. Lancet Oncol. 2015;16(8):979–89. ePub July 2015
18. Schmoll HJ, Haustermans K, Price T, et al. Preoperative chemoradiotherapy and postoperative chemotherapy with capecitabine and oxaliplatin versus capecitabine alone in locally advanced rectal cancer: response to the local treatment after chemoradiation and surgery as secondary endpoint. Eur J Cancer. 2013;49:S482–2.
19. Nijkamp J, Kusters M, Beets-tan RH, et al. Three-dimensional analysis of recurrence patterns in rectal cancer: the cranial border in hypofractionated preoperative radiotherapy can be lowered. Int J Radiat Oncol Biol Phys. 2011;80(1):103–10.
20. Syk E, Torkzad M, Blomqvist P, et al. Local recurrence in rectal cancer: anatomic localization and effect on radiation target. Int J Radiat Oncol Biol Phys. 2008;73(3):658–64.
21. Myerson RJ, Garofalo MC, El Naqa I, et al. Elective clinical target volumes for conformal therapy in anorectal cancer: a radiation therapy oncology group consensus panel contouring atlas. Int J Radiat Oncol Biol Phys. 2009;74:824–30.
22. Camma C, Giunta M, Fiorica F, Paglioaro L, Craxi A, Cottone M. Preoperative radiotherapy for resectable rectal cancer. JAMA. 2000;284:1008–15.
23. Wong RKS, Tandan V, De Silva S, et al. Pre-operative radiotherapy and curative surgery for the management of localized rectal carcinoma. Cochrane Database Syst Rev. 2007;18(2):CD002102. John Wiley & Sons
24. Wiltshire KL, Ward IG, Swallow C, et al. Preoperative radiation with concurrent chemotherapy for resectable rectal cancer: effect of dose escalation on pathologic complete response, local recurrence-free survival, disease-free survival, and overall survival. Int J Radiat Oncol Biol Phys. 2006;64:709–16.
25. Ortholan C, Romestaing P, Chapet O, et al. Correlation in rectal cancer between clinical tumor response after neoadjuvant radiotherapy and sphincter or organ preservation: 10-year results of the Lyon R 96-02 randomized trial. Int J Radiat Oncol Biol Phys. 2012;83:165–71.
26. Jakobsen A, Ploen J, Vuong T, Appelt A, Lindeberg J, Rafaelsen RS. The dose-effect relationship in chemoradiation of locally advance rectal cancer. A randomized trial comparing two radiation doses. Int J Radiat Oncol Biol Phys. November 2012;84(4):950–4.
27. Gunderson L, Willettt C, Calvo FA, Harrison L. Intraoperative irradiation, Current clinical oncology. Second ed. New York: Humana Press.
28. Dubois J-B, Bussieres E, Richaud P, et al. Intra-operative radiotherapy of rectal cancer: results of the French multi-institutional randomized study. Radiother Oncol. 2011;98:298–303.
29. Garofalo M, Moughan J, Hong T, et al. RTOG 0822: a phase II study of preoperative (PREOP) chemoradiotherapy (CRT) utilizing IMRT in combination with capecitabine (C) and oxaliplatin (O) for patients with locally advanced rectal cancer. Int J Radiat Oncol Biol Phys. 2011;81(2):S3–4. abstract # 6
30. Vuong T, Niazi T, Letellier F, et al. A dose escalation phase II study using intensity modulated radiation therapy (IMRT) and concurrent chemotherapy for patients with advanced rectal

cancer and magnetic resonant imaging (MRI) defined positive circumferential radial margins (CRM+). Int J Radiat Oncol Biol Phys. 2011;81(2.) Abstract # 252

31. Vuong T, Belliveau PJ, Michel RP, et al. Conformal preoperative endorectal brachytherapy treatment for locally advanced rectal cancer: early results of a phase I/II study. Dis Colon Rectum. 2002;45:1486–93. discussion 1493-5
32. Vuong T, Richard C, Niazi T, et al. High dose rate endorectal brachytherapy for patients with curable rectal cancer. Semin Colon Rectal Surg. 2010;21:115–9.
33. Vuong T, Niazi T, Devic S: Role of endoluminal brachytherapy for rectal cancer: current status and challenges. Proceedings of ESTRO 3rd Forum, 24–28 April 2014.
34. Breugom AJ, Vermeer TA, van den Broek CBM, et al. Effect of preoperative treatment strategies on the outcome of patients with clinical T3, non-metastasized rectal cancer: a comparison between Dutch and Canadian expert centers. Eur J Surg Oncol. 2015;41(8):1039–44.

The Proper Treatment for the Complete Responder After Neoadjuvant Therapy

5

Angelita Habr-Gama, Maria Susana Bruzzi,
Maria Laura Morici, Guilherme Pagin São Julião,
and Rodrigo Oliva Perez

Abstract

The incorporation of new treatment modalities has significantly increased the complexity of decision-making for patients with locally advanced rectal cancer. Neoadjuvant chemoradiation (CRT) is considered one of the preferred treatment strategies for these patients. In addition, this treatment strategy may lead to significant tumor regression, ultimately leading to complete pathological response in up to 42% of patients. The assessment of tumor response following CRT and prior to radical surgery may identify patients with complete clinical response that could be managed nonoperatively with strict follow-up (watch and wait strategy) and thus avoiding unnecessary postoperative morbidity, including long-term urinary, sexual, and fecal continence dysfunctions and the frequent need for temporary or definitive stomas.

Avoiding immediate surgery for patients with complete clinical response may provide good long-term oncological outcomes and excellent functional results. In addition, close surveillance may allow early detection of local recurrences with salvage options avoiding any oncological compromise. This chapter deals

A. Habr-Gama, M.D. (✉)
Angelita & Joaquim Gama Institute, Rua Manoel da Nóbrega, 1564 São Paulo, Brazil

University of São Paulo School of Medicine, Av. Dr. Arnaldo, 455, Cerqueira César, São Paulo, Brazil
e-mail: gamange@uol.com.br

M.S. Bruzzi, M.D. • M.L. Morici, M.D. • G.P. São Julião, M.D.
Angelita & Joaquim Gama Institute, Rua Manoel da Nóbrega, 1564 São Paulo, Brazil

R.O. Perez, M.D. Ph.D.
Angelita & Joaquim Gama Institute, Rua Manoel da Nóbrega, 1564 São Paulo, Brazil

Colorectal Surgery Division, Department of Gastroenterology, University of São Paulo School of Medicine, São Paulo, Brazil

G. Dapri, J.H. Marks (eds.), *Surgical Techniques in Rectal Cancer*,
https://doi.org/10.1007/978-4-431-55579-7_5

with critical issues in appropriate selection of patients, details in follow-up, and management of local recurrences following a nonoperative approach to a patient with complete clinical response following neoadjuvant CRT.

Keywords
Rectal cancer • Neoadjuvant chemoradiation therapy • Complete clinical response • Watch and wait

5.1 Introduction

Rectal cancer management has become increasingly complex over the last few decades [1]. The widespread use of neoadjuvant therapies has introduced a new variable, tumor response, which may dramatically change ultimate surgical decision from radical surgery to local excision, transanal endoscopic microsurgery, or even no surgery at all for the management of these patients. In this setting, surgeons have to consider many aspects of the disease including primary assessment, optimal treatment strategy, assessment of response, and final management decision, prior to deciding on a definitive treatment approach.

5.2 Indications for Neoadjuvant Therapy

Standard indications for neoadjuvant therapy in rectal cancer are mostly derived from randomized controlled studies that showed a local control benefit among patients with cT3–4 or cN+ treated with radiation or chemoradiation followed by radical surgery [2, 3]. However, recent updates with longer follow-up of these same cohorts suggest that benefits in local disease control following neoadjuvant CRT and radical surgery are marginal or even outweighed by treatment-related toxicities [4–6]. In this setting, the use of routine neoadjuvant CRT or RT to all patients with cT3–4 or cN+ has been replaced by a more selective use based on specific radiological features. Based on the outcomes of the MERCURY study, patients at higher risk for the development of local recurrence were those with threatened circumferential resection margin, extramural vascular invasion, N2 disease, and pelvic nodal disease [1, 7]. Therefore, considering neoadjuvant approaches for the improvement of local disease control, only high-risk patients would benefit the most instead of all cT3 or cN+ rectal cancers.

On the other hand, neoadjuvant radiation alone, chemoradiation, or even chemotherapy alone may lead to significant tumor regression resulting in significant changes in tumor size, depth of penetration, nodal sterilization, and even complete tumor disappearance, also known as complete pathological response (pCR) [8, 9]. This latter group of patients with pCR is associated with improved oncological outcomes. In addition, considering there is no residual cancer in the resected specimen, there would be an opportunity for these patients to avoid radical surgery and its associated immediate morbidity, mortality, functional disorders, and need for stomas [10, 11].

If neoadjuvant therapy is offered only for advanced stage disease patients (high-risk patients for local recurrence), very few will develop complete tumor response (up to 30%). Neoadjuvant therapy may be extremely useful for the selection of those patients that may safely avoid a radical operation and thus may be used more effectively if more widely adopted to include patients with earlier disease stages. If earlier diseases stages are offered this treatment strategy (including cT2N0), complete response may develop more frequently, reaching up to 40–50% of patients and would allow more patients to benefit from avoiding radical surgery and associated morbidities [12–16]. In fact, this may be even more relevant for the patients with increased age and associated comorbidities. Taking into consideration that more recent data on postoperative mortality are studied following colorectal surgery, it is estimated that elderly and comorbid patients have inferior 1-year survival in the setting of a complete pathological response following radical surgery when compared to patients managed nonoperatively [17].

5.3 Types of Neoadjuvant Therapy

Considering neoadjuvant therapy will be used for the purpose of tailoring surgical therapy for patients based on tumor response, strategies associated with significant tumor regression are preferred [18]. Therefore, combined association of chemotherapy and radiation (i.e., long course with hyper-fractionated RT doses) has been shown to result in greater tumor regression rates and increased chance of a complete response [13, 19]. In contrast, short-course RT alone may only lead to significant tumor regression if longer intervals between RT completion and assessment of response are allowed [20]. The standard 1 week interval will lead to virtually no chance of developing a pCR [18].

Several dose escalation studies seem to suggest that additional RT doses to the rectum may increase the pCR and cCR rates. Therefore, strategies have included the combination of external beam and intrarectal RT boosts to maximize response rates. Intrarectal radiation may be delivered by means of contact radiation (also known as the Papillon technique) or with high-dose endorectal brachytherapy (HDBR). These strategies are currently being investigated in the setting of organ-preserving strategies for the management of complete clinical responders [21, 22].

Even though most studies have dealt with radiation or chemoradiation therapies in the neoadjuvant setting, there is a suggestion that chemotherapy alone could provide similar outcomes in terms of rates of pathological response. This strategy would allow to spare patients from potentially unnecessary radiation-related toxicities [8]. Interesting long-term data from the Swedish rectal cancer trials have suggested that patients undergoing neoadjuvant RT were more likely to develop second malignancies and hospital readmissions due to small bowel obstruction and abdominal pain [23, 24].

An alternative regimen with radiation and increased number of cycles of chemotherapy has resulted in surprisingly high rates of complete tumor regression [25]. In this study, patients received 54 Gy of radiation (external beam) and concomitant 5-FU-based chemotherapy. However, instead of the two cycles given in the beginning and end of radiation, additional cycles are delivered every 21 days not only during radiation but also during the resting period after RT completion. After the completion of six cycles (in total) with this regimen, ≥50% of patients with baseline cT2/cT3 rectal cancer developed complete clinical response and avoided radical surgery after a ≥ median 50 months of follow-up [26]. One question could be whether the improved rates of cCR in comparison with historical controls is a consequence of the "modest" increase in radiation therapy (from 50.4 to 54 Gy) or the increased number of cycles of chemotherapy (2–6 cycles). In fact, even though the credit for this significant increase in cCR rates may be quickly attributed to the increase in the number of 5-FU cycles, the radiation therapy dose escalation may have played a significant role.

Alternative neoadjuvant strategies have been considered with the use of different chemotherapy agents and schedules to improve the rates of complete tumor regression without compromising treatment-related toxicity. Even though the addition of a second drug (to 5-fluorouracil-based regimens) has been considered a predictive factor for complete tumor regression, studies have failed to demonstrate any increase in complete pathological response with the addition of oxaliplatin or cetuximab.

Another strategy would be the delivery of chemotherapy prior to CRT, also known as induction chemotherapy. The rationale of this regimen is to deal with micrometastatic disease of patients at higher risk for systemic dissemination by delivering systemic chemotherapy upfront (in addition to adjuvant chemotherapy after radical surgery). Different induction chemotherapy regimens with capecitabine/oxaliplatin (CAPOX) or cetuximab + CAPOX (CAPOX-C) have been studied in this setting [27]. In one of the first studies using this treatment strategy offered to patients at higher risk for systemic recurrence, pCR rates were not substantially improved [27]. Even though patients undergoing induction chemotherapy with CAPOX-C did show improved tumor response, pCR rates were not significantly increased, even among *KRAS/BRAF* wild-type tumors. A recent update of 5-year follow-up, reported that the addition of cetuximab was not associated with a statistically significant improvement in survival regardless of *KRAS/BRAF* status [28]. In a similar study recently reported using upfront FOLFOX followed by standard CRT in a broader patient population (not exclusively restricted to high-risk patients) resulted in surprising 38% complete response (either pathological or clinical response) [29]. This considerably high pCR and cCR rates led the authors to suggest that this regimen could be the ideal platform for an organ-preserving strategy [29].

The understanding of the effects of systemic chemotherapy alone on primary rectal cancer in the absence of RT led to the idea of a phase II trial with neoadjuvant chemotherapy alone without the use of preoperative radiation. In a recent preliminary report of this study, after six cycles of FOLFOX + bevazicumab followed by radical surgery, the observed pCR rate was 25% [30]. These findings supported the idea that perhaps radiation therapy could be omitted in selected patients.

This particular issue is currently under investigation in a prospective randomized trial (PROSPECT) where patients are randomized to CRT versus chemotherapy upfront and selective CRT for poor responders. There is a chance that RT may be ultimately be omitted to a significant proportion of patients that respond well to chemotherapy alone and therefore may potentially avoid the long-term detrimental effects of RT.

5.4 Assessing Tumor Response: Why?

The rationale for assessing tumor response after neoadjuvant therapy is to define final treatment strategy based upon the current status of the tumor, that is, after therapy. The assessment of tumor response is important even if you are not ultimately changing the type of resection. After neoadjuvant therapy, tumors present significant changes in size, depth, and proximity to the mesorectal fascia. Even if total mesorectal excision will be the definitive treatment strategy, it may be considerably useful to know ahead of time what challenges are expected during surgical resection.

In up to 42% of patients undergoing neoadjuvant CRT, however, complete tumor regression may develop. The problem is that most of the times, radical surgery is required to appropriately confirm the presence of complete pathological response. In an effort to spare patients from potentially unnecessary surgery, colorectal surgeons have attempted to assess tumor response in order to estimate pathological response by clinical, endoscopic, and radiological means. In this setting, the term complete clinical response has been used for patients with no clinical evidence of residual cancer after neoadjuvant therapy. However, the features of a complete clinical response may be quite subjective and dependent on surgeon's experience, different diagnostic tools, and treatment-related factors. Attempts to standardize the definition of a complete clinical response are already available, particularly with the use of endoscopic and radiological imaging [31]. Still, clinical assessment remains highly subjective and surgeon dependent.

It has been suggested that patients with complete clinical response (*using very stringent criteria*) could be offered no immediate radical surgery. Instead, a strict surveillance program, also known as the "watch and wait" strategy, with frequent visits to the colorectal surgeon, and the use of multiple staging modalities could provide safe follow-up. Initial studies trying to estimate the accuracy of clinical assessment in predicting pathological response were disappointing [32]. However, more recent studies have shown that clinical assessment can accurately detect pathological response when stringent criteria are used [33]. In a recent retrospective study, surgeons were asked to indicate the presence of pCR based on photographs of resected specimens without any information on radiological imaging or digital rectal examination (Table 5.1) [31]. Curiously, negative and positive predictive values were ≥90% using these stringent criteria. On one hand, this means that using these criteria would be considerably safer to offer no immediate surgery to these patients [33, 34]. On the other hand, the low overall specificity of these features in identifying a pCR will inevitably lead to a significant proportion of patients that still undergo radical surgery. Altogether,

Table 5.1 Clinical and endoscopic features of clinical complete response [31]

Complete response	Incomplete response
Whitening of the mucosa	Any residual deep ulcer
Telangiectasia	Any residual superficial ulcer
Subtle loss of pliability	Palpable nodule
No tumor felt or seen	Stenosis

these data suggest that there is significant room for improvement to allow a more substantial proportion of patients to avoid unnecessary radical surgery after achieving a complete pathological response [35].

5.5 Assessing Tumor Response: When and How?

Intervals between CRT completion and assessment of response may also be relevant. Studies suggest that longer intervals are associated with higher pCR rates [36–38]. The only randomized study comparing two different intervals between CRT completion and surgery demonstrated that patients undergoing a 6-week interval developed more significant tumor regression when compared to a 2-week interval. Even though no survival benefit or differences in sphincter preservation were observed, 6 weeks shortly became the standard of care to patients undergoing neoadjuvant CRT followed by surgery. Retrospective data has further suggested that longer than 6 weeks intervals could be associated with even higher rates of tumor regression [36, 37, 39, 40]. In fact, several small series reported on higher rates of pCR after 7 weeks of CRT. Finally, one study suggested that pCR rates would only plateau after 12 weeks from CRT completion [36, 37, 39, 40]. There are ongoing randomized studies to address these issues that will provide us further information on the ideal interval between CRT and assessment of response, in an effort to maximize the chance of a patient developing complete response [39]. There is a chance, however, that intervals will need to be tailored or individualized for each patient, as tumors may respond differently as a function of time to treatment [41]. It has been our practice to assess tumor response at least 8 weeks from CRT completion. As said, longer intervals (up to 12 weeks) have been used for the majority of patients unless there is worsening of symptoms or radiological evidence of disease progression. Even though progression is rarely seen, it is not impossible.

Response assessment always begins with the characterization of symptoms. Symptomatic patients rarely have complete tumor regression, even though this feature has very low specificity. Digital rectal examination is perhaps one of the most relevant tools in tumor response assessment. There is currently no single diagnostic tool that can possibly replace the information given by digital rectal examination (DRE). Very frequently, irregularities of the rectal wall are better felt than seen, and should be considered as highly suspicious for residual cancer (Fig. 5.1). *No patient is considered for nonoperative approach in the presence of rectal wall irregularities, mass ulceration, or stenosis.* In terms of DRE, a complete clinical response is the absence of any irregularity of the rectal wall. The area can be thickened and firm,

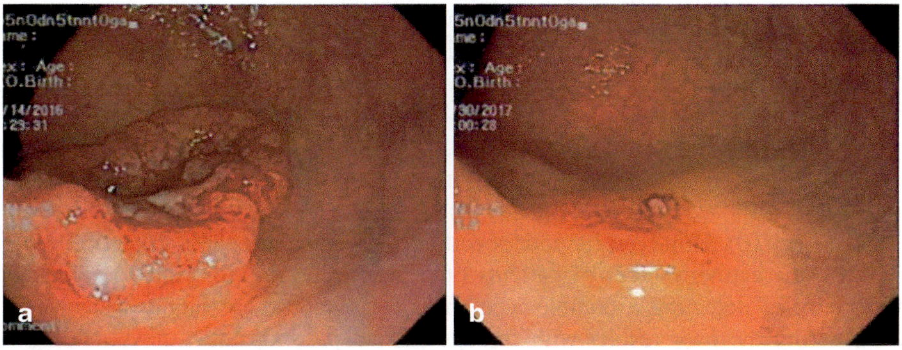

Fig. 5.1 Endoscopic view of a patient with a rectal cancer managed by neoadjuvant chemoradiation. Pretreatment endoscopic view shows an ulcerated lesion with elevated borders of approximately 3 cm in diameter. (**a**) Post chemoradiation endoscopic assessment reveals incomplete clinical response. (**b**) There is still a residual ulcer covered with fibrin and with slightly elevated borders

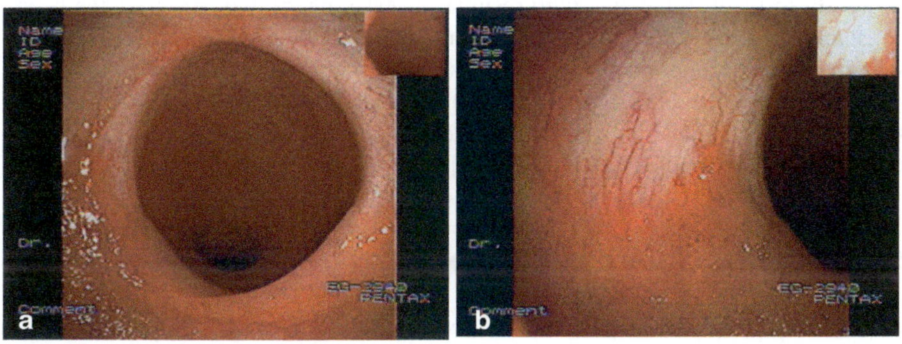

Fig. 5.2 Endoscopic view of a patient with complete clinical response following neoadjuvant chemoradiation. There is whitening of the mucosa (**a**) and the presence of telangiectasia (**b**) in the area where the tumor was

but to be considered a complete clinical response, the surface has to be regular and smooth [31].

Endoscopic assessment is also very important. Whitening of the mucosa and telangiectasia are usually seen in patients with a complete clinical response (Fig. 5.2).

The presence of any ulceration or mucosal irregularity missed on DRE should prompt additional investigations and usually rule out a complete clinical response. Frequently, DRE may have to be reassessed after endoscopic guidance of any findings suggestive of residual cancer. During flexible or rigid proctoscopy, biopsies are frequently considered for the assessment of response. If there is clinical evidence (DRE and endoscopic) of a cCR, forceps biopsies rarely add clinically relevant information [42]. On the other hand, in the presence of clinical evidence of residual cancer (incomplete response), endoscopic biopsies are also rarely useful, except for convincing patients there is residual disease there. Even in the presence of negative endoscopic biopsies, patients with incomplete clinical response should not be offered a nonoperative approach [42]. As cited previously, one study suggested that clinical criteria are associated with high negative and positive predictive values for the detection of pCR. In fact, the finding of clinical features consistent with cCR was statistically associated with a complete pathological response (ypT0). However, its poor specificity indicates that these criteria underestimate the actual number of patients of pCR. In this setting, tools to enhance specificity of detecting a complete pathological response are highly warranted. Considering the poor results with forceps endoscopic biopsies, a novel strategy using incisional biopsies in an ex vivo model has been attempted. After completion of proctectomy, specimens were opened, and an incisional biopsy was performed to assess primary tumor regression to CRT. In the presence of an incomplete pathological response, incisional biopsies were able to detect only 55%. As such, incisional biopsy is certainly not suitable as a stand-alone method to deem patients fit for watch and wait. The potential utility of incisional biopsy may be restricted in its ability to identify patients with residual disease that may otherwise have been considered for a watch and wait approach. It is likely that the reason for the poor sensitivity for residual disease using incisional biopsy was due to the fragmented and scattered distribution of some residual tumors [43]. Ultimately, these findings support that incisional biopsies are not likely to provide sufficient accuracy for the identification of complete responders [44].

5.6 Local Excision of the Tumor Site

In the presence of an incomplete clinical response and patients are resistant to radical resection or medically unfit, the least we would offer is a full-thickness excisional biopsy, preferably with the use of transanal endoscopic microsurgery. This "excisional biopsy," otherwise referred to as a local excision, is primarily considered as a diagnostic procedure and may be appropriate for patients with small (≤3 cm) lesions that are restricted to the bowel wall (ycT1/2N0). However, we would restrict this to patients with low residual lesions that would otherwise require an abdominal-perineal excision or a coloanal intersphincteric resection as a definitive procedure [45]. Appropriate pathological information regarding ypT classification, tumor regression grade, lymphovascular/perineural invasion and resection margins may allow final decision regarding the need for total mesorectal excision and protectomy.

It has been our policy to offer strict follow-up to patients with final pathological specimen showing ypT0 after this "diagnostic" transanal local excision. This is due to the fact that the risk of lymph node metastases among these patients has been shown to be very low in the setting of neoadjuvant CRT and long (≥8 weeks) intervals. This is already true for unselected patients with ypT0, where the risk of nodal metastases are well under 10% and in most cases less than 5% [46–48]. However, with the significant improvements in radiological imaging, particularly with high-resolution magnetic resonance (MR) with the use of diffusion-weighted series and other lymphotropic agents, selection of patients with ycT0N0 is expected to further improve [49]. On the other end of the spectrum, patients with unsuspected residual ≥ypT3, lymphovascular invasion, positive resection margins, and more than 10% of viable residual cancer cells have been recommended immediate radical surgery.

Equally challenging cases are those with intermediate residual cancers: ypT1 or early ypT2 (restricted to the superficial muscular layer) cancers without lymphovascular invasion or other unfavorable pathological features. In the presence of negative margins (≥5 mm), it has been our policy to follow-up these patients without immediate radical surgery, only if they would otherwise require an abdominal-perineal excisions or coloanal anastomosis. This strategy of offering patients with small superficial residual cancers, radiologically staged as ycN0, a local procedure is quite appealing. However, there are at least three main drawbacks to this treatment strategy. First, the healing of the rectal defects determined by local excision after neoadjuvant CRT are quite challenging and painful, particularly those closer to anal verge [50, 51]. Healing problems are much more frequent and may take as long as 8 weeks to completely heal. Even though severe complications are not frequent, pain may be quite significant requiring readmission to the hospital. The second drawback is that sphincter preservation may be compromised after the performance of full-thickness local excision in this setting. A few studies have addressed this issue and reported that patients requiring radical resection after FTLE frequently ended up with an APR, even though they originally were considered candidates for a sphincter-preserving procedure [45, 52]. Finally, the completion of total mesorectal excision in this setting may provide an imperfect mesorectal specimen for the pathologist. A recent review of patients undergoing completion TME indicated that previous TEM was a risk factor for poor quality of the TME specimen [53]. All of these issues should be kept in mind when offering patients "diagnostic" or "therapeutic" local excision after partial response.

5.6.1 Why Not Offer Patients with a cCR Transanal Local Excision for the Histological Confirmation of ypT0?

As mentioned above, the healing of local excision defects following neoadjuvant CRT is not as simple as after local excision alone. The rates of wound dehiscence may be quite significant. In this setting, not only is pain an issue but also significant scarring following delayed healing may develop which will make patient follow-up even more difficult. Even though ypT0 may be associated with lower risk of local failures, the risk is not zero, and the patient still requires appropriate follow-up. The distinction between local recurrences in a rectal wall following wound dehiscence after a local excision with or without rectal stenosis may be quite challenging. Therefore, we believe that follow-up is considerably facilitated by the preservation of rectal wall integrity with the "watch and wait" approach allowing for earlier detection of possible recurrences in addition to superior functional outcomes.

5.7 Radiological Imaging

Radiological assessment of response is of paramount importance to appropriately select patients for an alternative treatment strategy such as the "watch and wait" approach following a complete clinical response. As a matter of fact, the developments in radiological imaging, including both PET/CT and MR, have been quite significant. Proper magnetic resonance imaging with the use of diffusion-weighted techniques is now used routinely for the assessment of response in these patients. Currently, we would only consider a true complete responder (1) in a patient showing low signal intensity area replacing the area of the previous tumor or (2) in a patient with no detectable abnormalities in standard MR associated with no evidence of disease on clinical and endoscopic examination (Fig. 5.3). A recent publication has reported three different patterns of low signal intensity that are compatible with a complete clinical response: minimal fibrosis, transmural fibrosis, and irregular fibrosis [54]. Others have attempted to estimate tumor regression grades (as described for pathological assessment) [55] by standard MR imaging [56]. In addition, diffusion-weighted MR series may provide evidence of the absence of restriction to diffusion to fulfill the criteria for a radiological complete response [57]. In our previously reported experiences with this "watch and wait" treatment strategy, MR imaging was not available to a significant proportion of patients [58]. Therefore, there is a hope that the incorporation of these findings for the selection of patients with complete clinical response will significantly impact the outcomes of the watch and wait strategy. The presence of mixed signal intensity (Fig. 5.4) within the area of the previous cancer should raise a suspicion of an incomplete clinical response (Fig. 5.5). In addition to the assessment of the rectal wall, the mesorectum is also at

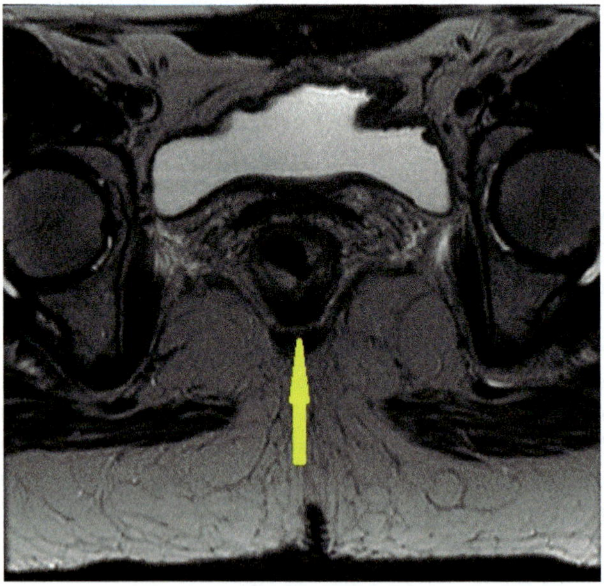

Fig. 5.3 Post chemoradiation high-resolution magnetic resonance shows low signal intensity (mrTRG1) of the rectal wall where the tumor previously was. Additional findings include absence of metastatic nodes or extramural venous invasion

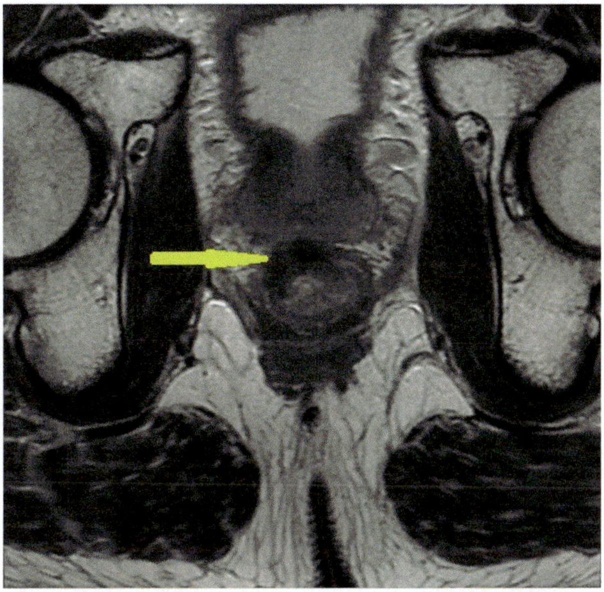

Fig. 5.4 Post chemoradiation high-resolution magnetic resonance shows mixed signal intensity of the rectal wall in the area of the residual tumor

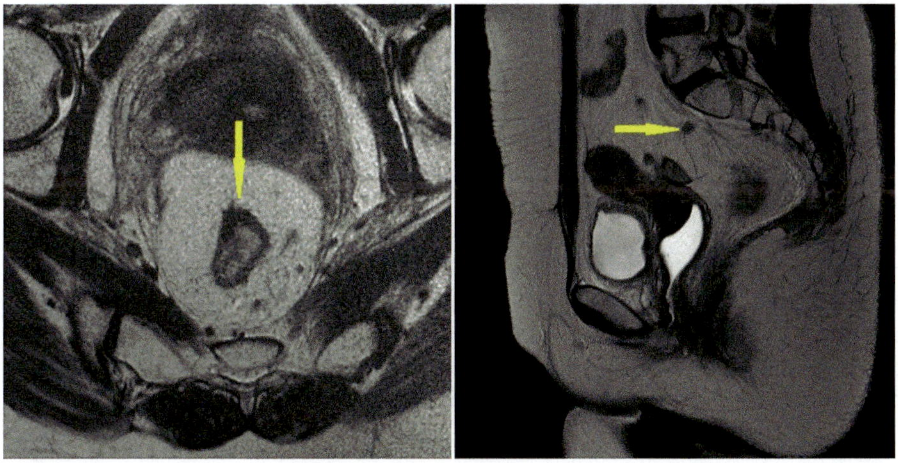

Fig. 5.5 Post chemoradiation high-resolution magnetic resonance shows complete radiological response in the primary lesion indicated by a low signal intensity area (mrTRG1) but evidence of residual cancer in an upper mesorectal node with mixed signal intensity

risk for the presence of residual cancer despite complete primary regression (ypT0N1). Therefore, MR imaging should also provide the colorectal surgeon with information regarding possible mesorectal (or even lateral node) involvement regardless of primary tumor response (Fig. 5.6).

Molecular imaging may also play a role in the assessment of tumor response. PET/CT imaging offers information on tumor metabolism in addition to standard

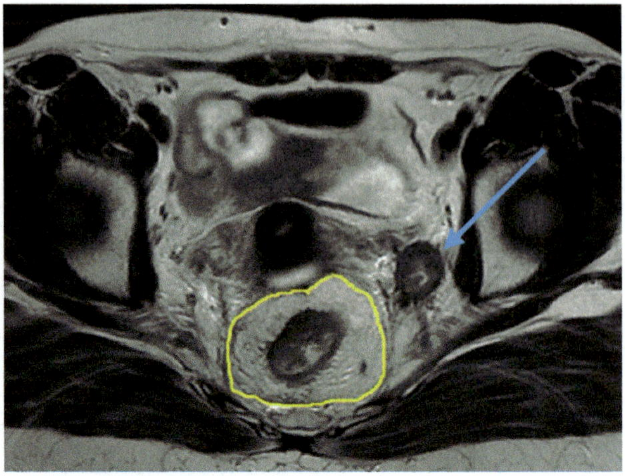

Fig. 5.6 Post chemoradiation high-resolution magnetic resonance shows nodal metastasis (*blue arrow*) in the lateral compartment outside of the mesorectum (*yellow line*)

radiological anatomical features. In this setting, PET/CT has been used for the assessment of tumor response to neoadjuvant chemoradiation therapy [12, 59]. In addition to the visual identification of FDG uptake within the area of the rectal wall harboring the tumor or within the mesorectum, PET/CT allows the estimation of the metabolism profile. Standard uptake values are direct estimations of tissue metabolism and may be used for the distinction of residual inflammatory changes and residual cancer. The measurement of SUV in two different intervals from FDG injection is routinely performed (at 1 and 3 h) and allows two distinct patterns (dual time) of metabolism. Increases in SUVs (between 1 and 3 h) suggest the presence of residual cancer, whereas decreases suggest inflammatory or fibrotic changes [41]. Even though we have used PET/CT to distinguish between complete and incomplete responses in the setting of a prospective study with acceptable overall accuracy (85%), PET/CT may not be appropriate for routine use for this purpose, mainly due to increased cost and need for multiple studies with significant radiation exposure [12]. Instead, the use of this molecular imaging modality should perhaps be considered for patients with significant discordant results between studies, particularly between clinical and radiological findings.

5.8 Carcinoembryonic Antigen (CEA)

Pretreatment CEA levels have been shown to be predictors of response to neoadjuvant CRT and ultimately survival [55, 60]. Posttreatment CEA levels are also relevant, and normal levels after CRT have been associated with increase complete clinical response rates [61]. Abnormal CEA levels before or after CRT should raise the suspicion of incomplete response to CRT and/or metastatic dissemination. In this setting, abnormal CEA levels should lead to a more liberal use of PET/CT imaging for the assessment of tumor response since it may also allow the detection of unsuspected metastatic disease in addition to the diagnosis of incomplete response.

5.9 Final Decision Management

Patients are usually assessed for tumor response to neoadjuvant chemoradiation at least 8–10 weeks from treatment completion regardless of the exact treatment regimen used. Clinical and endoscopic features are assessed in the clinic using digital rectal examination and rigid proctoscopy. Flexible proctoscopy is used solely for video documentation or for situations where endoscopic biopsies are required. Again, endoscopic biopsies are rarely useful due to the considerably low negative predictive values. Still, they may be useful to convince the patient that there is residual cancer. Colorectal surgeons should not be obsessed for the obtainment of positive biopsies prior to the indication for radical surgery. Clinical assessment showing incomplete response should suffice. CEA levels should be normal both before and after treatment; otherwise additional studies are strongly recommended.

If a patient has clinical evidence of a complete response, radiological assessment should be performed for two purposes. First, confirmation of findings consistent with a complete response within the rectal wall should be present; second, confirmation of the absence of dissemination to the mesorectal/lateral nodes is also required. Usually, MR with diffusion-weighted series is sufficient for most cases. In patients with an incomplete clinical response due to subtle mucosal irregularities, radiological staging that indicates complete response, and a normal CEA (prior to and after CRT), transanal local excision (preferably using TEM) may be used primarily as a diagnostic procedure. In patients with a complete clinical response but with radiological evidence of residual disease on MRI or abnormal CEA levels (pre- or posttreatment), PET/CT may be a useful assessment tool. A normal PET/CT may still allow consideration of a nonoperative approach in selected cases after discussion with the patient. Abnormal PET/CT in this setting should be viewed as highly suspicious for residual cancer. Incomplete clinical response (gross residual cancer or ulceration) should prompt restaging to allow proper determination of final surgical approach, but never to suggest a nonoperative approach.

5.10 Follow-Up

Patients suspected for a complete clinical response are closely followed and reassessed for tumor response every 1–2 months for the first year, every 3 months for the second year, and every 6 months thereafter. If initial radiological assessment of response is normal (MR) or consistent with a complete response, radiological reassessment may be performed at 6 months from initial assessment.

In this recent report, patients with cCR were not routinely treated by adjuvant systemic therapy regardless of their baseline staging features. As cited earlier, follow-up included visits every 1–2 months to a single experienced colorectal surgeon, with clinical and digital rectal examination [62]. In addition, rigid proctoscopy and CEA levels were performed every 2–3 months. After 1 year of follow-up, patients were examined every 3 months similarly and every 6 months after 3 years. A radiologic imaging modality (preferably MRI) was used to rule out mesorectal disease at the initial assessment of response; if this radiological assessment of response was normal or consistent with a complete response, radiological reassessment would be performed at 6 months from initial assessment and yearly thereafter. Distant metastases surveillance was performed as recommended for usual colorectal cancer with regular CT scans.

5.11 Additional Therapy

Until now, patients with a complete clinical response have not been offered adjuvant systemic therapy of any kind following nonoperative management. However, the risk of systemic recurrence among these patients is still significant and may ultimately justify its use in selected patients according to baseline radiological features such as nodal positivity. Therefore, even though high-risk patients (cT3N+ at baseline staging) may still be considered for a nonoperative approach after a cCR following CRT, adjuvant systemic chemotherapy may prove to be beneficial. Even though this may sound appropriate, it warrants further investigation in properly designed prospective studies.

Patients with pCR managed by radical surgery are still at risk for developing systemic recurrences. In a pooled analysis of ≥2000 patients with pCR, with nearly 40% receiving adjuvant systemic therapy, 11% developed systemic recurrences. Among patients with cCR managed nonoperatively without any adjuvant systemic therapy, distant metastases rate was 18%. Differences in adjuvant therapy between these studies may have accounted for these differences in distant metastases rates [9].

One explanation for the good prognosis after pCR is that a pCR after chemoradiation is indicative of a prognostically favorable biological tumor profile, with less propensity for local recurrence and distant metastases and a better survival than for patients with less response.

Finally, the use of neoadjuvant therapy regimens incorporating additional cycles of chemotherapy during or prior to radiation may have the advantage of providing additional systemic control to patients with rectal cancer irrespective of final primary tumor response.

5.12 Local Recurrence and Salvages

5.12.1 Definition of Early Regrowth and Late Recurrence

A major limitation of this nonoperative approach would be the impossibility of salvage in the event of a local recurrence. It is recognized that the majority of these recurrences are developed in the first year after completion of CRT. In previous reports, an arbitrarily defined cutoff of 12 months following CRT finalization has been suggested to distinguish between early regrowths (≤12 months) and late recurrences (>12 months). Even though these local failures may not be distinguishable from the oncological point of view, early recurrences may have distinct biological behavior and represent more rapidly growing residual cancer cells when compared to late recurrences making this subdivision clinically relevant [62].

5.12.2 Salvage

In a recent report of 183 patients undergoing standard neoadjuvant CRT, 49% developed an initial complete clinical response. When early tumor regrowths (<12 months of follow-up) and late recurrences were considered together, 28 patients (31%) experienced local recurrence (after a median follow-up time of 60 months). More than half of these recurrences developed within the first 12 months of follow-up. Of the 28, 26 patients underwent salvage therapy. In four patients, local re-recurrence was detected following salvage. The overall salvage rate for local recurrence was 93%, and the local recurrence-free survival at 5 years was 94%. Seventy-eight percent of patients ultimately underwent an organ-preserving procedure [62].

In conclusion, "watch and wait" with no immediate resection and rigorous follow-up after a cCR to neoadjuvant CRT leads to good long-term oncological outcomes and represents an attractive organ-preserving strategy for rectal cancer management. Close surveillance allows early recognition of local recurrence, resulting in the possibility of salvage for the majority of patients (>90%) and excellent local disease control (94%).

References

1. Kosinski L, Habr-Gama A, Ludwig K, Perez R. Shifting concepts in rectal cancer management: a review of contemporary primary rectal cancer treatment strategies. CA Cancer J Clin. 2012;62:173–202.
2. Sauer R, Becker H, Hohenberger W, Rodel C, Wittekind C, Fietkau R, et al. Preoperative versus postoperative chemoradiotherapy for rectal cancer. N Engl J Med. 2004;351:1731–40.
3. Kapiteijn E, Marijnen CA, Nagtegaal ID, Putter H, Steup WH, Wiggers T, et al. Preoperative radiotherapy combined with total mesorectal excision for resectable rectal cancer. N Engl J Med. 2001;345:638–46.
4. Sauer R, Liersch T, Merkel S, Fietkau R, Hohenberger W, Hess C, et al. Preoperative versus postoperative chemoradiotherapy for locally advanced rectal cancer: results of the German CAO/ARO/AIO-94 randomized phase III trial after a median follow-up of 11 years. J Clin Oncol. 2012;30:1926–33.
5. Peeters KC, van de Velde CJ, Leer JW, Martijn H, Junggeburt JM, Kranenbarg EK, et al. Late side effects of short-course preoperative radiotherapy combined with total mesorectal excision for rectal cancer: increased bowel dysfunction in irradiated patients–a Dutch colorectal cancer group study. J Clin Oncol. 2005;23:6199–206.
6. van Gijn W, Marijnen CA, Nagtegaal ID, Kranenbarg EM, Putter H, Wiggers T, et al. Preoperative radiotherapy combined with total mesorectal excision for resectable rectal cancer: 12-year follow-up of the multicentre, randomised controlled TME trial. Lancet Oncol. 2011;12:575–82.
7. Taylor FG, Quirke P, Heald RJ, Moran B, Blomqvist L, Swift I, et al. Preoperative high-resolution magnetic resonance imaging can identify good prognosis stage I, II, and III rectal

cancer best managed by surgery alone: a prospective, multicenter, European study. Ann Surg. 2011;253:711–9.
8. Schrag D, Weiser MR, Goodman KA, Gonen M, Cercek A, Reidy DL, et al. Neoadjuvant FOLFOX-bev, without radiation, for locally advanced rectal cancer. J Clin Oncol. 2010;28:3511. (suppl; abstr)
9. Maas M, Nelemans PJ, Valentini V, Das P, Rodel C, Kuo LJ, et al. Long-term outcome in patients with a pathological complete response after chemoradiation for rectal cancer: a pooled analysis of individual patient data. Lancet Oncol. 2010;11:835–44.
10. Smith FM, Waldron D, Winter DC. Rectum-conserving surgery in the era of chemoradiotherapy. Br J Surg. 2010;97:1752–64.
11. Habr-Gama A, Perez RO. Non-operative management of rectal cancer after neoadjuvant chemoradiation. Br J Surg. 2009;96:125–7.
12. Perez RO, Habr-Gama A, Gama-Rodrigues J, Proscurshim I, Juliao GP, Lynn P, et al. Accuracy of positron emission tomography/computed tomography and clinical assessment in the detection of complete rectal tumor regression after neoadjuvant chemoradiation: long-term results of a prospective trial (National Clinical Trial 00254683). Cancer. 2012;118:3501–11.
13. Sanghera P, Wong DW, McConkey CC, Geh JI, Hartley A. Chemoradiotherapy for rectal cancer: an updated analysis of factors affecting pathological response. Clin Oncol (R Coll Radiol). 2008;20:176–83.
14. Garcia-Aguilar J, Shi Q, Thomas CR Jr, Chan E, Cataldo P, Marcet J, et al. A phase II trial of neoadjuvant chemoradiation and local excision for T2N0 rectal cancer: preliminary results of the ACOSOG Z6041 trial. Ann Surg Oncol. 2012;19:384–91.
15. Lezoche E, Baldarelli M, Lezoche G, Paganini AM, Gesuita R, Guerrieri M. Randomized clinical trial of endoluminal locoregional resection versus laparoscopic total mesorectal excision for T2 rectal cancer after neoadjuvant therapy. Br J Surg. 2012;99:1211–8.
16. Habr-Gama A, Perez RO, Nadalin W, Sabbaga J, Ribeiro U Jr, Silva e Sousa AH Jr, et al. Operative versus nonoperative treatment for stage 0 distal rectal cancer following chemoradiation therapy: long-term results. Ann Surg. 2004;240:711–7. discussion 7-8
17. Smith FM, Rao C, Oliva Perez R, Bujko K, Athanasiou T, Habr-Gama A, et al. Avoiding radical surgery improves early survival in elderly patients with rectal cancer, demonstrating complete clinical response after neoadjuvant therapy: results of a decision-analytic model. Dis Colon Rectum. 2015;58:159–71.
18. Bujko K, Nowacki MP, Nasierowska-Guttmejer A, Michalski W, Bebenek M, Kryj M. Long-term results of a randomized trial comparing preoperative short-course radiotherapy with preoperative conventionally fractionated chemoradiation for rectal cancer. Br J Surg. 2006;93:1215–23.
19. Bosset JF, Calais G, Mineur L, Maingon P, Radosevic-Jelic L, Daban A, et al. Enhanced tumorocidal effect of chemotherapy with preoperative radiotherapy for rectal cancer: preliminary results–EORTC 22921. J Clin Oncol. 2005;23:5620–7.
20. Radu C, Berglund A, Pahlman L, Glimelius B. Short-course preoperative radiotherapy with delayed surgery in rectal cancer–a retrospective study. Radiother Oncol. 2008;87:343–9.
21. Gerard JP, Chapet O, Ortholan C, Benezery K, Barbet N, Romestaing P. French experience with contact X-ray endocavitary radiation for early rectal cancer. Clin Oncol (R Coll Radiol). 2007;19:661–73.
22. Vuong T, Devic S, Podgorsak E. High dose rate endorectal brachytherapy as a neoadjuvant treatment for patients with resectable rectal cancer. Clin Oncol (R Coll Radiol). 2007;19:701–5.
23. Birgisson H, Pahlman L, Gunnarsson U, Glimelius B. Occurrence of second cancers in patients treated with radiotherapy for rectal cancer. J Clin Oncol. 2005;23:6126–31.
24. Birgisson H, Pahlman L, Gunnarsson U, Glimelius B. Adverse effects of preoperative radiation therapy for rectal cancer: long-term follow-up of the Swedish rectal cancer trial. J Clin Oncol. 2005;23:8697–705.
25. Habr-Gama A, Perez RO, Sabbaga J, Nadalin W, Sao Juliao GP, Gama-Rodrigues J. Increasing the rates of complete response to neoadjuvant chemoradiotherapy for distal rectal cancer:

results of a prospective study using additional chemotherapy during the resting period. Dis Colon Rectum. 2009;52:1927–34.

26. Habr-Gama A, Sabbaga J, Gama-Rodrigues J, Sao Juliao GP, Proscurshim I, Bailao Aguilar P, et al. Watch and wait approach following extended neoadjuvant chemoradiation for distal rectal cancer: are we getting closer to anal cancer management? Dis Colon Rectum. 2013;56:1109–17.
27. Chua YJ, Barbachano Y, Cunningham D, Oates JR, Brown G, Wotherspoon A, et al. Neoadjuvant capecitabine and oxaliplatin before chemoradiotherapy and total mesorectal excision in MRI-defined poor-risk rectal cancer: a phase 2 trial. Lancet Oncol. 2010;11:241–8.
28. Dewdney A, Cunningham D, Tabernero J, Capdevila J, Glimelius B, Cervantes A, et al. Multicenter randomized phase II clinical trial comparing neoadjuvant oxaliplatin, capecitabine, and preoperative radiotherapy with or without cetuximab followed by total mesorectal excision in patients with high-risk rectal cancer (EXPERT-C). J Clin Oncol. 2012;30:1620–7.
29. Cercek A, Goodman KA, Hajj C, Weisberger E, Segal NH, Reidy-Lagunes DL, et al. Neoadjuvant chemotherapy first, followed by chemoradiation and then surgery, in the management of locally advanced rectal cancer. J Natl Compr Cancer Netw. 2014;12:513–9.
30. Schrag D, Weiser MR, Goodman KA, Gonen M, Hollywood E, Cercek A, et al. Neoadjuvant chemotherapy without routine use of radiation therapy for patients with locally advanced rectal cancer: a pilot trial. J Clin Oncol. 2014;32:513–8.
31. Habr-Gama A, Perez RO, Wynn G, Marks J, Kessler H, Gama-Rodrigues J. Complete clinical response after neoadjuvant chemoradiation therapy for distal rectal cancer: characterization of clinical and endoscopic findings for standardization. Dis Colon Rectum. 2010;53:1692–8.
32. Hiotis SP, Weber SM, Cohen AM, Minsky BD, Paty PB, Guillem JG, et al. Assessing the predictive value of clinical complete response to neoadjuvant therapy for rectal cancer: an analysis of 488 patients. J Am Coll Surg. 2002;194:131–5. discussion 5-6
33. Smith FM, Chang KH, Sheahan K, Hyland J, O'Connell PR, Winter DC. The surgical significance of residual mucosal abnormalities in rectal cancer following neoadjuvant chemoradiotherapy. Br J Surg. 2012;99:993–1001.
34. Habr-Gama A, Perez RO. The surgical significance of residual mucosal abnormalities in rectal cancer following neoadjuvant chemoradiotherapy (Br J Surg 2012; 99: 993-1001). Br J Surg. 2012;99:1601. author reply -2
35. Smith FM, Wiland H, Mace A, Pai RK, Kalady MF. Clinical criteria underestimate complete pathological response in rectal cancer treated with neoadjuvant chemoradiotherapy. Dis Colon Rectum. 2014;57:311–5.
36. Kalady MF, de Campos-Lobato LF, Stocchi L, Geisler DP, Dietz D, Lavery IC, et al. Predictive factors of pathologic complete response after neoadjuvant chemoradiation for rectal cancer. Ann Surg. 2009;250:582–9.
37. Tulchinsky H, Shmueli E, Figer A, Klausner JM, Rabau M. An interval >7 weeks between neoadjuvant therapy and surgery improves pathologic complete response and disease-free survival in patients with locally advanced rectal cancer. Ann Surg Oncol. 2008;15:2661–7.
38. Francois Y, Nemoz CJ, Baulieux J, Vignal J, Grandjean JP, Partensky C, et al. Influence of the interval between preoperative radiation therapy and surgery on downstaging and on the rate of sphincter-sparing surgery for rectal cancer: the Lyon R90-01 randomized trial. J Clin Oncol. 1999;17:2396.
39. Evans J, Tait D, Swift I, Pennert K, Tekkis P, Wotherspoon A, et al. Timing of surgery following preoperative therapy in rectal cancer: the need for a prospective randomized trial? Dis Colon Rectum. 2011;54:1251–9.
40. Wolthuis AM, Penninckx F, Haustermans K, De Hertogh G, Fieuws S, Van Cutsem E, et al. Impact of interval between neoadjuvant chemoradiotherapy and TME for locally advanced rectal cancer on pathologic response and oncologic outcome. Ann Surg Oncol. 2012;19:2833–41.
41. Perez RO, Habr-Gama A, Sao Juliao GP, Gama-Rodrigues J, Sousa AH Jr, Campos FG, et al. Optimal timing for assessment of tumor response to neoadjuvant chemoradiation in patients

with rectal cancer: do all patients benefit from waiting longer than 6 weeks? Int J Radiat Oncol Biol Phys. 2012;84:1159–65.
42. Perez RO, Habr-Gama A, Pereira GV, Lynn PB, Alves PA, Proscurshim I, et al. Role of biopsies in patients with residual rectal cancer following neoadjuvant chemoradiation after downsizing: can they rule out persisting cancer? Colorectal Dis. 2012;14:714–20.
43. Perez RO, Habr-Gama A, Smith FM, Kosinski L, Sao Juliao GP, Grzona E, et al. Fragmented pattern of tumor regression and lateral intramural spread may influence margin appropriateness after TEM for rectal cancer following neoadjuvant CRT. J Surg Oncol. 2014;109:853–8.
44. Smith FM, Wiland H, Mace A, Pai RK, Kalady MF. Assessment of a novel, full-thickness incisional biopsy model to restage rectal tumours after neoadjuvant chemoradiotherapy: results of an ex vivo pilot study. Tech Coloproctol. 2015;19:159–64.
45. Perez RO, Habr-Gama A, Lynn PB, Sao Juliao GP, Bianchi R, Proscurshim I, et al. Transanal endoscopic microsurgery for residual rectal cancer (ypT0-2) following neoadjuvant chemoradiation therapy: another word of caution. Dis Colon Rectum. 2013;56:6–13.
46. Mignanelli ED, de Campos-Lobato LF, Stocchi L, Lavery IC, Dietz DW. Downstaging after chemoradiotherapy for locally advanced rectal cancer: is there more (tumor) than meets the eye? Dis Colon Rectum. 2010;53:251–6.
47. Bujko K, Nowacki MP, Nasierowska-Guttmejer A, Kepka L, Winkler-Spytkowska B, Suwinski R, et al. Prediction of mesorectal nodal metastases after chemoradiation for rectal cancer: results of a randomised trial: implication for subsequent local excision. Radiother Oncol. 2005;76:234–40.
48. Kim DW, Kim DY, Kim TH, Jung KH, Chang HJ, Sohn DK, et al. Is T classification still correlated with lymph node status after preoperative chemoradiotherapy for rectal cancer? Cancer. 2006;106:1694–700.
49. Lambregts DM, Beets GL, Maas M, Kessels AG, Bakers FC, Cappendijk VC, et al. Accuracy of gadofosveset-enhanced MRI for nodal staging and restaging in rectal cancer. Ann Surg. 2011;253:539–45.
50. Marks JH, Valsdottir EB, DeNittis A, Yarandi SS, Newman DA, Nweze I, et al. Transanal endoscopic microsurgery for the treatment of rectal cancer: comparison of wound complication rates with and without neoadjuvant radiation therapy. Surg Endosc. 2009;23:1081–7.
51. Perez RO, Habr-Gama A, Sao Juliao GP, Proscurshim I, Scanavini Neto A, Gama-Rodrigues J. Transanal endoscopic microsurgery for residual rectal cancer after neoadjuvant chemoradiation therapy is associated with significant immediate pain and hospital readmission rates. Dis Colon Rectum. 2011;54:545–51.
52. Bujko K, Richter P, Kolodziejczyk M, Nowacki MP, Kulig J, Popiela T, et al. Preoperative radiotherapy and local excision of rectal cancer with immediate radical re-operation for poor responders. Radiother Oncol. 2009;92:195–201.
53. Hompes R, McDonald R, Buskens C, Lindsey I, Armitage N, Hill J, et al. Completion surgery following transanal endoscopic microsurgery: assessment of quality and short- and long-term outcome. Colorectal Dis. 2013;15:e576–e81.
54. Lambregts DM, Maas M, Bakers FC, Cappendijk VC, Lammering G, Beets GL, et al. Long-term follow-up features on rectal MRI during a wait-and-see approach after a clinical complete response in patients with rectal cancer treated with chemoradiotherapy. Dis Colon Rectum. 2011;54:1521–8.
55. Restivo A, Zorcolo L, Cocco IM, Manunza R, Margiani C, Marongiu L, et al. Elevated CEA levels and low distance of the tumor from the anal verge are predictors of incomplete response to chemoradiation in patients with rectal cancer. Ann Surg Oncol. 2013;20:864–71.
56. Patel UB, Taylor F, Blomqvist L, George C, Evans H, Tekkis P, et al. Magnetic resonance imaging-detected tumor response for locally advanced rectal cancer predicts survival outcomes: MERCURY experience. J Clin Oncol. 2011;29:3753–60.
57. Lambregts DM, Vandecaveye V, Barbaro B, Bakers FC, Lambrecht M, Maas M, et al. Diffusion-weighted MRI for selection of complete responders after chemoradiation for locally advanced rectal cancer: a multicenter study. Ann Surg Oncol. 2011;18:2224–31.

58. Habr-Gama A, Perez RO, Nadalin W, Nahas SC, Ribeiro U Jr, Silva ESAH Jr, et al. Long-term results of preoperative chemoradiation for distal rectal cancer correlation between final stage and survival. J Gastrointest Surg. 2005;9:90–9. discussion 9-101
59. Kristiansen C, Loft A, Berthelsen AK, Graff J, Lindebjerg J, Bisgaard C, et al. PET/CT and histopathologic response to preoperative chemoradiation therapy in locally advanced rectal cancer. Dis Colon Rectum. 2008;51:21–5.
60. Das P, Skibber JM, Rodriguez-Bigas MA, Feig BW, Chang GJ, Wolff RA, et al. Predictors of tumor response and downstaging in patients who receive preoperative chemoradiation for rectal cancer. Cancer. 2007;109:1750–5.
61. Perez RO, Sao Juliao GP, Habr-Gama A, Kiss D, Proscurshim I, Campos FG, et al. The role of carcinoembriogenic antigen in predicting response and survival to neoadjuvant chemoradiotherapy for distal rectal cancer. Dis Colon Rectum. 2009;52:1137–43.
62. Habr-Gama A, Gama-Rodrigues J, Sao Juliao GP, Proscurshim I, Sabbagh C, Lynn PB, et al. Local recurrence after complete clinical response and watch and wait in rectal cancer after neoadjuvant chemoradiation: impact of salvage therapy on local disease control. Int J Radiat Oncol Biol Phys. 2014;88:822–8.

Adjuvant Chemotherapy

6

Erik L. Zeger and Richard M. Goldberg

Abstract

Adjuvant chemotherapy in the treatment of rectal cancer is controversial. While current guidelines recommend adjuvant chemotherapy following TME, the benefit in the setting of neoadjuvant chemoradiation may be limited. Recommended regimens include single-agent fluoropyrimidines and an oxaliplatin combination regimen with either with infusional fluoropyrimidine (FOLFOX) or capecitabine (CAPEOX). Assumptions that the benefits noted in large colon cancer adjuvant studies are translatable to the treatment of patients with rectal cancer may or may not be justified. Other agents commonly used in metastatic colorectal cancer, including irinotecan, bevacizumab, and cetuximab, have not been shown beneficial in the adjuvant setting in colorectal cancer. Longer time to the initiation of adjuvant chemotherapy appears to result in worse survival. Patients with a pathologic complete response to neoadjuvant chemoradiation may not benefit from adjuvant chemotherapy, whereas partial responders appear to have better outcomes. Further trials are necessary to answer important questions in rectal cancer adjuvant chemotherapy—including whether oxaliplatin improves outcomes, if neoadjuvant chemotherapy would improve compliance and outcomes in rectal cancer.

Keywords

Adjuvant • Chemotherapy • Rectal cancer

E.L. Zeger, M.D. (✉)
Lankenau Medical Center, 100 Lancaster Avenue, Wynnewood, PA 19096, USA
e-mail: zegere@mlhs.org

R.M. Goldberg, M.D.
Division of Medical Oncology, The Ohio State University James Comprehensive Cancer Center and Solove Research Institute, 460 West Tenth Avenue, Suite D920, Columbus, OH 43210, USA

G. Dapri, J.H. Marks (eds.), *Surgical Techniques in Rectal Cancer*,
https://doi.org/10.1007/978-4-431-55579-7_6

Abbreviations

95% CI	95% confidence interval
aCT	Adjuvant chemotherapy
CRT	Chemoradiation therapy
DFS	Disease-free survival
HR	Hazard ratio
OS	Overall survival
pCR	Pathologic complete response
TME	Total mesorectal excision

6.1 Introduction

Adjuvant chemotherapy is both a routine and controversial component of the multimodality treatment of locally advanced (T3–4 or N+) rectal cancer [1, 2]. Most patients will receive neoadjuvant chemoradiation followed by total mesorectal excision (TME) and adjuvant chemotherapy with a fluoropyrimidine with or without oxaliplatin.

Today, adjuvant chemotherapy is standardly recommended for patients with stage II–III rectal cancers, stage III colon cancers, and some stage II colon cancers with high-risk features [3–5]. Specifically in clinical stage II/III rectal cancer, the NCCN recommends adjuvant chemotherapy in patients following neoadjuvant chemoradiation and surgery irrespective of the findings on surgical pathology at the time of definitive surgery that incorporates total mesorectal excision [3]. Recommended regimens include single-agent fluoropyrimidines and an oxaliplatin combination regimen with either with infusional fluoropyrimidine (FOLFOX) or capecitabine (CAPEOX).

This chapter will focus on adjuvant chemotherapy in rectal cancer, specifically in patients who had been treated preoperatively with neoadjuvant chemoradiation.

6.2 Adjuvant Chemotherapy Options

Various 5-FU-based regimens are acceptable including weekly bolus 5-FU (Roswell Park regimen) [6], short-term infusional 5-FU with leucovorin (de Gramont regimen) [7], oral capecitabine [8], and oxaliplatin-based regimens [9].

5-FU can be administered as a bolus or via continuous infusion. Various schedules of fluoropyrimidine administration have been developed. Side effect profiles differ depending on the method of administration. Bolus 5-FU typically results in more myelosuppression and mucositis, while infusional 5-FU results in more gastrointestinal toxicity in the form of diarrhea and hand-foot syndrome. Most studies including the large PETACC-02 trial found no difference in recurrence-free survival or overall survival for bolus versus infusional approaches [10]. Short-term infusional 5-FU with leucovorin regimens such as the de Gramont schedule also known as LV5FU2 (5-FU 600 mg/m^2 infusion over 22 h, 5-FU bolus 400 mg/m^2, and leucovorin 200 mg/m^2 on two consecutive days every 2 weeks) and modified regimens with a 46 h continuous infusion are used in combination with oxaliplatin (FOLFOX). Central venous catheters are required for these infusional 5-FU regimens as they are with any regimen containing oxaliplatin since oxaliplatin can be associated with pain on infusion if administered via a peripheral vein.

Oral fluoropyrimidines include capecitabine and uracil and tegafur or UFT (UFT is not commercially available in the USA). The convenience of oral compared to infusional 5-FU therapy is obvious. For patients who are considered to be highly compliant, oral therapy is an attractive and effective option. Capecitabine is absorbed and converted through three enzymatic steps into active 5-FU. The third enzyme, thymidine phosphorylase, is present in higher concentrations in tumor compared to normal cells. Capecitabine was compared to bolus Mayo regimen 5-FU therapy in the X-ACT study of 1987 patients with stage III colon cancer. It was administered at 1250 mg/m^2 twice daily for 14 of 21 days for 6 months. Capecitabine was deemed to be at least as effective as bolus 5-FU with disease-free survival (DFS) (64–61%, $p = 0.05$) and overall survival (81–78%, $p = 0.07$). Side effects were similar except patients treated with capecitabine who had an increased risk of hand-foot syndrome [8]. Hand-foot syndrome is characterized by palmar and plantar erythema and pain followed by desquamation in some patients. The application of hydrating skin lotion and dose reduction of capecitabine can help reduce the severity of hand-foot syndrome. In the X-ACT study, nearly half of patients required a dose reduction in capecitabine. Regional differences in capecitabine tolerability have been noted with North American patients having increased side effects compared to European and Asian patients [11]. In clinical practice it is not uncommon for oncologists to reduce the starting dose of capecitabine from the standard 1250 mg/m^2 twice daily to assess tolerability and to escalate to the recommended dose if toxicity is not seen. The elderly are more prone to capecitabine toxicity, in part due to the diminished renal function commonly seen with aging, and care should be taken in this population for potential serious diarrhea. Capecitabine is cleared by the kidneys and should be avoided in patients with significantly reduced creatinine clearance [12].

Oxaliplatin is an effective agent when combined with a fluoropyrimidine in the adjuvant treatment of colorectal cancer. Evidence is limited to the ARO/CAO/AIO-04 in rectal cancer treatment, and much of the presumed benefit is extrapolated from large colon cancer trials including NSABP C-07 and MOSAIC [13, 14].

The NSABP C-07 study compared over 2400 patients treated with bolus weekly 5-FU (Roswell Park regimen) with or without oxaliplatin. Oxaliplatin was administered at 85 mg/m^2 in weeks 1, 3, and 5 of an 8 week cycle (FLOX regimen). While DFS at 5 years favored FLOX, there was no statistically significant overall survival advantage (80 compared to 78%, HR 0.88). The side effect profile of the FLOX group was significant—including gastrointestinal toxicity, diarrhea, and dehydration, resulting in five deaths. Nausea, emesis, and sensory neuropathy were more prominent in the FLOX arm [14, 15]. Consequently, the FLOX regimen is infrequently recommended by most oncologists.

The MOSAIC study randomized over 2240 patients with stage II and III colon cancer to adjuvant therapy with infusional 5-FU (de Gramont regimen) with or without oxaliplatin (85 mg/m^2 every 14 days—FOLFOX4) [9]. Five year DFS was higher in the FOLFOX arm compared to infusional 5-FU (73 versus 67%, HR 0.80). Overall survival was also significantly prolonged at 6 years (79 versus 76%, HR 0.84, $p = 0.046$). Disease-free survival was also higher in the FOLFOX arm for stage III patients (66 versus 59%, HR 0.78, $p = 0.05$) but not in stage II patients. The toxicity profile of FOLFOX includes diarrhea, febrile neutropenia, and neuropathy. Febrile neutropenia was present in 1.8 versus 0.2%. Grades 3–4 diarrhea was also more common in the FOLFOX arm (10.8 versus 6.6%). The main limiting side effect of oxaliplatin following FOLFOX is peripheral sensory neuropathy. Nearly all patients develop temporary dysesthesias aggravated by cold exposure during treatment with oxaliplatin. The cold sensitivity starts immediately after oxaliplatin infusion and lasts typically 3–7 days. Peripheral sensory neuropathy is a cumulative effect of oxaliplatin treatment and presents with gradual hypoesthesia of the finger tips and plantar aspect of feet symmetrically. This can in some patients be long-lasting and permanent and when severe can impact the sensory aspects of activities of daily living including balance. In the MOSAIC study, peripheral neuropathy was grade 3 in 13% of patients receiving oxaliplatin. As expected, it gradually improved in most patients resulting in grades 1, 2, and 3 sensory neuropathy in 12, 3, and 0.7%, respectively after 1 year following treatment cessation [13].

5-FU-based adjuvant therapy either as a single agent or combined with oxaliplatin is an acceptable option. The favorable toxicity profile of infusional to bolus 5-FU have led most oncologists to utilize FOLFOX as the preferred adjuvant combination regimen. Various modifications have been made to FOLFOX4. FOLFOX6 is the present standard regimen due to convenience (which modification eliminates the second day of leucovorin). Another modification has been utilized, FOLFOX7, which removes the 5-FU bolus thus reducing myelosuppression [16].

Combining capecitabine with oxaliplatin is another option for adjuvant therapy in colorectal cancer. Many patients wish to avoid the inconvenience of 2 days of 5-FU infusion delivered via a pump as part of adjuvant FOLFOX therapy. A phase III trial of over 1800 patients with stage III colon cancer compared bolus 5-FU/leucovorin (either Mayo or Roswell Park regimens) to capecitabine with oxaliplatin [17]. Capecitabine was administered at 1000 mg/m^2 twice daily for 14 days of a 21 day cycle with oxaliplatin 130 mg/m^2 IV on day 1 of each cycle. Results favored the capecitabine/oxaliplatin combination over the 5-FU bolus regimens with improved DFS (HR 0.80, 95% CI 0.69–0.93) and overall survival (HR 0.83, 95% CI 0.70–0.99) [17, 18]. The capecitabine/oxaliplatin combination was less myelosuppressive than the 5-FU bolus regimens; however, it was associated with higher rates of neuropathy, hand-foot syndrome, and diarrhea.

6.3 Adjuvant Chemotherapy Trials in Rectal Cancers

The evidence for adjuvant chemotherapy in rectal cancer is not definitive and leads to a number of controversies. Assumptions that the benefits noted in large colon cancer adjuvant studies are translatable to the treatment of patients with rectal cancer may or may not be justified. While evidence from meta-analyses such as the Cochrane review [19] is supportive of adjuvant chemotherapy in rectal cancer, there is a growing body of randomized trials with less optimistic results.

Adjuvant chemotherapy results in increased survival following curative rectal cancer surgery based on a meta-analysis of 21 trials compared 4854 patients who received fluoropyrimidine-based chemotherapy with 4367 patients who did not receive chemotherapy [19]. These studies were completed in the era before preoperative chemoradiotherapy or TME were routinely performed and before the addition of oxaliplatin to adjuvant therapy regimens. Adjuvant chemotherapy in that setting resulted in both a significantly reduced risk of disease relapse (hazard ratio [HR] 0.75 95% CI 0.68–0.83) and death (HR 0.83, 95% CI 0.76–0.91).

There is only one published trial in patients with rectal cancer that randomized patients after preoperative chemoradiation and TME to adjuvant therapy versus none. The EORTC 22921 study prescribed 45 cGY plus or minus 5-FU followed by surgery with TME and then randomized enrolled patients to no postoperative treatment or adjuvant 5-FU plus leucovorin for 4 months. Chemotherapy consisted of fluorouracil 350 mg/m^2 daily bolus and leucovorin 20 mg/m^2 in weeks 1 and 5 during radiation and four cycles every 3 weeks in the adjuvant group. The overall survival for the patients enrolled in the no treatment arm was 49.7% compared to 50.7% in the treatment arm. These survival outcomes are not as good as those seen in other contemporary trials, and the study was felt not to be definitive due to the fact that there were substantial dose reductions and because less than 43% of patients received treatment as planned by the protocol [20, 21].

The German ARO/CAO/AIO-04 study randomized patients to either 5-FU or FOLFOX during neoadjuvant and adjuvant therapy. For patients on the 5-FU-alone arms the preoperative treatment called for the delivery of 5-FU with standard radiation at 50.4 cGy over 5.5 weeks followed after surgery by 5-FU given days 1–5 every month according to the Mayo Clinic regimen. The other cohort received 5-FU with oxaliplatin over 5.5 weeks with a 1 week treatment break in the midst of treatment followed by TME surgery and then the modified FOLFOX6 regimen. The primary endpoint was DFS at 3 years. For the 5-FU arms, this was 71.2%, and for the oxaliplatin-containing arms was 75.9% ($p < 0.03$). Overall survival was not reported in this manuscript although overall survival was reported as not being significantly different between the two arms in an ASCO 2014 presentation by Rodel et al. [22, 23]. These data are suggestive of benefit from the addition of oxaliplatin but are not definitive due to the lack of a defined survival advantage leading to the need for consideration of data from adjuvant trials in colon cancer as supportive but indirect evidence of benefit for combination therapy. The Cancer Genome Atlas analysis of tumors from patients with both colon and rectal cancer showed that the genomic profile of tumors from both sites were similar suggesting the validity of such an approach [24].

The CHRONICLE study [25] randomized patients to neoadjuvant chemoradiation to 6 months of adjuvant chemotherapy with capecitabine and oxaliplatin or observation. Poor accrual of only 113 patients led to early study closure. Overall survival at 3 years was 87.8% in chemotherapy arm compared to 88.8% in observation arm ($p = 0.55$) [25].

The Italian study by Cionini [26] randomized 655 patients with cT3–4 rectal cancer to adjuvant 5-FU or observation following chemoradiation and surgery followed by 5-FU 325 mg/m^2 and leucovorin 20 mg/m^2 on days 1–5 every 3 weeks for six cycles. Overall survival at 5 years was 68% in the adjuvant arm and 69.8% in the observation arm. Local recurrence was 7.4% in adjuvant chemotherapy arm and 8.7% in observation arm. Similar rates of distant metastatic disease were noted with 24.3 and 23.9% manifesting this in the cohorts assigned to the adjuvant chemotherapy and observation arms, respectively.

Another randomized study performed by the Dutch Colorectal Cancer Group [27] assessed adjuvant therapy with 5-FU/leucovorin or capecitabine in 470 patients with rectal cancer following chemoradiation and TME. DFS and overall survival were not different between the adjuvant chemotherapy and observation groups [26].

One criticism of these studies is the relatively small patient numbers that were enrolled when compared to those accrued to colon cancer adjuvant studies. Larger patient numbers are necessary to detect subtle DFS and survival differences especially between stage II and III rectal cancer. The second criticism would be the lack of oxaliplatin-containing adjuvant therapy in most of these studies.

The ADORE study [28] evaluated adjuvant therapy with either 5-FU/leucovorin or FOLFOX for 4 months in patients after neoadjuvant chemoradiation and TME with ypT3–4 or ypN+ disease. DFS at 3 years was 71.6% in the FOLFOX arm and 62.9% in the 5-FU/leucovorin arm (HR 0.657, 95% CI 0.43–0.99, $p = 0.047$). Toxicity was more common for all grades in the FOLFOX group; however, no significant difference was found at grade 3 or 4.

6.4 Agents Not Effective in the Adjuvant Setting

Other agents commonly used in metastatic colorectal cancer unfortunately have not shown benefit in the adjuvant setting. These agents include irinotecan, bevacizumab, and cetuximab. Irinotecan while effective in the metastatic setting has no role in the adjuvant setting based on three negative randomized trials. CALGB 89803 compared bolus 5-FU/leucovorin to irinotecan with bolus 5-FU/leucovorin (IFL regimen). The IFL regimen was noted to have increased myelosuppression, neutropenic fever, and death (2.8 versus 1%) [27]. Two subsequent studies assessed irinotecan with infusional 5-FU/leucovorin (FOLFIRI: irinotecan 180 mg/m^2 IV, 5-FU bolus 400 mg/m^2, leucovorin 400 mg/m^2, 2400 mg/m^2 46 h continuous 5-FU infusion) [28, 29]. PETACC-3 compared treatment with FOLFIRI and infusional 5-FU/leucovorin in 3278 patients, 2094 of which had stage III colon cancer. There was no difference in disease-free survival or overall survival (74 versus 71%) [28].

Bevacizumab is a monoclonal antibody to vascular endothelial growth factor (VEGF), a potent regulator of tumor angiogenesis. When added to fluoropyrimidine-containing regimens with oxaliplatin or irinotecan, bevacizumab prolongs DFS and overall survival in stage IV colon cancer. In the NSABP C-08 study [30], 2672 patients with stage II/III colon cancer received FOLFOX for 6 months with or without bevacizumab (5 mg/kg IV every 2 weeks for 12 months). No improvements in the 3 year disease-free (78 versus 75%, HR 0.93, 95% CI 0.81–1.08) or 5 year overall survival (83 versus 81%, HR for death 0.95% CI 0.79–1.13) were noted. Common side effects of bevacizumab were noted in the investigational arm including hypertension, proteinuria, and inhibited wound healing. There was no increase reported in bowel perforation or hemorrhage/thrombotic complications [31]. Two other trials, AVANT and QUASAR2, have likewise not shown any benefit to use of bevacizumab in the adjuvant setting in colon cancer [30, 32].

Epidermal growth factor receptor (EGFR) inhibition is another target in stage IV colorectal cancer treatment. Cetuximab (chimeric mouse/human antibody) and panitumumab (human antibody) are approved agents in patients with wild-type/nonmutated RAS genes. Cetuximab has been tested in the adjuvant treatment of stage III colon cancer in the N0147 and PETACC8 studies with FOLFOX, but unfortunately there was no additive benefit, and toxicity was enhanced [33, 34].

Outside of a clinical trial, these drugs should not be used in the adjuvant setting.

6.5 Time to Initiation of Adjuvant Chemotherapy

There is no standard optimal time following colorectal cancer surgery to initiate adjuvant chemotherapy. Most colon cancer trials have required starting adjuvant therapy by 6–8 weeks following surgery. Delays beyond 8 weeks are not uncommon and due to variety of reasons including surgical complications [35, 36] and disorganization in the health-care system [37]. An active area of debate is whether a delay to initiate adjuvant chemotherapy in colorectal cancer impacts outcome [38]. While no randomized trials have addressed this issue in colorectal cancer, there are several retrospective studies offering differing conclusions. Limitations of the studies would include inclusion of only stage III patients and fluoropyrimidine-only regimens (not containing oxaliplatin). Three studies noted decreased overall survival with delays beyond 8 weeks [39, 40] and 12 weeks [41]. Another study found no difference in disease-free or overall survival [42]. A meta-analysis of eight studies [43] in colorectal cancer reviewed outcomes between patients initiating adjuvant chemotherapy before and after 8 weeks from surgery. Patients with a delay beyond 8 weeks had poorer outcomes including higher death rates (relative risk 1.2, 95% CI 1.15–1.26) [44]. A second meta-analysis [45] compared ten studies on 15,410 patients. Nine of the studies were population-based or cohort designs, and one was a randomized trial. This study noted a 4 week increase in time to start of adjuvant chemotherapy resulted in both a decrease in disease-free survival (HR 1.14, 95% CI 1.10–1.18) and overall survival (HR 1.14, 95% CI 1.10–1.17). Each 4 week delay in starting adjuvant chemotherapy resulted in a 14% decrease in overall survival [46].

As mentioned earlier, the studies reviewed were in the era of fluoropyrimidine adjuvant therapy without oxaliplatin. Extrapolations of the data to oxaliplatin-containing chemotherapy may not be valid.

Another common assumption is that a 12 week delay negates any benefit of adjuvant chemotherapy. There is no direct evidence in the published literature that this is in fact true.

These results would encourage improved referral efficiency of the patient following surgery to their medical oncologist to discuss and initiate adjuvant chemotherapy [43]. Future clinical trials should better control for time to the initiation of adjuvant chemotherapy. Since many patients are currently treated with preoperative chemotherapy and radiation followed by TME, the initiation of postoperative adjuvant therapy can be delayed by the need to recover from the effects of the prior treatments, and the safe deliverable doses of adjuvant therapy may be compromised by the marrow-related toxicity that can follow pelvic irradiation. Also, the administration of combination chemotherapy that is advantageous in the control of systemic disease is frequently begun 16 or more weeks from the time that treatment is initiated. These considerations have led to the consideration of moving at least some component of combination chemotherapy ahead of the other interventions so that not only chemoradiation but also combination chemotherapy becomes a part of preoperative therapy.

The optimal length of adjuvant chemotherapy for rectal cancer is not defined. Most adjuvant studies in colon cancer patients have utilized 6 months as standard including the MOSAIC study [9]. Others recommend a total of 6 months of chemotherapy including the 6 weeks of neoadjuvant chemoradiation which would reduce the length of adjuvant therapy to approximately 4 months.

6.6 Selecting Patients for Adjuvant Chemotherapy Based on Chemoradiation Response

Improved parameters beyond clinical staging are needed for the selection of patients with rectal cancer who might benefit from adjuvant chemotherapy [45, 47, 48]. In colorectal cancer pathologic factors including lymph node involvement, lymphovascular, and perineural invasion, obstruction/perforation influences the use of adjuvant chemotherapy. Adjuvant chemotherapy decisions in rectal cancer are complicated by the use of neoadjuvant chemoradiation [49]. Endorectal ultrasound and pelvic MRI have improved the pretreatment evaluation in rectal cancer, but these modalities are far from perfect [50]. This leads to the consideration of should the decision on whether to administer adjuvant chemotherapy be based upon clinical or pathologic staging? One approach would be to treat all patients with adjuvant chemotherapy if they received neoadjuvant chemoradiation regardless of the findings at the time that the pathologist examines the surgical specimen as recommended by the NCCN guidelines [3]. Another approach is to use pathologic staging after chemoradiation. Both methods have potential pitfalls with the former leading to overtreatment and the later to undertreatment of some cases.

Can the response to chemoradiation identify subgroups which benefit/do not benefit from adjuvant chemotherapy? Early reports identified potential benefit in responders [51] but not in complete pathologic responders [52, 53]. The largest study to address this question was a pooled analysis of 3313 patients from 13 datasets (five prospective/eight retrospective) [54]. Adjuvant chemotherapy was 5-FU and leucovorin in nearly all patients. Patients were subdivided into pathologic staging categories based on response: pCR defined as ypT0N0, ypT1–2, and ypT3–4. A second analysis of lymph node status impact on aCT divided patients into two categories: ypN0 and ypN+. The primary outcome was recurrence-free survival (RFS) defined as a local and/or distant recurrence. 1723 of 3313 (52%) received adjuvant chemotherapy. HR for RFS with 95% CI for adjuvant chemotherapy patients based on stage: pCR 1.25 (0.68–2.29), ypT1–2 0.58 (0.37–0.89), and ypT3–4 0.83 (0.66–1.10). DFS and overall survival were also analyzed based on response group showing benefit in ypT1–2, ypT3–4, and ypN0 but not in pCR or ypN+ groups. These data support the notion that the potential benefit of adjuvant chemotherapy in rectal cancer can be predicted by postchemoradiation pathologic stage. pCR patients appear to have a good prognosis with or without adjuvant chemotherapy. Improved outcomes are noted in patients who respond to chemoradiation (ypT1–2). Weaknesses of this analysis include the fact that it used nonrandomized individual patient data. Another concern is the adjuvant chemotherapy in most patients was 5-FU and leucovorin without oxaliplatin. A randomized trial or pooled data from randomized trials would better answer these questions [55].

6.7 Neoadjuvant Chemotherapy

Noncompliance with adjuvant chemotherapy is common in solid tumor oncology. Better compliance has been noted with the delivery of neoadjuvant combination chemotherapy, and several studies are now investigating this approach. Grupo Cancer de Recto 3 reinforced this theory where patients were assigned to chemoradiation with neoadjuvant or adjuvant chemotherapy with capecitabine and oxaliplatin [56]. Compliance with neoadjuvant chemotherapy was much higher than in the adjuvant group (94 versus 57%). Ongoing studies assessing neoadjuvant chemotherapy include the PROSPECT trial in the USA comparing standard infusional 5-FU or capecitabine-based chemoradiation to six cycles of FOLFOX. CRT is reserved in the FOLFOX arm for patients with less than 20% decrease in the dimensions of the primary rectal tumor. All patients undergo TME, and adjuvant FOLFOX is recommended for all patients.

The European RAPIDO trial is comparing standard neoadjuvant chemoradiation delivered over 5 weeks followed by surgery and adjuvant capecitabine/oxaliplatin to short-course radiation and neoadjuvant capecitabine/oxaliplatin followed by surgery [54]. Unfortunately, these studies do not include arms without adjuvant chemotherapy and will not help to clarify whether there is a benefit to adjuvant therapy among the various subgroups who show complete or partial responses versus those few who manifest progressive disease during neoadjuvant treatment.

Conclusion

Precisely which patients with rectal cancer benefit from adjuvant chemotherapy and the best treatment to deliver is controversial. Conflicting study results, small trials, and imbalances in the ability to deliver planned postoperative chemotherapy continue to make it difficult to draw definitive conclusions from clinical trials. Clearly further randomized clinical trials to assess and select patients likely to benefit from adjuvant chemotherapy are needed. Advancements in rectal cancer management as a consequence of better imaging, better surgery, and refinements in radiation therapy techniques have significantly reduced local recurrence rates; however, systemic metastatic rates remain unacceptably high. Improved pathologic and biologic markers are needed to help clarify which patients warrant and which can benefit from adjuvant chemotherapy. Additional research is needed to expand the armamentarium of chemotherapeutic agents and to discover the utility of biologics that could be beneficial in the adjuvant setting in rectal cancer.

References

1. Beets G, Glimelius B. Adjuvant chemotherapy for rectal cancer still controversial. Lancet Oncol. 2014;15:130–1.
2. Palata M, Czito B, Willett C. Adjuvant chemotherapy for rectal cancer-an unresolved issue. Nat Rev Clin Oncol. 2014;11:182–4.
3. Rectal Cancer. NCCN Clinical Practice Guidelines in Oncology. 2015. [Cited 1 June 2015]. www.nccn.org.
4. Benson A, Schrag D, Somerfield M, et al. American Society of Clinical Oncology recommendations on adjuvant chemotherapy for stage II colon cancer. J Clin Oncol. 2004;22(16):3408–19.
5. Figueredo A, Charette M, Maroun J, Brouwers M, Zuraw L. Adjuvant therapy for stage II colon cancer: a systematic review from the cancer care Ontario program in evidence-based care's gastrointestinal cancer disease site group. J Clin Oncol. 2004;22(16):3395–407.
6. Haller D, Catalano P, macdonald J, et al. Phase III study of fluorouracil, leucovorin, and levamisole in high-risk stage II and III colon cancer: final report of intergroup 0089. J Clin Oncol. 2005;23:8671.
7. Andre T, Quinaux E, Louvet C, et al. Phase II study comparing a semimonthly with a monthly regimen of fluorouracil and leucovorin as adjuvant treatment for stage II and III colon cancer patients: final results of GERCOR C96.1. J Clin Oncol. 2007;25:3732.
8. Twelves C, Wong A, Nowalski M, et al. Capecitabine as adjuvant treatment for stage III colon cancer. N Engl J Med. 2005;352:2696–704.
9. Andre T, Boni C, Mounedji-Boudiaf L, Navarro M, Tabernero J. Oxaliplatin, fluorouracil, and leucovorin as adjuvant treatment for colon cancer. N Engl J Med. 2004;350(23):2343–51.
10. Kohne C, Bedenne L, Carrato A, et al. A randomised phase III intergroup trial comparing high-dose infusional 5-fluorouracil with or without folinic acid with standard bolus 5-fluouracil/folinic acid in the adjuvant treatment of stage III colon cancer: the pan-European trial in adjuvant colon. Eur J Cancer. 2013;49:1868.
11. Haller D, Cassidy J, Clarke S, et al. Potential regional differences for the tolerability profiles of fluoropyrimidines. J Clin Oncol. 2008;26:2118.
12. Poole C, Gardiner J, Twelves C, Johnston P, Harper P, et al. Effect of renal impairment on the pharmokinetics and tolerability of capecitabine in cancer patients. Cancer Chemother Pharmacol. 2002;49(7):225–34.
13. Andre T, Boni C, Navarro M, et al. Improved overall survival with oxaliplatin, fluorouracil, and leucovorin as adjuvant treatment in stage II or III colon cancer in the MOSAIC trial. J Clin Oncol. 2009;27:3109.

14. Yothers G, O'Connell M, Allegra C, et al. Oxaliplatin as adjuvant therapy for colon cancer: updated results for NSABP C-07 trial, including survival and subset analyses. J Clin Oncol. 2011;29:3768.
15. Kuebler J, Wieand H, O'Connell M, et al. Oxaliplatin combined with weekly bolus fluorouracil and leucovorin as surgical adjuvant chemotherapy for stage II and III colon cancer: results from NSABP C-07. J Clin Oncol. 2007;25:2198.
16. Maindrault-Goebel F, de Gramont A, Louvet C, André T, Carola E, et al. High-dose intensity oxaliplatin added to the simplified bimonthly leucovorin and 5-fluorouracil regimen as second-line therapy for metastatic colorectal cancer (FOLFOX 7). Eur J Cancer. 2001;37(8):1000–5.
17. Haller D, Tabernero J, Maroun J, et al. Capecitabine plus oxaliplatin compared with fluorouracil and folinic acid as adjuvant therapy for stage III colon cancer. J Clin Oncol. 2011; 29:1465.
18. Schmoll H, Tabernero J, Maroun J, et al. Capecitabine plus oxaliplatin versus bolus 5-fluorouracil/leucovorin as adjuvant therapy for stage III colon cancer: survival follow-up of study NO16968. J Clin Oncol. 2012;30(4):388.
19. Petersen S, Harling H, Kirkeby L, Wille-Jorgensen P, Mocellin S. Postoperative adjuvant chemotherapy in rectal cancer operated for cure. Cochrane Collab. 2012;3:1–51.
20. Hong T, Ryan D. Adjuvant chemotherapy for locally advanced rectal cancer: is it a given? J Clin Oncol. 2015;33(17):1878–990.
21. Bosset J, Calais G, Mineur L, Maingon P, Stojanovic-Rundic S, et al. Fluorouracil-based adjuvant chemotherapy after preoperative chemoradiotherapy in rectal cancer: long-term results of the EORTC 22921 randomised study. Lancet Oncol. 2014;15:184–90.
22. Rodel C, Graeven U, Fietkau R, Hohenberger W, Hothorn T, et al. Oxaliplatin added to fluorouracil-based preoperative chemoradiotherapy and postoperative chemotherapy of locally advanced rectal cancer (the German CAO/ARO/AIO-04 study): final results of the multicentre, open-label randomised, phase 3 trial. Lancet Oncol. 2015;16:979–89.
23. Rodel C, Liersch T, Fietkau R, Hohenberger W, Graeven U, et al. Preoperative chemoradiotherapy and postoperative chemotherapy with 5-fluorouracil and oxaliplatin versus 5-fluorouracil alone in locally advanced rectal cancer: results of the German CAO/ARO/AIO-04 randomized phase III trial. J Clin Oncol. 2014;32(Suppl; abst 3500):5s.
24. Cancer Genome Atlas Network. Comprehensive molecular characterization of human colon and rectal cancer. Nature. 2012;487:330–7.
25. Glynne-Jones R, Counsell N, Quirke P, et al. Chronicle: results of a randomised phase III trial in locally advanced rectal cancer after neoadjuvant chemoradiation randomising postoperative adjuvant capecitabine plus oxaliplatin (XELOX) versus control. Ann Oncol. 2014;25:1356–62.
26. Breugom A, an Gijn W, Muller E, et al. Adjuvant chemotherapy for rectal cancer patients treated with preoperative (chemo) radiotherapy and total mesorectal excision: a Dutch colorectal cancer group (DCCG) randomized phase III trial. Ann Oncol. 2015;26:696–701.
27. Saltz L, Niedzwiecki D, Hollis D, et al. Irinotecan fluorouracil plus leucovorin is not superior to fluorouracil plus leucovorin alone as adjuvant treatment for stage III colon cancer: results of CALGB 89803. J Clin Oncol. 2007;25:3456.
28. Van Cutsem E, Labianca R, Bodoky G, et al. Randomized phase III trial comparing biweekly infusional fluorouracil/leucovorin alone or with irinotecan in the adjuvant treatment of stage III colon cancer: PETACC-3. J Clin Oncol. 2009;27:3117.
29. Ychou M, Raoul J, Douillard J, et al. A phase III randomised trial of LV5FU2 + irinotecan versus LV5FU2 alone in adjuvant high-risk colon cancer (FNCLCC Accord02/FFCD9802). Ann Oncol. 2009;20:674.
30. Midgley R, Love S, Tomolinson I, et al. 2015. Final results from QUASAR2, a multicenter international randomized phase III trial of capecitabine+/− bevacizumab in the adjuvant setting of stage II/III colorectal cancer. ESMO cCongress.
31. Allegra C, Yothers G, O'Connell M, et al. Bevacizumab in stage II-III colon cancer: 5-year update of the NSABP C-08 trial. J Clin Oncol. 2013;31:359.
32. de Gramont A, Van Cutsem E, Schmoll H, et al. Bevacizumab plus oxaliplatin-based chemotherapy as adjuvant treatment for colon cancer (AVANT): a phase 3 randomised controlled trial. Lancet Oncol. 2012;13:1225.

33. Alberts S, Sargent D, Nair S, et al. Effect of oxaliplatin, fluorouracil, and leucovorin with or without cetuximab on survival among patients with resected stage III colon cancer: a randomized trial. JAMA. 2012;307:1383.
34. Taieb J, Tabernero J, Mini E, et al. Oxaliplatin, fluorouracil, and leucovorin with or without cetuximab in patients with resected stage III colon cancer (PETACC-8): an open-label, randomised phase 3 trial. Lancet Oncol. 2014;15:862.
35. Merkow R, Bentrem D, Mulcahy M, et al. Effect of postoperative complications on adjuvant chemotherapy use for stage III colon cancer. Ann Surg. 2013;248:847.
36. Hendren S, Birkmeyer J, Yin H, et al. Surgical complications are associated with omission of chemotherapy use for stage III colon cancer. Dis Colon Rectum. 2010;53:1587.
37. Wasserman D, Boulos M, Hopman W, et al. Reasons for delay in time to initiation of adjuvant chemotherapy for colon cancer. J Oncol Pract. 2015;11(1):e28–35.
38. Bayraktar U, Chen E, Bayraktar S, et al. Does delay of adjuvant chemotherapy impact survival in patients with resected stage II and III colon adenocarcinoma? Cancer. 2011;117:2364.
39. Czaykowski P, Gill S, Kennecke H, et al. Adjuvant chemotherapy for stage III colon cancer: does timing matter? Dis Colon Rectum. 2011;54:1082.
40. Dahl O, Flug O, Carlsen E, et al. Final results of a randomised phase III study on adjuvant chemotherapy with 5-FU and levamisole in colon and rectum cancer stage II and III by the Norwegian gastrointestinal cancer group. Acta Oncol. 2009;48:368.
41. Lima I, Yasui Y, Scarfe A, Winget M. Association between receipt and timing of adjuvant chemotherapy and survival for patients with stage III colon cancer in Alberta, Canada. Cancer. 2011;117:3833.
42. Ahmed S, Ahmad I, Zhu T, et al. Early discontinuation but not the timing of adjuvant therapy affects survival of patients with high-risk colorectal cancer: a population-based study. Dis Colon Rectum. 2010;53:1432.
43. Mutch M. Surgeons play a central role in the utilization of adjuvant chemotherapy for colorectal cancer. Dis Colon Rectum. 2013;56(12):1327–9.
44. Des Guetz G, Nicolas P, Perret G, et al. Does delaying adjuvant chemotherapy after curative surgery for colorectal cancer impair survival? A meta-analysis. Eur J Cancer. 2010;46:1049.
45. Haynes A, You Y, Hu C, Eng C, Kopetz E, et al. Postoperative chemotherapy use after neoadjuvant chemoradiotherapy for rectal cancer: analysis of surveillance, epidemiology, and end results-medicare data, 1998-2007. Cancer. 2014;120(8):1162–70.
46. Biagi J, Raphael M, Mackillop W, Kong W, King W, et al. Association between time to initiation of adjuvant chemotherapy and survival in colorectal cancer. JAMA. 2011;305(22):2335–42.
47. Zhu J, Xu Y, Gu W, Peng J, Cai G, et al. Adjuvant therapy for T3N0 rectal cancer in the total mesorectal excision era-identification of the high risk patients. Radiat Oncol. 2010;5(118):1–8.
48. Wibe A, Law W, Fazio V, Delaney C. Tailored rectal cancer treatment-a time for implementing contemporary prognostic factors? Colorectal Dis. 2013;15:1333–44.
49. Sauer R, Becker H, Hohenberger W, et al. Preoperative versus postoperative chemoradiotherapy for rectal cancer. N Engl J Med. 2004;351:1731–40.
50. Bipat S, Glas A, Slors F, et al. Rectal cancer: local staging and assessment of lymph node involvement with endoluminal US, CT and MR imaging—a meta-analysis. Radiology. 2004;232:773–83.
51. Collette L, Bosset J, den Dulk M, et al. Patients with curative resection of cT3–4 rectal cancer after preoperative radiotherapy or radiochemotherapy: does anybody benefit from adjuvant fluorouracil-based chemotherapy? A trial of the EORTC. J Clin Oncol. 2007;25:4379–86.
52. Capirci C, Valentini V, Cionini L, et al. Prognostic value of pathologic complete response after neoadjuvant therapy in locally advanced rectal cancer: long-term analysis of 566 ypCR patients. Int J Radiat Oncol Biol Phy. 2008;72:99–107.
53. Maas M, Nelemans P, Valentini V, et al. Long-term outcome in patients with a pathological complete response after chemoradiation for rectal cancer: a pooled analysis of individual patient data. Lancet Oncol. 2010;11:835–44.
54. Dienstmann R. Personalizing colon cancer adjuvant therapy: selecting optimal treatments for individual patients. J Clin Oncol. 2015;33:1787–96.

55. Maas M, Nelemans P, Valentini V, Crane C, Capirici C, et al. Adjuvant chemotherapy in rectal cancer: defining subgroups who may benefit after neoadjuvant chemoradiation and resection. Int J Cancer. 2015;137:212–20.
56. Fernandez-Martos C, et al. Phase II, randomized study of concomitant chemoradiotherapy followed by surgery and adjuvant capecitabine plus oxaliplatin (CAPOX) compared with induction CAPOX followed by comcomitant chemoradiotherapy and surgery in magnetic resonance imaging-defined. J Clin Oncol. 2010;28:859–65.
57. Breugom A, Swets M, Bosset J, Collette L, Sainato A, et al. Adjuvant chemotherapy after preoperative (chemo)radiotherapy and surgery of patients with rectal cancer: a systematic review and meta-analysis of individual patient data. Lancet Oncol. 2015;16:200–7.

Future Therapies in Medical Oncology

7

Jason Paik, Cindy Kin, and George A. Fisher Jr.

Abstract

Antibodies to EGFR (cetuximab and panitumumab) and VEGF-A (bevacizumab) that are routinely used for treating metastatic colorectal cancer have failed to find a role in the management of localized rectal cancer. Other molecular targets worth considering include Her2/neu, BRAF, the PI3 kinase pathway, HSP90, and most recently the hypermutated phenotype of MSI tumors. Here we review selected trials using targeted agents in localized rectal cancer and propose other targeted strategies that have not yet been tested. In this era of molecular profiling, rectal cancer is an ideal opportunity to test the biological effects and clinical outcomes of preoperative molecularly targeted therapy.

Keywords

Rectal • Neoadjuvant • Targeted therapy • Immunotherapy • Defective DNA repair

J. Paik, M.D., Ph.D. • G.A. Fisher Jr., M.D., Ph.D. (✉)
Department of Medicine (Oncology), Stanford University Comprehensive Cancer Center,
875 Blake Wilbur Drive, Stanford, CA 94305, USA
e-mail: georgeaf@stanford.edu

C. Kin, M.D.
Department of Surgery (Colorectal), Stanford University Comprehensive Cancer Center,
875 Blake Wilbur Drive, Stanford, CA 94305, USA

G. Dapri, J.H. Marks (eds.), *Surgical Techniques in Rectal Cancer*,
https://doi.org/10.1007/978-4-431-55579-7_7

7.1 Introduction

Despite the success of molecularly "targeted" agents in metastatic colon and other cancers, the management of localized rectal cancer remains limited to preoperative cytotoxic chemotherapy and radiation with controversies regarding optimal doses, frequency, and sequencing. Both pre- and post-operative chemotherapy treatments for rectal cancer are thoroughly discussed in previous chapters of this book. We will review novel agents and targets that have been tested or are in development as preclinical concepts or trials for rectal cancer. We will first discuss antibodies to EGFR and VEGF that have been proven to be effective in metastatic colon cancer and their lack of efficacy when combined with chemoradiation regimens for rectal cancer. We will then present early data suggesting efficacy of Her2/neu and BRAF targeted therapies that are approved for breast cancer and melanomas, respectively, but have yet to be approved in colon cancers or tested in localized rectal cancer. Though alterations in Her2/neu and BRAF are rare in localized rectal cancer (<10%), genomic alterations in the PI3K pathway can occur in up to 40% of colorectal patients. A number of investigational agents target this pathway, though none have been approved for any cancer yet. Preclinical studies suggest that inhibition of heat shock proteins (HSP90) may have radiosensitizing properties, and early clinical results are encouraging. Finally, the immune modulating checkpoint inhibitors in MSI or hypermutated colon cancers, albeit rare in rectal cancer, have had such impressive clinical responses that testing these agents in locally advanced rectal cancers would be worthwhile.

7.2 EGFR

One of the first targeted therapies used in oncology is the monoclonal antibody against the human epidermal growth factor receptor (EGFR1, ErBB1, Her1) cetuximab. Cetuximab, an IgG1 chimeric antibody against EGFR, has been shown to increase the response rate and progression-free survival of patients with RAS wild-type metastatic colorectal cancers [1]. The success of cetuximab in combination with radiation in head and neck cancers [2] in improving locoregional control and overall survival suggested that cetuximab in combination with radiation might be effective for rectal cancer as well. However, trials incorporating cetuximab into neo-adjuvant chemoradiation regimens yielded disappointing results. Two randomized phase II trials failed to show a statistically significant benefit of cetuximab [3, 4]. In the study by Dewdney [4], patients either received CAPOX (capecitabine and oxaliplatin) for four cycles followed by chemoradiation with capecitabine or the identical therapy in combination with weekly cetuximab. Pathologic complete response (pCR) rates (11 vs. 7%), R0 resection rates (96 vs. 90%), and disease-free survival rates (HR 0.65; 95% CI, 0.3–2.16; $P = 0.36$) were numerically superior for the cetuximab arm versus the no cetuximab arm, yet failed to reach statistical significance. Curiously, there was a survival advantage for cetuximab-treated patients (HR 0.27; 95% CI, 0.07–0.99; $P = 0.034$) though this is difficult to explain

Table 7.1 Potential targets for therapy in rectal cancer

Target	Estimated prevalence	Potential agents	References
EGFR (in RAS WT)	~50%	Cetuximab	[3, 4]
		Panitumumab	[5, 6]
		Nimotuzumab	[7]
Her2/neu	2.8–25.3%	TrastuzumabPertuzumab Trastuzumab emtansine Lapatinib	[8–10]
BRAF	2.1%	Vemurafenib	[11–14]
		Dabrafenib	
		Encorafenib	[15]
PI3K/Akt	40%	Nelfinavir	[16, 17]
		Aspirin	[18]
		Alpelisib	[7]
Hsp90	–	Ganetespib	[19]
Hypermutated/MSI	1.3–4.3%	Pembrolizumab	[20]

given that there was no difference in the rate of deaths due to metastatic disease. A smaller phase II trial randomized rectal cancer patients to capecitabine and irinotecan (CAPIRI) with concurrent radiation or that same regimen with weekly cetuximab. In that trial, pCR rates (8 vs. 19%), R0 resection rates (97 vs. 98%), and 5-year disease-free survival rates (79 vs. 82%) for treatment without and with cetuximab, respectively, showed no benefit in any clinical endpoint for cetuximab-treated patients (Table 7.1).

Panitumumab, an IgG2 fully humanized antibody against EGFR, was also tested in the neoadjuvant setting in rectal cancer. The Swiss group [5] investigated the addition of panitumumab to chemoradiation with capecitabine in locally advanced disease. While rates of pathologic response were better in the panitumumab arm, no difference was seen in pCR, at the cost of an increased rate of diarrhea and anastomotic leak. Similar findings were also reported by Belgian investigators [6]. Despite significant experience using two well-characterized monoclonal antibodies against EGFR in metastatic disease, these small phase II studies have shown no clinical benefit of these agents in the neoadjuvant setting and have stalled any further trials of EGFR inhibitors in rectal cancer [3–5].

7.3 Angiogenesis

Bevacizumab, a monoclonal antibody directed against the vascular endothelial growth factor A (VEGF-A), is approved for use in metastatic colorectal cancer and improves progression-free and overall survival when used in combination with chemotherapy [21]. Willett and colleagues initially described a complete pathologic response in a large T4 N1 rectal cancer treated with bevacizumab combined with chemoradiation with 5-FU [22]. However, subsequent trials did not bear out this early success. A recent update of a phase II trial using CAPOX, bevacizumab, and concurrent radiation for 57 patients with rectal cancer failed to meet its primary endpoint of pathologic complete response and reported only a pCR rate of 17% [23]. Furthermore, this regimen was associated with significant acute toxicity, including higher than expected rates of wound infection and wound dehiscence. Though distant recurrence rates were low, the lack of improvement in pCR rate, significant postsurgical complications, and the failure of adjuvant bevacizumab to improve disease-free survival in randomized phase III trials of stage III colon cancer have eliminated bevacizumab from further trials with chemoradiation. A randomized phase II trial of capecitabine with concurrent radiation with or without bevacizumab reported a pCR rate of 16% vs. 11% ($P = 0.54$) [24]. Though this failed to reach statistical significance, serial biopsies showed that a decrease in angiopoietin-2 (Ang-2) in the bevacizumab arm correlated with downstaging while levels of Ang-2 increased in the control arm. Unless a predictive biomarker is validated to predict benefit from bevacizumab therapy, it is unlikely that the future trials will pursue this strategy. However, with increasing interest in preoperative chemotherapy alone (i.e., omitting radiation), there may be a role for the addition of bevacizumab in that setting, though concerns for increased risks for post-operative complications may dictate a longer interval between bevacizumab and surgical resection.

7.4 Her2/neu

Inhibition of human epidermal growth factor receptor 2 (Her2/neu) may also be of benefit in patients with rectal cancer. Several studies have indicated variable prevalence of Her2/neu amplification and overexpression in colorectal cancers [25–28]. Ramanathan and colleagues [29], in a small phase II trial examining irinotecan and trastuzumab as second-line therapy for metastatic colon and rectal cancers, found limited utility due to low prevalence of Her2 overexpression as measured via immunohistochemistry (IHC).

In contrast, studies examining archived specimens exclusively from rectal cancers have shown higher rates of overexpression of Her2/neu. Liming and colleagues [30] showed that 31 out of 302 tumor specimens demonstrated at least 2+ expression of Her2/neu via IHC. Examination of 264 archived biopsy and resection specimens from patients under protocol at the German Rectal Cancer Study Group [31] revealed 12.4% of biopsies, and 26.7% of resected specimens were positive for Her2 overexpression either by 3+ grading on IHC or in situ hybridization (ISH) ratio greater than 2.0. Two studies from China also examined samples from patients with locally advanced rectal cancer; Meng and colleagues [32] showed that samples from 22 of 119 patients demonstrated IHC staining of 2–3+ with positive confirmatory FISH studies, while Yao and colleagues [33] showed that in resection specimens from 142 patients receiving preoperative radiation therapy, 15 (10.6%) and 21 (14.8%) showed IHC 2+ and 3+ staining, respectively. Finally, a Korean study of

539 newly diagnosed colorectal cancers showed an increase in Her2 expression in 8% of rectal cancers as measured by both ISH and IHC, a phenomenon which was not seen in either left- or right-sided colon cancers [34]. In contrast to these studies, in specimens from the EXPERT-C study in patients receiving neoadjuvant chemoradiation with capecitabine and oxaliplatin with or without cetuximab, only 3 out of 104 specimens were found to have IHC staining of 3+ and ISH ratio greater than 2.0. Treatment with cetuximab appeared to have no bearing on Her2/neu expression [35]. While the absolute proportion of rectal cancer patients with Her2/neu overexpression is low, prevalence is comparable to Her2/neu overexpression in gastric adenocarcinomas [36]. However, there is no clear evidence that Her2/neu expression in rectal cancers is associated with poorer prognosis as it is in gastric adenocarcinoma.

There may be important therapeutic implications for Her2/neu expression in patients with rectal cancer. Trastuzumab is a monoclonal antibody directed against the Her2/neu receptor that is approved for use in breast and gastric cancers. In breast cancer, trastuzumab is approved for use in the neoadjuvant, adjuvant, and metastatic settings for patients with Her2 overexpressing or amplified breast cancer [37, 38]. In particular, the use of trastuzumab combined with chemotherapy in the neoadjuvant setting leads to an increased pCR rate, lower relapse rates, and better disease-free and overall survival when compared to chemotherapy alone [39, 40]. The use of the anti-Her2 dimerization antibody pertuzumab may also be of benefit in the neoadjuvant setting, though relapse-free survival and overall survival data are lacking at this time [41]. Trastuzumab is also approved as first- and second-line therapy in patients with Her2 overexpressing or amplified metastatic gastric cancer. In patients with gastric adenocarcinoma with IHC staining of 3+ or ISH ratio greater than 2.0, trastuzumab combined with chemotherapy improved objective response rates and overall survival [42]. Studies of trastuzumab in neoadjuvant therapy of gastric cancer are ongoing.

The promising results in breast and gastric cancers lead to the question of whether patients with rectal cancer overexpressing Her2/neu would benefit from trastuzumab. Indeed, two case reports demonstrated significant response of patients with metastatic Her2-amplified rectal cancer to trastuzumab [8, 9]. Early data from the Italian HERACLES trial in which heavily pretreated patients with metastatic Her2-amplified, KRas wild-type colorectal cancer also showed promise, with objective responses seen in 8 of 23 patients [10]. The second phase of this trial, which completed accrual in July 2014, will assess the combination of trastuzumab and pertuzumab in this same population, as well as assess whether trastuzumab emtansine can be effective in the HERACLES-RESCUE trial, which is just beginning accrual. Taken together, trastuzumab and other agents targeting Her2/neu may improve response rates in metastatic rectal cancer. Whether these agents can also increase pCR rates in patients undergoing neoadjuvant chemoradiation and adjuvant radiation is also of significant interest as well.

In summary, Her2/neu targeted agents may be effective in patients whose tumors have Her2/neu overexpression (IHC 3+) or amplification or when there is an activating mutation of the Her2/neu gene. The actual incidence of each in rectal cancer is still unclear, but cumulatively, there may be between 5 and 20% of patients with rectal cancer who might be eligible to test a Her2/neu targeted strategy. Though current trials focus on metastatic disease, it would be reasonable to consider a trial of a trastuzumab/pertuzumab combination as part of a neoadjuvant regimen for localized rectal cancer.

7.5 BRAF

A small subset of KRAS mutation-negative rectal cancers contains mutations in the oncogene BRAF – most commonly the V600E mutation, which imbues constitutive kinase activity that drives cellular proliferation [43–45]. Patients with BRAF mutation-positive colorectal cancer carry a significantly worse prognosis [46, 47]. Given this, the BRAF V600E inhibitor vemurafenib, an agent with effectiveness for other malignancies associated with this mutation, including melanoma and thyroid cancers, was investigated in metastatic, BRAF mutation-positive, colorectal cancer. Results from the phase I study showed at most a 5% objective response rate [11–13, 48]. Unlike in melanoma, concurrent MEK inhibition appeared to be inadequate [49].

Subsequently, preclinical data revealed that inhibition of BRAF V600E leads to feedback activation of EGFR and that concurrent inhibition of EGFR with cetuximab, gefitinib, or erlotinib was effective at inhibiting growth of colon cancers in vitro and in mouse models [50]. This observation was subsequently translated to phase 1 clinical trials, with encouraging evidence of activity when vemurafenib and cetuximab were coadministered to patients with BRAF mutant colorectal cancer [13, 14]. Based on this work, the SWOG1406 trial randomizes patients with metastatic BRAF mutation colorectal cancers to receive irinotecan and cetuximab with or without vemurafenib [51]. Encorafenib, another Raf inhibitor, is also under investigation in colorectal cancers together with cetuximab [52]. However, in comparison to colon cancer, BRAF mutations in rectal cancer appear to be less common (2–3%); therefore, there may not be a substantial impact overall for BRAF inhibition in patients with rectal cancer.

7.6 PI3K/Akt

Approximately 40% of colorectal cancers contain alterations that activate the phosphatidylinositide-3-kinase (PI3K)/Akt pathway, an important pathway whose constitutive activation leads to reduced apoptosis and increased cellular proliferation and survival [25, 53]. Multiple different components of this pathway are known to be overexpressed or mutated in colorectal and other cancers [54]; for example, many patients with Peutz-Jeghers syndrome are caused by mutations in STK11, a tumor suppressor that activates TSC2, a downstream target of Akt [55]. As discussed above, EGFR, Her2/neu, and BRAF are also participants in this pathway. Resistance to radiation due to increasing cellular survival in the face of hypoxia is at least in part mediated by this pathway [56, 57]. Therefore, perturbation of this pathway may increase the effectiveness of neoadjuvant chemotherapy and radiation in rectal cancers.

Several agents have been developed toward that goal and have been assessed in early-stage clinical trials. Perifosine, an oral nonspecific inhibitor of Akt, was assessed in phase II trial of patients with heavily pretreated metastatic colorectal cancer in combination with capecitabine; both progression-free survival and overall survival were significantly increased [58]. Unfortunately, phase III data were reported the following year, showing no difference in both PFS and OS for perifosine and capecitabine versus capecitabine alone [59]. Nelfinavir, a protease inhibitor used in the treatment of HIV, also appears to inhibit Akt phosphorylation [60] and increase blood flow to tumors with concomitant reduction in hypoxia. A phase I trial of patients with locally advanced rectal cancer receiving chemoradiation with capecitabine and also receiving nelfinavir showed acceptable toxicity [16]. The SONATINA trial, administered by the University of Oxford, combined nelfinavir with hypofractionated radiation and also showed an encouraging toxicity profile [17]. Further studies will be required to show an improvement in the rate of pCR and overall survival.

PIK3CA mutations are also known to be associated with colorectal cancers. Approximately 10–15% of all colorectal cancers contain PIK3CA mutations [25]; in a separate study of archived tissue from patients undergoing TME in the Netherlands, PIK3CA mutations were found in 7.9% of samples tested and furthermore were found to be a predictor for local recurrence [45]. Inhibition of PTGS2 (also known as COX2) by aspirin, a downstream target of the PI3K pathway, appears to be correlated with improvement in mortality of patients with colorectal cancer harboring PIK3CA mutations, while this effect was not seen in patients with wild-type PIK3CA [18]; however rofecoxib did not appear to have the same effect [61], and the same phenomenon was not seen in a different patient cohort from Florida and Australia [62]. Whether aspirin can reduce local recurrence in patients with resected rectal cancers has yet to be determined in a prospective study, but would be of great interest given that PTGS2 expression is significantly elevated in rectal cancers as compared to colon cancers [63].

Because of the importance of the PI3K/Akt pathway to cellular growth and proliferation, there is likely to be multiple modes of feedback upregulation of signaling to compensate for pharmacologic inhibition of a single member of the pathway, leading some investigators to assess combinatorial approaches. For example, Tabenero and colleagues [15, 64] recently presented data from a phase I trial showing concurrent inhibition of EGFR, BRAF, and PI3Kα using cetuximab, encorafenib, and alpelisib in patients with advanced BRAF mutant colorectal cancers; 23% of patients with dual EGFR and BRAF inhibition and 32% of patients with triple inhibition had at least partial responses, while the majority of patients receiving triple inhibition had at least stable disease. A phase 1/2 trial of dabrafenib, panitumumab, and the MEK inhibitor trametinib is also in progress [65]. However, other efforts have not been as successful, as demonstrated by the absence of clinical activity of the pan-Akt inhibitor MK-2206 with the MEK inhibitor selumetinib in advanced colorectal cancers [66].

7.7 Hsp90

Heat shock proteins (Hsp) are molecular chaperones critical for folding of proteins; one member of the Hsp family, Hsp90, plays an important role in multiple pathways in cellular proliferation and apoptosis, where it stabilizes what otherwise would be unstable mutated oncoproteins, including Her2/neu and Akt [67]. The discovery of a highly active Hsp90 conformation that is associated with cancer, which has increased activity and can be inhibited specifically by small molecular inhibitors [68], has led to the development of multiple drugs that are under investigation in a variety of tumors [69]. Further investigations lead to the observation that pharmacologic inhibition of Hsp90 could potentiate radiation in multiple tumor types [70, 71]. One Hsp90 inhibitor, ganetespib, showed anecdotal response as a single agent in phase 1 studies [72], leading to preclinical investigations that revealed synergy against colon cancer in vitro and in mouse models when combined with irradiation and capecitabine [73]. This preclinical data lead to phase 1 trial in stages II and III rectal cancers where ganetespib was administered together with radiation and capecitabine in the neoadjuvant setting; in this small study, 3 of 12 patients undergoing resection had a pCR [19]. It would be interesting to see if patients that have mutations of proteins known to be involved in rectal cancer tumorigenesis such as KRas, Her2, or BRAF are particularly sensitive to inhibition of Hsp90.

7.8 Hypermutator Phenotype and Microsatellite Instability

A small subset of patients with rectal cancer also have evidence of microsatellite instability, a phenotype most commonly associated with mutations in mismatch repair proteins as in Lynch syndrome or sporadic hypermethylation of the promoter of the gene MLH1. Prevalence of the MSI-H phenotype was measured in 3 of 165 (2%) tissue samples tested from a cohort in Sweden, with all samples deemed MSI+ associated with patients with known hereditary cancer-predisposing disorders [74], while in an assessment of 465 tissue samples from patients with rectal cancer in Korea, 4.3% of samples were deemed to be MSI-H [75]. The seminal TCGA study showed that only 1 of 75 tissue samples from patients with rectal cancer was characterized as MSI-H [25]. This study also identified a hypermutator phenotype, characterized by mutations in mismatch repair, CpG island methylation leading to silencing of MLH1 expression, or mutations in the polymerase polE; in contrast to colon cancers, only 3 of 75, including the single MSI-H patient sample, demonstrated significant hypermutability. This is consistent with the observation that MSI more commonly occurs in more proximal colorectal tumors, though a pathophysiologic explanation remains unknown. Despite this low prevalence of the hypermutator phenotype in rectal cancer, testing for MSI in a patient with rectal cancer according to the Bethesda guidelines may increase the pretest probability for a determination of an MSI-H genotype.

MSI-H colorectal tumors demonstrate a mutational burden 10–50 times that of microsatellite-stable tumors [76] and as such may have a substantially higher burden of neoantigens to which the immune system can respond [77]. Given this observation, Le and colleagues [20] sought to test the efficacy of immune checkpoint inhibition in patients with advanced colorectal cancer with and without mismatch repair deficiency by the PD-1 blocking monoclonal antibody pembrolizumab. Consistent with phase 1 data suggesting the lack of efficacy of pembrolizumab in colorectal patients, none of the patients with microsatellite-stable disease responded to PD-1 inhibition; however, in those patients with HNPCC or Lynch syndrome, 4 of 10 patients had objective responses, with progression-free survival at 78% versus 11% in microsatellite-stable disease. Despite the small sample size and early data, this study makes the tantalizing suggestion that immune checkpoint inhibition can release the immune system to act against the large burden of neoantigens that can be found in the tumors of these patients, providing for a modality of treatment completely different from the inhibition of oncogenic growth factor pathways described above. Patients with rectal cancer continue to be evaluated under this trial [78], and other trials are planned using this checkpoint inhibitor in the neoadjuvant setting as well as using other immune checkpoint inhibitors in metastatic disease. Furthermore, given that BRAF mutations are associated with sporadic microsatellite instability, combination therapy with BRAF inhibitors could also be considered [79]. It would also be interesting to see if patients with advanced KRAS wild-type colorectal cancers in the phase 3 trial using cetuximab together with Imprime PGG, a carbohydrate that putatively enhances anti-tumor antibody-dependent cytotoxicity, demonstrate differences in response depending on MSI status [80].

Conclusions

Despite the modest success of agents targeting the EGFR and VEGF pathways in metastatic colon cancer, neither strategy has made a significant impact on the management of localized rectal cancer. However, other molecular targets are present in rectal cancers, albeit at low frequencies of expression. Impressive clinical responses have been reported for metastatic colorectal cancers using Her2/neu targeted agents for those with Her2/neu amplification or overexpression. Similarly, in MSI colorectal cancers treated with PD-1 checkpoint inhibitors, dramatic and durable remissions have been reported. These responses underscore the need to explore molecularly targeted therapies in rectal cancer and to test other agents that target heat shock proteins, the PI3K pathway, BRAF, and other targets as they are discovered.

The acceptance of preoperative therapy of rectal cancer offers the opportunity to assess the biological effects of molecularly targeted agents by obtaining serial biopsies and ultimately the entire specimen for in-depth molecular analysis. Using rectal cancers as an in vivo test of new agents could significantly accelerate drug development in colorectal cancer as a whole. The rarity of distinct molecularly defined subsets that might respond to targeted agents will be challenging, but with well-designed multi-institutional basket trials, we believe the effectiveness of new agents can be validated.

References

1. Van Cutsem E, Köhne CH, Láng I, Folprecht G, Nowacki MP, Cascinu S, et al. Cetuximab plus irinotecan, fluorouracil, and leucovorin as first-line treatment for metastatic colorectal cancer: updated analysis of overall survival according to tumor KRAS and BRAF mutation status. J Clin Oncol. 2011;29(15):2011–9. doi:10.1200/JCO.2010.33.5091.
2. Bonner JA, Harari PM, Giralt J, Azarnia N, Shin DM, Cohen RB, et al. Radiotherapy plus cetuximab for squamous-cell carcinoma of the head and neck. N Engl J Med. 2006;354(6):567–78. doi:10.1056/NEJMoa053422.
3. Dewdney A, Cunningham D, Tabernero J, Capdevila J, Glimelius B, Cervantes A, et al. Multicenter randomized phase II clinical trial comparing neoadjuvant oxaliplatin, capecitabine, and preoperative radiotherapy with or without cetuximab followed by total mesorectal excision in patients with high-risk rectal cancer (EXPERT-C). J Clin Oncol. 2012;30(14):1620–7. doi:10.1200/JCO.2011.39.6036.
4. Kripp M, Horisberger K, Mai S, Kienle P, Gaiser T, Post S, et al. Does the addition of Cetuximab to Radiochemotherapy improve outcome of patients with locally advanced rectal cancer? Long-term results from phase II trials. Gastroenterol Res Pract. 2015;2015:273489. doi:10.1155/2015/273489.
5. Helbling D, Bodoky G, Gautschi O, Sun H, Bosman F, Gloor B, et al. Neoadjuvant chemoradiotherapy with or without panitumumab in patients with wild-type KRAS, locally advanced rectal cancer (LARC): a randomized, multicenter, phase II trial SAKK 41/07. Ann Oncol. 2013;24(3):718–25. doi:10.1093/annonc/mds519.
6. Mardjuadi FI, Carrasco J, Coche JC, Sempoux C, Jouret-Mourin A, Scalliet P, et al. Panitumumab as a radiosensitizing agent in KRAS wild-type locally advanced rectal cancer. Target Oncol. 2015;10(3):375–83. doi:10.1007/s11523-014-0342-9.
7. Jin T, Zhu Y, Luo JL, Zhou N, Li DC, Ju HX, et al. Prospective phase II trial of nimotuzumab in combination with radiotherapy and concurrent capecitabine in locally advanced rectal cancer. Int J Color Dis. 2015;30(3):337–45. doi:10.1007/s00384-014-2097-2.
8. Sorscher SM. Marked response to single agent trastuzumab in a patient with metastatic HER-2 gene amplified rectal cancer. Cancer Investig. 2011;29(7):456–9. doi:10.3109/07357907.2011.590569.
9. Disel U, Germain A, Yilmazel B, Abali H, Bolat FA, Yelensky R, et al. Durable clinical benefit to trastuzumab and chemotherapy in a patient with metastatic colon adenocarcinoma harboring ERBB2 amplification. Oncoscience. 2015;2(6):581–4.
10. Siena S, Sartore-Bianchi A, Lonardi S, Trusolino L, Martino C, Bencardino K, et al. Trastuzumab and lapatinib in HER2-amplified metastatic colorectal cancer patients (mCRC): The HERACLES trial. ASCO Meeting Abstracts. 2015;33(15 Suppl):3508.
11. Kopetz S, Desai J, Chan E, Hecht JR, O'Dwyer PJ, Maru D, et al. Phase II pilot study of Vemurafenib in patients with metastatic BRAF-mutated colorectal cancer. J Clin Oncol. 2015;33(34):4032–8. doi:10.1200/JCO.2015.63.2497.
12. Falchook GS, Long GV, Kurzrock R, Kim KB, Arkenau TH, Brown MP, et al. Dabrafenib in patients with melanoma, untreated brain metastases, and other solid tumours: a phase 1 dose-escalation trial. Lancet. 2012;379(9829):1893–901. doi:10.1016/S0140-6736(12)60398-5.
13. Hyman DM, Puzanov I, Subbiah V, Faris JE, Chau I, Blay JY, et al. Vemurafenib in multiple Nonmelanoma cancers with BRAF V600 mutations. N Engl J Med. 2015;373(8):726–36. doi:10.1056/NEJMoa1502309.
14. Hong DS, Morris VK, El Osta BE, Fu S, Overman MJ, Piha-Paul SA, et al. Phase Ib study of vemurafenib in combination with irinotecan and cetuximab in patients with BRAF-mutated metastatic colorectal cancer and advanced cancers. ASCO Meeting Abstracts. 2015;33(15 Suppl):3511.
15. Tabernero J, van Geel R, Bendell JC, Spreafico A, Schuler M, Yoshino T, et al. 11LBA Phase I study of the selective BRAFV600 inhibitor encorafenib (LGX818) combined with cetuximab and with or without the α-specific PI3K inhibitor alpelisib (BYL719) in patients with advanced

BRAF mutant colorectal cancer. European Journal of Cancer. 2014;50:199. doi:10.1016/S0959-8049(14)70732-4.

16. Buijsen J, Lammering G, Jansen RL, Beets GL, Wals J, Sosef M, et al. Phase I trial of the combination of the Akt inhibitor nelfinavir and chemoradiation for locally advanced rectal cancer. Radiother Oncol. 2013;107(2):184–8. doi:10.1016/j.radonc.2013.03.023.
17. Hill EJ, Enescu M, West N, Franklin JM, Chu K-Y, Li J, et al. Oral nelfinavir before and during radiation therapy for rectal cancer: Changes in tumor perfusion and correlation between tissue and radiological markers of response. ASCO Meeting Abstracts. 2014;32(3 Suppl):491.
18. Liao X, Lochhead P, Nishihara R, Morikawa T, Kuchiba A, Yamauchi M, et al. Aspirin use, tumor PIK3CA mutation, and colorectal-cancer survival. N Engl J Med. 2012;367(17):1596–606. doi:10.1056/NEJMoa1207756.
19. El-Rayes BF, Staley CA, Diaz R, Sullivan PS, Shaib WL, Landry JC. Phase I study of ganetespib (G), capecitabine (C), and radiation (RT) in rectal cancer. ASCO Meeting Abstracts. 2015;33(15 Suppl):3596.
20. Le DT, Uram JN, Wang H, Bartlett BR, Kemberling H, Eyring AD, et al. PD-1 blockade in tumors with mismatch-repair deficiency. N Engl J Med. 2015;372(26):2509–20. doi:10.1056/NEJMoa1500596.
21. Hurwitz H, Fehrenbacher L, Novotny W, Cartwright T, Hainsworth J, Heim W, et al. Bevacizumab plus irinotecan, fluorouracil, and leucovorin for metastatic colorectal cancer. N Engl J Med. 2004;350(23):2335–42. doi:10.1056/NEJMoa032691.
22. Willett CG, Duda DG, di Tomaso E, Boucher Y, Czito BG, Vujaskovic Z, et al. Complete pathological response to bevacizumab and chemoradiation in advanced rectal cancer. Nat Clin Pract Oncol. 2007;4(5):316–21. doi:10.1038/ncponc0813.
23. Marechal R, Vos B, Polus M, Delaunoit T, Peeters M, Demetter P, et al. Short course chemotherapy followed by concomitant chemoradiotherapy and surgery in locally advanced rectal cancer: a randomized multicentric phase II study. Ann Oncol. 2012;23(6):1525–30. doi:10.1093/annonc/mdr473.
24. Salazar R, Capdevila J, Laquente B, Manzano JL, Pericay C, Villacampa MM, et al. A randomized phase II study of capecitabine-based chemoradiation with or without bevacizumab in resectable locally advanced rectal cancer: clinical and biological features. BMC Cancer. 2015;15:60. doi:10.1186/s12885-015-1053-z.
25. Network CGA. Comprehensive molecular characterization of human colon and rectal cancer. Nature. 2012;487(7407):330–7. doi:10.1038/nature11252.
26. Park DI, Kang MS, Oh SJ, Kim HJ, Cho YK, Sohn CI, et al. HER-2/neu overexpression is an independent prognostic factor in colorectal cancer. Int J Color Dis. 2007;22(5):491–7. doi:10.1007/s00384-006-0192-8.
27. Kavanagh DO, Chambers G, O'Grady L, Barry KM, Waldron RP, Bennani F, et al. Is overexpression of HER-2 a predictor of prognosis in colorectal cancer? BMC Cancer. 2009;9:1. doi:10.1186/1471-2407-9-1.
28. Cancer Genome Atlas N. Comprehensive molecular characterization of human colon and rectal cancer. Nature. 2012;487(7407):330–7. doi:10.1038/nature11252.
29. Ramanathan RK, Hwang JJ, Zamboni WC, Sinicrope FA, Safran H, Wong MK, et al. Low overexpression of HER-2/neu in advanced colorectal cancer limits the usefulness of trastuzumab (Herceptin) and irinotecan as therapy. A phase II trial. Cancer Investig. 2004;22(6):858–65.
30. Liming S, Yuan Z, Qinghua D, Lei W, Qifeng J, Haojie L. Human epidermal growth factor receptor-2 and topoisomerase II alpha expressions in rectal cancer. Hepato-Gastroenterology. 2011;58(106):359–63.
31. Conradi LC, Styczen H, Sprenger T, Wolff HA, Rödel C, Nietert M, et al. Frequency of HER-2 positivity in rectal cancer and prognosis. Am J Surg Pathol. 2013;37(4):522–31. doi:10.1097/PAS.0b013e318272ff4d.
32. Meng X, Wang R, Huang Z, Zhang J, Feng R, Xu X, et al. Human epidermal growth factor receptor-2 expression in locally advanced rectal cancer: association with response to neoadjuvant therapy and prognosis. Cancer Sci. 2014;105(7):818–24. doi:10.1111/cas.12421.

33. Yao YF, Du CZ, Chen N, Chen P, Gu J. Expression of HER-2 in rectal cancers treated with preoperative radiotherapy: a potential biomarker predictive of metastasis. Dis Colon Rectum. 2014;57(5):602–7. doi:10.1097/DCR.0000000000000107.
34. Seo AN, Kwak Y, Kim DW, Kang SB, Choe G, Kim WH, et al. HER2 status in colorectal cancer: its clinical significance and the relationship between HER2 gene amplification and expression. PLoS One. 2014;9(5):e98528. doi:10.1371/journal.pone.0098528.
35. Sclafani F, Roy A, Cunningham D, Wotherspoon A, Peckitt C. Gonzalez de Castro D et al. HER2 in high-risk rectal cancer patients treated in EXPERT-C, a randomized phase II trial of neoadjuvant capecitabine and oxaliplatin (CAPOX) and chemoradiotherapy (CRT) with or without cetuximab. Ann Oncol. 2013;24(12):3123–8. doi:10.1093/annonc/mdt408.
36. Park DI, Yun JW, Park JH, Oh SJ, Kim HJ, Cho YK, et al. HER-2/neu amplification is an independent prognostic factor in gastric cancer. Dig Dis Sci. 2006;51(8):1371–9. doi:10.1007/s10620-005-9057-1.
37. Smith I, Procter M, Gelber RD, Guillaume S, Feyereislova A, Dowsett M, et al. 2-year follow-up of trastuzumab after adjuvant chemotherapy in HER2-positive breast cancer: a randomised controlled trial. Lancet. 2007;369(9555):29–36. doi:10.1016/S0140-6736(07)60028-2.
38. Slamon DJ, Leyland-Jones B, Shak S, Fuchs H, Paton V, Bajamonde A, et al. Use of chemotherapy plus a monoclonal antibody against HER2 for metastatic breast cancer that overexpresses HER2. N Engl J Med. 2001;344(11):783–92. doi:10.1056/NEJM200103153441101.
39. Petrelli F, Borgonovo K, Cabiddu M, Ghilardi M, Barni S. Neoadjuvant chemotherapy and concomitant trastuzumab in breast cancer: a pooled analysis of two randomized trials. Anti-Cancer Drugs. 2011;22(2):128–35.
40. Gianni L, Romieu GH, Lichinitser M, Serrano SV, Mansutti M, Pivot X, et al. AVEREL: a randomized phase III trial evaluating bevacizumab in combination with docetaxel and trastuzumab as first-line therapy for HER2-positive locally recurrent/metastatic breast cancer. J Clin Oncol. 2013;31(14):1719–25. doi:10.1200/JCO.2012.44.7912.
41. Gianni L, Pienkowski T, Im YH, Roman L, Tseng LM, Liu MC, et al. Efficacy and safety of neoadjuvant pertuzumab and trastuzumab in women with locally advanced, inflammatory, or early HER2-positive breast cancer (NeoSphere): a randomised multicentre, open-label, phase 2 trial. Lancet Oncol. 2012;13(1):25–32. doi:10.1016/S1470-2045(11)70336-9.
42. Bang YJ, Van Cutsem E, Feyereislova A, Chung HC, Shen L, Sawaki A, et al. Trastuzumab in combination with chemotherapy versus chemotherapy alone for treatment of HER2-positive advanced gastric or gastro-oesophageal junction cancer (ToGA): a phase 3, open-label, randomised controlled trial. Lancet. 2010;376(9742):687–97. doi:10.1016/S0140-6736(10)61121-X.
43. Chen J, Guo F, Shi X, Zhang L, Zhang A, Jin H, et al. BRAF V600E mutation and KRAS codon 13 mutations predict poor survival in Chinese colorectal cancer patients. BMC Cancer. 2014;14:802. doi:10.1186/1471-2407-14-802.
44. Saridaki Z, Tzardi M, Sfakianaki M, Papadaki C, Voutsina A, Kalykaki A, et al. BRAFV600E mutation analysis in patients with metastatic colorectal cancer (mCRC) in daily clinical practice: correlations with clinical characteristics, and its impact on patients' outcome. PLoS One. 2013;8(12):e84604. doi:10.1371/journal.pone.0084604.
45. He Y, Van't Veer LJ, Mikolajewska-Hanclich I, van Velthuysen ML, Zeestraten EC, Nagtegaal ID, et al. PIK3CA mutations predict local recurrences in rectal cancer patients. Clin Cancer Res. 2009;15(22):6956–62. doi:10.1158/1078-0432.CCR-09-1165.
46. Samowitz WS, Sweeney C, Herrick J, Albertsen H, Levin TR, Murtaugh MA, et al. Poor survival associated with the BRAF V600E mutation in microsatellite-stable colon cancers. Cancer Res. 2005;65(14):6063–9. doi:10.1158/0008-5472.CAN-05-0404.
47. Clancy C, Burke JP, Kalady MF, Coffey JC. BRAF mutation is associated with distinct clinicopathological characteristics in colorectal cancer: a systematic review and meta-analysis. Color Dis. 2013;15(12):e711–8. doi:10.1111/codi.12427.
48. Falchook GS, Lewis KD, Infante JR, Gordon MS, Vogelzang NJ, DeMarini DJ, et al. Activity of the oral MEK inhibitor trametinib in patients with advanced melanoma: a phase 1 dose-escalation trial. Lancet Oncol. 2012;13(8):782–9. doi:10.1016/S1470-2045(12)70269-3.

49. Corcoran RB, Atreya CE, Falchook GS, Kwak EL, Ryan DP, Bendell JC, et al. Combined BRAF and MEK inhibition with Dabrafenib and Trametinib in BRAF V600-mutant colorectal cancer. J Clin Oncol. 2015;33(34):4023–31. doi:10.1200/JCO.2015.63.2471.
50. Prahallad A, Sun C, Huang S, Di Nicolantonio F, Salazar R, Zecchin D, et al. Unresponsiveness of colon cancer to BRAF(V600E) inhibition through feedback activation of EGFR. Nature. 2012;483(7387):100–3. doi:10.1038/nature10868.
51. S1406 Phase II Study of Irinotecan and Cetuximab With or Without Vemurafenib in BRAF Mutant Metastatic Colorectal Cancer. 2014. https://clinicaltrials.gov/ct2/show/study/NCT02164916.
52. Study of LGX818 and Cetuximab or LGX818, BYL719, and Cetuximab in BRAF Mutant Metastatic Colorectal Cancer. 2012. https://clinicaltrials.gov/ct2/show/NCT01719380/.
53. Johnson SM, Gulhati P, Rampy BA, Han Y, Rychahou PG, Doan HQ, et al. Novel expression patterns of PI3K/Akt/mTOR signaling pathway components in colorectal cancer. J Am Coll Surg. 2010;210(5):767–76, 76–8. doi:10.1016/j.jamcollsurg.2009.12.008.
54. Danielsen SA, Eide PW, Nesbakken A, Guren T, Leithe E, Lothe RA. Portrait of the PI3K/AKT pathway in colorectal cancer. Biochim Biophys Acta. 2015;1855(1):104–21. doi:10.1016/j.bbcan.2014.09.008.
55. Hemminki A, Markie D, Tomlinson I, Avizienyte E, Roth S, Loukola A, et al. A serine/threonine kinase gene defective in Peutz-Jeghers syndrome. Nature. 1998;391(6663):184–7. doi:10.1038/34432.
56. Bussink J, van der Kogel AJ, Kaanders JH. Activation of the PI3-K/AKT pathway and implications for radioresistance mechanisms in head and neck cancer. Lancet Oncol. 2008;9(3):288–96. doi:10.1016/S1470-2045(08)70073-1.
57. Schuurbiers OC, Kaanders JH, van der Heijden HF, Dekhuijzen RP, Oyen WJ, Bussink J. The PI3-K/AKT-pathway and radiation resistance mechanisms in non-small cell lung cancer. J Thorac Oncol. 2009;4(6):761–7. doi:10.1097/JTO.0b013e3181a1084f.
58. Bendell JC, Nemunaitis J, Vukelja SJ, Hagenstad C, Campos LT, Hermann RC, et al. Randomized placebo-controlled phase II trial of perifosine plus capecitabine as second- or third-line therapy in patients with metastatic colorectal cancer. J Clin Oncol. 2011;29(33):4394–400. doi:10.1200/JCO.2011.36.1980.
59. Bendell JC, Ervin TJ, Senzer NN, Richards DA, Firdaus I, Lockhart AC, et al. Results of the X-PECT study: A phase III randomized double-blind, placebo-controlled study of perifosine plus capecitabine (P-CAP) versus placebo plus capecitabine (CAP) in patients (pts) with refractory metastatic colorectal cancer (mCRC). ASCO Meeting Abstracts. 2012;30(18 Suppl):LBA3501.
60. Gupta AK, Cerniglia GJ, Mick R, McKenna WG, Muschel RJ. HIV protease inhibitors block Akt signaling and radiosensitize tumor cells both in vitro and in vivo. Cancer Res. 2005;65(18):8256–65. doi:10.1158/0008-5472.CAN-05-1220.
61. Domingo E, Church DN, Sieber O, Ramamoorthy R, Yanagisawa Y, Johnstone E, et al. Evaluation of PIK3CA mutation as a predictor of benefit from nonsteroidal anti-inflammatory drug therapy in colorectal cancer. J Clin Oncol. 2013;31(34):4297–305. doi:10.1200/JCO.2013.50.0322.
62. Kothari N, Kim R, Jorissen RN, Desai J, Tie J, Wong HL, et al. Impact of regular aspirin use on overall and cancer-specific survival in patients with colorectal cancer harboring a PIK3CA mutation. Acta Oncol. 2015;54(4):487–92. doi:10.3109/0284186X.2014.990158.
63. Dimberg J, Samuelsson A, Hugander A, Söderkvist P. Differential expression of cyclooxygenase 2 in human colorectal cancer. Gut. 1999;45(5):730–2.
64. Dienstmann R, Patnaik A, Garcia-Carbonero R, Cervantes A, Benavent M, Roselló S, et al. Safety and activity of the first-in-class Sym004 anti-EGFR antibody mixture in patients with refractory colorectal cancer. Cancer Discov. 2015;5(6):598–609. doi:10.1158/2159-8290.CD-14-1432.
65. BRAF/MEK/EGFR Inhibitor Combination Study in Colorectal Cancer (CRC). 2012. https://clinicaltrials.gov/ct2/show/NCT01750918.
66. Do K, Speranza G, Bishop R, Khin S, Rubinstein L, Kinders RJ, et al. Biomarker-driven phase 2 study of MK-2206 and selumetinib (AZD6244, ARRY-142886) in patients with colorectal cancer. Investig New Drugs. 2015;33(3):720–8. doi:10.1007/s10637-015-0212-z.

67. Trepel J, Mollapour M, Giaccone G, Neckers L. Targeting the dynamic HSP90 complex in cancer. Nat Rev Cancer. 2010;10(8):537–49. doi:10.1038/nrc2887.
68. Kamal A, Thao L, Sensintaffar J, Zhang L, Boehm MF, Fritz LC, et al. A high-affinity conformation of Hsp90 confers tumour selectivity on Hsp90 inhibitors. Nature. 2003;425(6956):407–10. doi:10.1038/nature01913.
69. Neckers L, Workman P. Hsp90 molecular chaperone inhibitors: are we there yet? Clin Cancer Res. 2012;18(1):64–76. doi:10.1158/1078-0432.CCR-11-1000.
70. Russell JS, Burgan W, Oswald KA, Camphausen K, Tofilon PJ. Enhanced cell killing induced by the combination of radiation and the heat shock protein 90 inhibitor 17-allylamino-17-demethoxygeldanamycin: a multitarget approach to radiosensitization. Clin Cancer Res. 2003;9(10 Pt 1):3749–55.
71. Camphausen K, Tofilon PJ. Inhibition of Hsp90: a multitarget approach to radiosensitization. Clin Cancer Res. 2007;13(15 Pt 1):4326–30. doi:10.1158/1078-0432.CCR-07-0632.
72. Goldman JW, Raju RN, Gordon GA, El-Hariry I, Teofilivici F, Vukovic VM, et al. A first in human, safety, pharmacokinetics, and clinical activity phase I study of once weekly administration of the Hsp90 inhibitor ganetespib (STA-9090) in patients with solid malignancies. BMC Cancer. 2013;13:152. doi:10.1186/1471-2407-13-152.
73. He S, Smith DL, Sequeira M, Sang J, Bates RC, Proia DA. The HSP90 inhibitor ganetespib has chemosensitizer and radiosensitizer activity in colorectal cancer. Investig New Drugs. 2014;32(4):577–86. doi:10.1007/s10637-014-0095-4.
74. Nilbert M, Planck M, Fernebro E, Borg A, Johnson A. Microsatellite instability is rare in rectal carcinomas and signifies hereditary cancer. Eur J Cancer. 1999;35(6):942–5.
75. Hong SP, Min BS, Kim TI, Cheon JH, Kim NK, Kim H, et al. The differential impact of microsatellite instability as a marker of prognosis and tumour response between colon cancer and rectal cancer. Eur J Cancer. 2012;48(8):1235–43. doi:10.1016/j.ejca.2011.10.005.
76. Llosa NJ, Cruise M, Tam A, Wicks EC, Hechenbleikner EM, Taube JM, et al. The vigorous immune microenvironment of microsatellite instable colon cancer is balanced by multiple counter-inhibitory checkpoints. Cancer Discov. 2015;5(1):43–51. doi:10.1158/2159-8290.CD-14-0863.
77. Xiao Y, Freeman GJ. The microsatellite instable subset of colorectal cancer is a particularly good candidate for checkpoint blockade immunotherapy. Cancer Discov. 2015;5(1):16–8. doi:10.1158/2159-8290.CD-14-1397.
78. Phase 2 Study of MK-3475 in Patients With Microsatellite Unstable (MSI) Tumors. 2013. https://clinicaltrials.gov/ct2/show/NCT01876511/.
79. Weisenberger DJ, Siegmund KD, Campan M, Young J, Long TI, Faasse MA, et al. CpG island methylator phenotype underlies sporadic microsatellite instability and is tightly associated with BRAF mutation in colorectal cancer. Nat Genet. 2006;38(7):787–93. doi:10.1038/ng1834.
80. Study of Imprime PGG® in Combination With Cetuximab in Subjects With Recurrent or Progressive KRAS Wild Type Colorectal Cancer (PRIMUS). 2011. https://clinicaltrials.gov/ct2/show/NCT01309126.

Surgical Anatomy of the Rectum

8

David Moszkowicz, David Fuks, and Brice Gayet

Abstract

The goal of infraperitoneal rectal resection for cancer is complete mesorectal excision, including the rectal visceral fascia that envelops the mesorectum (with "extra-fascial" excision), with lymphadenectomy of the inferior mesenteric lymphatic drainage system. If the proper plane of dissection is respected, this also guarantees preservation of genitourinary function by sparing the autonomic innervation of the detrusor muscles, the smooth muscle urethral sphincter, the glandular and smooth muscle components of the vaginal wall, and the erectile bodies. While the oncologic goal of surgery for rectal cancer is complete removal of all tumoral tissues, it is also important to spare the nerves, in women as well as in men. There is risk of nerve injury throughout the procedure. Dissection must be guided by the planes of the perirectal fascia, the so-called "nerve guardians" of the pelvis. Detailed knowledge of the anatomy of the rectum and its fascial relationships is one major prerequisite for both accurate diagnostic imaging and successful treatment.

Keywords

Surgical anatomy • Rectum • Pelvic innervation

D. Moszkowicz, M.D., Ph.D
Service de Chirurgie Digestive, Oncologique et Métabolique, Hôpital Ambroise-Paré, AP—HP, 9, Avenue Charles-de-Gaulle, 92104 Boulogne-Billancourt, France

UVSQ/Université Paris Saclay, UFR des Sciences de la Santé Simone-Veil, 2 Avenue de la Source de la Bièvre, 78180 Montigny-Le-Bretonneux, France

D. Fuks, M.D., Ph.D • B. Gayet, M.D., Ph.D (✉)
Département de Chirurgie Digestive, Oncologique et Métabolique, Institut Mutualiste Montsouris, Université Paris Descartes, 42 Boulevard Jourdan, 75014 Paris, France

UFR Paris Descartes, Paris, France
e-mail: brice.gayet@imm.fr

G. Dapri, J.H. Marks (eds.), *Surgical Techniques in Rectal Cancer*,
https://doi.org/10.1007/978-4-431-55579-7_8

8.1 Introduction

The goal of infraperitoneal rectal resection for cancer is complete mesorectal excision (the mesorectum corresponds to the inferior rectal ligament for anatomists), including the rectal visceral fascia that envelops the mesorectum ("extra-fascial" excision), with lymphadenectomy of the inferior mesenteric lymphatic drainage system [1–3]. If the proper plane of dissection is respected, this also guarantees preservation of genitourinary function by sparing the autonomic innervation of the detrusor muscles, the smooth muscle urethral sphincter, the glandular and smooth muscle components of the vaginal wall, and the erectile bodies (corpus cavernosum and corpus spongiosum) [4]. While the oncologic goal of surgery is complete removal of all tumoral tissues, it is also important to spare the nerves, in women as well as in men [5]. There is risk of nerve injury throughout the procedure. Dissection must be guided by the planes of the perirectal fascia, the so-called "nerve guardians" of the pelvis. Detailed knowledge of the anatomy of the rectum and its fascial relationships is one major prerequisite for both accurate diagnostic imaging and successful treatment.

8.2 Descriptive Anatomy and Limits of the Rectum

The rectum, terminal portion of the digestive tract, is interposed between the sigmoid colon and the anal verge. It has a curved shape and occupies the sacral hollow from the level of S3 down to the coccyx [6]. The rectum is composed of a pelvic portion, or rectal ampulla, and a perineal portion, or anal canal. They are responsible for the storage and controlled evacuation of feces through sophisticated neuromuscular sphincter mechanisms [7].

The precise locations of both the proximal and distal end of the rectum are debatable. Although not anatomically distinct, delineating the sections of the rectum is of great importance to the surgeon for the surgical treatment of rectal cancer (Fig. 8.1a). The rectosigmoid junction is considered to be at the level of S3 by anatomists and at the sacral promontory, after mobilization, by surgeons (Fig. 8.1b). The distal limit is regarded as the muscular anorectal ring by surgeons and as the dentate line by anatomists [8]. The rectum is 15 to 20 cm long and can be divided into three parts: the upper, middle, and lower rectum. From the anal verge, these three parts are anatomically defined as follows: the lower rectum, 0–5 cm; the middle rectum, 5–10 cm; and the upper rectum, 10–15 cm [7].

Most parts of the rectum are extraperitoneal, although anteriorly the upper rectum is covered by the visceral peritoneum around the front and sides down to the peritoneal reflection [9]. Although the measures of the distances from the anal verge are quite variable, the peritoneal reflection is normally found between 7 and 9 cm from the anal verge. In women it may be lower, at 7.5 to 5 cm from the anal verge at the anterior rectal wall [8]. At the posterior rectal wall, the rectosigmoid junction can be found between 18 and 19 from the anal verge.

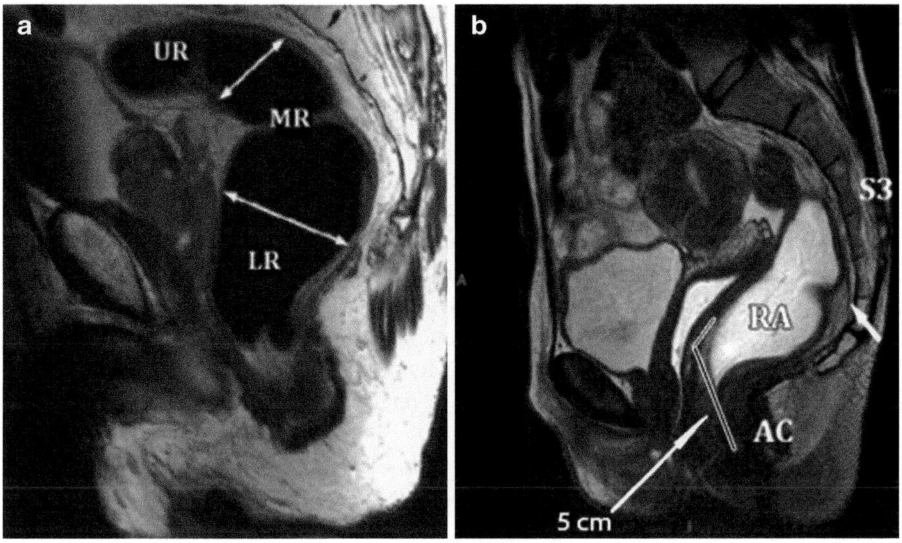

Fig. 8.1 (**a**, **b**) Rectosigmoidal junction and limits of the rectum. On the sagittal MRI images, the rectosigmoidal junction is located at the anterior border of S3. The recto-sacral ligament (*thick arrow*) is formed by dense connective tissue between the rectal visceral fascia and presacral fascia at the level of the third and fourth sacral vertebrae. The 5 cm measure illustrates the approximate length of the lower rectum at the anterior rectal surface. *UR* upper rectum, *MR* middle rectum, *LR* lower rectum, *RA* rectal ampulla, *AC* anal canal

At its lower end, the rectum is angled forward by the puborectalis sling, forming the anorectal junction. Anteriorly, in women, the rectum is related to the posterior vaginal wall; in men, the rectum lies behind the prostate, seminal vesicles, vas deferens, and urinary bladder. The rectum exhibits lateral curves, which correspond on the intraluminal aspect to Houston's valves. There are usually three: two on the left side (at 7–8 cm and 12–13 cm) and one at 9–11 cm on the right side. The middle valve is the most consistent [8]. The sigmoid colon is differentiated from the rectum by the segmentation of the complete longitudinal muscle layer to form the taenia coli and by its diameters (6–8 cm for the sigmoid, 1.5–3.5 for the rectum). Shafik et al. found the rectosigmoid junction to be a large bowel segment 2.8 ± 0.9 cm in length [10] with electrophysiological properties of a rectosigmoid sphincter [11]. During surgery, a Hegar bougie may be used to better demonstrate the diameter transition at the level of the rectosigmoid junction.

In adults, the rectal wall is composed of the mucosa, submucosa, and muscularis propria. The muscularis propria has an inner circular layer and an outer longitudinal layer. The longitudinal muscle of the rectum fuses with striated fibers of the levator ani and puborectalis muscle at the level of the anorectal ring, forming the conjoined longitudinal muscle. At the level of the puborectalis portion of the levator ani muscle, the rectal adventitia constitutes a thin, microscopic layer that is interposed between the outer longitudinal muscular layer and the inner fascia of the levator ani muscle. The wall of the anal canal is composed of the mucosa, submucosa, and muscularis. The muscularis is composed of a thick inner circular layer (the internal sphincter) and an outer longitudinal layer that is composed of a small layer of connective tissue (the intersphincteric space). The latter separates the longitudinal layer from the striated muscle of the external sphincter [12]. The sphincter muscles form an anteroposterior slit, which is the anal canal. The anal valves and the distal end of the ampullary part of the rectum mark the proximal margin of the anal canal. The proximal 10 mm of the anal canal are lined by columnar, rectal-type mucosa. The following 15 mm, including the valves, are lined by stratified epithelium. Distal to that is approximately 10 mm of thick, nonciliated stratified epithelium. The most distal 5–10 mm is lined by hairy skin [11]. Histological measurements of the length of the surgical anal canal (anorectal ring to anal verge) demonstrated an average length of 4.2 cm [7].

8.3 Pararectal and Paraanal Spaces

The anorectum comprises clinically relevant spaces [13].

The *ischiorectal* fossa is subdivided by a thin horizontal fascia into two spaces: the perianal and the ischiorectal space. The *ischiorectal space* occupies the upper two-thirds of the ischiorectal fossa. It forms a pyramid-shaped space between the anal canal and the lower part of the rectum medially and the pelvic sidewall and ischial tuberosity laterally. The superior aspect of this space is bounded by the levator complex. The *perianal space* envelops the lower portion of the anal canal. It runs laterally with the subcutaneous fat of the buttocks and extends medially into the intersphincteric space.

The *intersphincteric space* is a virtual space between the internal and external anal sphincter muscles that could be dissected for sphincter-saving proctectomy in case of very low rectal cancer respecting the external anal sphincter [14].

The *superficial postanal space* is between the anococcygeal ligament and the skin, and the *deep postanal space* lies between the anococcygeal ligament and the anococcygeal raphe.

The *supralevator spaces* are between the peritoneum superiorly and the levator ani muscle inferiorly. These bilateral spaces are lateral to the rectum and medial to the obturator fascia. The *retrorectal or presacral space* is located between the rectal visceral fascia anteriorly and the presacral fascia posteriorly. It is bordered anteriorly by the subperitoneal rectum, posteriorly by the presacral fascia, laterally by the parietal leaflet of the pelvic fascia that covers the bony and muscular walls of the pelvic cavity, superiorly by the peritoneum of the recto-genital pouch (*Douglas pouch*), and inferiorly by the anococcygeal levator muscles that form the pelvic diaphragm (Fig. 8.2).

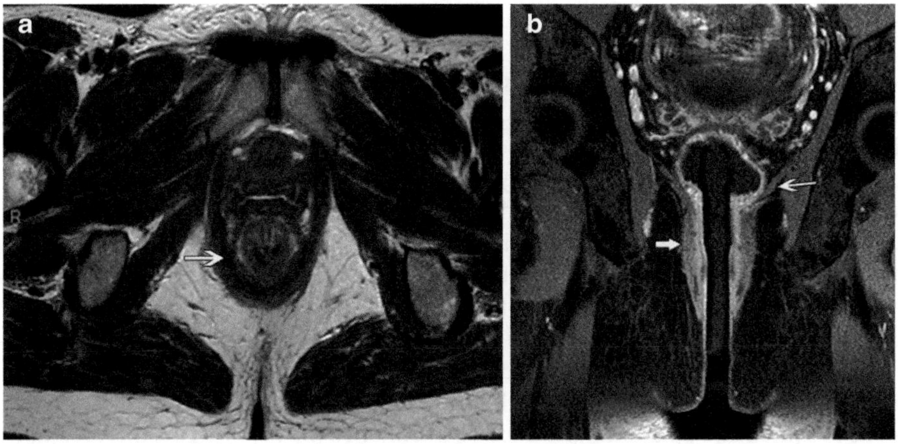

Fig. 8.2 Levator ani muscles. Para-axial (**a**) and frontal (**b**) views of the rectum at the level of the pelvic diaphragm (*thins arrows*) and the external anal sphincter (*thick arrow*)

The *posterior perineum* (or anal perineum) consists of the ensemble of soft tissues lying below the levators, bordered anteriorly by the line joining the two ischial tuberosities (palpable in the genitofemoral fold) and posteriorly by the tip of the coccyx in the intergluteal fold [15]. The structures within this space are identical in both males and females: the ischiorectal fossae are divided into supra- and infralevator portions by the pelvic diaphragm. Posterior to the anal canal, the coccygeal muscles, the posterior bundles of the puborectalis sling, and the iliococcygeal muscles all insert into the anococcygeal ligament in the midline. A second muscular diaphragm, the deep transverse perineal muscle, lies anterior to the rectum, stretching from the internal aspect of the ischial ramus to the central tendon of the perineum (perineal body); it is covered superiorly and inferiorly by the superior and inferior fascias of the urogenital diaphragm. It is sometimes reinforced by the superficial transverse perineal muscle, but this anatomy is not constant. The superficial perineal fascia overlies this entire area in the subcutaneous fat and continues anteriorly to join the superficial abdominal fascia [16].

8.4 Mesorectum and Fascial Structures

The pelvis is supported by the endopelvic fascia, which has two components: a visceral and a parietal layer. The visceral layer of the endopelvic fascia (rectal visceral fascia) lines the rectum. The parietal layer of the endopelvic fascia covers the sacrum dorsally (presacral fascia) and the pelvic wall (obturator internus and pyriformis muscles) laterally.

8.4.1 The Mesorectum and the Rectal Visceral Fascia

Within the envelope of the rectal visceral fascia lie the terminal branches of the inferior mesenteric artery (IMA), the associated veins and lymphatics, and a variable pad of supporting fat (the mesorectum for surgeons, the inferior rectal ligament for anatomists). This fat may be very thick and bulky or thin but usually almost nonexistent in the 2 cm of its most distal portion [17]. This structure completely surrounds the rectum over most of its length and extends from the level of the peritoneal reflection down to the puborectalis muscle sling. There, the rectal visceral fascia fuses with the superior fascia of the pelvic diaphragm (the covering fascia of the levator ani muscle) [18] (Fig. 8.3). On histologic and electron microscopy examination, rectal visceral fascia appeared as a multilayered structure of variable thickness ranging from 20 to 1000 μm with an average thickness (measured in vitro) of about 150 μm made up of multiple bundles of collagen fibers [19]. This mesorectum fascial envelope, so-called fascia recti by surgeons, should be removed intact in rectal cancer surgery to prevent local recurrence [20].

8.4.2 The Parietal Pelvic Fascia and the Recto-sacral Ligament

The parietal pelvic fascia is the loose, multilayered fascia lining the pelvic walls. The pelvic plexuses are closely applied on it, and when intact after surgery, the parietal fascia provides protection to the presacral veins and nerves lying within it.

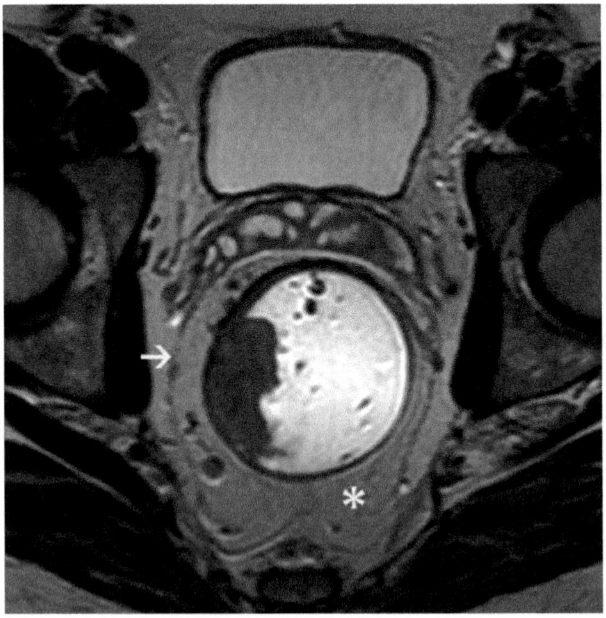

Fig. 8.3 Mesorectum. Para-axial view of the mesorectum (*star*) in a rectal cancer patient. The mesorectum is surrounded by the rectal visceral fascia (fascia recti, *arrow*)

Recently, histological examinations demonstrated a fascial retrorectal multilaminar structure. Hypogastric nerves are bordered anteriorly by a prehypogastric fascia between the nerve trunk and the rectal visceral fascia and by the parietal presacral fascia posteriorly [21, 22]. Crapp and Cuthbertson described what they called the recto-sacral ligament as an attachment between the parietal fascia and the rectal visceral fascia at the level of the body of S4, 3–5 cm proximal to the anorectal junction [23]. While applying firm pressure and anterior traction on the rectum, the operating surgeon observes fusion of the rectal visceral fascia and the parietal fascia near the S4 level in most patients. The retrorectal space is the avascular plane of loose areolar tissue lying between the parietal fascia posteriorly and the rectal visceral fascia anteriorly. It is the "holy plane" referred to by Heald [24]. This space is continuous superiorly with the retroperitoneal space and inferiorly to where these fasciae are connected on the sacrum ventral aspect with a dense area of fibers: the recto-sacral ligament (Fig. 8.1). After division of the recto-sacral ligament, a similar space continues below the horizontal rectum to the anorectal junction [20, 25].

8.4.3 Recto-genital Fascia or Denonvilliers' Fascia

The fascia of Denonvilliers (or recto-prostatic septum in male/rectovaginal septum in female) lies anterior to the rectal visceral fascia, passing from the peritoneum of the recto-vesical pouch above to the pelvic floor in the region of the perineal body below [12, 26, 27]. Its lateral edges were recently clearly defined [28]. The recto-vaginal septum was found, in women, to be composed of multiple connective tissue layers that were closely applied to the vagina and contained smooth muscle fibers from the vagina and the inferior segment of the uterus (Fig. 8.4 a, b, c). Ventrocranially, it formed an incomplete anatomic partition between the posterior and the middle compartments of the pelvis. The multiple connective tissue layers were separated laterally and made a "Y"-shaped extension that joined the lateral vaginal wall anteriorly and the visceral fascia of the rectum posteriorly. It had a close relationship with the neurovascular bundles (cf. infra).

8.5 Blood Supply

The rectum, which is part of the distal portion of the hindgut, is mainly supplied by the superior rectal artery, arising as the terminal branch from the inferior mesenteric artery (IMA). Similarly, the venous drainage of the hindgut, and therefore of the rectum, is to the inferior mesenteric vein into the portal system [9]. Veins from the upper two-thirds of the rectum are drained by the superior rectal vein. Veins from the lower third of the rectum are drained by the middle and inferior rectal veins into the internal iliac veins. The rectum is additionally supplied by the middle and inferior rectal arteries.

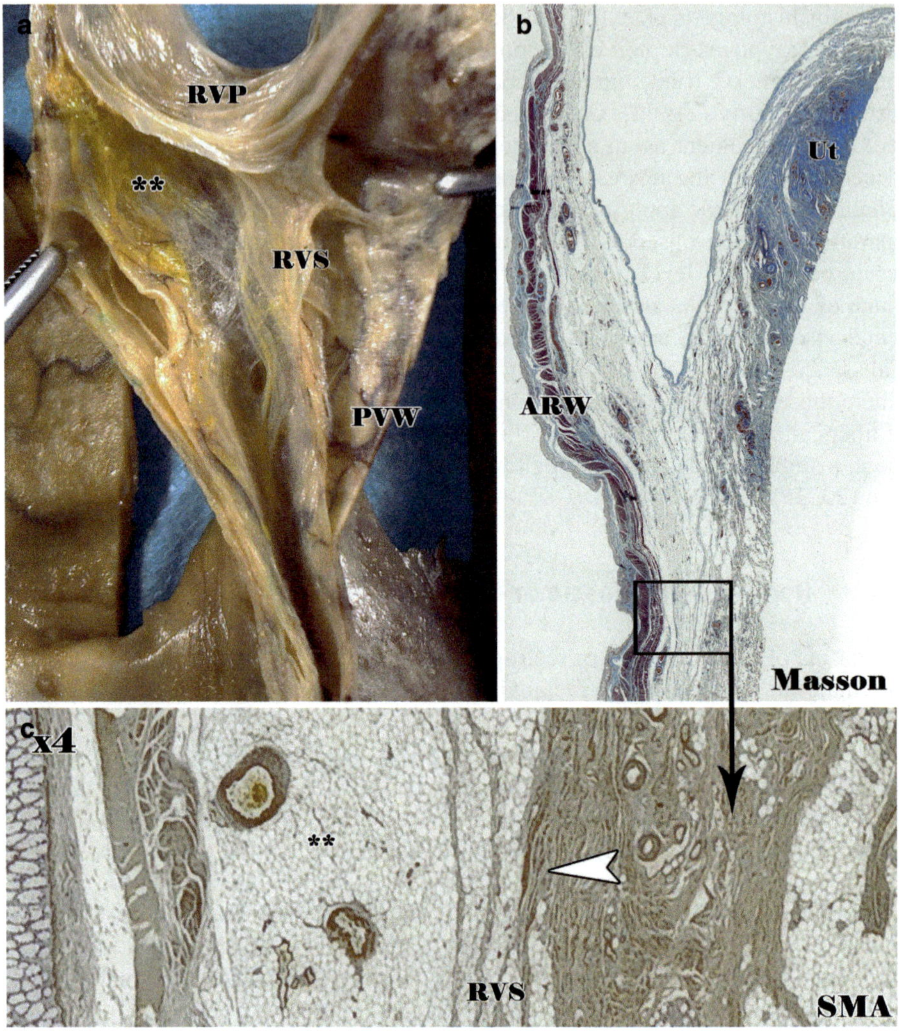

Fig. 8.4 Adult rectovaginal septum (RVS). (**a**) Macroscopic dissection of midsagittal section of a 78-year-old old adult cadaver showing the RVS located between the posterior vaginal wall (PVW) and anterior rectal wall (ARW). (**b**) RVS stained with Masson trichrome. (**c**) *Black square*, x4 magnification. Immunolabeled with anti-smooth muscle actin (SMA) the RVS contains smooth muscle fibers (white arrowhead). originated from the vagina and uterus (Ut). *RUP* rectouterine pouch; bold asterisks anterior mesorectum. Adapted from [28]

8.5.1 Superior Rectal Artery

The superior rectal artery typically continues in the same downward course as the IMA to reach the back of the upper third of the rectum. At this point, it bifurcates into two vessels, adjacent to the inferior portion of the recto-genital pouch and opposite the level of S3 [29]. The larger right branch supplies the posterior and lateral surface of the rectum. It divides into two main branches, which run down to the right anterior and posterior aspects of the rectum. The smaller left branch supplies the anterior surface of the rectum and continues undivided down the left lateral aspect of the rectum. These branches generally break up into smaller vessels that finally penetrate the muscle layer to reach the submucosa. Here they proceed downward as straight vessels, which terminate usually above the anal valves as a capillary plexus.

8.5.2 Middle Rectal Artery

The middle rectal arteries originate from the anterior divisions of the internal iliac arteries or from their inferior vesical branches. They proceed medially and forward below the pelvic peritoneum, in the tissue of the so-called lateral ligaments, to reach the rectal wall [30, 31]. Here they anastomose with the branches of the superior and inferior rectal arteries. However, the MRA may be absent [29, 32].

8.5.3 Inferior Rectal Artery

The inferior rectal arteries spring from the internal pudendal arteries in pudendal canal in the obturator internus fascia of the outer walls of the ischiorectal fossa. They run medially and slightly forward, dividing into branches that penetrate the external and internal anal sphincters, and finally reach the submucosa of the anal canal.

8.5.4 Medial Sacral Artery

The medial sacral artery originates from the aortic bifurcation, proceeds distally posterior to the presacral fascia, and inconstantly reaches the anal canal at the level of the coccyx.

8.5.5 Sacral Foraminal Veins

Presacral veins form a venous plexus on the surface of the lower sacrum. They are mistakenly considered at risk during rectal dissection [33]. As a matter of fact, hemorrhage comes more frequently from the sacral basivertebral veins connecting the presacral venous plexus to the intrasacral canal venous plexus at the level of anterior sacral foramina. The historically performed blunt dissection with stripping of the connective tissue between recto-sacral ligament and presacral fascia with the underlying periosteum off the sacrum can lead, on one hand, to rupture of these connecting veins that then retract into the sacral foramina and bleed profusely and, on the other hand, to mesorectal rupture and cancer spreading.

However, the advent of laparoscopy and the spreading of TME technique have allowed improved surgical technique and results [34, 35].

8.6 Lymphatic Drainage

Numerous small nodes are located adjacent to the bowel wall. They drain to the larger nodes along the mesenteric vessels and subsequently to clustered nodes around the origins of the IMA.

8.6.1 Intramural Lymphatics

In the submucous and subserous layer of the rectal wall, there are continuous lymphatic plexuses, which drain into the extramural lymphatics.

8.6.2 Extramural Lymphatics

The extramural lymphatics follow the blood vessels supplying the rectum and anal canal. Lymph from the parts of the rectum that receive blood supply from the superior rectal artery drains to superior rectal nodes after transversing pararectal nodes. From superior rectal nodes, lymph passes to inferior mesenteric nodes.

Between 5 and 10% of lymphatics can pass directly through the rectal visceral fascia at the level of the middle rectum and reach internal iliac nodes [16].

The lymphatic drainage of the remainder of the rectum and anal canal is dependent on its relationship to the mucocutaneous junction. The area proximal to the mucocutaneous junction either drains superiorly (parallel to the middle rectal arteries on the corresponding pelvic sidewall) or traverses the levator ani muscle to follow the inferior rectal arteries. These two possible pathways lead to internal iliac nodes, common iliac nodes, and the lumbar trunk. Lymphatic drainage below the mucocutaneous junction is not parallel to blood vessels. The collecting ducts pass anteriorly and superiorly in the perineum. Together with lymphatic channels from the perianal skin, they pass to superficial inguinal nodes.

8.7 Pelvic-Perineal Innervation: Nerve-Oriented Rectal Cancer Excision Steps

Optimal treatment of rectal adenocarcinoma involves total mesorectal excision with nerve-preserving dissection. Improved knowledge of pelvic nerve anatomy may help reduce this and define the key anatomical zones at risk [36]. Pelvic nerve damage may occur during ligation of the inferior mesenteric artery, at every point of total mesorectal excision and through the perineal dissection of abdominoperineal resection. Recently, the transanal total mesorectal excision was described as an alternative to conventional low anterior resection. Magnificated view of the pelvic might enhance nerve preservation and functional results [37].

8.7.1 Inferior Mesenteric Lymphadenectomy: Preservation of the Inferior Mesenteric Plexus (IMP)

High ligation of the inferior mesenteric artery (IMA) at its origin from the aorta is intended to achieve complete removal of regional lymph nodes [38, 39]. The IMA should then be ligated 1.5 cm from its origin, thus preserving the nerve fibers of the inferior mesenteric plexus that lie on the anterior aspect of the aorta (Fig. 8.5). The relationship of the ureters to the IMA and superior rectal artery is of particular importance to the surgeon. Because the trunk deviates to the left, it passes close to the left ureter and left gonadic vessels, which are in danger during ligation of the IMA [29].

8.7.2 Retrorectal Dissection: Preservation of the Superior Hypogastric Plexus and the Hypogastric Nerves

8.7.2.1 Anatomical Basis

The superior hypogastric plexus (SHP) is a network of pre- and postganglionic fibers anterior to the body of L5 arising from T10–L3 and is a continuation of the preaortic sympathetic trunks [41]. It is mostly in an inter-iliac position and accompanies the inferior mesenteric and superior rectal arteries between the posterior aspect of the sigmoid and the anterior surface of the lowest lumbar vertebra. It forms the origin of two hypogastric nerves (HNs) that run over the sacral promontory situated 1 cm on either side of the midline and 2 cm medial to the ureter and iliac artery

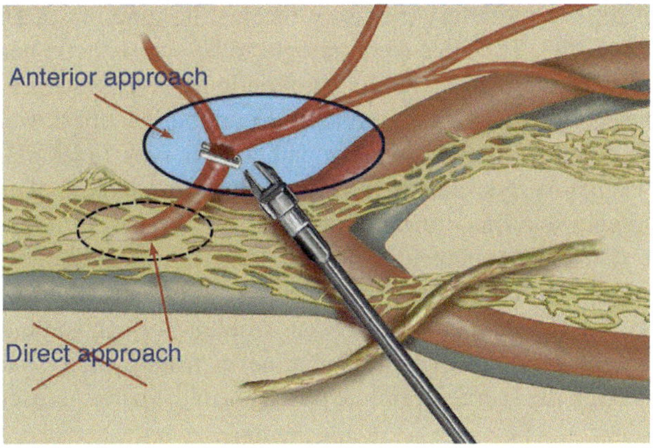

Fig. 8.5 Inferior mesenteric lymphadenectomy: preservation of the inferior mesenteric plexus. Adapted from [40]

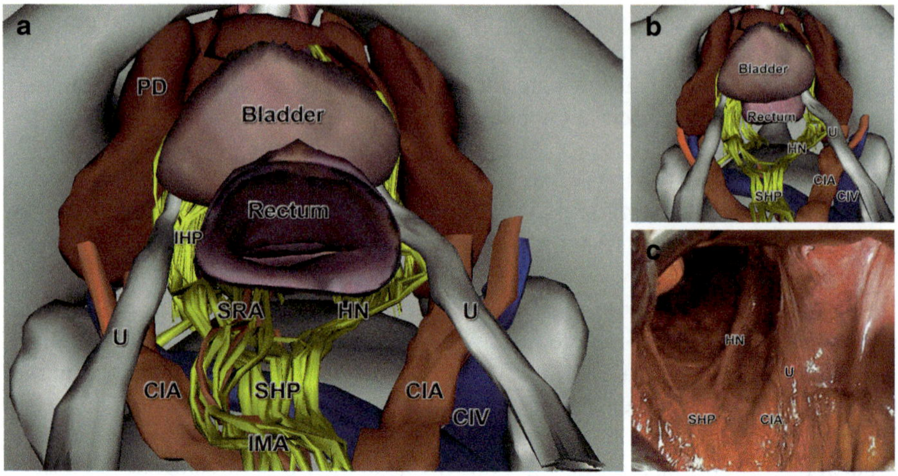

Fig. 8.6 (**a**) Intra-abdominal view of fetal pelvic tridimensional reconstruction using CAAD with immunolabeled pelvic nerves. Same reconstructed view (**b**) and intraoperative view (**c**) after rectal resection during total mesorectal excision (TME). Nerves fibers destined to the rectum and accompanying the inferior mesenteric artery (IMA) and superior rectal artery (SRA) are resected during IMA ligation, but the superior hypogastric plexus (SHP) and hypogastric nerves (HNs) must be preserved. Other abbreviations: common iliac artery and vein (CIA, CIV), inferior hypogastric plexus (IHP), pelvic diaphragm (PD), and ureter (U). Adapted from [36]

[42] (Fig. 8.6). They vary in gross anatomy, sometimes consisting of fine filaments that spread out over a width of about 1 cm and sometimes being 5–8 mm wide [25, 43]. HNs travel posterolaterally to the posterior rectal wall behind the ureters and medially to the posterior division branches of internal iliac arteries. Some fibers split from HNs and are destinated to the posterolateral rectal wall, bladder wall, and ureterovesical junction. Most fibers of HNs then accompany the ureter on its dorsal side. When the ureter is about to join the wall of the bladder, the HNs come to lie at the ventral edge of the lateral rectal wall, and this initiates the formation of the inferior hypogastric plexus (IHP). The intersection of the ureter with the posterior wall of the uterine artery precisely locates the junction of HNs and IHP at its superior angle [21]. The HNs were thought to be sympathetic nerves. However, it's recently been shown that the pelvic autonomic nervous system is more complex than previously thought, as adrenergic and cholinergic fibers were found to coexist within "sympathetic" and "parasympathetic" nerves [44]. SHP and HN damage causes ejaculatory dysfunction (retrograde ejaculation, loss of ejaculation) [45] and urinary urgency and incontinence [46–48].

The pelvic splanchnic nerves (PSNs) or erectile nerves (Eckard) have been considered to be parasympathetic nerves and generally arise from the ventral roots of S3 to S4 in men and S2 to S4 in women [49]. In some exceptional cases, branches may originate from S5 [50], but never from S1 [51]. These nerves enter the pelvis through the sacral foramina, posterior to the parietal fascia that covers the piriformis muscle and crosses the retrorectal space, to enter the visceral compartment through the visceral fascia about 4 cm from the midline [42, 51]. Small branches of the PSNs that run medially to enter the mesorectum have been identified. These contain the specific parasympathetic fibers of the rectum and make up the medial segment of the IHP. They lie in the lateral ligament that joins the parietal fascia overlying the pelvic sidewall to the rectal visceral fascia medially [25]. Sato and Sato showed that the superoanterior part of the "lateral ligaments" contained the middle rectal artery and the inferoposterior part contained the PSNs [52]. However, other authors do not consider the "lateral ligaments" to exist and report that the middle rectal artery is a small, inconstant, and frequently unilateral vessel [53]. Rutegard et al. have clarified the issue by showing that the main components of the lateral ligament are autonomic nerves passing from the pelvic plexus to the rectum within a condensation of connective tissue [43].

These mainly sympathetic fibers are responsible for detrusor contractility and vaginal lubrication and genital swelling during sexual arousal [54]. Damage to these nerves causes erectile dysfunction and decreased blood flow to the vagina and vulva, which can reduce vaginal lubrication.

8.7.2.2 Surgical Consequences

Then, the peritoneal incision is continued distally down to the junction between the mesosigmoid and mesorectum. The retrorectal space is entered at the level of the sacral promontory in the plane that separates the prehypogastric plexus behind from the hypogastric nerves (HNs) in the rectal visceral fascia, in front (Fig. 8.7).

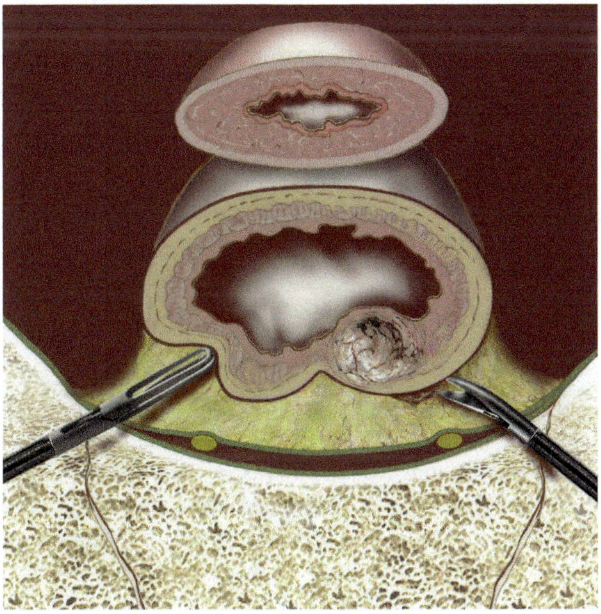

Fig. 8.7 Retrorectal dissection: preservation of the superior hypogastric plexus and the hypogastric nerves. Adapted from [40]

Dissection begins in the bifurcation at the origin of the HNs and continues downward along the midline and then laterally. The correct plane is when dissection stays in front of, not within, the alveolar tissue that separates the two conjunctive tissue planes, so not to dissect behind the HNs. At the level of S4, the rectal visceral leaf and the posterior parietal presacral leaf join to form the recto-sacral ligament, the division of which opens the terminal part of the posterior dissection of the lower rectum, exposing the levator muscles. Danger: one should not try to dissect and control the nerve structures as if they were somatic nerves—the autonomous nerves can be seen by transparency but should remain distant from the plane of dissection behind the fascia that covers them. Beware of dissection behind the presacral fascia, which endangers both the HNs and the foraminal sacral veins.

8.7.3 Anterior Dissection of the Subperitoneal Rectum: Preservation of the Innervation of the Prostate/Posterior Wall of the Vagina (e.g., in the Case of a Posterior Tumor)

After incision of the peritoneum at the bottom of the rectouterine pouch, dissection is continued anterior to the rectum preserving the nerve branches arising from the inferior hypogastric plexus (IHP) that innervate the vagina [28]. The rectovaginal septum, separating the posterior aspect of the vagina from the anterior aspect of the rectum, cannot be identified independently, but, rather, corresponds to fine layers of conjunctive tissue and smooth muscle fibers, in front of which the nerves run. Classically, this septum is resected, but, when oncologic conditions permit, can actually be preserved without modifying the circumferential margin, leading to dissection in contact with the rectal visceral fascia (plane of the mesorectum) [55, 56] (Fig. 8.8). Danger: dissection performed in contact with the vaginal posterior wall (extra-mesorectal dissection) can lead to bleeding and is associated with injury to the autonomous nerves and vaginal parietal arteries. Nonetheless, this dissection may be necessary if the circumferential margin is involved [55].

8.7.4 Laterorectal Dissection: Preservation of the Inferior Hypogastric Plexus

8.7.4.1 Anatomical Basis

The inferior hypogastric plexus (IHP) is a network of sympathetic and parasympathetic fibers arising from hypogastric nerves (HNs) and pelvic splanchnic nerves (PSNs) [57]. It is a quadrangular-shaped plaque of nervous tissue with two aspects (visceral and parietal), four edges (superior "cranial," anterior "ventral," posterior "dorsal," and inferior "caudal"), and four angles (superior, anteroinferior, anterosuperior, and posteroinferior). It lies between the rectal visceral fascia and the parietal

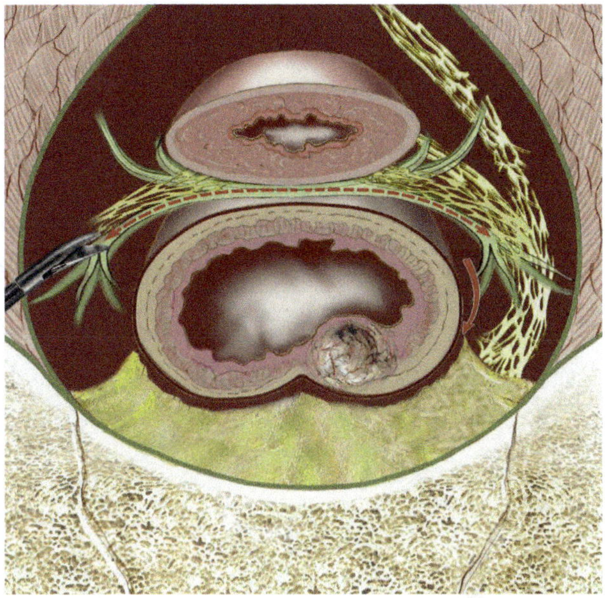

Fig. 8.8 Anterior dissection of the subperitoneal rectum: preservation of the innervation of the posterior wall of the vagina. Laterorectal dissection: preservation of the inferior hypogastric plexus. Adapted from [40]

fascia (Fig. 8.9). The IHP measures 3–4 cm and is located retroperitoneally and laterally on both sides of the rectum close to the prostate and seminal vesicle in men. In females, it radiates from an area anterolateral to the rectum, passes lateral to the cervix and the vaginal fornix and extends to the lateral vaginal wall and base of the bladder. The cranial portion of the IHP is situated directly beneath the lateral margin of the recto-genital pouch, where the HNs join the plexus. The bulk of the plexus is localized at the level of the vaginal fornix. At this site, fibers and ganglia of the IHP are both sympathetic and parasympathetic [59]. Adrenergic positivity is stronger in the anterior part of the plexus, whereas cholinergic positivity is stronger in its posterior third [59]. Because the IHP consists of both sympathetic and parasympathetic efferent fibers, any damage to this plexus may cause severe disturbances in urogenital and sexual function including erection and ejaculation.

8.7.4.2 Surgical Consequences

Then, the lateral peritoneal incision is completed joining together the anterior and posterior incisions (Fig. 8.8). Dissection continues in contact with the rectal visceral fascia and encounters only the distal portion of the branches of the IHP as they form the inferior rectal nerve plexus running to the posterolateral wall of the rectum and the involuntary internal anal sphincter, most often accompanied by the middle rectal artery. This artery can be simply coagulated, avoiding any traumatic maneuvers of dissection or ligation. Injury to the afferent splanchnic nerves of the IHP is unlikely at this level unless extended lateral lymphadenectomy is performed in contact with or removing the parietal leaf of the pelvic fascia that covers the muscles of the lateral pelvic wall (internal obturator and piriformis muscles). Danger: the term

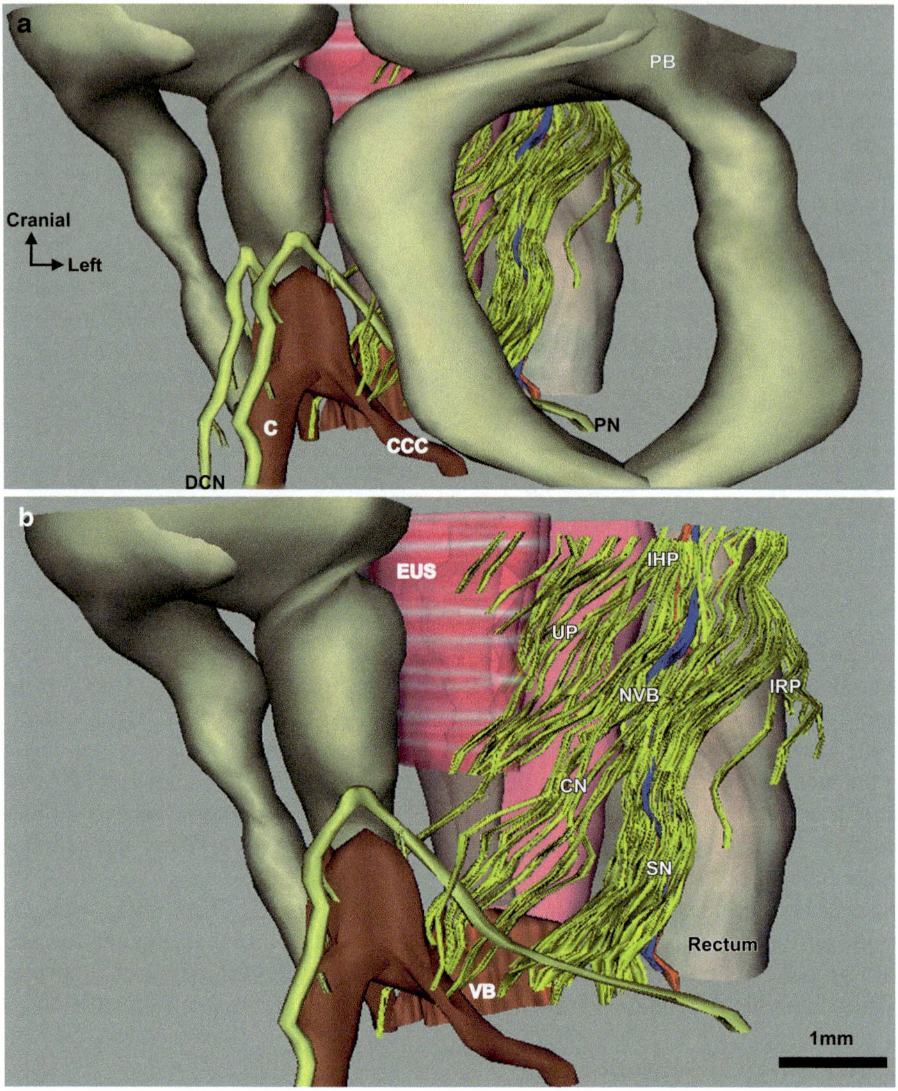

Fig. 8.9 Computer-assisted three-dimensional reconstruction of a 19-week-old female fetal pelvis and perineum. Anterolateral view of the pelvic and perineal organs (**a**) with left coxal bone and right innervation complete transparency (**b**). The neurovascular bundle (NVB) originates from the inferior hypogastric plexus (IHP) and successively gives three major projections: the urethral plexus (UP) for the urethral sphincter, the cavernous nerve (CN) for the corpus cavernosum, and the spongious nerve (SN) for vestibular bulbs (VB). *DNC* dorsal clitoris nerve, *PB* pubic bone, *PN* pudendal nerve, *C* clitoris body, *EUS* external urethral sphincter, *IRP* inferior rectal plexus. Adapted from [58]

"lateral stalk" (or wing or ligament) of the rectum does not correspond to any real anatomic structure and should be discarded. Performing any dissection outside the parietal leaf of the pelvic fascia in contact with the piriformis or internal obturator muscles risks injuring the IHP or its branches.

8.7.5 Anterolateral "Interfascial" Dissection of the Lower Rectum: Preservation of the Neurovascular Bundles

8.7.5.1 Anatomical Basis

The anteroinferior part of the inferior hypogastric plexus (IHP) converges in a caudal direction and reaches down to the pelvic floor. The closer the levator ani muscle is to the rectum, the more the distal plexus is pushed into a small triangular space bordered by the levator ani muscle laterally, the rectum dorsally, and the vagina ventrally. These anteroinferior fibers are gathered in neural bundles forming neurovascular bundles (NVBs) with the vaginal pedicle. The NVBs are situated at the 2 o'clock and 10 o'clock positions around the anterior rectum and at the 5 o'clock and 7 o'clock positions around the posterior vaginal wall [21] (Figs. 8.9 and 8.10). These bundles then form two major perineal projections: an anterior projection for the urethral sphincter complex and an inferior projection for the perineal erectile bodies. The last four collateral branches of the NVBs are medial to the posterior vaginal wall, anterior to the urethral sphincter (urethral plexus), anterolateral to the clitoris corpora cavernosa (cavernous nerve), and posterolateral to the clitoris bulbs (spongious nerve) [58]. The trunk of the NVBs

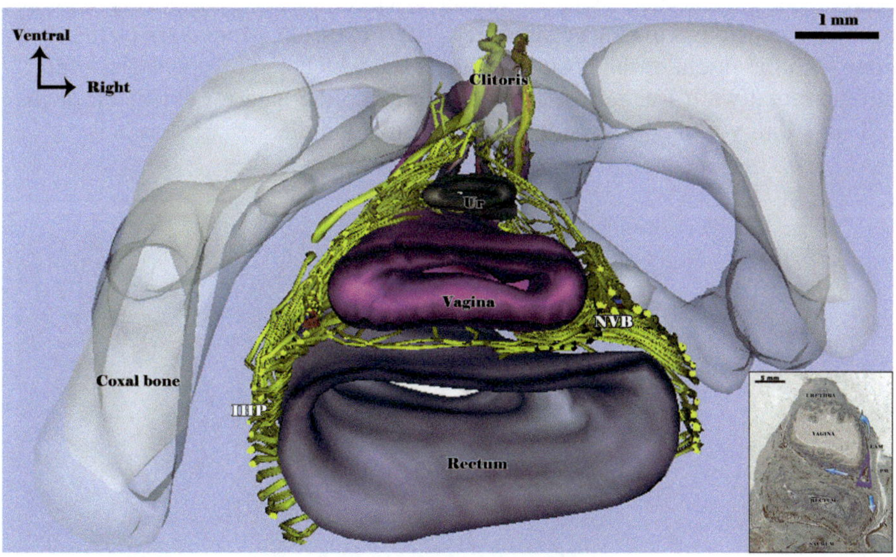

Fig. 8.10 Three-dimensional (3D) view of fetus intrapelvic organs with pelvic nerves. Superior infraperitoneal 3D view of a 30-week-old female fetus: intrapelvic organs with immunolabeled pelvic nerves showing the position of the inferior hypogastric plexus (IHP) on the lateral aspects of the rectum. From the IHP, efferent branches rise in distal directions: posteroinferior for the rectal wall, lateral for the levator ani muscles, and anteroinferior to form the NVBs. Some fibers from the NVBs branch medially to innervate the posterior vaginal wall. More caudally, the bundle puts out fibers in three major projections: an anterior projection for the urethral sphincter complex, an anterolateral projection (the cavernous nerve) that travels anterolaterally to the vagina to reach the corpora cavernosa, and a posterolateral projection (the spongious nerve) that continues posterolaterally to the vagina to innervate the corpus spongiosum. In inset, *blue arrows* show the directions of the IHP and NVB main terminal efferences. *Ur* urethra. Adapted from [58]

is situated between the anterolateral and posterolateral extension of the rectovaginal septum (RVS)—i.e., between "the two arms of the elongated Y"—and all the nerves of the NVBs are scattered in the loose connective tissue. Posterolateral extension of the RVS separates the NVBs from the rectal visceral fascia [28].

In men, recent data in opposition with the classical conception of Walsh [60] suggest that periprostatic nerve fibers are dispersed around the prostate on all sides with a significant percentage of these fibers present in the anterior and anterolateral sectors [61]. At the prostate apex and the urethral levels, the NVBs have two divisions: cavernous nerves (CNs) and spongious nerves (SNs). The CNs are a continuation of the anterior and anterolateral fibers around the apex of the prostate, traveling toward the corpora cavernosa. The SNs are a continuation of the posterolateral NVBs, and they reach the corpus spongiosum [61].

8.7.5.2 Surgical Consequences

Then, the last step of the rectal dissection is where the risk of nerve injury is highest. Dissection should remain in contact with the rectal wall covered by its visceral fascia, in the area devoid of mesorectal fatty tissue. In this way, the posterior extension of the RVS is respected, protecting the nerve bundle. Likewise, dissection remains "interfascial," between the rectal visceral fascia, posteriorly, and the posterior extension of the RVS, anteriorly [40] (Fig. 8.11). More distally, the RVS unites with the fascia of the levator ani muscles, which can be opened in contact with the rectal wall. Danger: dissection anterior to the anterior extension of the RVS risks injury to the trunk of the neurovascular bundle.

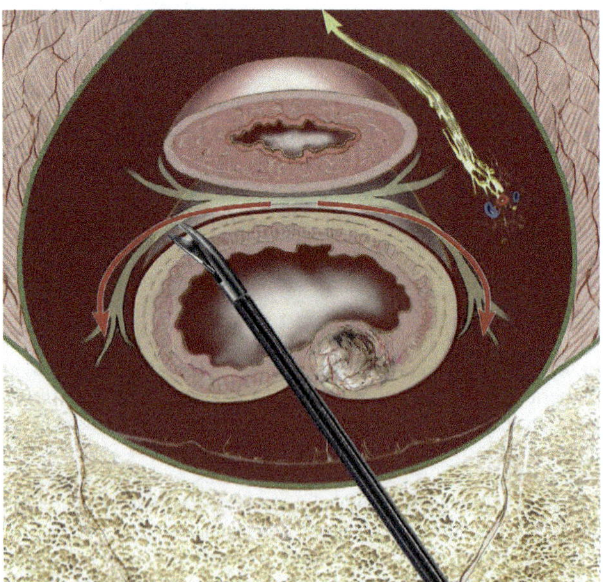

Fig. 8.11 Anterolateral "interfascial" dissection of the lower rectum: preservation of the neurovascular bundles. Adapted from [40]

8.7.6 Nerve Pathways of the Infralevator Compartment

The pudendal nerve is a mixed nerve, containing both somatic (sensory and motor) and autonomic sympathetic fibers [58]. It originates from the sacral plexus, frequently from roots S2 to S4 [62–64], sometimes L5 [50], and rarely from S1 to S5 [65]. These come through the anterior sacral foramina and unite to form the nerve trunk. This runs deep in the pudendal canal and deep in the pelvic floor musculature and passes through the ischioanal fossa where it gives off three terminal branches: (1) the perineal nerve that supplies sensory innervation to the perineal skin and motor innervation to the ischiocavernosus, bulbocavernosus, and superficial transverse perineal muscles and to the striated urethral rhabdosphincter; (2) the inferior rectal nerve that provides motor innervation to the external anal sphincter and sensory innervation to the perianal skin; and (3) the dorsal penis nerve or clitoris nerve that is also a mixed nerve that supplies the corpus cavernosum [58]. Damage to the pudendal nerve may cause urinary incontinence and sensory sexual impotence because of its role in orgasm [66–68]. Fecal incontinence after rectal cancer surgery has been linked to pudendal nerve injury, even when the anal sphincter is not damaged [69].

References

1. Heald RJ, Husband EM, Ryall RD. The mesorectum in rectal cancer surgery – the clue to pelvic recurrence? Br J Surg. 1982;69(10):613–6.
2. MacFarlane JK, Ryall RD, Heald RJ. Mesorectal excision for rectal cancer. Lancet. 1993;341(8843):457–60.
3. Carlsen E, Schlichting E, Guldvog I, Johnson E, Heald RJ. Effect of the introduction of total mesorectal excision for the treatment of rectal cancer. Br J Surg. 1998;85(4):526–9.
4. Lindsey I, Mortensen NJ. Iatrogenic impotence and rectal dissection. Br J Surg. 2002;89(12):1493–4.
5. da Silva GM, Hull T, Roberts PL, Ruiz DE, Wexner SD, Weiss EG, et al. The effect of colorectal surgery in female sexual function, body image, self-esteem and general health: a prospective study. Ann Surg. 2008;248(2):266–72.
6. Moran BJ, Jackson AA. Function of the human colon. Br J Surg. 1992;79(11):1132–7.
7. Salerno G, Sinnatamby C, Branagan G, Daniels IR, Heald RJ, Moran BJ. Defining the rectum: surgically, radiologically and anatomically. Color Dis. 2006;8(Suppl 3):5–9.
8. Jorge JM, Wexner SD. Anatomy and physiology of the rectum and anus. Eur J Surg. 1997;163(10):723–31.
9. Heald RJ, Moran BJ. Embryology and anatomy of the rectum. Semin Surg Oncol. 1998;15(2):66–71.
10. Shafik A, Doss S, Asaad S, Ali YA. Rectosigmoid junction: anatomical, histological, and radiological studies with special reference to a sphincteric function. Int J Color Dis. 1999;14(4–5):237–44.
11. Bharucha AE. Pelvic floor: anatomy and function. Neurogastroenterol Motil. 2006;18(7):507–19.
12. Aigner F, Zbar AP, Ludwikowski B, Kreczy A, Kovacs P, Fritsch H. The rectogenital septum: morphology, function, and clinical relevance. Dis Colon Rectum. 2004;47(2):131–40.
13. Schäfer A-O, Langer M. MRI of rectal cancer [Internet]. Berlin, Heidelberg: Springer; 2010 [cited 2015 Jun 5]. Available from: http://link.springer.com/10.1007/978-3-540-72833-7
14. Rullier E, Laurent C, Bretagnol F, Rullier A, Vendrely V, Zerbib F. Sphincter-saving resection for all rectal carcinomas: the end of the 2-cm distal rule. Ann Surg. 2005;241(3):465–9.

15. Moszkowicz D, Valverde A, Mosnier H. Transperineal retro-anal resection of retro-rectal tumors. J Visc Surg. 2013;150(5):345–8.
16. Baqué P. Manuel pratique d'anatomie. Paris: Ellipses; 2008.
17. Peschaud F, Benoist S, Julie C, Penna C, Nordlinger B. The mesorectum: an anatomical entity that is difficult to evaluate with MRI. Morphologie. 2005;89(286):126–30.
18. Muntean V. The surgical anatomy of the fasciae and the fascial spaces related to the rectum. Surg Radiol Anat. 1999;21(5):319–24.
19. Kulaylat MN. Mesorectal excision: surgical anatomy of the rectum, mesorectum, and pelvic fascia and nerves and clinical relevance. World J Surg Proced. 2015;5(1):27.
20. Bisset IP, Chau KY, Hill GL. Extrafascial excision of the rectum: surgical anatomy of the fascia propria. Dis Colon Rectum. 2000;43(7):903–10.
21. Moszkowicz D, Alsaid B, Bessede T, Penna C, Benoit G, Peschaud F. Female pelvic autonomic neuroanatomy based on conventional macroscopic and computer-assisted anatomic dissections. Surg Radiol Anat. 2011;33(5):397–404.
22. Kinugasa Y, Murakami G, Suzuki D, Sugihara K. Histological identification of fascial structures posterolateral to the rectum. Br J Surg. 2007;94(5):620–6.
23. Crapp AR, Cuthbertson AM. William Waldeyer and the rectosacral fascia. Surg Gynecol Obstet. 1974;138(2):252–6.
24. Heald RJ. The 'holy plane' of rectal surgery. J R Soc Med. 1988;81(9):503–8.
25. Bissett IP, Hill GL. Extrafascial excision of the rectum for cancer: a technique for the avoidance of the complications of rectal mobilization. Semin Surg Oncol. 2000;18(3):207–15.
26. Lindsey I, Guy RJ, Warren BF, Mortensen NJ. Anatomy of Denonvilliers' fascia and pelvic nerves, impotence, and implications for the colorectal surgeon. Br J Surg. 2000;87(10):1288–99.
27. Zhai LD, Liu J, Li YS, Yuan W, He L. Denonvilliers' fascia in women and its relationship with the fascia propria of the rectum examined by successive slices of celloidin-embedded pelvic viscera. Dis Colon Rectum. 2009;52(9):1564–71.
28. Peschaud F, Moszkowicz D, Alsaid B, Bessede T, Penna C, Benoit G. Preservation of genital innervation in women during total mesorectal excision: which anterior plane? World J Surg. 2012;36(1):201–7.
29. Goligher JC, Duthie HL, Nixon HH. Surgery of the anus, rectum, and colon. Springfield: Thomas; 1967. p. 1140.
30. Church JM, Raudkivi PJ, Hill GL. The surgical anatomy of the rectum – a review with particular relevance to the hazards of rectal mobilisation. Int J Color Dis. 1987;2(3):158–66.
31. Liang JT, Chang KJ, Wang SM. Lateral rectal ligaments contain important nerves. Br J Surg. 1998;85(8):1162.
32. Lin PH, Chaikof EL. Embryology, anatomy, and surgical exposure of the great abdominal vessels. Surg Clin North Am. 2000;80(1):417–33, xiv.
33. Baque P, Karimdjee B, Iannelli A, Benizri E, Rahili A, Benchimol D, et al. Anatomy of the presacral venous plexus: implications for rectal surgery. Surg Radiol Anat. 2004;26(5):355–8.
34. Havenga K, Enker WE, Norstein J, Moriya Y, Heald RJ, van Houwelingen HC, et al. Improved survival and local control after total mesorectal excision or D3 lymphadenectomy in the treatment of primary rectal cancer: an international analysis of 1411 patients. Eur J Surg Oncol. 1999;25(4):368–74.
35. Søreide O, Norstein J. Local recurrence after operative treatment of rectal carcinoma: a strategy for change. J Am Coll Surg. 1997;184(1):84–92.
36. Moszkowicz D, Alsaid B, Bessede T, et al. Where does pelvic nerve injury occur during rectal surgery for cancer? Color Dis. 2011;13:1326–34.
37. Tuech J-J, Karoui M, Lelong B, De Chaisemartin C, Bridoux V, Manceau G, et al. A step toward NOTES total mesorectal excision for rectal cancer: endoscopic transanal proctectomy. Ann Surg. 2015;261(2):228–33.
38. Adachi Y, Inomata M, Miyazaki N, Sato K, Shiraishi N, Kitano S. Distribution of lymph node metastasis and level of inferior mesenteric artery ligation in colorectal cancer. J Clin Gastroenterol. 1998;26(3):179–82.

39. Kanemitsu Y, Hirai T, Komori K, Kato T. Survival benefit of high ligation of the inferior mesenteric artery in sigmoid colon or rectal cancer surgery. Br J Surg. 2006;93(5):609–15.
40. Moszkowicz D, Peschaud F. Step-by-step nerve-preserving mesorectal excision in the female. J Visc Surg. 2014;151(2):137–40.
41. Lu S, YQ X, Chang S, Zhang YZ, Shi JH, Ding ZH, et al. Clinical anatomy study of autonomic nerve with respective to the anterior approach lumbar surgery. Surg Radiol Anat. 2009;31(6):425–30.
42. Daniels IR, Woodward S, Taylor FG, Raja A, Toomey P. Female urogenital dysfunction following total mesorectal excision for rectal cancer. World J Surg Oncol. 2006;4:6.
43. Rutegard J, Sandzen B, Stenling R, Wiig J, Heald RJ. Lateral rectal ligaments contain important nerves. Br J Surg. 1997;84(11):1544–5.
44. Zaitouna M, Alsaid B, Diallo D, Benoit G, Bessede T. Identification of the origin of adrenergic and cholinergic nerve fibers within the superior hypogastric plexus of the human fetus. J Anat. 2013;223(1):14–21.
45. Havenga K, Maas CP, DeRuiter MC, Welvaart K, Trimbos JB. Avoiding long-term disturbance to bladder and sexual function in pelvic surgery, particularly with rectal cancer. Semin Surg Oncol. 2000;18(3):235–43.
46. Maas CP, Moriya Y, Steup WH, Kiebert GM, Kranenbarg WM, van de Velde CJ. Radical and nerve-preserving surgery for rectal cancer in The Netherlands: a prospective study on morbidity and functional outcome. Br J Surg. 1998;85(1):92–7.
47. Kim NK, Aahn TW, Park JK, Lee KY, Lee WH, Sohn SK, et al. Assessment of sexual and voiding function after total mesorectal excision with pelvic autonomic nerve preservation in males with rectal cancer. Dis Colon Rectum. 2002;45(9):1178–85.
48. Akasu T, Sugihara K, Moriya Y. Male urinary and sexual functions after mesorectal excision alone or in combination with extended lateral pelvic lymph node dissection for rectal cancer. Ann Surg Oncol. 2009;16(10):2779–86.
49. Havenga K, DeRuiter MC, Enker WE, Welvaart K. Anatomical basis of autonomic nerve-preserving total mesorectal excision for rectal cancer. Br J Surg. 1996;83(3):384–8.
50. Baader B, Herrmann M. Topography of the pelvic autonomic nervous system and its potential impact on surgical intervention in the pelvis. Clin Anat. 2003;16(2):119–30.
51. Mundy AR. An anatomical explanation for bladder dysfunction following rectal and uterine surgery. Br J Urol. 1982;54(5):501–4.
52. Sato K, Sato T. The vascular and neuronal composition of the lateral ligament of the rectum and the rectosacral fascia. Surg Radiol Anat. 1991;13(1):17–22.
53. Jones OM, Smeulders N, Wiseman O, Miller R. Lateral ligaments of the rectum: an anatomical study. Br J Surg. 1999;86(4):487–9.
54. Trimbos JB, Maas CP, Deruiter MC, Peters AA, Kenter GG. A nerve-sparing radical hysterectomy: guidelines and feasibility in Western patients. Int J Gynecol Cancer. 2001;11(3):180–6.
55. Kinugasa Y, Murakami G, Uchimoto K, Takenaka A, Yajima T, Sugihara K. Operating behind Denonvilliers' fascia for reliable preservation of urogenital autonomic nerves in total mesorectal excision: a histologic study using cadaveric specimens, including a surgical experiment using fresh cadaveric models. Dis Colon Rectum. 2006;49(7):1024–32.
56. Lindsey I, Warren BF, Mortensen NJ. Denonvilliers' fascia lies anterior to the fascia propria and rectal dissection plane in total mesorectal excision. Dis Colon Rectum. 2005;48(1):37–42.
57. Mauroy B, Demondion X, Bizet B, Claret A, Mestdagh P, Hurt C. The female inferior hypogastric (= pelvic) plexus: anatomical and radiological description of the plexus and its afferences – applications to pelvic surgery. Surg Radiol Anat. 2007;29(1):55–66.
58. Moszkowicz D, Alsaid B, Bessede T, Zaitouna M, Penna C, Benoit G, et al. Neural supply to the clitoris: immunohistochemical study with three-dimensional reconstruction of cavernous nerve, spongious nerve, and dorsal clitoris nerve in human fetus. J Sex Med. 2011;8(4):1112–22.
59. Alsaid B, Bessede T, Karam I, Abd-Alsamad I, Uhl JF, Benoit G, et al. Coexistence of adrenergic and cholinergic nerves in the inferior hypogastric plexus: anatomical and immunohistochemical study with 3D reconstruction in human male fetus. J Anat. 2009;214(5):645–54.

60. Walsh PC, Lepor H, Eggleston JC. Radical prostatectomy with preservation of sexual function: anatomical and pathological considerations. Prostate. 1983;4(5):473–85.
61. Alsaid B, Bessede T, Diallo D, Moszkowicz D, Karam I, Benoit G, et al. Division of autonomic nerves within the neurovascular bundles distally into corpora cavernosa and corpus spongiosum components: immunohistochemical confirmation with three-dimensional reconstruction. Eur Urol. 2011;59(6):902–9.
62. Gagnard C, Godlewski G, Prat D, Lan O, Cousineau J, Maklouf Y. The nerve branches to the external anal sphincter: the macroscopic supply and microscopic structure. Surg Radiol Anat. 1986;8(2):115–9.
63. Matzel KE, Schmidt RA, Tanagho EA. Neuroanatomy of the striated muscular anal continence mechanism. Implications for the use of neurostimulation. Dis Colon Rectum. 1990;33(8):666–73.
64. Shafik A, el-Sherif M, Youssef A, Olfat ES. Surgical anatomy of the pudendal nerve and its clinical implications. Clin Anat. 1995;8(2):110–5.
65. Schraffordt SE, Tjandra JJ, Eizenberg N, Dwyer PL. Anatomy of the pudendal nerve and its terminal branches: a cadaver study. ANZ J Surg. 2004;74(1–2):23–6.
66. Connell K, Guess MK, La Combe J, Wang A, Powers K, Lazarou G, et al. Evaluation of the role of pudendal nerve integrity in female sexual function using noninvasive techniques. Am J Obstet Gynecol. 2005;192(5):1712–7.
67. Wallner C, Lange MM, Bonsing BA, Maas CP, Wallace CN, Dabhoiwala NF, et al. Causes of fecal and urinary incontinence after total mesorectal excision for rectal cancer based on cadaveric surgery: a study from the cooperative clinical investigators of the Dutch total mesorectal excision trial. J Clin Oncol. 2008;26(27):4466–72.
68. Wallner C, van Wissen J, Maas CP, Dabhoiwala NF, DeRuiter MC, Lamers WH. The contribution of the levator ani nerve and the pudendal nerve to the innervation of the levator ani muscles; a study in human fetuses. Eur Urol. 2008;54(5):1136–42.
69. Tomita R, Igarashi S, Ikeda T, Koshinaga T, Fujisaki S, Tanjoh K. Pudendal nerve terminal motor latency in patients with or without soiling 5 years or more after low anterior resection for lower rectal cancer. World J Surg. 2007;31(2):403–8.

Laparoscopic Exposure of Critical Anatomy in Rectal Cancer Surgery: Techniques and Examples

9

Haane Massarotti and Steven D. Wexner

Abstract

Laparoscopic colorectal surgery has considerably evolved over the past 20 years, with the development of an organized approach to performing laparoscopic colorectal surgery. During the past few decades, there have been significant improvements in outcome for rectal cancer with the introduction of total mesorectal excision (TME) for resection of low and mid rectal cancers. While laparoscopic colectomy for colon cancer is highly accepted, there has been a slower progression to acceptance of laparoscopic proctectomy for rectal cancer. Laparoscopic resection of rectal cancer has been primarily performed by highly experienced laparoscopic colorectal surgeons and has achieved acceptable short-term outcomes and long-term safety. However, with the proper technique and experience, laparoscopy offers superb visualization of the pelvic cavity, allowing for meticulous rectal mobilization and resection.

Keywords

Laparoscopy • Critical anatomy • Rectal cancer surgery • Total mesorectal excision

H. Massarotti, M.D. • S.D. Wexner, M.D., Ph.D. (Hon.) (✉)
Department of Colorectal Surgery, Cleveland Clinic Florida,
2950 Cleveland Clinic Boulevard, Weston, FL 33331, USA
e-mail: wexners@ccf.org

G. Dapri, J.H. Marks (eds.), *Surgical Techniques in Rectal Cancer*,
https://doi.org/10.1007/978-4-431-55579-7_9

9.1 Introduction

Laparoscopic colorectal surgery has considerably evolved over the past 20 years. The twentieth century saw the development of an organized approach to performing laparoscopic colorectal surgery. The first laparoscopic colon resection was reported by Moises Jacobs in Miami, Florida, in June of 1990 [1]. Patrick Leahy resected a proximal rectal cancer using lower anterior resection [2–4]. During the past few decades, there have been significant improvements in outcome for rectal cancer with the introduction of the total mesorectal excision (TME) technique for resection of low and mid rectal cancer. While laparoscopic colectomy for colon cancer is highly accepted, there has been a slower progression to acceptance of laparoscopic proctectomy for rectal cancer. Laparoscopic resection of rectal cancer has been primarily performed by highly experienced laparoscopic colorectal surgeons and has achieved acceptable short-term outcomes and long-term safety. Due to the complexity of the anatomic structures in the pelvis, laparoscopic rectal resection is often perceived to be more technically challenging. However, with proper technique and experience, laparoscopy offers superb visualization of the pelvic cavity, allowing for meticulous rectal mobilization and cancer resection.

9.2 Components of an Adequate Rectal Cancer Resection

Overall survival, quality of life, and disease-free survival are the primary goals of surgery for rectal cancer. The secondary goal is sphincter preservation. While long-term outcomes may be determined by patient factors, biology of the cancer, and tumor characteristics, appropriate technique will help optimize patient outcomes [5]. The adequacy of a proctectomy for rectal cancer is determined by the proximal, distal, and circumferential margins, the completeness of the mesorectum and number of lymph nodes harvested [6–9]. Initially, a 5 cm distal margin was thought to be necessary. Currently, </=1 cm distal margin is considered adequate for most rectal cancers when combined with TME, and a smaller distal margin is acceptable for certain patients for whom there is no other option for sphincter preservation. For cancers located at or below the mesorectal margin, a 1 cm or even negative distal mural margin is acceptable [10–12]. The concept of TME refers to the sharp dissection of the rectum between the visceral and parietal layers of the endopelvic fascia, thus ensuring en bloc removal of the primary rectal cancer and associated mesentery, lymphatics, and vascular and perineural deposits [10, 13]. TME is an accepted surgical technique for mid- and low rectal cancers while controversial for upper and rectosigmoid cancers. When the rectum is mobilized such that an intact perirectal fascial envelope is preserved, the risk of local recurrence is reduced, while preserving autonomic nerves and reducing intraoperative bleeding [14–21]. The prognosis of patients with rectal cancer has been directly associated with macroscopic assessment of the completeness of the TME specimen, where patients with an incomplete mesorectum have increased recurrence compared to patients with a complete mesorectum [22]. Lymph node metastasis is a well-recognized prognostic factor in rectal cancer; a minimum of 12 nodes are needed to perform an adequate evaluation. However, this caveat, does not always apply after chemoradiation therapy as the radiation may

destroy lymph nodes. Collecting as many lymph nodes as possible is necessary due to the variability in available lymph nodes among patients [23, 24]. Thus, an adequate specimen after a proctectomy for rectal cancer will have a complete TME, with a 5 cm proximal margin, a negative distal margin, and 12 or more lymph nodes, even following preoperative neoadjuvant chemoradiotherapy (Fig. 9.1a, b).

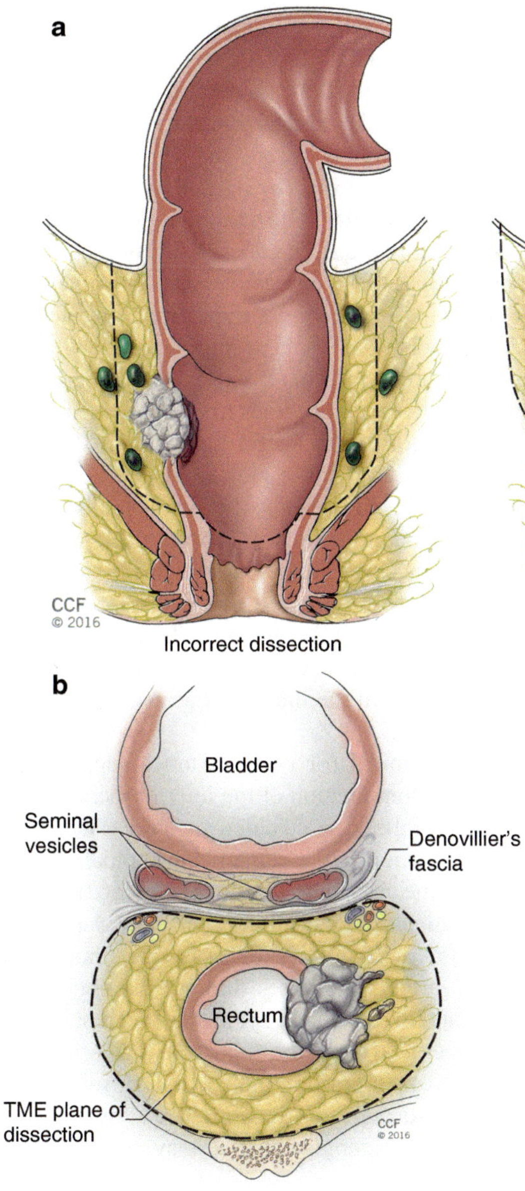

Fig. 9.1 TME schematic. (**a**) Incorrect dissection and correct dissection. (**b**) TME cross-section. Reprinted with permission, Cleveland Clinic Center for Medical Art & Photography © 2003–2016. All Rights Reserved

9.3 Anatomy

The rectum is the fixed terminal portion of the large intestine. Its proximal portion is marked by the convergence of the taeniae coli and the disappearance of the appendices epiploicae. The rectum is 15 cm in length. Anatomists define the extent of the rectum from the level of the sacral promontory to the dentate line, whereas surgeons define the rectum from the convergence of the taenia coli to the level of the anorectal ring [25]. The posterior surface of the rectum is completely extraperitoneal and is adherent to the presacral tissues. The proximal third of the rectum is anteriorly and laterally covered by peritoneum. The middle third of the rectum is covered by only the peritoneum on the anterior surface, while the lower third is completely extraperitoneal. The anterior peritoneal reflection is where the junction of the parietal peritoneal covering of the rectum meets the bladder in men and the uterus in women; this space is known as the pouch of Douglas. The rectum has three lateral curves: the upper and lower curves are convex to the right and middle curve is convex to the left. During flexible sigmoidoscopy, these curves are seen as valves of Houston. The posterior aspect of the rectum is invested in a thick, adherent mesorectum. A thin layer of investing fascia, known as the fascia propria, lines the lateral and posterior aspect of the rectum and mesorectum. This fascia is a distinct layer from the presacral fascia. Technically, this difference becomes important when performing a TME. Distally, the fascia propria forms the lateral ligaments or lateral stalks of the rectum. The middle rectal artery and pelvic plexus are both closely related. Because the middle rectal artery provides branches to the lateral stalks in up to 25% of individuals, arterial bleeding may occur during mobilization [25]. Both ureters should be identified during rectal cancer surgery. The ureters rest on the psoas muscle in their inferomedial course. They are crossed by the spermatic vessels anteriorly and the genitofemoral nerve posteriorly. In the pelvis, the ureter crosses the pelvic brim a little lateral to and anterior to the bifurcation of the common iliac artery. The ureter then descends between the internal iliac artery and the peritoneum (Fig. 9.2) [26].

The superior, middle, and inferior hemorrhoidal (or rectal) arteries supply the rectum. The superior hemorrhoidal artery is a continuation of the inferior mesenteric artery (IMA). It lies posterior and to the right of the sigmoid colon and comes in close proximity to the bowel at the rectosigmoid junction. The middle hemorrhoidal artery arises from the internal iliac arteries or, in some cases, the inferior gluteal arteries. It is variable and can be absent in 40–80% of patients. It enters the rectum anterolaterally and passes alongside the lateral stalks. The inferior hemorrhoidal artery is a branch of the pudendal artery from the internal iliac artery. It courses through the obturator canal, obturator fascia, ischiorectal fascia, and external anal sphincter. It can be seen during the perineal portion of an abdominoperineal resection (Fig. 9.3), [25].

Understanding pelvic innervation is critical to minimizing the risk of injury to the bladder or causing erectile dysfunction during mobilization. The sympathetic supply of the rectum arises from L1 to L3. Preganglionic fibers synapse in the

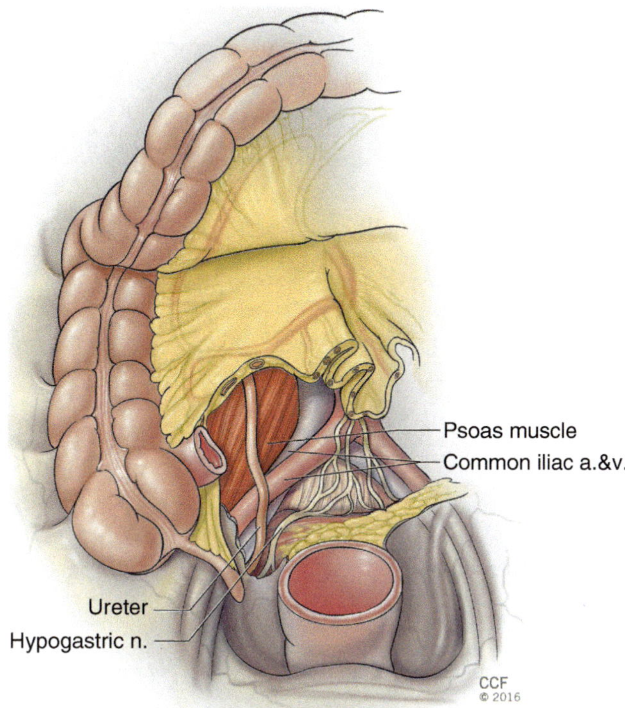

Fig. 9.2 The course of the ureters in relationship to vessels, nerve, and psoas muscle. Reprinted with permission, Cleveland Clinic Center for Medical Art & Photography © 2003–2016. All Rights Reserved

preaortic plexus. Postganglionic fibers from the preaortic plexus follow the branches of the IMA and superior rectal artery to the upper rectum. The lower rectum is innervated by the presacral nerves, which are formed by fusion of the aortic plexus and lumbar splanchnic nerves. Immediately below the sacral promontory, the presacral nerves form the hypogastric plexus (also called the superior hypogastric plexus). Two main hypogastric nerves (right and left) carry sympathetic innervation from the hypogastric plexus to the pelvic plexus, which lies adjacent to the lateral stalks. The branches of the superior hypogastric nerves can be identified while retracting the sigmoid colon anteriorly and entering the areolar plane. The areolar plane lies between the posterior aspect of the superior rectal artery and the branches of the hypogastric nerves. The parasympathetic nerves (pelvic splanchnic or erectile nerves) are not as easily identifiable as the hypogastric nerves. They arise from the ventral roots of S2–S4 and pass laterally to join the sympathetic hypogastric nerves at the pelvic plexus. Small branches of these parasympathetic nerves are in the lateral ligaments. From the pelvic plexus, combined sympathetic and parasympathetic fibers enter the upper rectum, lower rectum, and anal canal. The periprostatic plexus, a subdivision of the pelvic plexus, is located on Denonvilliers' fascia and supplies the prostate, seminal vesicles, ejaculatory ducts, and bulbourethral glands [13, 25, 26].

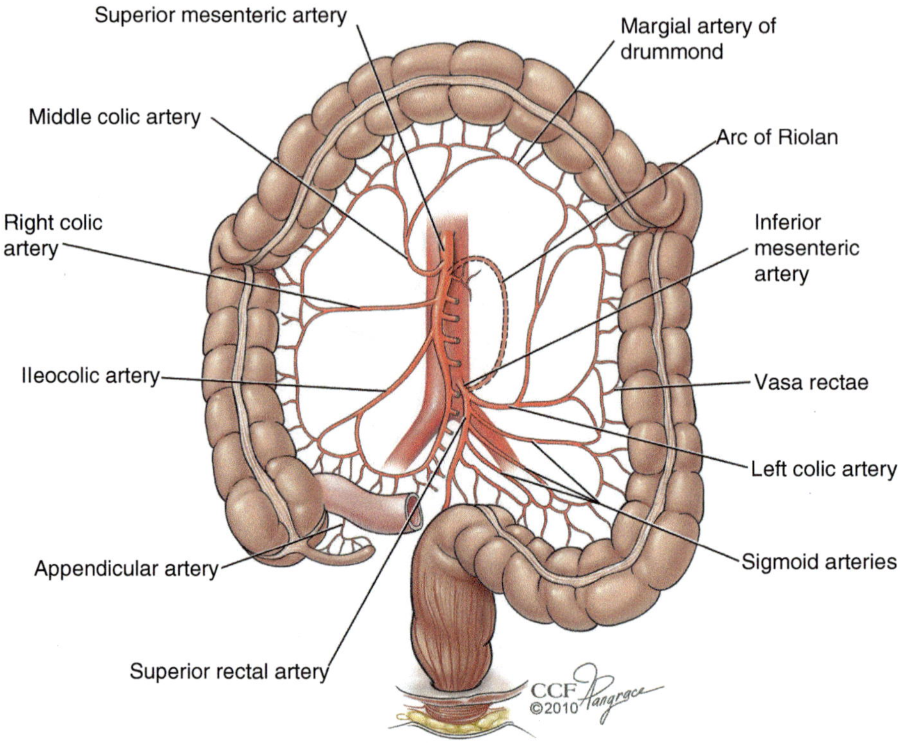

Fig. 9.3 Arterial supply of the rectum. Reprinted with permission, Cleveland Clinic Center for Medical Art & Photography © 2003–2016. All Rights Reserved

Trauma to the autonomic nerves may occur during several distinct points of rectal cancer surgery. During high ligation of the IMA near the aorta, the sympathetic preaortic nerves may be injured. During dissection at the level of the sacral promontory or in the presacral region, division of both the superior hypogastric plexus and hypogastric nerves may occur. Sympathetic denervation with intact parasympathetic innervation results in retrograde ejaculation and bladder dysfunction. Injury to the parasympathetic nerves (or nervi erigentes) may occur during excessive lateral traction of the rectum or during division of the lateral stalks; these nerves are closely related to the middle hemorrhoidal artery. Division of the nervi erigentes will result in erectile dysfunction. Finally, dissection near the prostate may damage the periprostatic plexus, which is composed of both sympathetic and parasympathetic nerves. Injury to this plexus may be avoided by starting the anterior mobilization of the rectum in the midline between the rectum and the seminal vesicles. The incision is carried to the lateral border of the seminal vesicles and curved downward and posteriorly. Injury can result in erectile impotence and a flaccid bladder (Fig. 9.4) [25, 26].

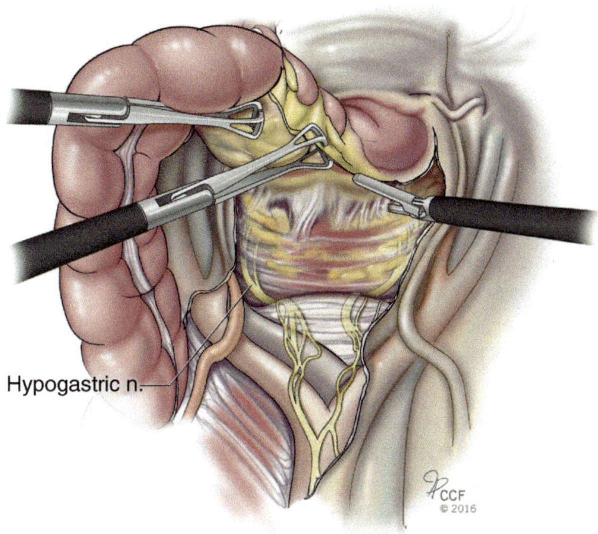

Fig. 9.4 Hypogastric nerves over the pelvic brim, just posterior to rectum. Reprinted with permission, Cleveland Clinic Center for Medical Art & Photography © 2003–2016. All Rights Reserved

9.4 Indications and Contraindications to Laparoscopic Rectal Cancer Surgery

Indications for a laparoscopic low anterior resection (LAR) with stapled or handsewn coloanal or colorectal anastomosis are:

- Middle rectal tumors (5–10 cm) from the anal verge
- Low rectal tumors (0–5 cm) from anal verge, with a distal margin of >1 cm, with an extra 1 cm of rectum required for a stapled anastomosis

Note: The surgeon should perform an intersphincteric restorative proctocolectomy with handsewn coloanal anastomosis for rectal cancer if any of the following situations occur:

- Extension of the distal edge of the tumor or to the cephalad aspect of the internal sphincter on preoperative imaging
- Inability to obtain a negative distal margin

Relative contraindications for a laparoscopic LAR:

- Unable to perform laparoscopy due to anatomic circumstances and are largely contingent upon surgical expertise [27]

Note: a patient would not be a candidate for an LAR, open or laparoscopic, and would be better served with an abdominoperineal resection if any of the following conditions are present:

- Fixation of the tumor on digital rectal examination
- Involvement of the external sphincter by tumor
- Inadequate distal margin possible even with an intersphincteric dissection
- Severe preoperative fecal incontinence
- Poor preoperative (or anticipated preoperative) sphincter function
- Patient preference
- Initial pre-neoadjuvant T3 or T4 lesion with external sphincter complex involvement [28]

9.5 Laparoscopic Surgical Techniques

9.5.1 Patient Positioning

After induction of general anesthesia, intubation, and placement of an orogastric tube, the patient is placed in the modified lithotomy position on a beanbag with the lower extremities oriented such that the toes, knee, and contralateral shoulder are in line. The knees should be slightly flexed and the thighs should be completely parallel to the ground. The arms are carefully tucked in the adducted position with the help of a beanbag, and the chest is strapped to the table to allow for safe steep tilting of the table. All bony prominences, areas of potential bodily injury, and intravenous sites should be padded. The patient should be placed such that 3–4 cm of the perineum rests below the inferior edge of the operating table. This position allows for rapid access for irrigation, examination, endoscopy, and anastomosis creation. Our practice is to ask urologists to routinely place bilateral ureteral stents after induction of anesthesia to facilitate safe laparoscopic pelvic dissection by providing tactile and visual confirmation of the ureter. The rectum is irrigated with saline through a mushroom catheter until the effluent is clear; after which betadine is introduced into the catheter and the catheter is left in place. The preoperatively selected stoma site is marked with a light needle tip skin scratch. The abdomen is prepped and draped in the usual sterile manner, ensuring that the sterile field is wide enough for a laparotomy, if needed.

9.5.2 Equipment

One of the difficulties of mastering laparoscopic surgery is developing the psychomotor skills necessary to work in a three-dimensional space guided by a two-dimensional image [29, 30]. Three-dimensional imaging was developed as an adjunct to two-dimensional imaging to overcome the challenges of loss of depth perception

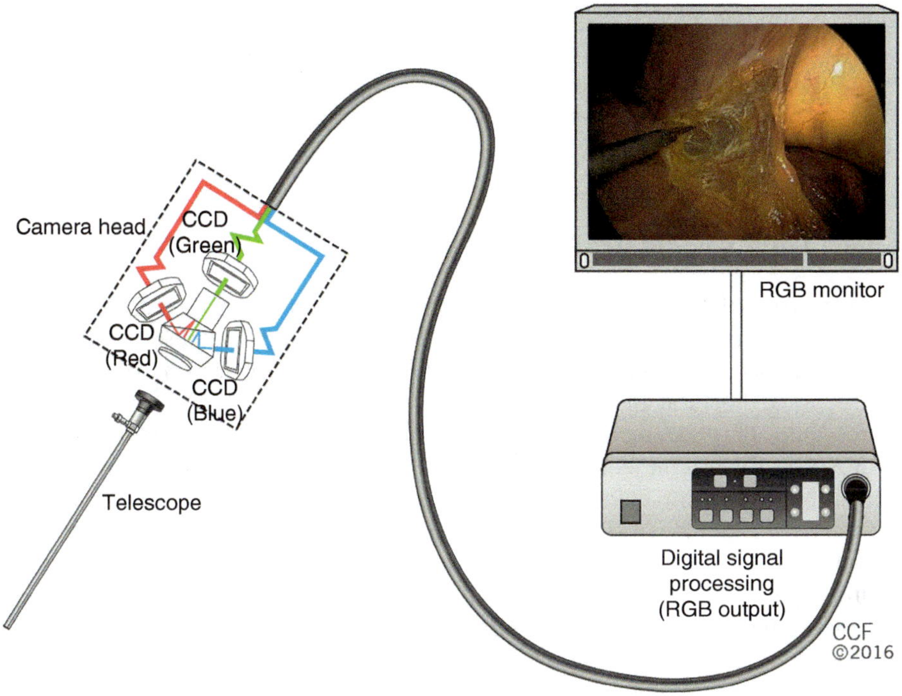

Fig. 9.5 Basic laparoscopic setup and connections. Reprinted with permission, Cleveland Clinic Center for Medical Art & Photography © 2003–2016. All Rights Reserved

and spatial orientation associated with laparoscopy. Functional high-quality camera equipment is essential to performing rectal cancer surgery. The following section will describe the basics of laparoscopic camera equipment.

The ability to clearly see the operating field is crucial in performing laparoscopic rectal cancer surgery (Fig. 9.5). The production of an excellent laparoscopic image requires the following equipment:

- Light source
- Fiber-optic light cable
- Laparoscope
- Camera head (with the imaging chip)
- Video signal processor
- Video cable
- Monitor [31]

If any of these components malfunction, the image and ability to operate will be compromised. The optical laparoscope, one of the first laparoscopes developed, has a visual channel and a fiber-optic light channel. In contrast, the digital laparoscope, which is used in modern laparoscopy, has the image sensor at the tip of the laparoscope. Today, high-definition video systems are available, providing the highest-quality image in modern laparoscopy [31]. The defining characteristic of these systems is the integration of the laparoscope, light cable, and interface to the digital signal processor.

9.5.3 Laparoscope Overview

A wide array of laparoscopes and different diameters and viewing angles are available. The rigid laparoscope contains a lens system that is housed in the core of the laparoscope and focuses and transmits light from the abdomen to the camera [32]. Optical fibers at the periphery of the scope transmit light from the light source into the abdomen. We generally recommend the standard 10 mm laparoscope for routine colorectal procedure, as this provides a wide overview that is mandatory for colorectal procedures requiring visualization of all four quadrants. A 5 mm laparoscope, when combined with a powerful light source and high-quality video camera, may be used in certain procedures such as diagnostic laparoscopy or stoma creation. We also recommend the 30° laparoscope, as opposed to the 0° laparoscope, as it provides an increased ability to view deeper structures [32]. The flexible laparoscope, originally developed for flexible endoscopy, is used by some laparoscopists. These laparoscopes offer more axis of rotation and flexion to possibly facilitate versatile viewing. The disadvantages of the flexible laparoscope include the requirement for an advanced operator and image degradation due to the deflected image in some systems. Its use is most applicable for single-port laparoscopy [31].

9.5.3.1 Two-Dimensional Vision

The standard for laparoscopic imaging is two-dimensional imaging. Two-dimensional imaging technology is well developed and has been available as long as laparoscopy has been utilized. The disadvantage of two-dimensional imaging is that the surgeon loses depth perception and spatial orientation [33]. Compared to standard laparotomy, laparoscopy using two-dimensional imaging requires the development of a special set of psychomotor skills to overcome the loss of depth perception and spatial orientation. The challenges of two-dimensional laparoscopy have been overcome through major advances in the development of brighter and higher-resolution images [34]. With experience, laparoscopic surgeons learn to compensate for the drawbacks of two-dimensional laparoscopy.

9.5.3.2 Three-Dimensional Vision

Three-dimensional technology for laparoscopic vision was introduced in the 1990s. The key to visual ergonomics of three-dimensional laparoscopy is to capture and magnify the small space of the abdominal cavity. The magnification in height and width of the intra-abdominal object is determined by the size of the three-dimensional monitor compared to the operative field. The magnification in depth is defined by the stereoptic ability of the camera, which records the left and right perspective. Most current three-dimensional systems (Storz, Schoelly/Intuitive Surgical/Aesculap) use a bichanneled laparoscope, in which imaging is obtained with a dual-lens system. Two separate lenses are present within a single laparoscope along with two cameras. Each camera captures their respective images, which are then displayed and synchronized on a video monitor. Currently, three-dimensional monitors are not commonly used in hospitals due to the ergonomic limitations, poor image resolution, the requirement to wear uncomfortable eyewear, and the high cost [33, 35].

9.5.4 Port Placement

Laparoscopic entry into the abdominal cavity can be performed via the closed (Veress) or open (Hasson) technique. We prefer the Hasson technique as it minimizes risk of injury to the peritoneal structures. A 12 mm vertical incision is made just below or above the umbilicus. An extension of this excision may be used for specimen extraction. The subcutaneous tissues are dissected to the level of the fascia. The fascia is grasped with Kocher clamps. Two anchoring sutures are placed on the lateral edges of the exposed fascia using 2–0 Vicryl to form handles for the Hasson trocar. A vertical fascial incision is made. The preperitoneal fat is spread to expose the peritoneum. The peritoneum is grasped with a smaller clamp and divided sharply, ensuring there is no exposed bowel. The 12 mm Hasson trocar is placed and secured using the anchor sutures. While the open approach to laparoscopic entry minimizes risk, there remains a risk of injury to any viscera that may be directly under the abdominal wall. This is especially true during reoperative surgery. The insufflation tube is attached and carbon dioxide pneumoperitoneum is established at a pressure of 15 mmHg. A 30° 10 mm camera is white balanced on a white surface and introduced into the abdominal cavity. A careful survey of the entire abdominal cavity is performed to note any adhesions or metastatic disease.

Port placement should be done carefully to allow for adequate triangulation of instruments and freedom of motion, unobstructed by the iliac spines and costal margins. Our preference is to place 10 mm trocars for all assistant ports to allow for flexibility of changing the laparoscope placement during the operation. A 10 mm right lower quadrant port should be placed about 2–3 cm medial and superior to the anterior superior iliac spine, while the 10 mm right upper quadrant port should be approximately 4–5 fingerbreadths superior to this. There should be a 1–2 cm margin between the right upper quadrant port and the lower ribs. A 10 mm left lower quadrant port, which should mirror image the right lower quadrant port, may be placed for the assistant (Fig. 9.6).

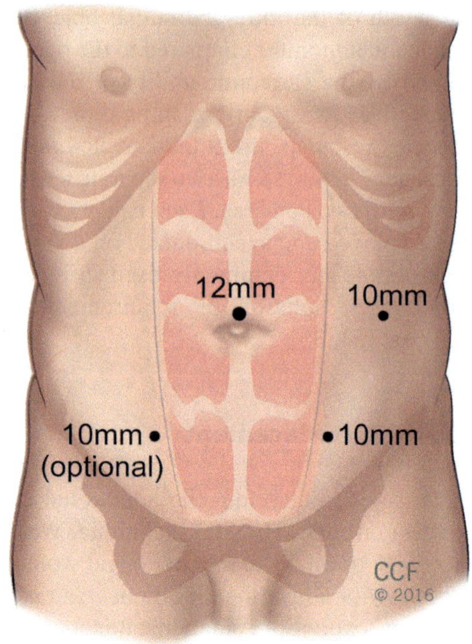

Fig. 9.6 Port placement. Reprinted with permission, Cleveland Clinic Center for Medical Art & Photography © 2003–2016. All Rights Reserved

9.5.5 Sigmoid and Descending Colon Mobilization

9.5.5.1 Medial to Lateral

The patient is placed in steep right-side-down and Trendelenburg position, allowing displacement of the omentum and small bowel loops to the right side of the abdomen and out of the pelvis. The left colon is grasped gently with 10 mm laparoscopic Babcock graspers, and traction is placed anteriorly. The IMA is identified and skeletonized cephalad to the left colic artery between 1.2 cm from th aorta. The IMA is then divided with a bipolar energy source. The bare area of the mesentery is divided toward the patient's head until the inferior mesenteric vein (IMV) is identified just lateral to the duodenum. The IMV is divided at the inferior edge of the pancreas and lateral aspect of the duodenum cephalad to the left colic vein (Fig. 9.7)**.** The colonic mesentery is dissected away from the retroperitoneum, ensuring the ureter is identified. This dissection is continued proximally and distally until the only remaining attachments are the lateral attachments to the abdominal sidewall, spleen, and omentum.

9.5.5.2 Lateral to Medial

The patient is placed in a steep right-side-down and Trendelenburg position, allowing displacement of the omentum and small loops to the right side of the abdomen and out of the pelvis. The left colon is gently grasped with nonlocking 10 mm laparoscopic Babcock graspers and medially and cranially retracted. The white line of Toldt in the left paracolic gutter is incised, and dissection is performed with the

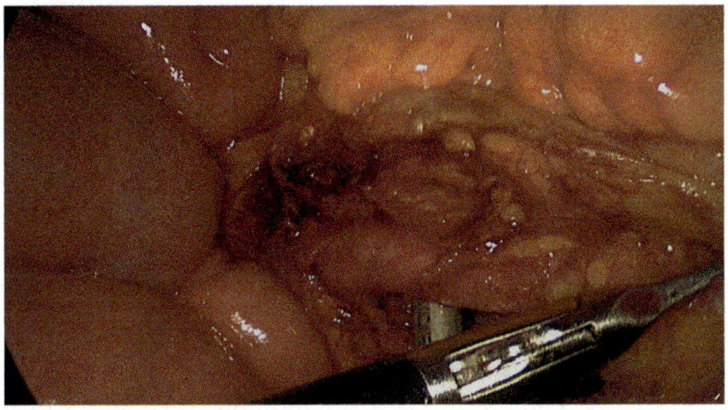

Fig. 9.7 Intraoperative photo of IMA and IMV branching from the aorta near the duodenum. P = pancreas, D = duodenum, IMV = inferior mesenteric vein

ultrasonic scalpel in the avascular plane between the mesocolon and retroperitoneum. Care must be taken so as not to dissect too laterally, therefore inadvertently mobilizing through or lateral to Gerota's fascia. Care must also be taken to stay in the plane anterior to the left ureter. This precaution helps ensure that the sigmoid mesentery is not entered and posteriorly lying small bowel is not injured. Mobilization is continued to the level of the root of the mesentery and the duodenum while continually identifying and protecting the left ureter.

9.5.6 Splenic Flexure Mobilization

The rationale for mobilizing the splenic flexure is to ensure adequate length of the proximal colon to perform a tension-free anastomosis. We routinely mobilize the splenic flexure during all operations for rectal cancer. Once the dissection is extended toward the splenic flexure as far as possible, the patient is repositioned in a reverse Trendelenburg position. The right-side-down position is maintained. The surgeon can stand between the patient's legs. The greater omentum is gently grasped, retracted anteriorly, and divided from the transverse colon. The lesser sac is entered by grasping the lesser omentum, retracting it anteriorly, and dividing it close to the transverse colon until the posterior aspect of the stomach is visualized. Once the lesser sac is opened, the first assistant standing on the left side of the patient can retract the transverse colon posteriorly while the surgeon uses the left hand grasper for anterior countertraction on the lesser omentum. A bipolar energy device in the right hand will divide the gastrocolic ligament, proceeding in an antegrade fashion. Care must be taken to avoid injuring the pancreatic tail, splenic vessels, and spleen [27, 36].

9.5.7 Rectal Mobilization

The patient is placed in a steep Trendelenburg position, and the small bowel and omentum are gently placed in the upper abdomen. The camera is directed toward the pelvis. Using an ultrasonic energy device, the avascular plane, between the mesorectum and the presacral fascia and posterior to the rectum, is entered [27]. This plane is entered by making a small incision in the line of reflection of the visceral peritoneum covering the right anterolateral aspect of the rectum and carried onto the parietal peritoneum lining the right pelvic wall [37]. Adequate proximal traction is retracting the rectum cranially and toward the left. Once the retrorectal space is entered, the right hypogastric nerve is identified anterior to the parietal fascia that lines the sacrum and lateral pelvic wall. The dissection proceeds anterior and medial to the nerve with the ultrasonic scalpel along the retrorectal space until the pelvic floor is identified. Maintaining the dissection in this avascular plane assures safety of the hypogastric nerve and presacral venous plexus [37]. The rectum is retracted anteriorly and toward the right to continue this dissection on the left posterior lateral aspect of the rectum. The lateral dissection may be the most difficult, as the plane between the mesorectum and endopelvic fascia is not as clear (Fig. 9.8a). The lateral ligaments and neurovascular bundle and middle hemorrhoidal artery (when present) are divided with the harmonic scalpel. Care must be taken to divide the ligaments and artery away from the parietal pelvic fascia, where injury to the sympathetic and parasympathetic plexus may result in urinary and sexual dysfunction [2, 3]. In thinner patients, the nervi erigentes may be seen running at the back of the lateral edge of the seminal vesicles, bladder neck, and prostate. If bleeding is encountered, the dissection is too medial in the mesorectum or lateral along the pelvic sidewall [2, 3]. During the lateral dissection, the ureters must once again be identified (Fig. 9.8b). Lateral dissection is facilitated by proper medial retraction. In our practice, we do not include a lateral lymph node dissection, as commonly performed in Japan. This resection increases surgical morbidity [2, 3].

Attention is then placed toward the anterior part of the rectum. In the line of reflection of the visceral peritoneum onto the back of the vagina or prostate, a small incision is made with the harmonic scalpel. The first assistant will place an open soft retractor (such as a bowel grasper or Babcock) on the vagina or Denonvilliers' fascia and place gentle anterior retraction. The anterior plane is developed as low as possible to allow full mobilization of the rectum down to its lower third portion, where perirectal fat is absent [37]. In males, adequate anterior retraction of Denonvilliers' fascia will allow the seminal vesicles to be separated from the mesorectum. In females, the first assistant may gently lift the uterus (if present) anteriorly to facilitate anterior rectal dissection. Retraction may be performed using the open jaws of a laparoscopic grasper, which simulates the use of a St. Mark's retractor in open surgery [2, 3]. Occasionally, retraction may require suspension of the uterus to the anterior abdominal wall using an extracorporeal suture with a straight Keith needle. An alternative is to use any curved needle that is introduced through a 10 mm trocar and used to suture through the uterine corpus or around the round ligaments in the avascular window just lateral to the uterus [27]. The principles of TME should be followed down to 1–2 cm distal to the tumor, but the mesorectal envelope should be mobilized to a level at least 5 cm distal to the distal edge of the tumor (Fig. 9.9).

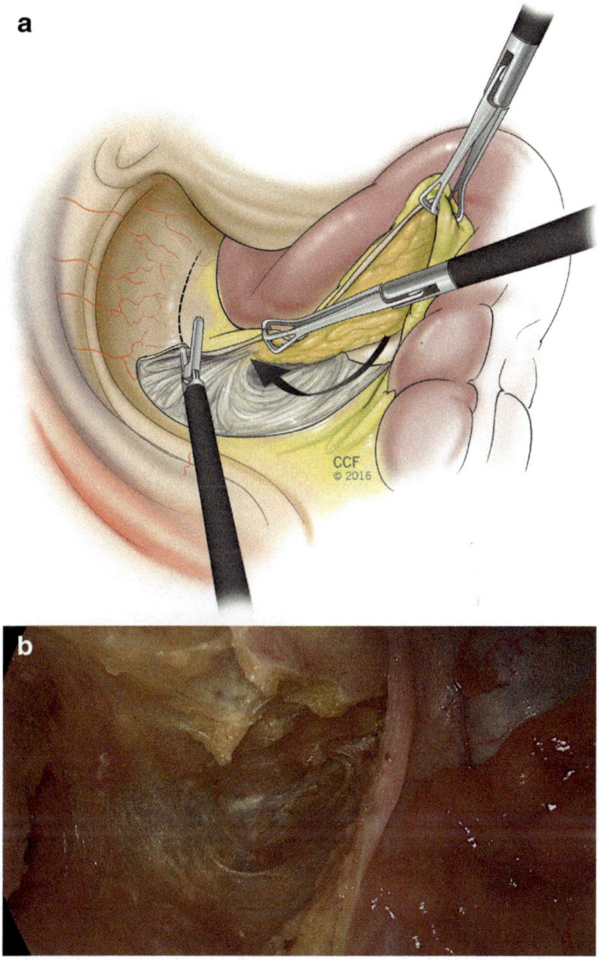

Fig. 9.8 (**a**) Areolar plane posterior to rectum during dissection. (**b**) Left ureter coursing lateral to rectum at level of iliac bifurcation. Reprinted with permission, Cleveland Clinic Center for Medical Art & Photography © 2003–2016. All Rights Reserved

9.5.8 Distal Rectal Transection

The rectum is clamped at the level of the desired transection, and an intraoperative flexible sigmoidoscopy is performed to confirm the distances from the dentate line and to the intended resection point and to the distal aspect of the tumor. Stapled transection of the distal rectum is performed using an articulating endoscopic stapler with a 3.5 mm staple height. More than one firing of the stapler should be avoided, as multiple stapler firings have been associated with anastomotic leaks. The stapler is usually articulated to create a perpendicular transection. The first assistant may elevate the anus to lift it and the distal rectum, facilitating placement of a straight staple line. The proximal colon is brought to the pelvis. The proposed level of proximal transection is identified, ensuring a tension-free anastomosis. Beginning proximally at the site of high ligation of the inferior mesenteric artery,

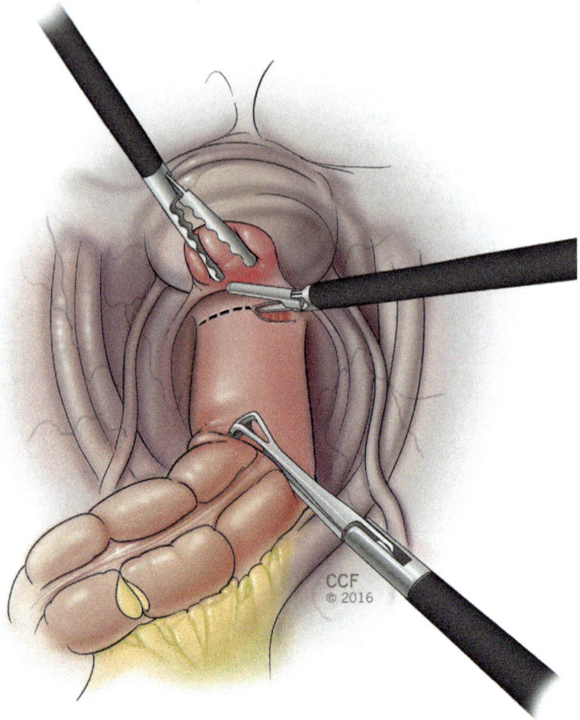

Fig. 9.9 Anterior retraction of the vagina (after hysterectomy) while incising the peritoneum. Reprinted with permission, Cleveland Clinic Center for Medical Art & Photography © 2003–2016. All Rights Reserved

the mesentery is transected with the bipolar device to the level of the descending and sigmoid colon junction. A suture or clip may be placed to mark the level. A locking laparoscopic clamp is placed on the distal specimen. The umbilical incision is extended to approximately 3 cm. Alternatively, a 3 cm left lower quadrant or Pfannenstiel incision can be made, or transanal specimen extraction may be performed. A wound protector is placed in the wound, and the distal specimen is delivered through the incision with the assistance of the clamped laparoscopic grasper. If a straight colorectal anastomosis is anticipated, the proximal level of transection is identified, ensuring the proximal colon reaches beyond the pubis extracorporeally to ensure a tension-free anastomosis. After division of the mesentery to the proximal margin of the colon, fluorescence imaging is used to confirm adequate mucosal perfusion to the proximal colonic margin of the anticipated anastomosis. This confirmation may be done by viewing the colon through an endoscopic fluorescence imaging infrared system after administration of intravenous indocyanine green by the anesthesiologist (Fig. 9.10). After satisfactory confirmation of blood supply, the proximal colon is clamped with a purse-string device after a purse-string suture is placed and the bowel is divided, the anvil of a circular 33 EEA™ stapler is secured in place. Care must be taken to ensure full-thickness bites with small amount of

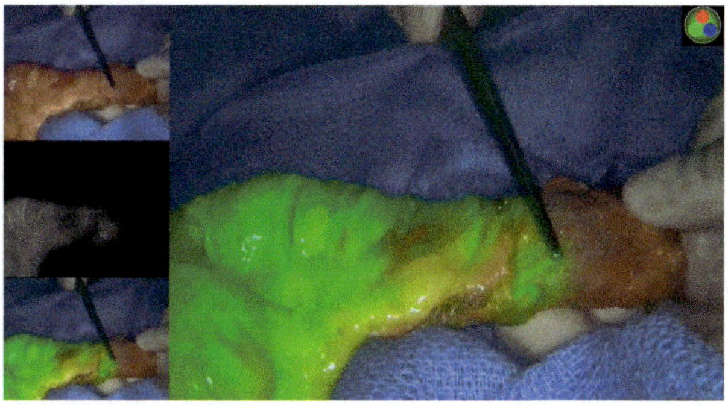

Fig. 9.10 Fluorescence imaging of colon prior to transection of proximal margin

mucosa are taken. The colon is prepared for the anastomosis by clearing the mesentery and the appendices epiploicae off the anvil. The proximal colon with the purse string and anvil returned to the abdominal cavity and pneumoperitoneum is reestablished. The wound protector cap with trocar facilitates reintroduction of pneumoperitoneum.

9.5.9 Stapled End-to-End Low Colorectal Anastomosis

After pneumoperitoneum is reestablished, the patient is positioned to steep Trendelenburg and left-side-up position; a circular 33 mm EEA™ stapler is introduced into the rectal remnant, gently dilating the muscles while communication is maintained between the surgeon and first assistant to ensure proper placement of the stapler. The spike of the stapler is slowly advanced through the rectal stump, preferably in the center near the staple line. Using an anvil grasper and an atraumatic grasper, the anvil is attached to the stapler, ensuring that the colon is properly oriented. The mesentery is proximally visualized to the level of the ligament of Treitz, ensuring that it is straight and without a 180 degree or 360 degree rotation. A digital examination of the vagina should be performed to insure the posterior wall is not included in the staple line. Indocyanine green perfusion assessment may be repeated prior to stapler firing. Under direct vision, the stapler is fired. The stapler is gently withdrawn from the rectum and proximal and distal "donuts" are inspected for completeness and sent to pathology. The pelvis is filled with saline, and routine intraoperative endoscopy is performed to both inspect the anastomosis for integrity and hemostasis and insufflate to perform an air leak test. The proximal colon should be gently occluded using an atraumatic grasper while performing the air leak test. If bubbles are encountered, options for remedy include suture repair or redoing the anastomosis. Indocyanine greek perfusion assessment is repeated with the custom designed rigid proctoscope and zero-degree near infrared light camera.

9.5.10 Anastomosis

9.5.10.1 Coloanal Anastomosis: Handsewn

A coloanal anastomosis may be performed using a handsewn technique. For this method, the rectum is not divided, although the mesentery is intracorporeally divided to the rectosigmoid junction. With the help of a Lonestar (TM) Cooper Surgical, Trumbull, CT device, an intersphincteric or submucosal dissection is performed from the perineum to enter the previously dissected retrorectal space. The rectum has been mobilized completely to the level of the dentate lane, and the specimen is extracted through the anus. The coloanal anastomosis is performed using interrupted 2–0 braided absorbable sutures, concomitantly transecting the proximal colon and performing the anastomosis one quadrant at a time to prevent proximal retraction of the colon (Fig. 9.11). Each subsequent suture is placed by bisecting the remainder of the anastomosis, ensuring evenly placed sutures. Alternatively, a circular-stapled anastomosis may be performed. Indocyanine green perfusion imaging is performed.

9.5.10.2 Coloanal Anastomosis: Double Stapled

A coloanal double-stapled anastomosis is performed by placing a purse-string suture in the proximal colon. The colon is pulled through the anus. The anvil of a 33 mm stapler is inserted, the suture is tied, and the colon is returned to the pelvis. A transanal purse-string suture is placed at the distal transection margin around the anal cuff. Under laparoscopic vision, the trocar is advanced through the anal cuff, and the suture is secured. The circular stapler and anvil are then re-engaged and the stapler is fired, carefully ensuring exclusion of the sphincter.

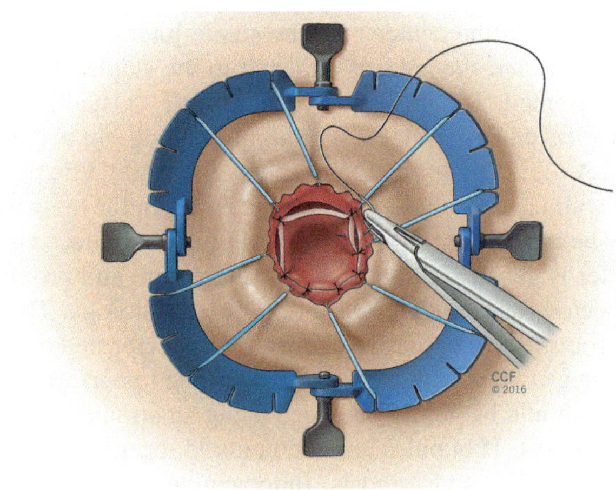

Fig. 9.11 Lonestar™ in place and placement of sutures during handsewn coloanal anastomosis. Reprinted with permission, Cleveland Clinic Center for Medical Art & Photography © 2003–2016. All Rights Reserved

9.5.10.3 Coloanal Anastomosis: Colonic J-Pouch Creation and Anastomosis

We prefer to use the colonic J-pouch as compared to straight anastomoses as it has better functional outcome, particularly relative to bowel frequency, urgency, fecal incontinence, and the use of antidiarrheal medications [38]. The relative superiority of a colonic J-pouch diminishes 2 years after surgery [38]. Coloplasty (longitudinal colostomy closed transversely) results in an increased number of anastomotic leaks in the perioperative period when compared to a colonic J-pouch and has been abandoned [38].

With the laparoscopic assisted technique, the colonic J-pouch is created extracorporeally after removal of the specimen and exteriorization of the proximal colonic staple line. A colonic J-pouch is created by folding a 6–8 cm portion of redundant colon back onto itself and creating a common channel using two firings of a 100 cm linear cutting stapler. Anastomosis of the colonic J-pouch to the anus is done from the apex of the J-pouch to the anus in a side-to-end manner using a 33 mm circular stapler in a similar fashion as described above. The same type of J-pouch and anastomosis can be transanally undertaken, either as a double-stapled, double purse-string, or handsewn anastomosis (Fig. 9.12).

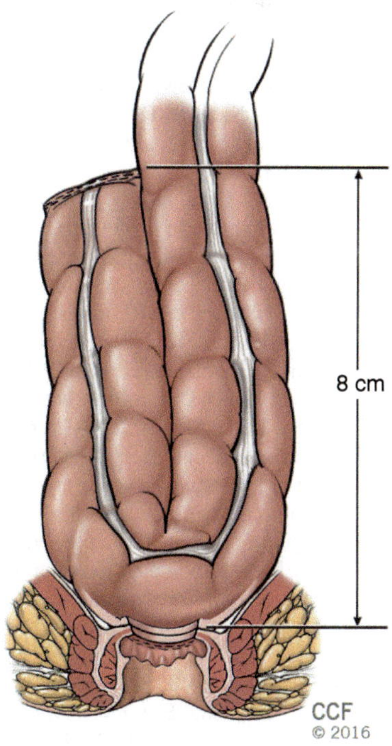

Fig. 9.12 Colonic J-pouch with measurements. Reprinted with permission, Cleveland Clinic Center for Medical Art & Photography © 2003–2016. All Rights Reserved

Creation of a diverting ileostomy is done according to the surgeon's preference. Accepted indications for fecal diversion following an LAR include colorectal anastomosis <610 cm, coloanal anastomosis, malnutrition, immunosuppression, hemodynamic instability, intraoperative blood loss, purulent peritonitis, pelvic sepsis, neoadjuvant chemotherapy, or a positive leak test [2, 3]. Additional risk factors include male gender, obesity, and multiple distal linear stapler firings. We routinely divert all high risk low anterior and low coloanal anastomoses.

References

1. Jacobs M, Verdeja JC, Goldstein HS. Minimally invasive colon resection (laparoscopic colectomy). Surg Laparosc Endosc. 1991;1(3):144–50.
2. Cologne KG, Senagore AJ. Development of Minimally invasive colorectal surgery: History, evidence, learning curve, and current adaptation. In: Bardakciglu O, editor. Advanced techniques in Minimally invasive and robotic colorectal surgery. New York, NY: Springer; 2015. p. 3–6.
3. Cologne KG, Senagore AJ. Proctectomy and rectopexy: laparoscopic approach. In: Bardakicioglu O, editor. Advanced techniques in minimally invasive and robotic colorectal surgery. New York, NY: Springer; 2015. p. 151–62.
4. Lau WY, Leow C, Li AK. Surgical history: history of endoscopic and laproscopic surgery. World J Surg. 1997;21:444–53.
5. Champagne BJ. Management of rectal cancer. In: Bailey R, editor. Colorectal surgery. Philadelphia, PA: Elsevier Saunders; 2013.
6. Pollett WG, Nicholls RJ. The relationship between the extent of distal clearance and survival and local recurrence rates after curative anterior resection for carcinoma of the rectum. Ann Surg. 1983;198:159–63.
7. Phillips RK, Hittinger R, Blesovsky L, Fry JS, Fielding LP. Local recurrence following curative surgery for large bowel cancer: the overall picture. Br J Surg. 1984;71:6–12.
8. Quirke P, Durdey P, Dixon MF, Williams NS. Local recurrence of rectal adenocarcinoma due to inadequate surgical resection. Lancet. 1986;328:996–9.
9. Williams NS, Dixon MF, Johnston D. Reappraisal of the 5 centimeter rule of distal excision due to inadequate surgical resection. Br J Surg. 1983;70(3):150–4.
10. Monson JRT, Weiser MR, Buie WD, et al. Practice parameters for the Management of Rectal Cancer (revised). Dis Colon Rectum. 2013;56(5):535–50.
11. Bernstein TE, Endreseth BH, Romundstad P, Wibe A. Norweigian colorectal cancer registry. What is a safe distal resection margin in rectal cancer patients treated by low anterior resection without preoperative radiotherapy? Color Dis. 2012;14(2):e48–55.
12. Fitzgerald TL, Brinkley J, Zervos EE. Pushing the envelope beyond a centimter in rectal cancer: oncologic implications of close, but negative margins. J Am Coll Surg. 2011;213(5):589–95.
13. Bokey EL. Carcinoma of the rectum. In: Corman RB, Corman ML, editors. Corman's colon and rectal surgery, Sixth Edition. 6th ed. Philadelphia, PA: Lippincott Williams and Wilkins; 2013.
14. Heald RJ, Ryall R. Recurrent cancer after restorative resection of the rectum. Br Med J (Clin Res Ed). 1982;284:826–7.
15. Heald RJ, Husband EM, Ryall RD. The mesorectum in rectal cancer surgery- the clue to pelvic recurrence? Br J Surg. 1982;69(10):613–6.
16. Martling AL, Holm T, Rutqvist LE, Moran BJ, Heald RJ, Cedemark B. Effect of surgical training programme on outcome of rectal cancer in the county of Stockholm. Stockholm colorectal cancer study group, Basingstoke bowel cancer research project. Lancet. 2000;356(9224):93–6.
17. Enker WE, Thaler HT, Cranor ML, Polyak T. Total mesorectal excision in the operative treatment of carcnoma of the rectum. J Am Coll Surg. 1995;181(4):335–46.
18. Hill GL, Rafique M. Extrafascial excision of the rectum for rectal cancer. Br J Surg. 1998;85(6):809–12.

19. Killingback M, Barron P, Dent OF. Local recurrence after curative resection of cancer of the rectum without total mesorectal excision. Dis Colon Rectum. 1991;44(4):473–83. discussion 483-486
20. Lindsey I, Mortensen NJ. Iatrogenic impotance and rectal dissection. Br J Surg. 2002;89(12):1493–4.
21. Moriya Y, Sugihara K, Akasu T, Fujita S. Nerve-sparing surgery with lateral node dissectoin for advanced low rectal cancer. Eur J Cancer. 1995;31A(7–8):1229–32.
22. Nagtegaal ID, van de Velde CJ, van der Worp E, Kapiteijn E, Quirke P, van Krieken JH. Cooperative clinical investigators of the Dutch colorectal cancer group. Macroscopic evaluation of rectal cancer resection specimen: clinical signifiance of the pathologist in quality control. J Clin Oncol. 2002;20:1729–34.
23. Goldstein NS. Lymph node recoveries from 2427 pT3 colorectal resection specimens spanning 45 yearsL recommendations for a minimum number of recovered lymph nodes based on predictive probabilities. Am J Surg Pathol. 2002;26(2):179–89.
24. Le Voyer TE, Sigurdson ER, Hanlon AL, Mayer RJ, Macdonald JS, Catalano PJ, Haller DG. Colon Cancer survival is associated with increasing number of lymph nodes analyzed: a second survey of intergroup trial INT-0089. J Clin Oncol. 2003;21:2912–9.
25. Araghizadeh F, Abdelnaby A. Anatomy and physiology. In: Bailey R, editor. Colorectal surgery. Philadelphia, PA: Elsevier Saunders; 2013.
26. Jorge J, Habr-Gama A. Anatomy and embryology. In: Beck DE, Roberts PL, editors. The ASCRS Textbook of colon and rectal surgery. 2nd ed. New York, NY: Springer; 2011.
27. Bashankaev B, Seo C, Wexner SD. Laproscopic low anterior resection. In: Wexner SD, Fleshman JW, editors. Master techniques in general surgery: colon and rectal surgery, abdominal operations. Philadelphia, PA: Lippincott Williams and Wilkins; 2012.
28. Landmann RG. Intersphincteric restorative proctocolectomy for malignant disease. In: Wexner SD, Fleshman JW, editors. Master technicques in general surgery: colon and rectal surgery, abdominal operations. Philadelphia, PA: Lippincott Williams and Wilkins; 2012.
29. Taffinder N, Smith SG, Huber J, Russell RC, Darzi A. The effect of a second-generation 3D endoscope on the laparoscopic precision of novices and experienced surgeons. Surg Endosc. 1999;13(11):1087–92.
30. Wilhelm D, Reiser S, Kohn N, Witte M, Leiner U, Muhlbach L, et al. Comparitive evaluation of HD 2D/3D laparoscopic monitors and benchmarking to a theoretical ideal 3D psuedodisplay: even well-experienced laparoscopists. Surg Endosc. 2014;28(8):2387–97.
31. Schwaitzberg SD. Imaging systems in minimially invasive surgery. In: Swantstrom LL, Soper NJ, editors. Mastery of endoscopic and laparoscopic surgery. Philadelphia, PA: Lippincott Williams and Wilkins; 2014. p. 47–61.
32. Nakajima K, Milsom JW, Bohm B. Equipment and instrumentation. In: Laparoscopic colorectal surgery. 2nd ed. New York, NY: Springer; 2006. p. 10–30.
33. Sorenson SM, Savran MM, Konge L, Bjerrum F. Three-dimensional versus two-dimensional vision in laparoscopy: a systematic review. Surg Endosc. 2016;30:11–23. ebut ahead of print
34. Wagner OJ, Hagen M, Kurmann A, Horgan S, Candinas D, Vorburger SA. Three-dimensional vision enhances task performance independently of the surgical method. Surg Endosc. 2012;26:2961–8.
35. Kunert W, Storz P, Kirschniak A. For 3D laparoscopy: a step toward advanced surgical navigation: how to get maximum benefit from 3D vision. Surg Endosc. 2013;27:696–9.
36. Bergamaschi RC, Larach SW, Pigazzi A, Marecik S, Valsdottir EB, Amrani S. Laparoscopic Colon and Rectal surgery. In: Corman ML, Bergamaschi RC, Nicholls RJ, Fazio VW, editors. Corman's colon and rectal surgery. 6th ed. Philadelphia, PA: Lippincott Williams and Wilkins; 2013.
37. Bleday R. Surgical treatment of rectal cancer. In: Beck DE, Roberts PL, Saclarides TJ, Senagore AJ, Stamos MJ, Wexner SD, editors. The ASCRS textbook of colon and rectal surgery. 2nd ed. New York, NY: Springer; 2011.
38. Brown CJ, Fenech D, McLeod RS. Reconstructive techniques after rectal resction for rectal cancer. Cochrane Database Syst Rev. 2008;16(2):CD006040.

Part II

Abdominal Laparoscopy and Robot-Assisted

Multiport Laparoscopic TME with Low Colorectal Anastomosis

10

Guy-Bernard Cadière

Abstract

Rectal cancer surgery has to be performed with total mesorectal excision.

Since the advent of minimally invasive surgery, nowadays, different techniques have been described. In this chapter the codified conventional laparoscopic technique with circular mechanical low colorectal anastomosis is described in step-by-step.

Keywords

Laparoscopic total mesorectal excision • Laparoscopy • TME • Rectal cancer • Minimal invasive surgery • Rectal surgery

10.1 Introduction

Rectal surgery has to be performed with total mesorectal excision (TME) [1]. There are two tricky dissections during TME. The first one is the opening of the presacral space, posteriorly [2]. The second one is the opening of the retrovesical space, anteriorly, which partly includes the Denonvilliers fascia, resected in its cranial position.

Anterior dissection: The incision of the peritoneal sheet starts 1 cm above the reflection of the Douglas pouch. This last one is held by atraumatic graspers in a way to allow the dissection of the retrovesical posteriorly to the seminal vesicle. The dissection continues anteriorly to the Denonvilliers fascia, dividing the adhesions crossing the retrovesical space. The Denonvilliers fascia is transected in an

G.-B. Cadière, M.D., Ph.D.
Department of Gastrointestinal Surgery, European School of Laparoscopic Surgery, Saint-Pierre University Hospital, 322, Rue Haute, 1000 Brussels, Belgium
e-mail: guy-bernard_cadiere@stpierre-bru.be

G. Dapri, J.H. Marks (eds.), *Surgical Techniques in Rectal Cancer*, https://doi.org/10.1007/978-4-431-55579-7_10

arc-shaped fashion 1 cm more distally to avoid, laterally, the section of the sacral (S2, S3) and hypogastric nerves.

Posterior dissection: The dissection starts with the incision of the peritoneal sheet 1 cm above the promontory, with the assistant holding tightly the rectum upward. The plane of dissection which opens naturally is the wrong one and leads to hemorrhage and hypogastric nerve lesions. It is mandatory to make an active dissection to find the right plane to get into, which generally corresponds to the vision of a different fat. The dissection ends when the levator muscles and internal sphincter comes up to your view.

10.2 Technique

10.2.1 Patient Positioning and Operative Setup

Patient is placed in a dorsal decubitus legs apart, left leg bent under a 40° flexion and right leg without flexion to keep the field free for the right hand movement of the surgeon. Surgeon stands on the right side of the patient with the camera assistant on the left side, the scrub nurse on the right side, and the assistant on the patient's left side. Surgeon's eyes, operative field (left colon), and the screen are on the same line (Fig. 10.1).

Pneumoperitoneum is obtained thanks to a Veress needle inserted in the left hypochondrium. This allows a safe approach as you are away from main anatomical structures.

Five trocars are needed:

- 11 mm in the umbilicus (place the optical trocar a bit above if the patient is small to avoid conflict with other instruments).
- 5 mm on the left flank for the exposition instrument managed by the assistant.

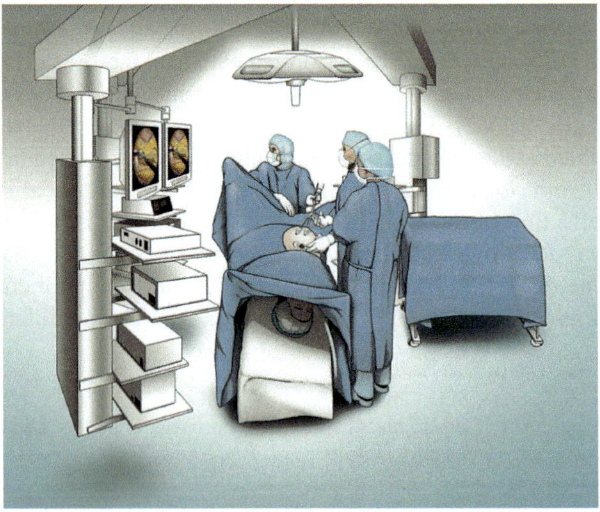

Fig. 10.1 Patient Positioning and Operative Setup

Fig. 10.2 Trocars disposition

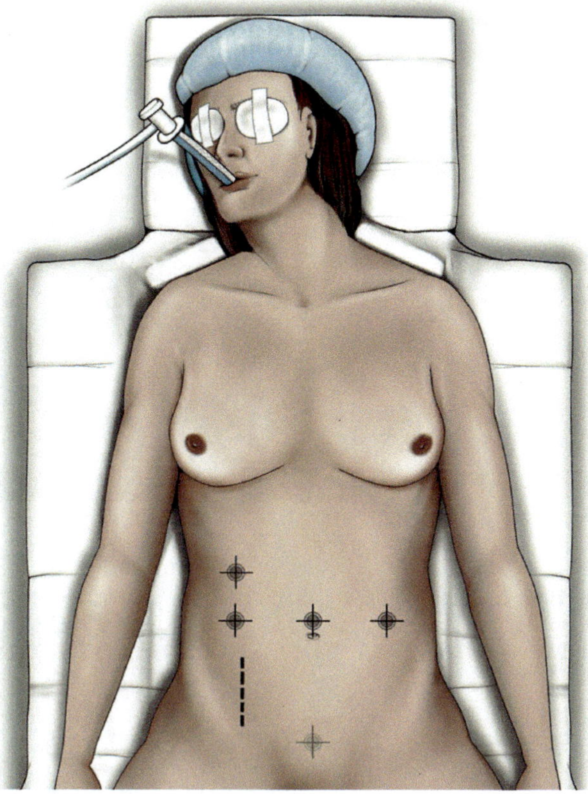

- 5 mm on the right flank for the left hand of the surgeon (as low as possible to avoid conflict with optical system but not too low to not get too tangentially on the operative field).
- 5 mm trocar in the right iliac fossa for the right hand of the surgeon.
- 12 mm trocar will later be inserted in the Pfannenstiel incision or replace the 5 mm trocar in the right iliac fossa to pass the stapler (Fig. 10.2).

10.2.2 Exposure

Patient is placed in a Trendelenburg position of at least 30° with a semilateral decubitus to the right (Fig. 10.3).

The first step of the operation is the clearing of the left colon view by pulling gently with atraumatic graspers the jejunum and the ileum in the right hypochondrium above the liver. This maneuver is facilitated by the Trendelenburg position of the patient (Fig. 10.4).

We should now be able to have our important surgical landmarks: the aorta with the emerging inferior mesenteric artery and the iliac bifurcation, the inferior mesenteric vein, the promontory, and the colorectal transition (Fig. 10.5).

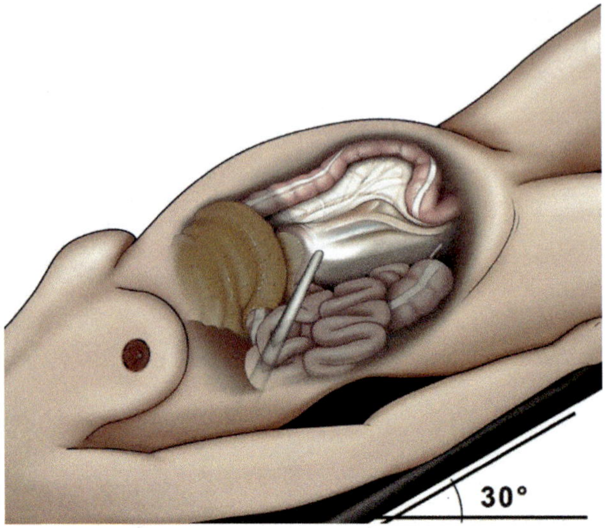

Fig. 10.3 Exposure of the left mesocolon

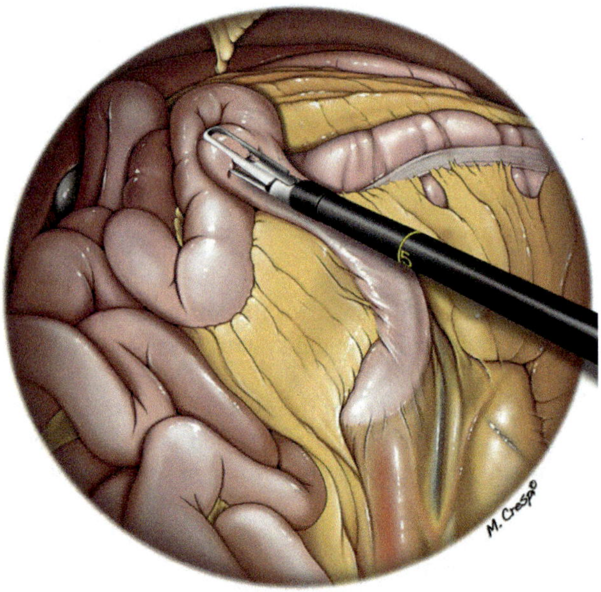

Fig. 10.4 Placement of the small bowel above the left liver

10.2.3 Dissection of Presacral Space

The dissection starts with the incision of the peritoneal sheet 1 cm above the promontory, with the assistant holding tightly the rectum upward. The plane of dissection which opens naturally is the wrong one and leads to hemorrhage and hypogastric nerve injury. It is mandatory to make an active dissection to find the right plane

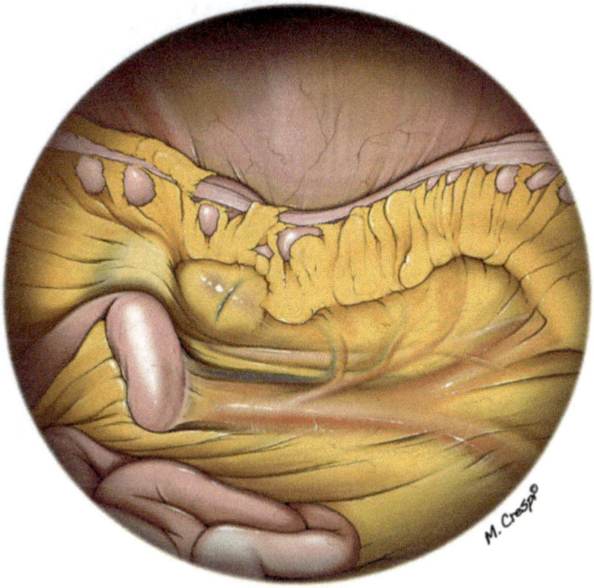

Fig. 10.5 Important surgical landmarks

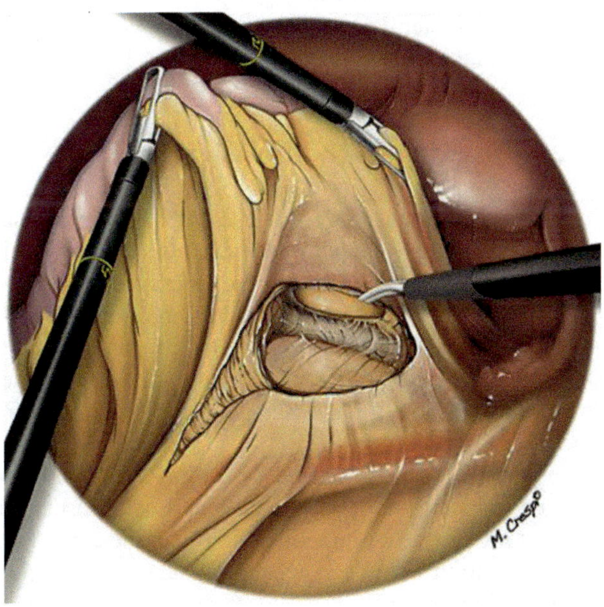

Fig. 10.6 Dissection of the fascia perirecti

(fascia perirecti) to get into, which generally corresponds to the vision of a different fat (Fig. 10.6).

This part might be tricky as you have to follow the plane covering the sacrum, the piriformis muscle, the coccygeal muscle, and finally the levator muscles without entering it as it contains presacral veins and hypogastric plexus and laterally the ureters.

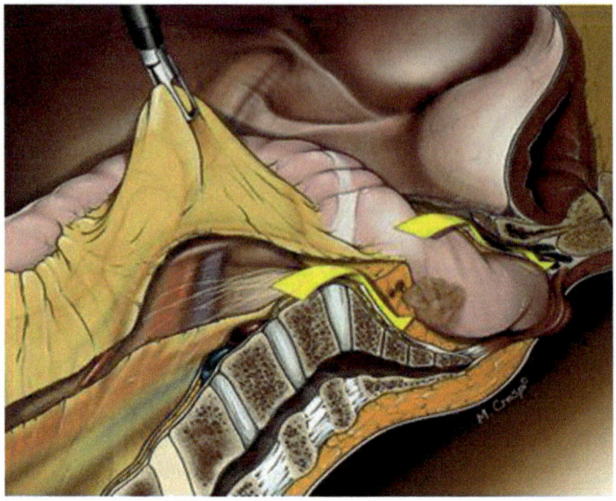

Fig. 10.7 Dissection of presacral space

Thanks to high pressure insufflation (14–15 mmHg), once inside the good plane, little coagulation is needed as you can dissect by gently pulling upward and laterally the rectum and its meso with a grasper.

The posterolateral dissection ends when you reached the levator muscles and the internal sphincter (Fig. 10.7).

10.2.4 Dissection of Retrovesical Space

The second important step is the opening of the retrovesical space, anteriorly, which partly includes the Denonvilliers fascia, resected in its cranial position. The dissection can be tricky as you might dissect to anteriorly in the seminal vesicle plane.

The incision of the peritoneal sheet starts 1 cm above the reflection of the Douglas pouch. This last one is held by atraumatic graspers in a way to allow the dissection of the retrovesical posteriorly to the seminal vesicle. The dissection continues anteriorly to the Denonvilliers fascia, dividing the adhesions crossing the retrovesical space (Fig. 10.8).

The dissection is facilitated by pulling upward the retrovesical fascia with the assistant grasper and downward the perirectal fascia with your left hand grasper, and then proceed to a blunt dissection with the curved side of your hook with minimal coagulation till you reach the plane of the levator muscles and the internal sphincter (Fig. 10.9).

The circumferential resection of the mesorectum should be complete and straightforward without coning, no bulk and no visualization of the muscularis propria. The circumferential resection is the most important factor to prevent

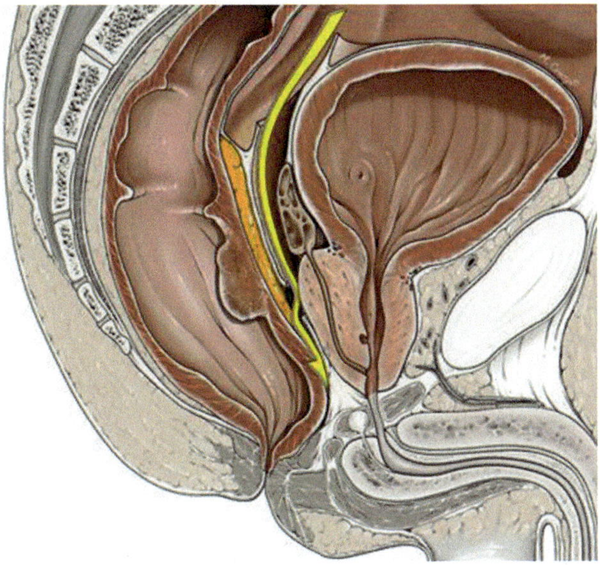

Fig. 10.8 Dissection of retrovesical space

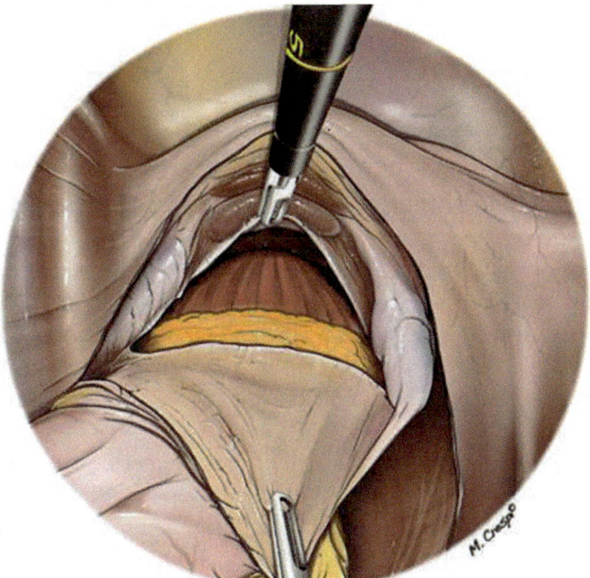

Fig. 10.9 Dissection of retrovesical space

local recurrence more than distal margins which have been shown now to be correct around 2 cm or less as the intramural dissemination rarely exceeds 2 cm (Fig. 10.10).

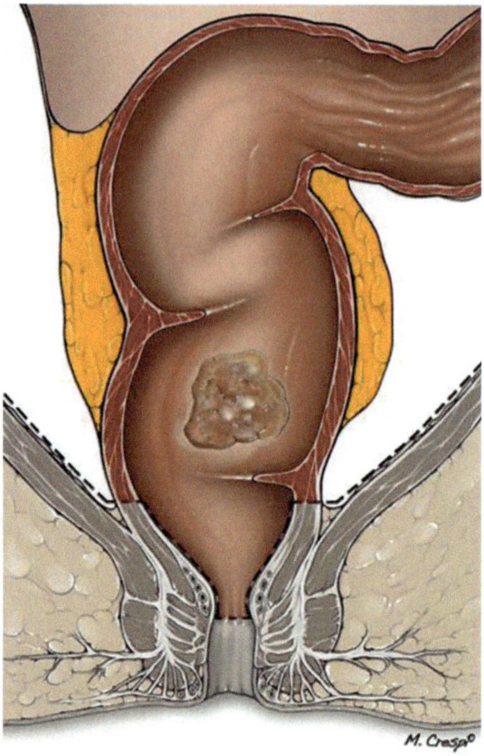

Fig. 10.10 Carcinologic rules

10.2.5 Mobilization of Descending Colon and Vascular Dissection

We now have to proceed to the mobilization of the descending colon and the splenic flexure if necessary as our goal is a tension-free anastomosis. To do so we incise the leaflet following a line along the aorta until we reach the angle of Treitz (Fig. 10.11).

While making the incision with the hook, care must be taken not to shave the aorta as the hypogastric plexus are running down anteriorly and laterally along the aorta (Fig. 10.12).

The dissection under the inferior mesenteric vein at its emergence from the inferior edge of the pancreas allows us to separate the Toldt's fascia (Fig. 10.13).

The assistant lifts up the inferior mesenteric vein and a blunt dissection progressively lower the Toldt's fascia which is recognizable by a white line at its reflection with the mesocolon. Care must be taken not to go too deep so as to not enter the Zuckerkandel fascia which contains the ureter. The dissection is done medially to laterally. A tent is slowly created. The tip of it is held by the assistant's grasper. We then dissect the inferior mesenteric artery at its emergence, clip it, and section it, but if the sigmoid is long enough, a preservation of the left colic artery is another option as there is no oncologic concern in this dissection (Fig. 10.14).

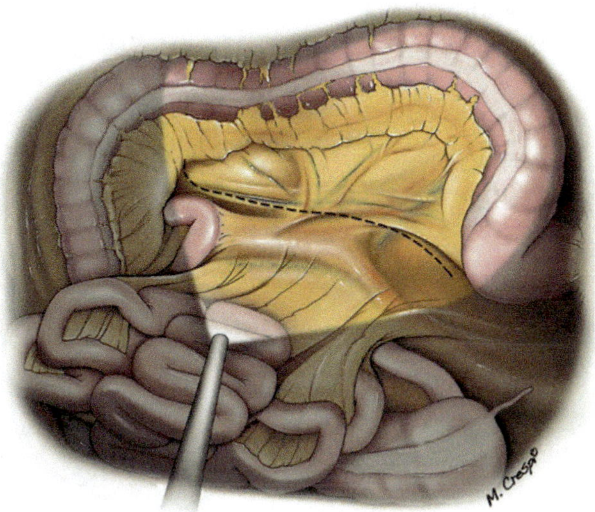

Fig. 10.11 Mobilization of the descending colon

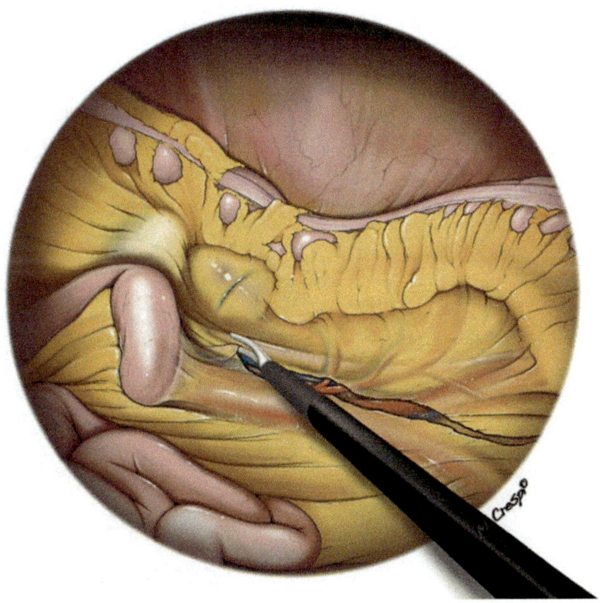

Fig. 10.12 Mobilization by medial to lateral approach

We then incise the left parietocolic gutter along our mesocolon to join our Toldt's fascia and our previous dissection (Fig. 10.15).

This way the colon should be able to be pulled down without any tension. In case not, additional severance of adhesions or mobilization of the splenic flexure is performed.

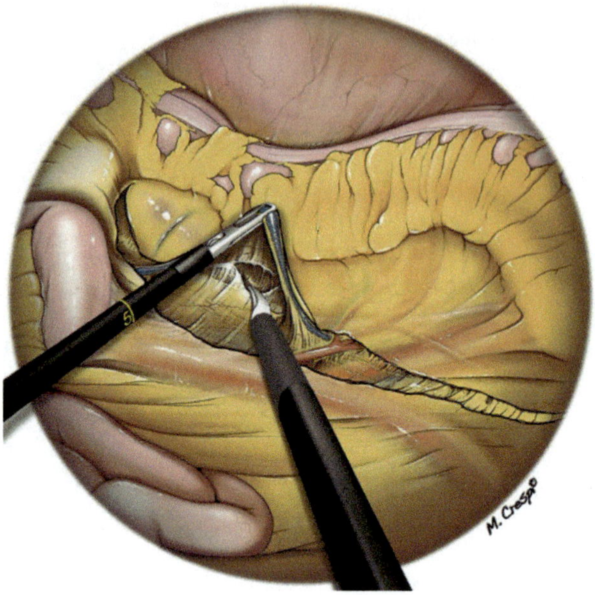

Fig. 10.13 Dissection of the Toldt's fascia

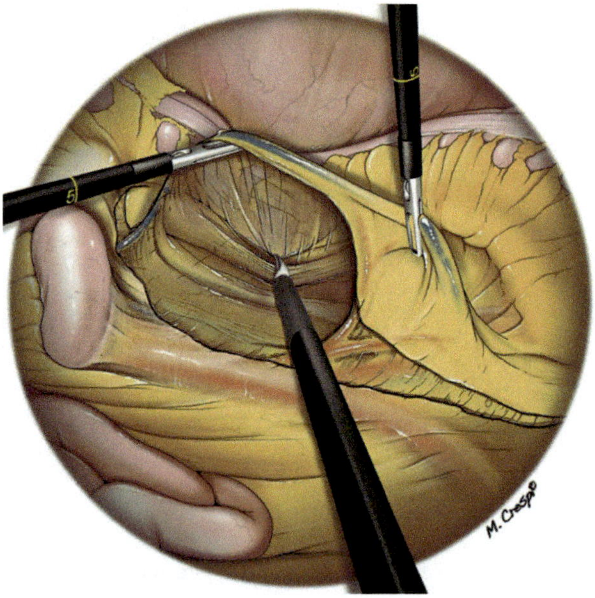

Fig. 10.14 Opening of the Toldt's fascia

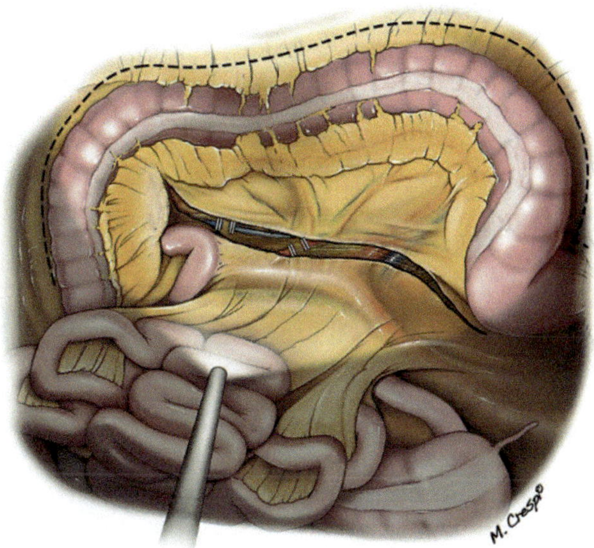

Fig. 10.15 Dissection of the left gutter

10.2.6 Rectal Transection and Specimen Extraction

The 12 mm trocar is inserted in the Pfannenstiel incision for the linear satpler. Since the axis of the colon and stapling device are not perpendicular to each other, this step can actually be quite difficult. Usually, several firings of the stapler are needed. Again the distal margins do not have to exceed 2 cm (Fig. 10.16).

The final view of the dissection shows a total resection of the mesorectum with a preservation of the sacral and hypogastric nerves and the elevator muscles on the bottom of the pelvis (Fig. 10.17).

A minilaparotomy is performed suprapubically on the midline by enlarging the stapler orifice. A wound protector is used. The bowel is extirpated and transected proximally.

10.2.7 Anastomosis

The anvil of the stapler is introduced inside the bowel and a pursestring performed in the usual fashion. The proximal colon is now ready for anastomosis and is reintroduced inside the abdomen. The minilaparotomy incision is closed hermetically in layers.

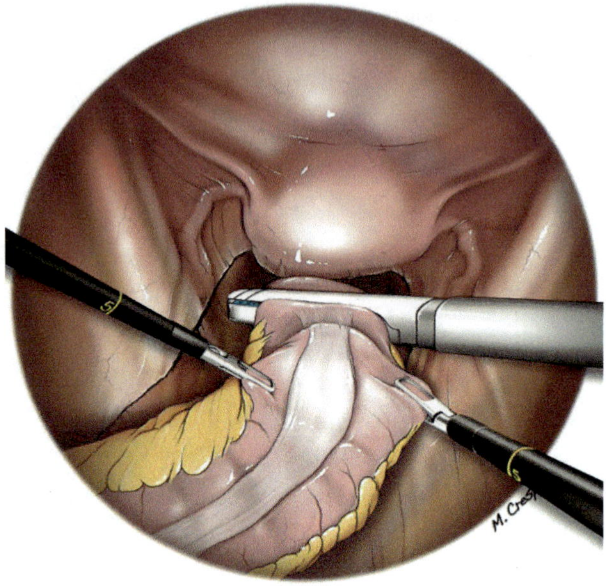

Fig. 10.16 Section of rectum

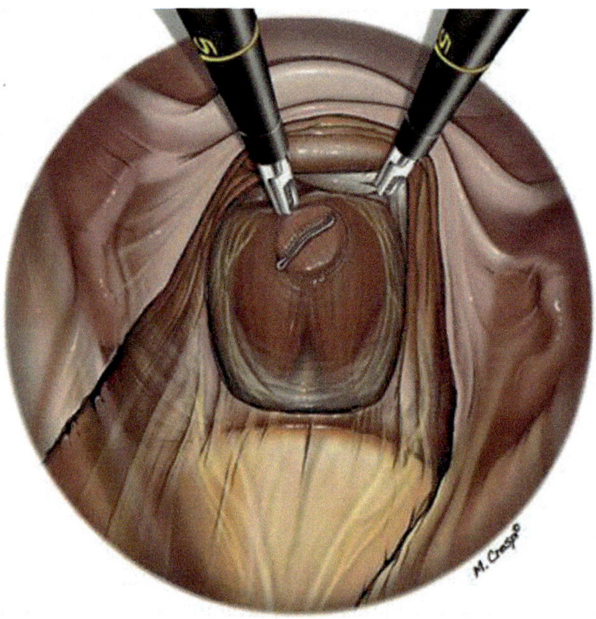

Fig. 10.17 Final view after resection of rectum

The colorectal anastomosis is performed as usual after transanal introduction of the circular stapler after checking the absence of rotation from the proximal colon (Figs. 10.18 and 10.19).

An air leak test is then performed and an external drainage is left in place (Fig. 10.20).

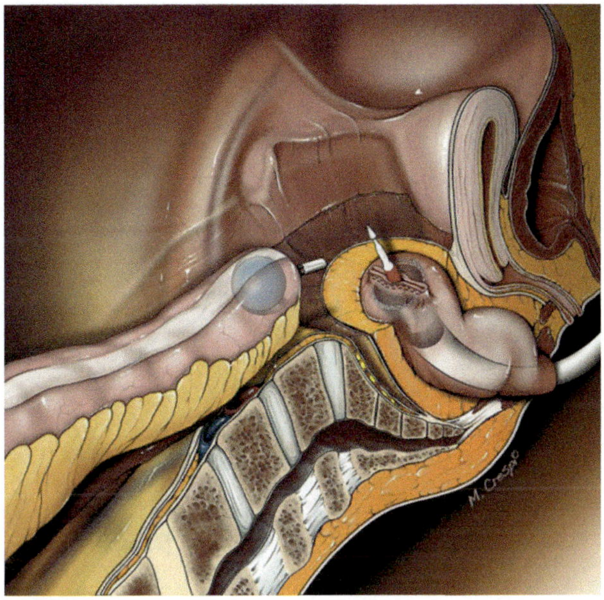

Fig. 10.18 Circular mechanical colorectal anastomosis

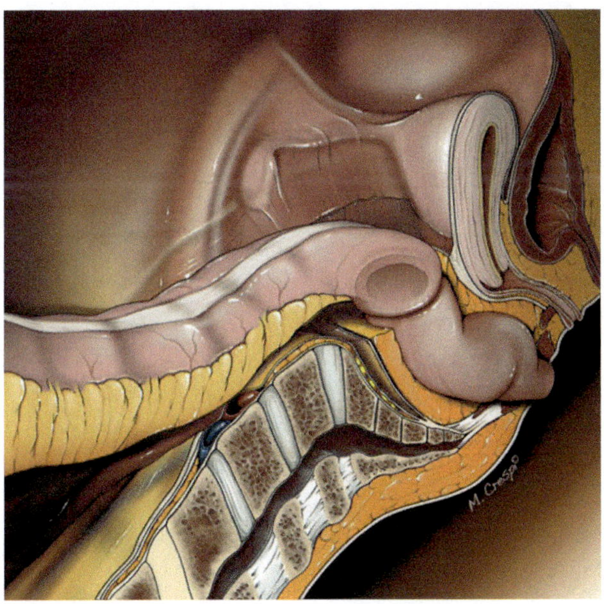

Fig. 10.19 Circular mechanical colorectal anastomosis

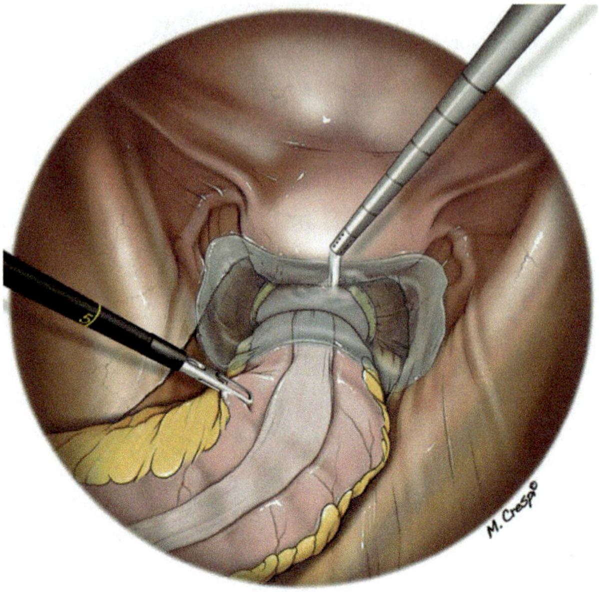

Fig. 10.20 Air leak test

References

1. Heald RJ. A new approach to rectal cancer. Br J Hosp Med. 1979;22(3):277–81.
2. Heald RJ. The 'Holy Plane' of rectal surgery. J R Soc Med. 1988;81(9):503–8.

Reduced Port Laparoscopic TME with Low Colorectal Anastomosis

11

Yasumitsu Hirano

Abstract

Recently, reduced port laparoscopic surgery (RPLS) including single-incision laparoscopic surgery (SILS) has been developed in many surgical procedures. However, rectal SILS is rare in colorectal lesions because of the difficulty to transect the lower rectum with sufficient distal margins from the umbilicus port with appropriate number of stapler firings. We have developed reduced port laparoscopic (SILS + 1 port) total mesenteric excision (TME) (RPLS-TME) in which we utilize the incision for pelvic drainage as an additional access route of the linear stapler at the transection of the lower rectum. A 2.5-cm transumbilical incision is made. A Lap protector is inserted through this incision, and the wound is protected. Next, an EZ-access is mounted, and three ports are placed. A 12-mm port is inserted in the right lower quadrant. All RPLS-TME procedures are performed with surgical techniques similar to those in our standard laparoscopic procedures. In this chapter, we explain how to perform our reduced port laparoscopic TME with low colorectal anastomosis for rectal cancer safely and reliably.

Keywords

Reduced port laparoscopic surgery • Total mesenteric excision • Single-incision laparoscopic surgery • Rectal cancer

Y. Hirano, M.D., Ph.D.
Department of Surgery, Mizonokuchi Hospital, Teikyo University School of Medicine, 5-1-1 Futago, Takatsu-ku, Kawasaki 213-8507, Japan
e-mail: yasumitsuhirano@gmail.com

G. Dapri, J.H. Marks (eds.), *Surgical Techniques in Rectal Cancer*,
https://doi.org/10.1007/978-4-431-55579-7_11

11.1 Introduction

Many surgeons have attempted to reduce the number and size of ports in laparoscopic surgery to decrease parietal trauma and improve cosmetic results; single-incision laparoscopic surgery (SILS) has been developed as the ultimate reduced port laparoscopic surgery (RPLS), which completed laparoscopic procedures by trocars located at one umbilical incision. However, the published studies of the SILS for colon and rectal surgery have limited almost in the right [1, 2] and sigmoid [3] colon, and the data in the literature about rectal SILS is sparse. This is mainly because the tip of the laparoscopic stapler is able to bend only 45 degrees in maximum which makes it very difficult to transect the lower rectum with sufficient distal margins from the umbilicus port with an appropriate number of staplers.

We routinely use pelvic drain as an early detector of anastomotic leaks and reduce the need for reoperation in selected patients undergoing rectal cancer surgery. Therefore in patients of lower rectal cancer, the small incision is required in the right or left lower quadrant of the abdomen for drainage. To utilize this incision, we have developed reduced port laparoscopic (SILS + 1 port) total mesenteric excision (TME) in which we use this incision as an additional access route for the linear stapler to transect the lower rectum [4]. This technique makes it possible to transect the lower rectum with one or two firings of laparoscopic stapler and brought us excellent outcomes. Furthermore, this incision is also used as the trocar for the operator's right-handed instrument which may decrease the conflict between the operative instruments and the camera caused by the limited space resulting from using only a single incision. In this chapter, we explain how to perform our reduced port laparoscopic TME with low colorectal anastomosis for rectal cancer safely and reliably.

11.2 Indications and Contraindications

Indication of this procedure is the rectal cancer that oncologically needs total mesenteric excision. Advanced T4 tumor, perforated tumor, stenosis with bowel distension, and severe comorbidity are contraindications.

11.3 Technique

11.3.1 Patient and Team Positioning

Under general anesthesia, the patient is placed on the operating table between side supports mounted on the table. The patient's arms are spread, and the feet are placed in boot-type leg holders with the legs spread apart and knees slightly flexed (Fig. 11.1). The surgeon and camera assistant stand at the patient's right side. The scrub nurse stands on the surgeon's right (Fig. 11.2a). The video monitor is placed on the left (Fig. 11.2b).

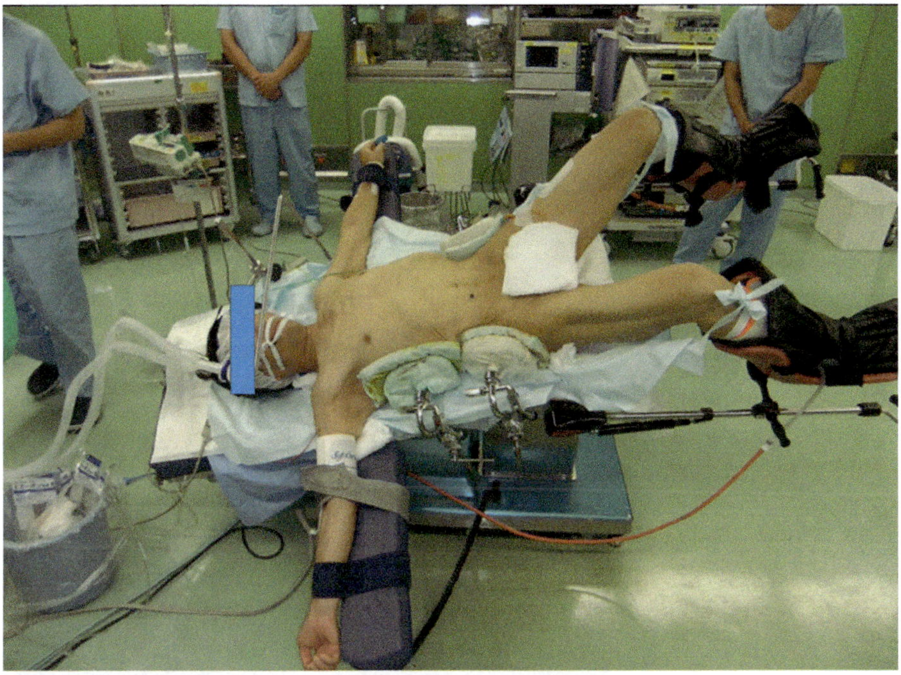

Fig. 11.1 Patient positioning

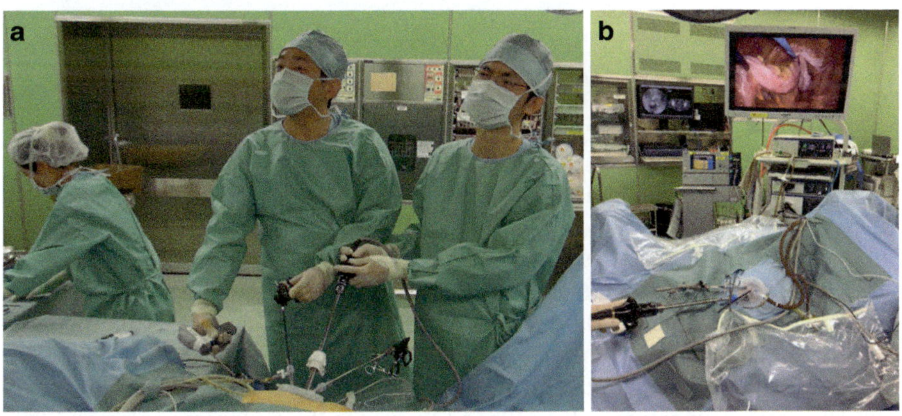

Fig. 11.2 (**a**) Positioning of the surgeon and assistant. (**b**) The video monitor is placed on the left

11.3.2 Port Position

First, a 2.5-cm transumbilical incision is made. A Lap protector (LP; Hakko Co., Nagano, Japan) is inserted through this incision (Fig. 11.1a), and the wound is protected. Next, an EZ access (Hakko Co., Nagano, Japan) is mounted to LP (Fig. 11.3), and one 12-mm port and two 5-mm ports are placed in EZ access. A 12-mm port is inserted in the right lower quadrant (Fig. 11.4).

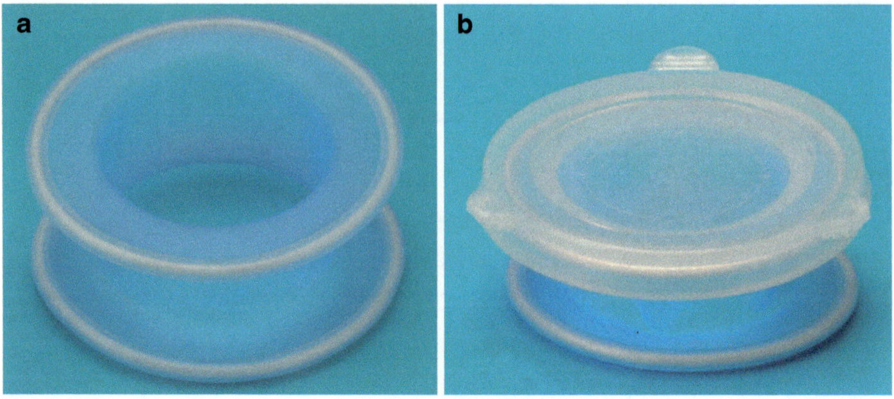

Fig. 11.3 The Lap protector FF10 (**a**) and EZ access (**b**) (Hakko Co., Nagano, Japan)

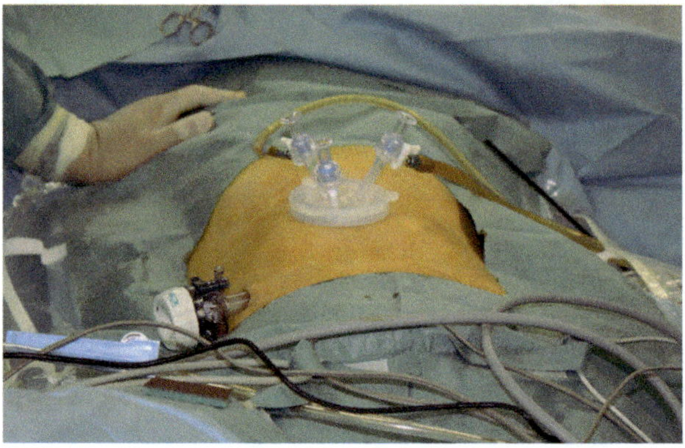

Fig. 11.4 External view of RPS TME. One 12-mm port and two 5-mm ports are placed in EZ access. A 12-mm port is inserted in the right lower quadrant

11.3.3 Operative Exposure

CO_2 pneumoperitoneum is established and maintained at 10 mmHg. After complete exploration of the abdomen to identify any metastatic nodules or superficial hepatic metastases with a 10mm flexible laparoscope, the patient is tilted into a deep Trendelenburg position and inclined to the right. The small intestine is moved into the right upper quadrant, exposing the root of the left colonic mesentery. The greater omentum is then flipped to expose the transverse colon and the splenic flexure.

11.3.4 Dissection of the Left Colonic Mesentery

By tenting the left colonic mesentery with atraumatic grasper held in the surgeon's left hand or with a retracting device such as the EndoGrab Retractor (Virtual Ports Ltd., Caesarea, Israel) (Fig. 11.5a). The left colonic mesentery is mobilized medial-to-lateral approach, keeping the right hypogastric nerve.

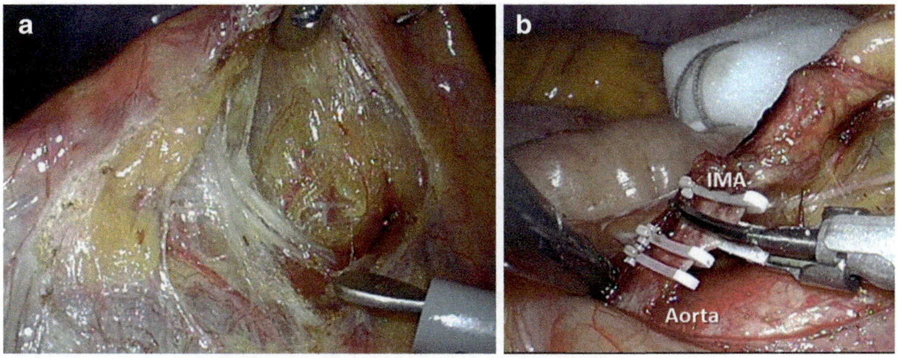

Fig. 11.5 The root of the left colonic mesentery is incised with an electric cautery (**a**), and the IMA is dissected between the clips (**b**)

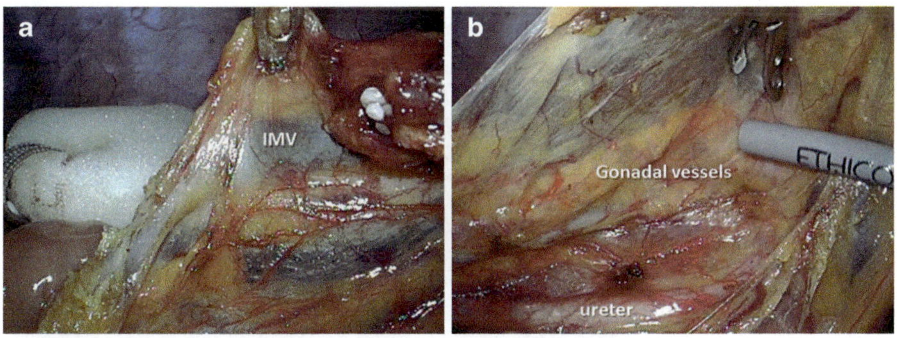

Fig. 11.6 The IMV (**a**). Dissection is performed sweeping down the retroperitoneal fascia to preserve the left ureter and the gonadal vessels in the prior plane (**b**)

11.3.5 Ligation of the Inferior Mesenteric Vessels

In a patient with advanced-stage cancer, the dissection is continued superiorly to the level of the root of the IMA. All of the soft tissue anterior to the IMA is completely removed, and the IMA is dissected between the clips slightly away from its aortic origin not to injure the lumber splanchnic nerves (Fig. 11.5b). In patients with early-stage cancer, the superior rectal artery is dissected between the clips to preserve the left colic artery. The IMV is dissected between two clips at the level of the IMA stump (Fig. 11.6a). Continuous dissection below the inferior mesenteric artery (IMA) is performed sweeping down the retroperitoneal fascia to preserve the left ureter and the gonadal vessels in the prior plane (Fig. 11.6b).

11.3.6 Mobilization of the Left Colon

The lateral attachments of the sigmoid colon are dissected until the previously dissected area (Fig. 11.7) and full mobilization of the sigmoid colon are completed.

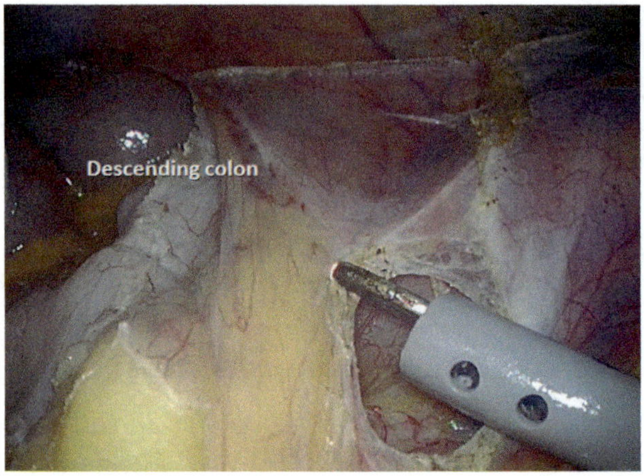

Fig. 11.7 The lateral attachments of the sigmoid colon are dissected until the previously dissected area

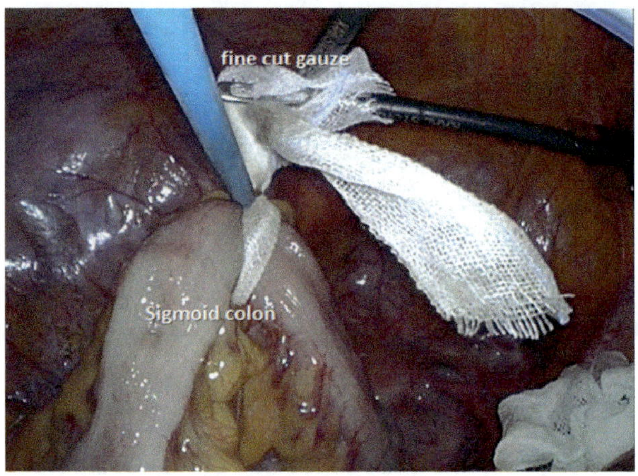

Fig. 11.8 The sigmoid colon is tightened with the fine cut gauze

11.3.7 Mobilization of the Rectum with Total Mesorectal Excision

Before starting the dissection of the mesorectum, the sigmoid colon is tightened with the fine cut gauze (Fig. 11.8), and the assistant retracts this gauze to make the operative field with the grasper inserted from umbilicus port. The rectum is posteriorly mobilized at first in front of the hypogastric nerve (Figs. 11.9 and 11.10).

In female patients, the straight needle with the 2-0 nylon thread is introduced by percutaneous puncture, directed through the uterus, withdrawn, and tied to retract the uterus (Fig. 11.11). In cases with male patients, we retract the peritoneum of the peritoneal reflection by similar methods. Thereafter anterior mobilization is performed at the plane immediately behind Denonvilliers' fascia not to injure the neurovascular bundle (Fig. 11.12). The lateral dissection of the rectum is performed afterward (Fig. 11.13), and the rectum enveloped within the fascia propria recti is completely removed.

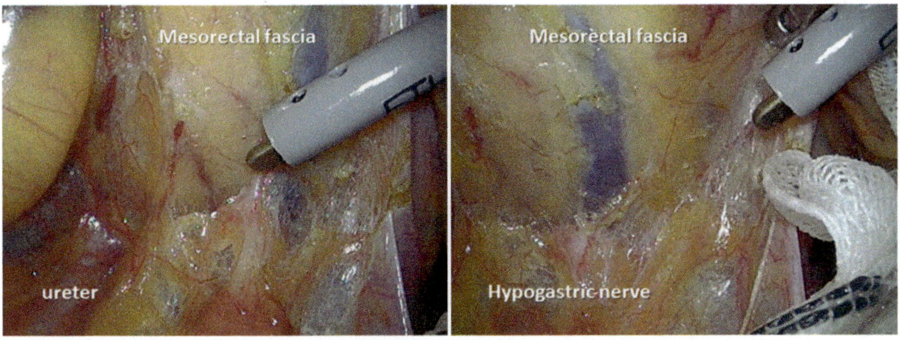

Fig. 11.9 The rectum is posteriorly mobilized at first in front of the hypogastric nerve

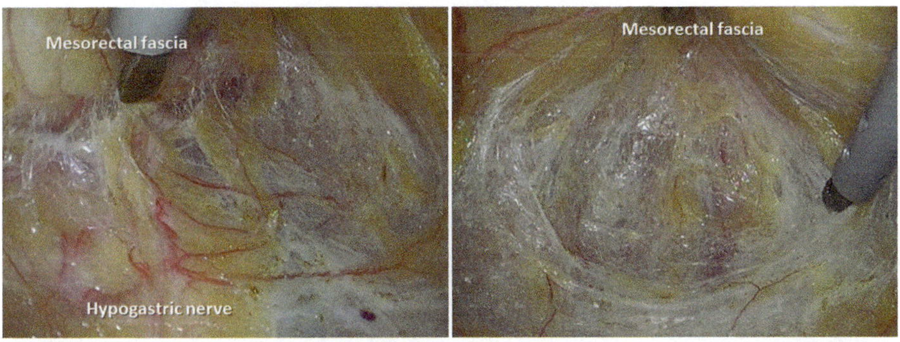

Fig. 11.10 The mesorectal fascia and the hypogastric nerve are preserved

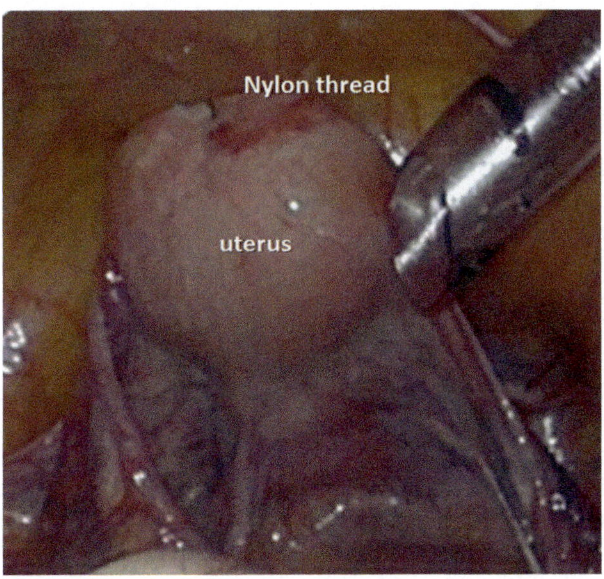

Fig. 11.11 The 2-0 nylon thread is introduced by percutaneous puncture, directed through the uterus, withdrawn, and tied to retract the uterus

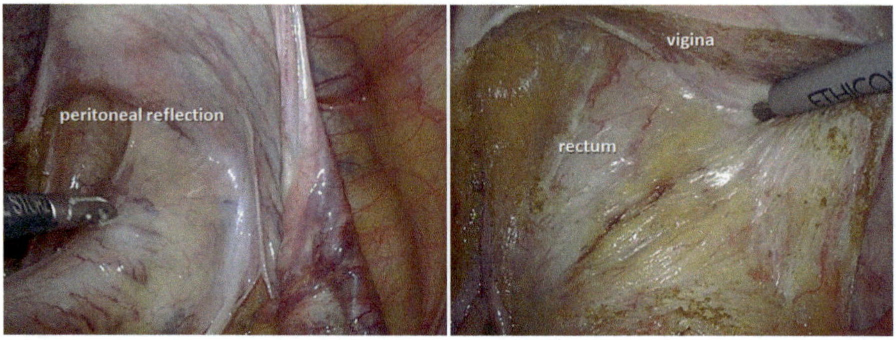

Fig. 11.12 Anterior mobilization is performed at the plane immediately behind Denonvilliers' fascia not to injure the neurovascular bundle

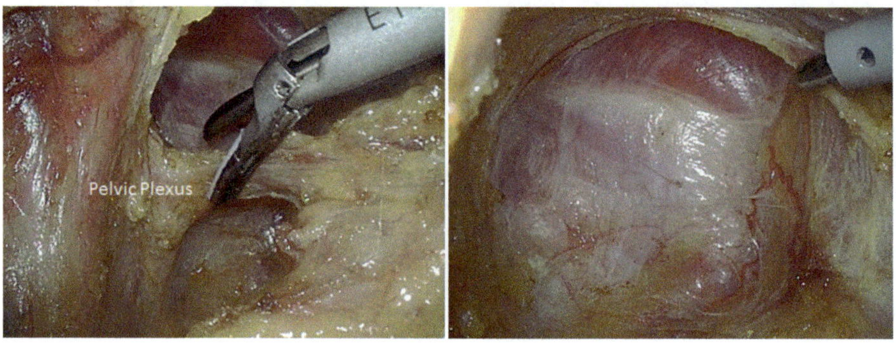

Fig. 11.13 The lateral dissection of the rectum is performed afterward

11.3.8 Transection of the Mesorectum and Rectum

The right side of rectal fascia is incised at the distal resection line, and the wall of the rectum is exposed, and mesorectal tissue is transected with laparoscopic coagulating shears (LCS). The distal rectum is then clamped with detachable forceps, and the rectum is transected normally using one or two endoscopic linear stapler inserted from the right lower quadrant port following after rectal lavage (Figs. 11.14 and 11.15).

11.3.9 Specimen Extraction and Anastomosis

The proximal colon is extracted through the umbilical incision. Resection is achieved following extracorporealization, and the anastomosis is performed with double-stapling technique using a transanally inserted circular stapler. After finishing the anastomosis, the surgeon inserts the transanal tube into the bowel lumen through the anus. The drainage part of the tube is placed above the anastomotic site. The transanal tube is sutured to the perianal skin for fixation. It was removed on the fifth postoperative day. A pelvic drainage tube is inserted from the right lower quadrant incision (Fig. 11.16). Normally diverting stoma is not performed.

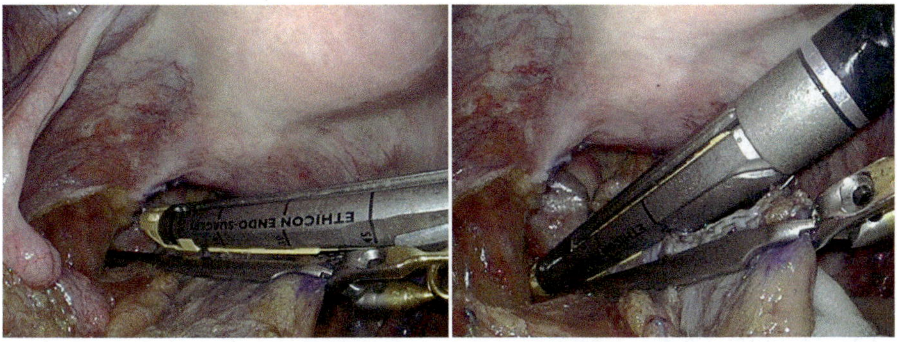

Fig. 11.14 The rectum is transected normally using one or two endoscopic linear stapler inserted from the right lower quadrant port

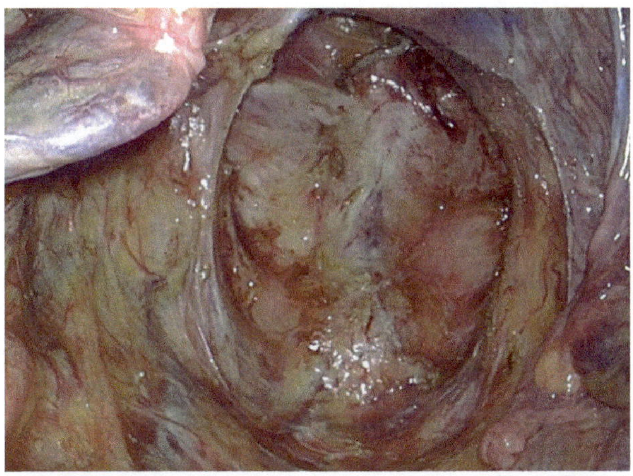

Fig. 11.15 The rectum enveloped within the fascia propria recti is completely removed

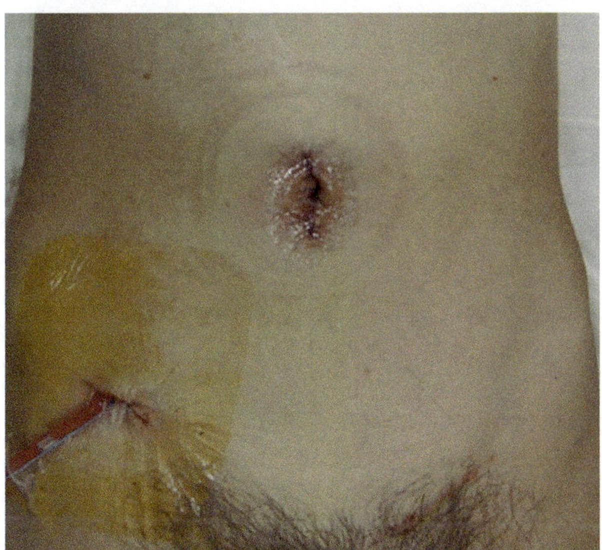

Fig. 11.16 Postoperative view. A pelvic drainage tube was inserted from the right lower quadrant incision

References

1. Curro G, Cogliandolo A, Lazzara S, La Malfa G, Navarra G. Single incision versus three-port conventional laparoscopic right hemicolectomy: is there any real need to go single? J Laparoendosci Adv Surg Tech A. 2012;22:621–4.
2. Yun JA, Yun SH, Park YA, Cho YB, Kim HC, Lee WY, Chun HK. Single-incision laparoscopic right colectomy compared with conventional laparoscopy for malignancy: assessment of perioperative and short-term oncologic outcomes. Surg Endosc. 2013;27:2122–30.
3. Kwag SJ, Kim JG, ST O, Kang WK. Single incision vs conventional laparoscopic anterior resection for sigmoid colon cancer: a casematched study. Am J Surg. 2013;206:320–5.
4. Hirano Y, Hattori M, Douden K, Shimizu S, Sato Y, Maeda K, Hashizume Y. Single-incision plus one port laparoscopic anterior resection for rectal cancer as a reduced port surgery. Scand J Surg. 2012;101:283–6.

Single-Port Laparoscopic TME with Low Colorectal Anastomosis

12

Léon Maggiori and Yves Panis

Abstract

Although single-port laparoscopy for colorectal resections was initially only performed for benign disease, there is now an increasing experience for colorectal malignancy. On the other hand, as with standard multiport laparoscopic approach in rectal cancer management, single-port laparoscopy for rectal procedures raises some concern about feasibility and safety of this technically demanding surgery. To date, only few studies reported the postoperative results of this minimally invasive approach, and no randomized control trial including rectal procedures is available. However, the results of these studies and of those of systematic reviews suggest that single-port rectal surgery may be associated with satisfactory postoperative morbidity rate and might even improve the postoperative recovery. However, long-term follow-up of single-port laparoscopic total mesorectal excision (SPLTME) for rectal cancer has not been reported in any study. In this chapter we will review the available literature on the topic and detail our surgical technique for SPLTME.

Keywords

Single port surgery • Rectal cancer • Laparoscopy • TAMIS

L. Maggiori, M.D., Ph.D. • Y. Panis, M.D., Ph.D. (✉)
Department of Colorectal Surgery, Pôle des Maladies de l'Appareil Digestif (PMAD), Beaujon Hospital, Assistance publique-Hôpitaux de Paris (AP-HP), University Denis Diderot (Paris VII), 100 boulevard du Général Leclerc, 92110 Clichy, France
e-mail: yves.panis@aphp.fr

G. Dapri, J.H. Marks (eds.), *Surgical Techniques in Rectal Cancer*,
https://doi.org/10.1007/978-4-431-55579-7_12

12.1 Introduction

Minimally invasive approach can be regarded as one of the major technical advances in surgery of the past 20 years. It has progressively become the standard approach for many benign and malignant diseases. As such, laparoscopy is now widely used for colorectal surgery. Compared to the open procedure, laparoscopic approach for colonic surgery provides various well-demonstrated benefits, including faster return of bowel function, less postoperative pain, shorter hospital stay, lower morbidity, and cosmetic advantage [1, 2]. Moreover, many studies have demonstrated the oncologic safety of laparoscopic colon cancer resection [3–5], as it is associated with similar results in terms of local control and survival, compared to standard open surgery. Furthermore, we have recently demonstrated, at a national level, that laparoscopy was independently associated with a lower postoperative mortality rate in colorectal cancer surgery [6].

On the other hand, the safety of laparoscopy for rectal cancer management was initially questioned, mainly because of high rates of conversion and postoperative morbidity in subgroup analyses of the first randomized control trial (CLASICC trial) comparing open to laparoscopic approaches [5]. More recently, additional randomized control trials, specifically focusing on rectal cancer, demonstrated the safety of this minimally invasive approach even in this indication [2, 7, 8].

Interest in laparoscopy led to the development of more minimally invasive surgical approaches such as mini-laparoscopy, NOTES (natural orifice transluminal endoscopic surgery), and more recently single-port laparoscopy (SPL). This latter technique is a technical refinement of the laparoscopic approach and consists of using a single multichannel port site, allowing the introduction of a camera and several instruments with only a 25–50 mm skin incision. In addition to the well-known advantages of laparoscopy, the main benefit of SPL might be improved postoperative pain, postoperative recovery, and cosmetic results. To date, SPL has been reported for various surgical procedures, and published experiences regarding more complex procedures such as colorectal surgery are rapidly growing. Although SPL for colorectal resections was initially only performed for benign disease, there is now an increasing experience for colorectal malignancy.

As for laparoscopic approach in rectal cancer management, SPL for rectal procedures raises some concern about feasibility and safety of this technically demanding surgery. In this chapter, we will review the published literature about SPL for low anterior resection and total mesorectal excision (TME), and we will describe our routine surgical technique for such cases.

12.2 Literature Review

Hamzaoglu et al. [9], in January 2011, were the first to publish their experience with SPL sphincter-saving excision for rectal cancer. They reported a series of four patients. Two of them underwent a partial mesorectal excision with colorectal anastomosis and two underwent a TME. Results were encouraging as additional laparoscopic port or conversion to laparotomy was required, intraoperative blood loss ranged from 50 to 200 mL, operative time ranged from 240 to 480 min, and no postoperative complication was observed.

Since, several studies were published on the topic. After reporting our two initial cases of TME for cancer by single port approach [10], we reported the results of 25 SPL colorectal procedures in a case-matched study, including three cases of proctectomy [11]. This study suggested the feasibility of this single-port approach, as we did not observe any difference of postoperative mortality and morbidity, as compared to the standard multiport laparoscopic approach. In 2011, Bulut et al. [12] reported ten consecutive cases of rectal cancer treated by SPL with good postoperative results. These results were recently updated, including 25 patients, with satisfactory results [13]. On the same way, Kim et al. [14] reported 73 colorectal cancer patients treated by SPL, including 32 rectal cancers. In this latter comparative study, although not randomized, postoperative morbidity was similar as compared to patients operated by multiport laparoscopy, but both return to normal bowel function and postoperative hospital stay were significantly shorter in SPL patients. Additionally, two other recent papers reported 19 [15] and 8 [16] patients, respectively, with rectal cancer treated by SPL, also with satisfactory postoperative results. Finally, very recently, Sourrouille et al. [17] reported their results of 13 patients who underwent a sphincter-saving rectal resection for rectal cancer through a single port. As compared to the outcomes of 32 patients who underwent the same procedure using a multiport laparoscopic approach, there was no difference in terms of oncological quality of the resection, postoperative morbidity, or length of hospital stay. However, postoperative pain was reduced in the single-port group.

In 2012, we performed a systematic review and meta-analysis on SPL colorectal surgery, including all studies published as of December 2011 [18]. We identified 20 studies [9–12, 16, 19–33], all of retrospective design, which reported a total of 105 rectal procedures, including 55 low anterior resections (52%), 4 abdominoperineal resections (4%), and 46 total proctocolectomies (with or without ileal pouch-anal anastomosis) (44%). Of these studies, only three were case-matched studies [11, 16, 30], all of them comparing single-port to standard multiport approaches. One of the main conclusions of this meta-analysis was the questioned technical feasibility of SPL rectal surgery, as only 67% were successfully completed through a SPL approach. Indeed, conversion to multiport laparoscopy was needed in 32 cases (30%) and conversion to laparotomy was needed in 3 cases (3%).

On the other hand, this meta-analysis demonstrated that postoperative outcomes of single-port laparoscopic rectal surgery were acceptable, as compared to the standard multiport approach. Pooled postoperative 30-day mortality rate was 0.2%, and meta-analysis of the comparative studies showed no difference of postoperative morbidity rates between SPL and multiport laparoscopic surgery (odds ratio, 0.84 [0.61, 1.15]; $p = 0.27$). Furthermore, we suggested that SPL might be associated with some benefits as compared to the multiport approach as the SPL was associated with a significantly shorter total skin incision (weighted mean difference, −0.52 [−0.79, −0.25]; $p < 0.001$) and a significantly shorter length of postoperative hospital stay (weighted mean difference, −0.75 [−1.30, −0.20]; $p = 0.008$), as compared to the multiport approach. Finally, this meta-analysis stressed the point that single-port laparoscopic surgery might be acceptable regarding the oncologic results obtained. Indeed, all reported surgical margins were negative (R0), and all studies reported a mean number of harvested lymph nodes of 12 or more. However, to date, long-term follow-up of SPLTME for rectal cancer was not reported in any study and both overall and disease-free survivals remain unknown.

Similarly, two additional literature reviews have recently been published on the same topic [34, 35]. The first one [34] suggested that SPL was feasible and safe when performed by surgeons highly experienced in laparoscopy. The authors concluded that, despite technical difficulties, SPL might be associated with potential benefits (i.e., size of the incision, hospital stay, operative time) as compared to its multiport counterpart, but those remain yet to be proven objectively. The second review, focusing only on colon cancer [35], suggested that SPL may be associated with a lower postoperative morbidity rate, as compared to the results of large randomized control trials of multiport laparoscopic approach.

More recently, two small-sampled randomized studies have been recently reported on SPL colonic surgery [36, 37], although they did not include rectal procedures. The first one, authored by Poon et al. [37], included 50 patients and demonstrated significantly shorter hospital stay and lower postoperative pain in patients operated by SPL. The second study in 32 patients demonstrated that operative results were similar in both single-port and standard laparoscopy groups [36].

12.3 Surgical Technique

We routinely perform transabdominal approach with stapled low colorectal anastomosis for SPL rectal cancer management, reserving the transanal-transabdominal with hand-sewn anastomosis for patients requiring either a standard coloanal anastomosis on the dentate line (rectal tumor located at less than 3 or 4 cm from the dentate line, for which stapled anastomosis will be very difficult by abdominal approach) of intersphincteric dissection for lesions located at less than 1 cm from the dentate line.

12.3.1 Transabdominal Approach and Stapled Low Colorectal Anastomosis

The surgeon and a first assistant are positioned on the right of the patient. A second assistant is placed on the left. As we always perform a diverting lateral ileostomy in rectal cancer cases, the single-port device is placed through a 25 mm skin incision in the right lower quadrant, at the precise stoma location. The procedure is performed using a 5 mm laparoscope with a 0° tip, a 5 mm Ultracision Harmonic scalpel (Ethicon Endosurgery, Spreitenbach, Switzerland), a 10 mm endoscopic linear stapler, and conventional straight 5 mm laparoscopic graspers. We routinely use the Octoport (Landanger, Paris, France) for SPL.

SPLTME is performed using the same technique as for standard laparoscopic TME with a medial-to-lateral approach. It begins by a medial approach (after placing the patient in 30° Trendelenburg with 20° right lateral tilt position, using one assistant grasper and the gravitational force) with vein division, dissection of the pancreas from below, mobilization of the transverse and left mesocolon, and after a clear identification of the left ureter, division of the inferior mesenteric artery. Then, splenic flexure mobilization and left colonic mobilization is finished laterally. During the step of splenic flexure mobilization, and because frequently the single port is too far for the splenic flexure, we add a 5 mm trocart on the left lower quadrant which helps for this step and which will be used for the suction drain left in place in the pelvis at the end of the operation. TME is then performed down to the pelvic floor. The rectum is distally transected using an endoscopic linear stapler using one or two cartridges.

The specimen is extracted through the single-port incision in the right lower quadrant. The colon is proximally transected and prepared, allowing the insertion of a circular stapler anvil. The colon is returned in the abdominal cavity, the single-port device is reinserted, and the pneumoperitoneum is reestablished. A low side-to-end colorectal anastomosis is then mechanically performed using a transanally inserted circular stapler. A pelvic suction drain is placed and the last ileal loop is exteriorized through the site of insertion of the single-port laparoscopic device.

Conclusion

Published studies regarding SPLTME are scarce, and no randomized control trial is available to date. However, review of the literature suggests that SPLTME is technically demanding but feasible and safe. Furthermore, it may be associated with improved postoperative outcomes as compared to the standard multiport approach. Long-term results of this procedure and well-designed prospective studies are eagerly waited, as they will allow complete demonstration of the outcomes associated with this novel minimally invasive approach.

Acknowledgment No financial disclosure.

References

1. Clinical Outcomes of Surgical Therapy Study Group. A comparison of laparoscopically assisted and open colectomy for colon cancer. N Engl J Med. 2004;350:2050–9.
2. Lujan J, Valero G, Hernandez Q, Sanchez A, Frutos MD, Parrilla P. Randomized clinical trial comparing laparoscopic and open surgery in patients with rectal cancer. Br J Surg. 2009;96:982–9.
3. Fleshman J, Sargent DJ, Green E, Anvari M, Stryker SJ, Beart RW Jr, et al. Laparoscopic colectomy for cancer is not inferior to open surgery based on 5-year data from the COST study group trial. Ann Surg. 2007;246:655–64.
4. Veldkamp R, Kuhry E, Hop WC, Jeekel J, Kazemier G, Bonjer HJ, et al. Laparoscopic surgery versus open surgery for colon cancer: short-term outcomes of a randomised trial. Lancet Oncol. 2005;6:477–84.
5. Guillou PJ, Quirke P, Thorpe H, Walker J, Jayne DG, Smith AM, et al. Short-term endpoints of conventional versus laparoscopic-assisted surgery in patients with colorectal cancer (MRC CLASICC trial): multicentre, randomised controlled trial. Lancet. 2005;365:1718–26.

6. Panis Y, Maggiori L, Caranhac G, Bretagnol F, Vicaut E. Mortality after colorectal cancer surgery: a French survey of more than 84,000 patients. Ann Surg. 2011;254:738–44.
7. Kang SB, Park JW, Jeong SY, Nam BH, Choi HS, Kim DW, et al. Open versus laparoscopic surgery for mid or low rectal cancer after neoadjuvant chemoradiotherapy (COREAN trial): short-term outcomes of an open-label randomised controlled trial. Lancet Oncol. 2010;11:637–45.
8. van der Pas MH, Haglind E, Cuesta MA, Furst A, Lacy AM, Hop WC, et al. Laparoscopic versus open surgery for rectal cancer (COLOR II): short-term outcomes of a randomised, phase 3 trial. Lancet Oncol. 2013;14:210–8.
9. Hamzaoglu I, Karahasanoglu T, Baca B, Karatas A, Aytac E, Kahya AS. Single-port laparoscopic sphincter-saving mesorectal excision for rectal cancer: report of the first 4 human cases. Arch Surg. 2011;146:75–81.
10. Gaujoux S, Bretagnol F, Au J, Ferron M, Panis Y. Single port access proctectomy with total mesorectal excision and intersphincteric resection with a primary transanal approach. Color Dis. 2011;13:e305–7.
11. Gaujoux S, Maggiori L, Bretagnol F, Ferron M, Panis Y. Safety, feasibility, and short-term outcomes of single port access colorectal surgery: a single institutional case-matched study. J Gastrointest Surg. 2012;16:629–34.
12. Bulut O, Nielsen CB, Jespersen N. Single-port access laparoscopic surgery for rectal cancer: initial experience with 10 cases. Dis Colon Rectum. 2011;54:803–9.
13. Bulut O, Aslak KK, Rosenstock S. Technique and short-term outcomes of single-port surgery for rectal cancer: a feasibility study of 25 patients. Scand J Surg. 2014;103:26–33. [Epub ahead of print]
14. Kim SJ, Ryu GO, Choi BJ, Kim JG, Lee KJ, Lee SC, et al. The short-term outcomes of conventional and single-port laparoscopic surgery for colorectal cancer. Ann Surg. 2011;254:933–40.
15. Vestweber B, Galetin T, Lammerting K, Paul C, Giehl J, Straub E, et al. Single-incision laparoscopic surgery: outcomes from 224 colonic resections performed at a single center using SILS. Surg Endosc. 2013;27:434–42.
16. Champagne BJ, Papaconstantinou HT, Parmar SS, Nagle DA, Young-Fadok TM, Lee EC, et al. Single-incision versus standard multiport laparoscopic colectomy: a multicenter, case-controlled comparison. Ann Surg. 2012;255:66–9.
17. Sourrouille I, Dumont F, Goere D, Honore C, Elias D. Resection of rectal cancer via an abdominal single-port access: short-term results and comparison with standard laparoscopy. Dis Colon Rectum. 2013;56:1203–10.
18. Maggiori L, Gaujoux S, Tribillon E, Bretagnol F, Panis Y. Single-incision laparoscopy for colorectal resection: a systematic review and meta-analysis of more than a thousand procedures. Color Dis. 2012;14:e643–54.
19. Gash KJ, Goede AC, Chambers W, Greenslade GL, Dixon AR. Laparoendoscopic single-site surgery is feasible in complex colorectal resections and could enable day case colectomy. Surg Endosc. 2011;25:835–40.
20. Geisler DP, Kirat HT, Remzi FH. Single-port laparoscopic total proctocolectomy with ileal pouch-anal anastomosis: initial operative experience. Surg Endosc. 2011;25:2175–8.
21. Chambers WM, Bicsak M, Lamparelli M, Dixon AR. Single-incision laparoscopic surgery (SILS) in complex colorectal surgery: a technique offering potential and not just cosmesis. Color Dis. 2011;13:393–8.
22. Chew MH, Wong MT, Lim BY, Ng KH, Eu KW. Evaluation of current devices in single-incision laparoscopic colorectal surgery: a preliminary experience in 32 consecutive cases. World J Surg. 2011;35:873–80.
23. Leblanc F, Makhija R, Champagne BJ, Delaney CP. Single incision laparoscopic total colectomy and proctocolectomy for benign disease: initial experience. Color Dis. 2011;13:1290–3.
24. Podolsky ER, Curcillo PG 2nd. Single port access (SPA) surgery--a 24-month experience. J Gastrointest Surg. 2010;14:759–67.
25. Ross H, Steele S, Whiteford M, Lee S, Albert M, Mutch M, et al. Early multi-institution experience with single-incision laparoscopic colectomy. Dis Colon Rectum. 2011;54:187–92.

26. Gash KJ, Goede AC, Kaldowski B, Vestweber B, Dixon AR. Single incision laparoscopic (SILS) restorative proctocolectomy with ileal pouch-anal anastomosis. Surg Endosc. 2011;25:3877–80.
27. van den Boezem PB, Sietses C. Single-incision laparoscopic colorectal surgery, experience with 50 consecutive cases. J Gastrointest Surg. 2011;15:1989–94.
28. Uematsu D, Akiyama G, Narita M, Magishi A. Single-access laparoscopic low anterior resection with vertical suspension of the rectum. Dis Colon Rectum. 2011;54:632–7.
29. Lauritsen ML, Bulut O. Single-port access laparoscopic abdominoperineal resection through the colostomy site: a case report. Tech Coloproctol. 2012;16:175–7.
30. Lee SW, Milsom JW, Nash GM. Single-incision versus multiport laparoscopic right and hand-assisted left colectomy: a case-matched comparison. Dis Colon Rectum. 2011;54:1355–61.
31. Geisler D, Garrett T. Single incision laparoscopic colorectal surgery: a single surgeon experience of 102 consecutive cases. Tech Coloproctol. 2011;15:397–401.
32. Bulut O, Nielsen CB. Single-incision laparoscopic low anterior resection for rectal cancer. Int J Color Dis. 2010;25:1261–3.
33. Geisler DP, Condon ET, Remzi FH. Single incision laparoscopic total proctocolectomy with ileopouch anal anastomosis. Color Dis. 2010;12:941–3.
34. Makino T, Milsom JW, Lee SW. Feasibility and safety of single-incision laparoscopic colectomy: a systematic review. Ann Surg. 2012;255:667–76.
35. Fung AK, Aly EH. Systematic review of single-incision laparoscopic colonic surgery. Br J Surg. 2012;99:1353–64.
36. Huscher CG, Mingoli A, Sgarzini G, Mereu A, Binda B, Brachini G, et al. Standard laparoscopic versus single-incision laparoscopic colectomy for cancer: early results of a randomized prospective study. Am J Surg. 2012;204:115–20.
37. Poon JT, Cheung CW, Fan JK, Lo OS, Law WL. Single-incision versus conventional laparoscopic colectomy for colonic neoplasm: a randomized, controlled trial. Surg Endosc. 2012;26:2729–34.

Robot-Assisted Multiport TME with Low Colorectal Anastomosis

13

Hye Jin Kim and Gyu-Seog Choi

Abstract

Rectal cancer, especially complex cases such as low-lying or irradiated cancer in a narrow pelvis, and cases involving men or obese patients, is one of the most common indications for the robotic approach. The surgical robot (da Vinci® surgical system, Intuitive Surgical, Sunnyvale, CA, USA) has the advantages of stable traction and countertraction, three-dimensional magnified vision, endowrist instrument function, simultaneous control of the instruments, and endoscope by the surgeon's intention. However, a limited range of surgical field, difficulty in manipulating redundant organs, and lack of tactile sense are some of disadvantages of the currently available surgical robot. Moreover, despite the mechanical advantages of robot over laparoscopy, at present, there are few evidences supporting the usefulness of robots for treating rectal cancer. This chapter will cover the basic operating room setup and techniques of standard total mesorectal excision (TME), with some modifications of the procedures on using robot. Hybrid fashion of laparoscopic mobilization of the left colon and robotic TME with prior version (da Vinci® S or Si system) and fully robotic low anterior resection with the latest da Vinci® Xi system are described here based on our experience.

Keywords

Robotic surgery • Rectal cancer • Total mesorectal excision

H.J. Kim • G.-S. Choi (✉)
Department of Surgery, Colorectal Cancer Center, Kyungpook National University Medical Center, School of Medicine, Kyungpook National University, 807 Hogukno, Buk-Gu, Daegu 702-210, South Korea
e-mail: kyuschoi@mail.knu.ac.kr

G. Dapri, J.H. Marks (eds.), *Surgical Techniques in Rectal Cancer*,
https://doi.org/10.1007/978-4-431-55579-7_13

13.1 Indications and Preoperative Preparation

The indications for robotic surgery are usually considered the same as those for laparoscopic surgery. However, the robotic approach is recommended mostly for middle or low rectal cancer due to the higher cost of robotic surgery (Tables 13.1 and 13.2) [1–12].

Preoperative assessment for pathologically diagnosed rectal cancer consists of pelvic magnetic resonance imaging and abdominopelvic and chest computed tomography (CT) scan with or without positron emission tomography-CT scan, along with routine laboratory tests. Routine mechanical bowel preparation depends on the surgeon's preference and does not differ in open and laparoscopic surgeries.

Intraoperative preparation includes shaving the patient from the lower chest to the pubic area. Anti-thromboembolic stockings and sequential compression devices are applied to prevent deep vein thrombosis. A Foley catheter is inserted after induction of anesthesia. Intravenous antibiotics are administered just before the skin incision. The use of a nasogastric tube is mostly omitted.

Table 13.1 Procedures of robotic rectal surgery

			No. of		Procedures		
Author	Study design		case	Totally/hybrid	AR/LAR	ISR	APR
Hellan [1]	Case series	Robot	39	Hybrid	22	11	6
Choi [2]	Case series	Robot	50	Totally	40	8	2
Pigazzi [3]	Case series multicenter	Robot	143	Totally/hybrid	80	32	31
deSousa [4]	Case series	Robot	44	Hybrid	30	6	8
Kang [5]	Case series	Robot	269/120	Totally/hybrid	265/118	NA/NA	4/2
Park [6]	Comparative	Robot Lap	41 82	Hybrid	29 63	12 18	0 1
Baek [7]	Comparative	Robot Lap	41 41	Hybrid	33 33	2 2	6 6
Baik [8]	Prospective comparative	Robot Lap	56 57	Hybrid	56 57	0 0	0 0
Kwark [9]	Comparative	Robot Lap	59 59	Totally	54 52	5 6	0 1
Park [10]	3-arm comparative	Robot Lap Open	52 123 88	Hybrid	52 121 82	NA NA NA	0 2 6
Kang [11]	3-arm comparative	Robot Lap Open	165 165 165	Totally	165 159 156	NA NA NA	1 6 9
Kim [12]	Comparative	Robot Open	100 100	Totally	100 100	NA NA	0 0

Lap, laparoscopic surgery; *AR*, anterior resection; *LAR*, low anterior resection; *ISR*, intersphincteric resection; *APR*, abdominoperineal resection; *NA*, not applicable

Table 13.2 Short-term outcomes

Author		Tumor height from the anal verge	Operation time [a] (min)	Blood loss[a] (ml)	LOS[a] (day)	Conversion (%)	Leak/PI (%)	Morbidity (%)	Mortality (%)
Hellan [1]	Robot	<7 cm (53.9%) 7–11 cm (41%) >11 cm (5.1%)	285 (180–540)	200 (25–6000)	4 (2–22)	2.6	12.1/NA	48.7	0
Choi [2]	Robot	Mean 7.3 (2–13) cm <8 cm (44%) 8–12 cm (50%) 12–15 cm (6%)	304.8 (190–485)	NA	9.2 (5–24)	0	8.3/33	18	0
Pigazzi [3]	Robot	<7 cm (58.7%) 7–11 cm (29.4%) >11 cm (9.8%	297 (90–660)	283(0–6000)	8.3 (2–33)	4.9	10.5/63.4	41.3	0
deSouza [4]	Robot	<7 cm (47.7%) 7–11 cm (41%) 11–15 cm (11.3%)	347 (155–510)	150 (50–1000)	5 (3–36)	4.5	5.6/100	45.4	2.3
Kang [5]	Robot	<6 cm (30.8%) 6–12 cm (51.4%) 12–15 cm (17.8%	311.8	NA	10.4	0.8	7/24.3	19	0
Park [6]	Robot Lap	1–4 cm (34.8%) 4–8 cm (65.2%)	231.9 168.6	NA	9.9 9.4	0 0	9.7/4.9 7.3/4.9	29.3 23.2	0 0
Baek [7]	Robot Lap	<7 cm/7–11 cm/>11 cm: 36.6%/51.2%/12.2% 24.4%/43.9%/31.7%	296 (150–520) 315 (174–584)	200 (20–2000) 300 (17–1000)	6.5 (2–33) 6.6 (3–20)	7.3 22	8.6/94.3 2.8/40	21.9 26.8	0 0

(continued)

Table 13.2 (continued)

Author		Tumor height from the anal verge	Operation time [a] (min)	Blood loss[a] (ml)	LOS[a] (day)	Conversion (%)	Leak/PI (%)	Morbidity (%)	Mortality (%)
Baik [8]	Robot	Mean 9.6(3–15) cm	190.1 (120–315)	NA	5.7 (5–10)	0	1.8/NA	10.7	0
	Lap	Mean 9.5(3–15) cm	191 (100–360)	NA	7.6 (4–16)	10.5	7.0/NA	19.3	0
Kwark [9]	Robot	Mean 8(6–10) cm	270 (241–325)	NA	NA	0	13.5/42.2	32.3	0
	Lap	Mean 8(6–10) cm	228 (177–254)	NA	NA	3.4	10.2/44.1	27.2	0
Park [10]	Robot	Mean 7.6 cm	232.6	NA	10.4	0	9.6/1.9	19.2	0
	Lap	Mean 8.7 cm	158.1	NA	9.8	0	5.1/4.1	12.2	0
	OS	Mean 8.9 cm	233.8	NA	12.8	–	9.1/4.5	20.5	1.1
Kang [11]	Robot	<6 cm/>6 cm:65.5% /34.5%	309.7	133	10.8	0.6	7.3/25	20.6	NA
	Lap	67.3%/32.7%	277.8	140.1	13.5	1.8	10.8/27.2	27.9	NA
	OS	59.4%/26.7%	252.6	275.4	16.0	–	3.4[a]/31.8	24.8	NA
Kim [12]	Robot	<6 cm /6–10 cm /10–14 cm: 44%/41%/15%	188	NA	7.1	0	2/22	26	0
	OS	47%/40%/13%	103	NA	6.9	–	4/8	27	0

[a]Values are mean (range); *Lap*, laparoscopic surgery; *OS*, open surgery; *LOS*, length of stay; *PI*, protective ileostomy; *NA*, not applicable

13.2 Position of the Patient, Port Setup, and Docking

13.2.1 Patient Position

The patient is placed in the lithotomy position and tilted right side down with the thighs below the level of the table and the knees slightly flexed. Both the patient's arms are placed alongside the body to prevent shoulder injury and to maximize working space for the surgical staff (Fig. 13.1).

13.2.2 Port Setup

13.2.2.1 Using the S or Si System

The unique concept of the "camera cone," a conical area that the robot can cover in a single docking, is important for placing the port in the robotic surgery (Fig. 13.2a). The port for a scope should be placed in the middle of the camera cone, which is located approximately 1–2 cm right lateral to and above the umbilicus. The other ports are placed along the margin of a curvilinear line that the camera cone would cover, at a minimum distance of 8 cm. It is important to remember that all port placement measurements must be made after full pneumoperitoneum is created by insufflation with a Veress needle that is inserted at the camera port site. The remote center (thick black bar) of the port is placed in the middle of the abdominal wall to minimize excessive friction during the procedure. For the hybrid laparoscopy-robotic approach, two additional 5-mm ports are placed on the upper midline and right upper quadrant of the abdomen for the assistant's use. If a diverting ileostomy is planned, a single-port access device can be placed at the right lower quadrant port site to utilize the robotic port and laparoscopic assistant instrument, to save the upper midline port (Fig. 13.2b).

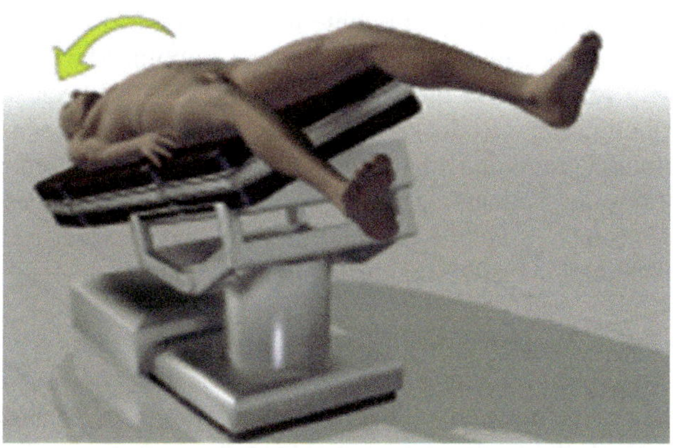

Fig. 13.1 Patient positioning

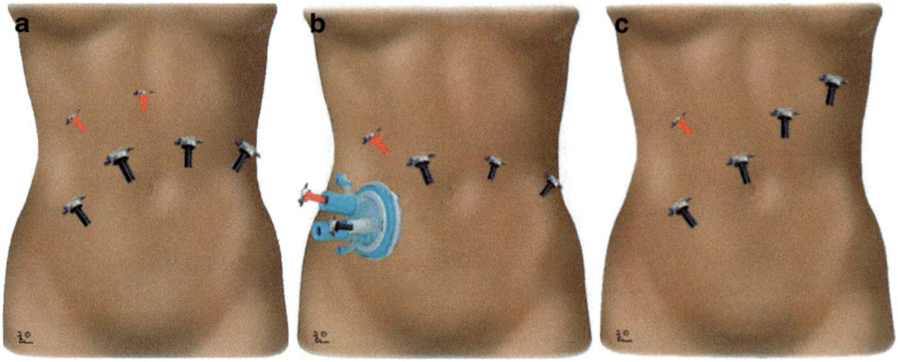

Fig. 13.2 (**a**) Port placement in the S or Si system, (**b**) port placement in case of using a single-port access, (**c**) port placement in the Xi system

13.2.2.2 Using the Xi System

The recent Xi system has a wider range of the camera cone, which enables the surgeon to facilitate mobilization of the left colon, including the splenic flexure, and simultaneous TME with a single docking. Port setup is easier than when using the S or Si system, as all ports are placed along a straight line from the left subcostal margin to the right lower quadrant at even distances of at least 6–8 cm. Similar to the S or Si system, an additional 5-mm laparoscopic port is placed on the right upper abdomen (Fig. 13.2c).

13.2.3 Patient Cart Docking

13.2.3.1 Using the S or Si System

The patient should be placed and tilted properly before docking. The entire small bowel should be shifted to the right upper abdomen, away from the surgical field, since once the robot is docked, the patient's position cannot be changed.

First, the inferior mesenteric artery (IMA) and the inferior mesenteric vein (IMV) are ligated, and the left colon is mobilized by laparoscopy. The robot is used only for TME, as the patient cart is placed between the patient's legs, while the robotic arms are docked to the trocars. If the surgeon plans to commence rectal mobilization with IMA division, the patient cart is recommended to be placed lateral to the patient's left thigh (Fig. 13.3a). This reduces arm collision during IMA ligation or sigmoid colon mobilization and provides a comfortable space for rectal examination or stapling during the procedure.

13.2.3.2 Using the Xi System

One of the advantages of the Xi system is the boom-arms, which can rotate independent of the position of the patient cart. Moreover, its automatic targeting mechanism suggests the optimal position of the robotic arms. Usually, docking from the patient's

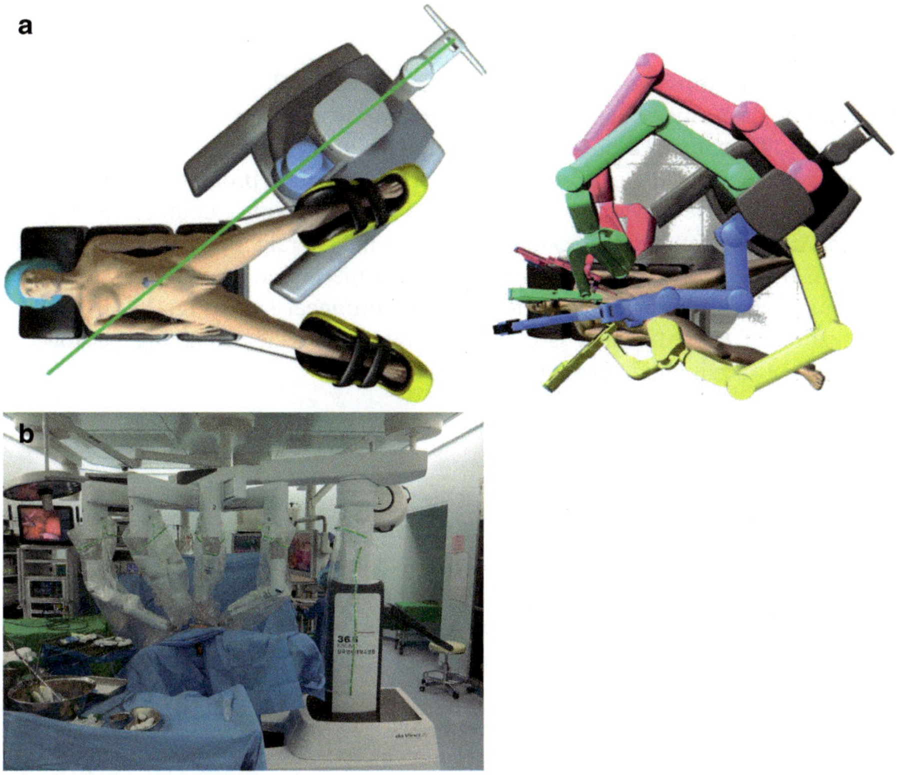

Fig. 13.3 (**a**) Docking the patient cart in the S or Si system. (**b**) Docking the patient cart in the Xi system

left side is recommended, but this depends on the working space available in the operating room (Fig. 13.3b).

13.3 Surgical Techniques

13.3.1 Hybrid Laparoscopic-Robotic Approach

As described in a previous report, during the laparoscopic phase of the takedown of the splenic flexure, the surgeon uses two trocars on the right side of the patient, while the assistant performs the remaining actions [6]. Briefly, dissection starts with IMA and IMV division, after which mobilization of full left colon is performed in a medial-to-lateral fashion. However, in young male patients, for achieving more precise preservation of the autonomic nerves around the aorta, the robotic approach is preferred for IMA ligation and division.

13.3.2 Totally Robotic Approach

After the robotic arms are docked to the trocars (Fig. 13.2c), a double fenestrated grasper, bipolar grasper, camera, and hot-shear are installed in arms 1, 2, 3, and 4, respectively. Then, the avascular space between the mesocolon and retroperitoneum is entered by incising the peritoneum in front of the sacral promontory, while the mesocolon along the superior rectal vessels is lifted up with a double fenestrated grasper. The dissection plane is extended upward and laterally up to the isolated and divided IMA (Fig. 13.4a) while sweeping down the ureter, gonadal vessels, and autonomic nerves along the aorta to the retroperitoneal side (Fig. 13.4b). Total mobilization of the left colon is completed by cutting the remaining peritoneal attachment of the sigmoid colon (Fig. 13.4c).

13.3.3 TME

13.3.3.1 Principal Techniques of Tractions

1. Major traction is maintained by the assistant by keeping the rectum in the appropriate tension so as to visualize the target area clearly.
2. Countertraction is handled by a double fenestrated grasper that is held in the third arm to create a wide surgical field, while it is lifting or pushing the pelvic wall or the rectum.
3. Minor traction is usually handled by surgeon's non-dominant hand with bipolar grasper that helps to adjust the dissection plane.
4. Finally, dissection itself is mostly carried out by the surgeon's dominant hand with monopolar scissors.

13.3.3.2 Sequence of TME

Mobilization of the rectum is commenced by incising the peritoneal membrane along the right pararectal sulcus with the assistant lifting up the mesocolon around the superior rectal vessels and a grasper through the third arm holding the upper part of the rectum. The right posterior aspect of the mesorectum is dissected through the thin inter-fascial space between the parietal and visceral pelvic fasciae till reaching the peritoneal reflection of the mid rectum. The hypogastric plexus and hypogastric nerves can be relatively easily identified and preserved, as long as inter-fascial dissection is maintained. However, excessive traction or thermal injury should be avoided. The peritoneal attachment on the left side of the rectum is then cut to complete the mobilization of the upper rectum.

As mobilization proceeds, the assistant grabs the cut edge of the mesorectum more distally and pulls it caudally, ventrally, and toward the left side. A double fenestrated grasper, with its jaws opened, then pushes the right anterior corner of the pelvic wall laterally. The surgeon's left hand gently pushes the mesorectum medially to continue mesorectal dissection through the "holy plane" (Fig. 13.5a). Dissection of the left side of the mid rectum is facilitated by the same maneuver

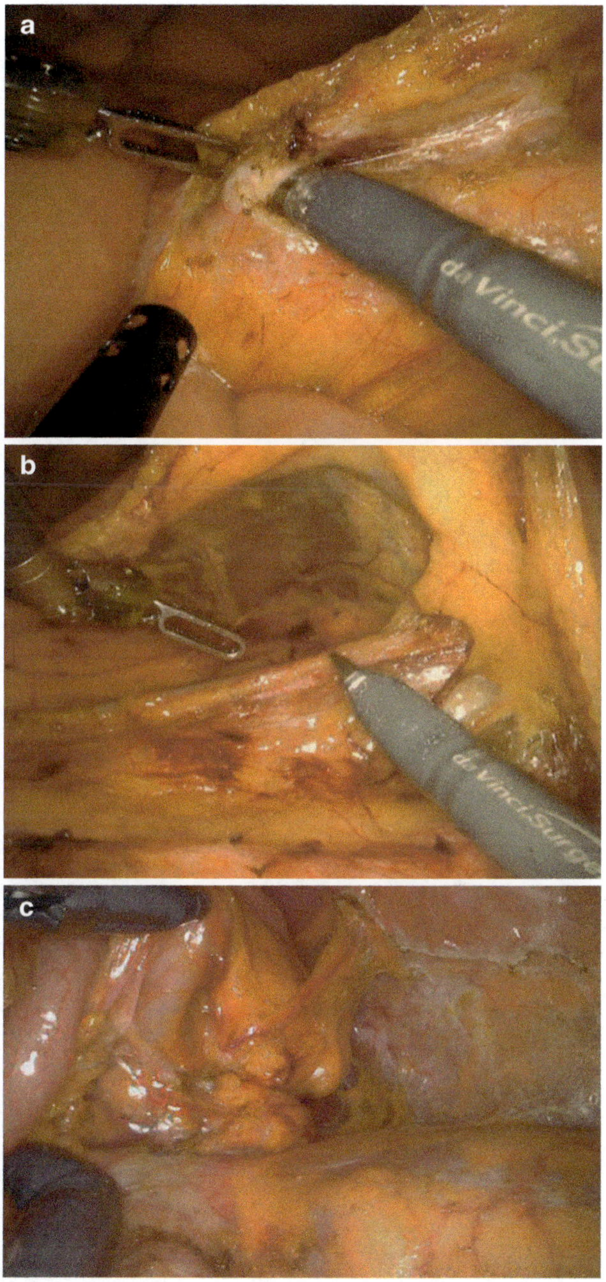

Fig. 13.4 (**a**) Identification and isolation of IMA, (**b**) avascular dissection plane with sweeping down ureter, gonadal vessels, and autonomic nerves, (**c**) mobilizing the full left colon

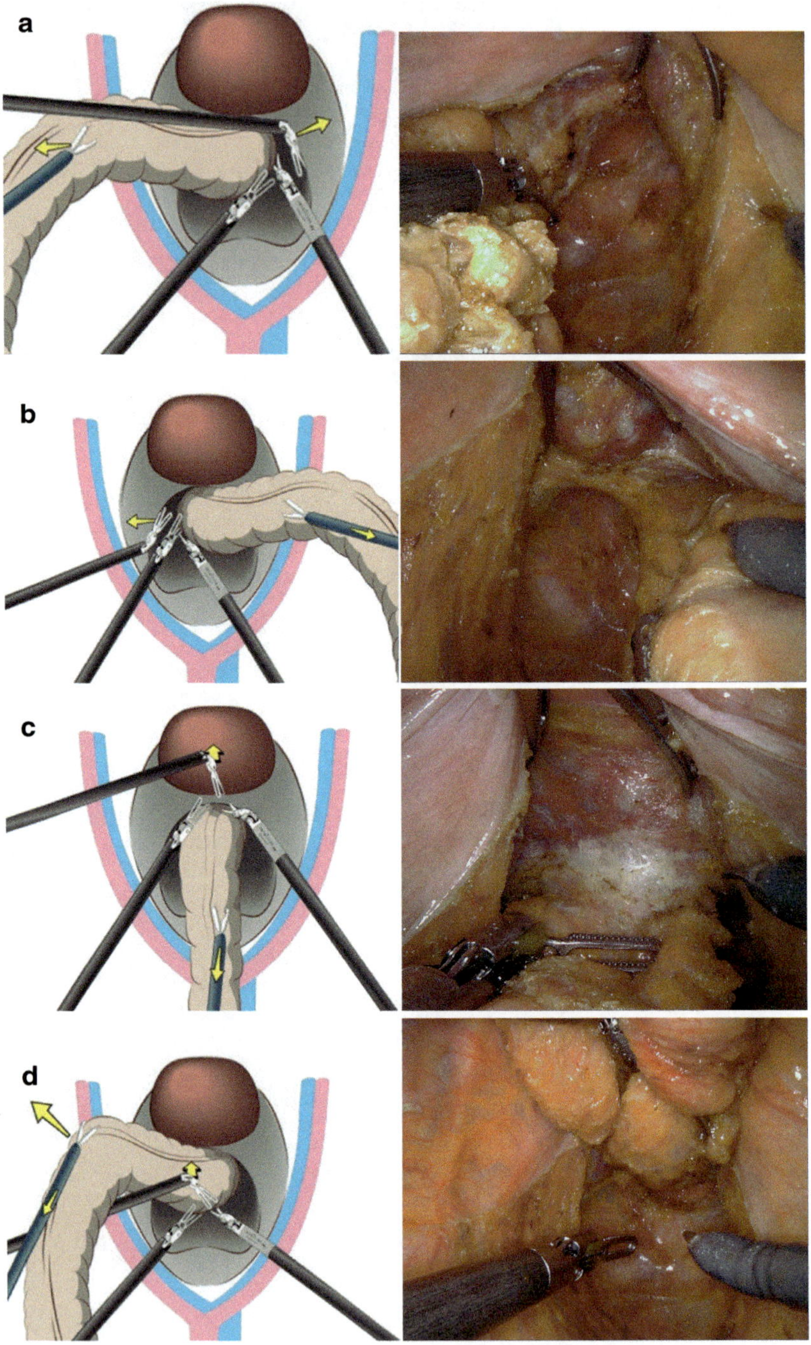

Fig. 13.5 (**a**) Right lateral dissection, (**b**) left lateral dissection, (**c**) anterior dissection, (**d**) posterior dissection by lifting up the posterior mesorectum with a double fenestrated grasper

to create circumferential mobilization (Fig. 13.5b). At this point, great care must be taken to preserve the pelvic nerves (parasympathetic predominant), which run perpendicularly and merge with the hypogastric nerves (sympathetic predominant) to form pelvic plexus (mixed autonomic).

For mobilization of the anterior side of the rectum, major traction by the assistant shifts the rectum back to the midline. Thereafter, a double fenestrated grasper lifts the anterior pelvic wall, while an instrument held in the surgeon's left hand pushes the rectum down to identify the fused peritoneal fascia (Denonvilliers fascia) (Fig. 13.5c). Depending on the tumor location, extra or intrafascial dissection is recommended. Generally, unless the tumor is on the anterior side, a dissection plane underneath Denonvilliers' fascia is preferred to safely preserve the neurovascular bundles, which contain the peripheral nerve endings of the pelvic plexus.

A very useful technique that we have developed for deep posterior dissection of the rectum is lifting up the posterior mesorectum with the third arm to secure the visual field between the rectum and sacrum (Fig. 13.5d). This maneuver enables the surgeon to use both hands to facilitate fine dissection around the last part of the rectum, even to enter the intersphincteric space.

Finally, the inferior hypogastric nerves and, distally, the pelvic nerve plexus can be identified and well preserved by these techniques (Fig. 13.6a–c).

13.3.4 Rectal Division and Anastomosis

When TME is completed using the abovementioned techniques, the rectum is clamped by applying a detachable clamp or manual ligation distal to the tumor, and the rectal stump is then irrigated with a tumoricidal solution per anus (Fig. 13.7a). The linear stapler is then introduced through the right lower quadrant by replacing the original trocar with a 12-mm one. If a robotic stapler is available, this step can be performed with ease and safety under the surgeon's control (Fig. 13.7b). The double fenestrated grasper can also be effectively used to clamp the rectum, irrigate the rectal stump, and adjust the rectal angle for stapling. (Fig. 13.7c).

A specimen can be delivered through the trans-umbilical incision or extension of the right lower quadrant trocar site (especially when a protective ileostomy is planned). After the anvil of the circular stapler is inserted into the proximal colon, the left colon is returned to the peritoneal cavity to create an anastomosis. At this time, it is recommended that the robotic third arm holding the anterior pelvic wall is retained till the end of surgery to retain envisioning of the pelvic cavity (Fig. 13.7d). A protective stoma is created or omitted according to the surgeon's preference.

13.4 Results

Most robotic rectal surgeries are recommended for mid or lower rectal cancer (Tables 13.1 and 13.2). Depending on the surgeons' preference and experience of previous laparoscopic surgery, a hybrid of laparoscopic left colon mobilization and robotic

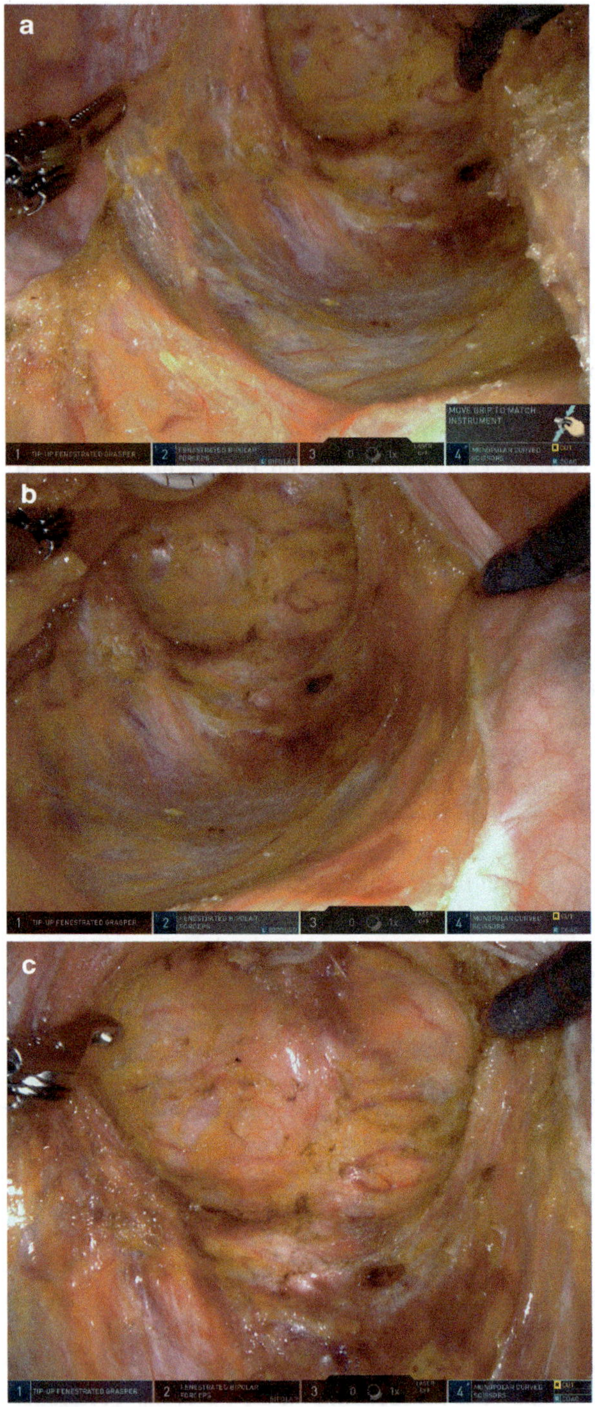

Fig. 13.6 (**a**) Rt. inferior hypogastric nerves, (**b**) Lt. inferior hypogastric nerves, (**c**) both pelvic plexus

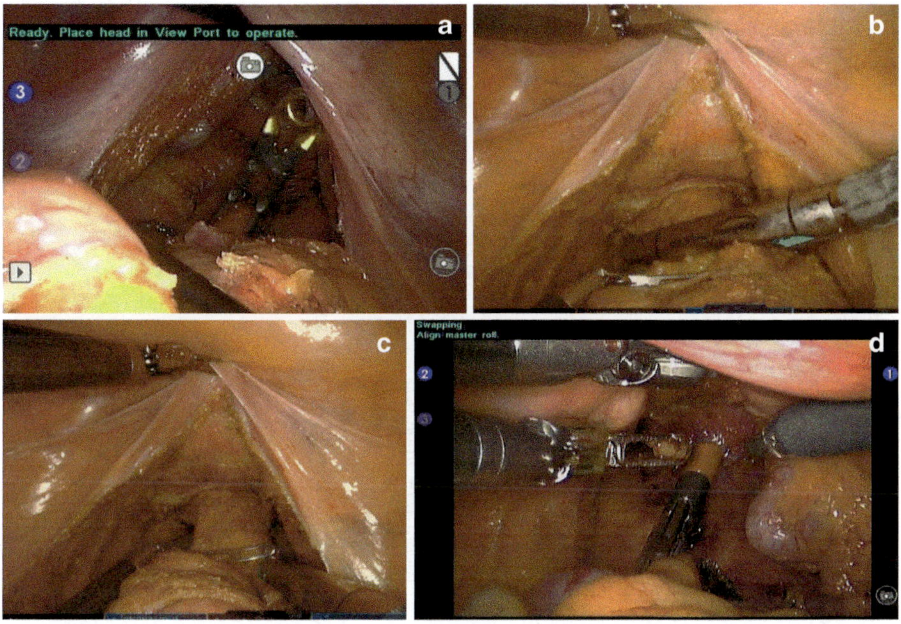

Fig. 13.7 (**a**) Clamping the rectum distal to the tumor and irrigating the rectal stump, (**b**) introducing robotic stapler under surgeon's control, (**c**) clamping the rectum by using the double fenestrated grasper, (**d**) robotic third arm holing the anterior pelvic wall till the end of surgery

rectal resection or a fully robotic approach are followed (Table 13.1). Regarding the learning curve for robotic rectal surgery, literatures have demonstrated that it could be shortened, compared to that of laparoscopic approach [13–16]. However, it is not clear whether shorter learning curve in robotic surgery is a real benefit or consequence of prior experience of laparoscopic surgery which most surgeons already had performed in many series of study. Currently, results from clinical randomized trials are lacking. However, it seems clear that higher cost and the longer operation time in the robotic group compared to the laparoscopic group are the most common obstacles for the spread of robotic surgery [17, 18]. A meta-analysis suggested that complex rectal cancer such as obesity, male patients, preoperative chemoradiation, and distal rectal cancer may be good indications for robotic approach [18, 19]. Other meta-analyses reported that the conversion rate could be reduced in the robotic group [20–24]. However, this phenomenon does not hold true in Korea and other Asian countries where laparoscopy for rectal cancer is extremely popular and more than 50–70% of patients with rectal cancer undergo minimally invasive surgery [2, 5, 6, 8–12]. Other short-term outcomes like recovery of bowel function, length of stay, morbidity, and mortality are almost the same in both groups (Table 13.2). The pathological parameters such as the number of lymph nodes harvested and surgical resection margins have been reported to be similar in both groups (Table 13.2). Oncologic outcomes are relatively rare due to small case volumes and short-term follow-up. Nonetheless, they might be regarded acceptable and similar to those of laparoscopy (Table 13.3).

Table 13.3 Oncologic outcomes

Author	Study design	No. of case	TNM stage	Follow-up [a](months)	Local recurrence	3-year DFS	3-year OS
Pigazzi [3]	Case series, multicenter	143	0–III	17.4 (0.1–52.5)	NA	77.6%	97%
Baek [29]	Case series	64	0–III	20.2 (1.7–52.5)	NA	73.7%	96.2%
Baik [30]	Case series	370	0–IV	26.5 ± 13.5	NA	79.2% 100/93.7/79.8/69.9/0 (stage: pCR/I/II/III/IV)	93.1% 100/99.2/97.0/90.0/48.4 (stage: pCR/I/II/III/IV)
Saklani [31]	Comparative (after CCRT)	74(Robot) 64(Lap)	0–III	30.1 (11–61)	2.7% 6.3%	77.7% 78.8%	90.0% 92.1%
Kang [11]	Comparative	104(Robot) 97(Lap) 110(OS)	0–III	22.4 (1–48)	NA NA NA	83.5% 81.9% 79.7%	NA NA NA
Choi (not published)	Case series	202	0–IV	22 (3–60)	4.1% (5 year)	78.8% 69.3% (5 year) 100/95.1/74.5/60/66.7 100/95.1/74.5/33.3(5 year) (pCR/I/II/III/IV)	99.4% 91.6% (5 year) 100/100/97.7/88.9/50 100/100/97.7/88.9/50(5 year) (pCR/I/II/III/IV)

[a]Values are mean (range); *Lap*, laparoscopic surgery; *OS*, open surgery; *CCRT*, chemoradiotherapy; *DFS*, disease-free survival; *OS*, overall survival; *pCR*, pathologic complete remission; *NA*, not applicable

One of the most promising advantages of robotic surgery for rectal cancer is the functional benefits such as preservation of urinary and sexual function after surgery. Several recent reports demonstrate that urinary and sexual functions, especially in male patients, have been better preserved in the robotic group [25–28].

In summary, despite higher cost and longer operation time, complex rectal surgery has been increasingly performed robotically. Robotic surgery manifests the favorable nature of minimally invasive surgery compared to open surgery. However, most reported short-term and long-term results are similar to those of laparoscopy. A lower conversion rate and better preservation of urinary and sexual function might be reliable potentials of robotic surgery in the treatment of rectal cancer. Looking back to how laparoscopic surgery has been evolving during the last several decades, it is optimistic that robotic surgery has a lot of room for improvement in the near future. Needless to say, further studies are necessary to demonstrate the real clinical benefits of robotic rectal surgery.

References

1. Hellan M, Anderson C, Ellenhorn JD, Paz B, Pigazzi A. Short-term outcomes after robotic-assisted total mesorectal excision for rectal cancer. Ann Surg Oncol. 2007;14(11):3168–73.
2. Choi DJ, Kim SH, Lee PJ, Kim J, Woo SU. Single-stage totally robotic dissection for rectal cancer surgery: technique and short-term outcome in 50 consecutive patients. Dis Colon Rectum. 2009;52(11):1824–30.
3. Pigazzi A, Luca F, Patriti A, Valvo M, Ceccarelli G, Casciola L, et al. Multicentric study on robotic tumor-specific mesorectal excision for the treatment of rectal cancer. Ann Surg Oncol. 2010;17(6):1614–20.
4. deSouza AL, Prasad LM, Marecik SJ, Blumetti J, Park J, Zimmern A, et al. Total mesorectal excision for rectal cancer: the potential advantage of robotic assistance. Dis Colon Rectum. 2010;53(12):1611–7.
5. Kang J, Min BS, Park YA, Hur H, Baik SH, Kim NK, et al. Risk factor analysis of postoperative complications after robotic rectal cancer surgery. World J Surg. 2011;35(11):2555–62.
6. Park JS, Choi GS, Lim KH, Jang YS, Jun SH. Robotic-assisted versus laparoscopic surgery for low rectal cancer: case-matched analysis of short-term outcomes. Ann Surg Oncol. 2010;17(12):3195–202.
7. Baek JH, Pastor C, Pigazzi A. Robotic and laparoscopic total mesorectal excision for rectal cancer: a case-matched study. Surg Endosc. 2011;25(2):521–5.
8. Baik SH, Kwon HY, Kim JS, Hur H, Sohn SK, Cho CH, et al. Robotic versus laparoscopic low anterior resection of rectal cancer: short-term outcome of a prospective comparative study. Ann Surg Oncol. 2009;16(6):1480–7.
9. Kwak JM, Kim SH, Kim J, Son DN, Baek SJ, Cho JS. Robotic vs laparoscopic resection of rectal cancer: short-term outcomes of a case-control study. Dis Colon Rectum. 2011;54(2):151–6.
10. Park JS, Choi GS, Lim KH, Jang YS, Jun SH. S052: a comparison of robot-assisted, laparoscopic, and open surgery in the treatment of rectal cancer. Surg Endosc. 2011;25(1):240–8.
11. Kang J, Yoon KJ, Min BS, Hur H, Baik SH, Kim NK, et al. The impact of robotic surgery for mid and low rectal cancer: a case-matched analysis of a 3-arm comparison--open, laparoscopic, and robotic surgery. Ann Surg. 2013;257(1):95–101.
12. Kim JC, Yang SS, Jang TY, Kwak JY, Yun MJ, Lim SB. Open versus robot-assisted sphincter-saving operations in rectal cancer patients: techniques and comparison of outcomes between groups of 100 matched patients. Int J Med Robot. 2012;8(4):468–75.
13. Kim YW, Lee HM, Kim NK, Min BS, Lee KY. The learning curve for robot-assisted total mesorectal excision for rectal cancer. Surg Laparosc Endosc Percutan Tech. 2012;22(5):400–5.

14. Sng KK, Hara M, Shin JW, Yoo BE, Yang KS, Kim SH. The multiphasic learning curve for robot-assisted rectal surgery. Surg Endosc. 2013;27(9):3297–307.
15. Kim HJ, Choi GS, Park JS, Park SY. Multidimensional analysis of the learning curve for robotic total mesorectal excision for rectal cancer: lessons from a single surgeon's experience. Dis Colon Rectum. 2014;57(9):1066–74.
16. Park EJ, Kim CW, Cho MS, Baik SH, Kim DW, Min BS, et al. Multidimensional analyses of the learning curve of robotic low anterior resection for rectal cancer: 3-phase learning process comparison. Surg Endosc. 2014;28(10):2821–31.
17. Keller DS, Senagore AJ, Lawrence JK, Champagne BJ, Delaney CP. Comparative effectiveness of laparoscopic versus robot-assisted colorectal resection. Surg Endosc. 2014;28(1):212–21.
18. Aly EH. Robotic colorectal surgery: summary of the current evidence. Int J Color Dis. 2014;29(1):1–8.
19. Scarpinata R, Aly EH. Does robotic rectal cancer surgery offer improved early postoperative outcomes? Dis Colon Rectum. 2013;56(2):253–62.
20. Antoniou SA, Antoniou GA, Koch OO, Pointner R, Granderath FA. Robot-assisted laparoscopic surgery of the colon and rectum. Surg Endosc. 2012;26(1):1–11.
21. Yang Y, Wang F, Zhang P, Shi C, Zou Y, Qin H, et al. Robot-assisted versus conventional laparoscopic surgery for colorectal disease, focusing on rectal cancer: a meta-analysis. Ann Surg Oncol. 2012;19(12):3727–36.
22. Trastulli S, Farinella E, Cirocchi R, Cavaliere D, Avenia N, Sciannameo F, et al. Robotic resection compared with laparoscopic rectal resection for cancer: systematic review and meta-analysis of short-term outcome. Color Dis. 2012;14(4):e134–56.
23. Mak TW, Lee JF, Futaba K, Hon SS, Ngo DK, Ng SS. Robotic surgery for rectal cancer: a systematic review of current practice. World J Gastrointest Oncol. 2014;6(6):184–93.
24. Memon S, Heriot AG, Murphy DG, Bressel M, Lynch AC. Robotic versus laparoscopic proctectomy for rectal cancer: a meta-analysis. Ann Surg Oncol. 2012;19(7):2095–101.
25. Luca F, Valvo M, Ghezzi TL, Zuccaro M, Cenciarelli S, Trovato C, et al. Impact of robotic surgery on sexual and urinary functions after fully robotic nerve-sparing total mesorectal excision for rectal cancer. Ann Surg. 2013;257(4):672–8.
26. Park SY, Choi GS, Park JS, Kim HJ, Ryuk JP. Short-term clinical outcome of robot-assisted intersphincteric resection for low rectal cancer: a retrospective comparison with conventional laparoscopy. Surg Endosc. 2013;27(1):48–55.
27. Broholm M, Pommergaard HC, Gogenur I. Possible benefits of robot-assisted rectal cancer surgery regarding urological and sexual dysfunction: a systematic review and meta-analysis. Color Dis. 2015;17(5):375–81.
28. Kim JY, Kim NK, Lee KY, Hur H, Min BS, Kim JHA. Comparative study of voiding and sexual function after total mesorectal excision with autonomic nerve preservation for rectal cancer: laparoscopic versus robotic surgery. Ann Surg Oncol. 2012;19(8):2485–93.
29. Baek JH, McKenzie S, Garcia-Aguilar J, Pigazzi A. Oncologic outcomes of robotic-assisted total mesorectal excision for the treatment of rectal cancer. Ann Surg. 2010;251(5):882–6.
30. Baik SH, Kim NK, Lim DR, Hur H, Min BS, Lee KY. Oncologic outcomes and perioperative clinicopathologic results after robot-assisted tumor-specific mesorectal excision for rectal cancer. Ann Surg Oncol. 2013;20(8):2625–32.
31. Saklani AP, Lim DR, Hur H, Min BS, Baik SH, Lee KY, et al. Robotic versus laparoscopic surgery for mid-low rectal cancer after neoadjuvant chemoradiation therapy: comparison of oncologic outcomes. Int J Color Dis. 2013;28(12):1689–98.

Robot-Assisted Reduced Port TME with Low Colorectal Anastomosis

14

Ichiro Takemasa, Emi Akizuki, Tomomi Ueki, Toshihiko Nishidate, Kenji Okita, and Tomohisa Furuhata

Abstract

Advances in minimally invasive laparoscopic surgery have grown to reduced-port surgery (RPS). Single-incision laparoscopic surgery (SILS) is considered the ultimate RPS for improving cosmesis and reducing postoperative pain and the risk of abdominal wall morbidities. Several reports have described both superior short-term and similar long-term results of SILS for colorectal malignancies when compared with standard laparoscopic surgery. However, there are some limitations such as instrument collision and insufficient countertraction. In a recent attempt to overcome the technical issues in SILS, by combining the use of the da Vinci robotic surgical system with the single-incision platform, the recognized challenges are somewhat simplified. Only a few reports of single-port robotic surgery for rectal disease have been conducted; however, the current robotic arm and equipment are still rather bulky and have a limited intrapelvic range of motion. Pure single approach may be not suited for sufficient oncological clearance.

We have developed the novel approach for minimally invasive surgery for rectal malignancies with combination of the da Vinci robotic surgical system and the concept of RPS, which is robot-assisted reduced-port total mesorectal excision (RARPTME). Our procedure is well suited for good countertraction and smooth maneuverability and can provide improved cosmesis and theoretically reduced postoperative pain when compared with standard robotic surgery that usually needs at least six or more scars.

I. Takemasa, M.D., Ph.D. (✉) • E. Akizuki, M.D., Ph.D. • T. Ueki, M.D., Ph.D.
T. Nishidate, M.D., Ph.D. • K. Okita, M.D., Ph.D. • T. Furuhata, M.D., Ph.D.
Department of Surgery, Surgical Oncology and Science, Sapporo Medical University, S1 W17, Chuo-ku, Sapporo 060-8556, Japan
e-mail: itakemasa@sapmed.ac.jp

G. Dapri, J.H. Marks (eds.), *Surgical Techniques in Rectal Cancer*,
https://doi.org/10.1007/978-4-431-55579-7_14

Herein, we describe our techniques for RARPTME with low colorectal anastomosis in detail. Our procedure makes standardization of safe and certain RARPTME possible.

Keywords
Robotic surgery • Reduced-port surgery • Rectal cancer • Low anterior resection

14.1 Introduction

Advances in minimally invasive treatment have moved toward decreasing trauma by reducing the number of ports and/or the size of the trocars [1]. The concept of reduced-port surgery (RPS) has been introduced to laparoscopic surgery for colorectal malignancies. Single-incision laparoscopic surgery (SILS) performed entirely through one extraction site is considered the ultimate RPS for improving cosmesis and reducing postoperative pain and the risk of abdominal wall morbidities including bleeding and hernia [2]. Several groups have reported the feasibility and benefits of SILS for colorectal malignancies including improved cosmesis, lower pain scores, and a shorter hospital stay, when compared with standard laparoscopic surgery [3–8]. Now a few reports have shown similar long-term oncological outcomes [9, 10]. Despite the increasing interest in SILS, the actual role of this novel approach for colorectal malignancies remains to be determined, because there are some limitations such as instrument collision, poor exposure, insufficient countertraction, and somewhat narrow patient applicability [7, 11]. Novel systems have been tested to offer intuitive instruments without external instrument collision, but their use remains experimental [12].

Introducing the da Vinci robotic surgical system (Intuitive Surgical, Inc., Sunnyvale, CA, USA) has innovated the field of minimally invasive surgery. The systems are designed to allow precise movements and careful dissection while providing a three-dimensional high-definition view, human wrist-like motion for the instruments, reduced physiological tremors, superior dexterity, and greater ergonomic comfort [13, 14]. These advantages may overcome several limitations of conventional laparoscopic surgery for colorectal malignancies. The da Vinci Surgical System has therefore been widely used for total mesorectal excision (TME) in patients with a narrow pelvis [15, 16]. But the standard robotic procedure usually needs at least six or more incisions on the patient's abdomen (Fig. 14.1a, b).

In a recent attempt to overcome the technical challenges in SILS, it has been postulated that the robotic surgical system could be applied to SILS [17, 18]. By combining the use of the robotic surgical system with the single-incision platform, the recognized challenges of SILS are simplified with maintaining potential advantages of this promising minimally invasive approach.

In 2009, the first successful case for humans, which was a single-port robotic partial nephrectomy, was reported [19]. Then the first attempt at single-port robotic colectomy were conducted with concept of chopstick surgery in 2010 [20–22] (Fig. 14.2).

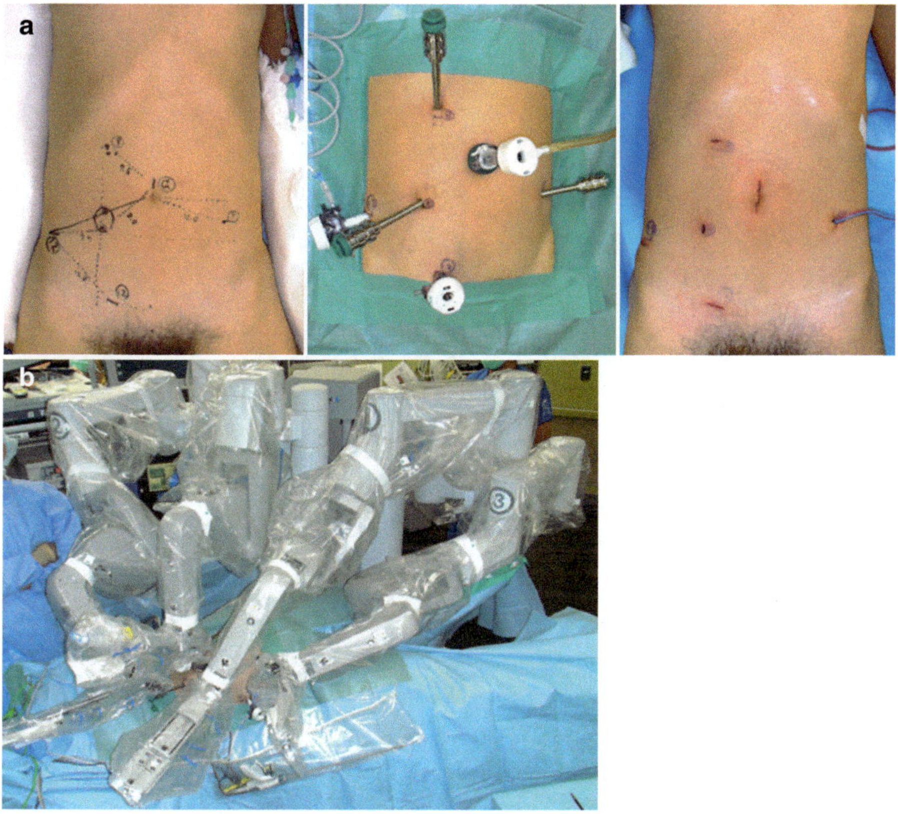

Fig. 14.1 (**a**) Trocar setting (six ports) in a standard robotic TME (three-arm approach) for rectal malignancies. (**b**) Robotic docking in a standard robotic TME (three-arm approach) for rectal malignancies

A significant advance was developed in the field of single-port robotic surgery, where the use of the da Vinci Single-Site Instrumentation platform was introduced (Fig. 14.3). The set includes a multichannel access port with four cannulas and an insufflation valve. Two curved cannulas are designed to cross within the access port for robotically controlled instruments. Significant differences in this platform are that the instrumentations are semirigid and non-wristed, and the surgeon's hand controls are electronically swapped by the computer interface.

Only a few reports of single-port robotic surgery for rectal disease have been published; however, the current robotic arm and equipment are still rather bulky and have a limited intrapelvic range of motion. It may be poorly suited for sufficient traction of the organ and smooth maneuverability. In the management of rectal malignancies, a certain oncologic clearance to maintain the principles of total mesorectal excision (TME) [23, 24] for rectal malignancies is the most important task. Thus, we have developed the novel approach for minimally invasive surgery for rectal malignancies with a combination of the da Vinci robotic surgical system and

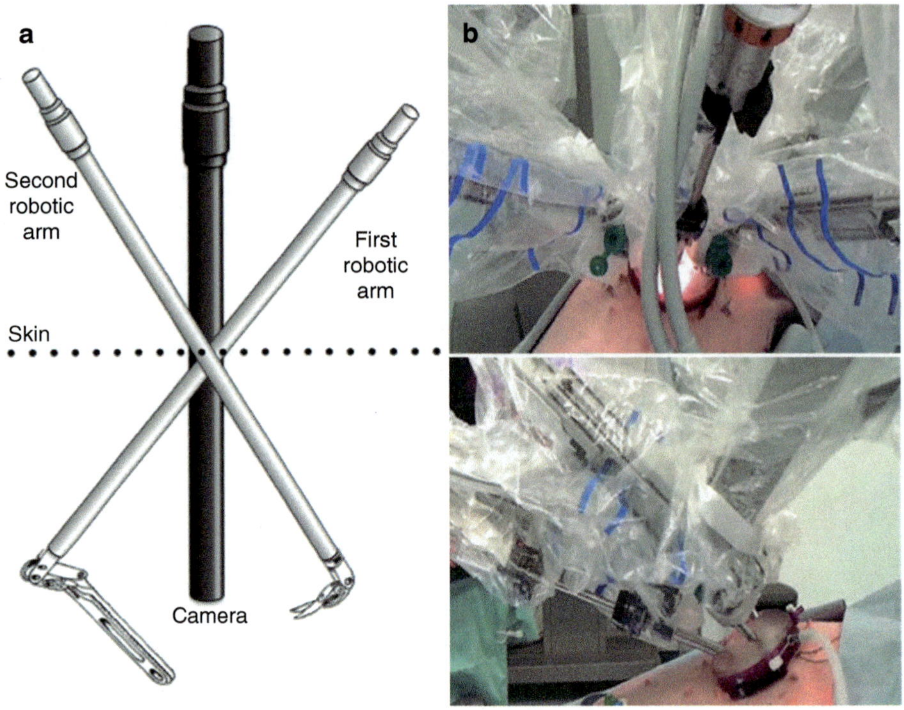

Fig. 14.2 *Left*: Robotic cross-arm "chopstick" technique (two-arm approach) for a single-incision surgery. *Right*: Robotic chopstick single-incision surgery (two-arm approach) in a porcine model

the concept of RPS, which is RARPTME. This procedure includes an initial 3-cm incision in the umbilicus and an 8-mm robotic trocar in the right lower quadrant with an additional 3-mm trocar in the right flank. Our robotic procedure is well suited for good countertraction and smooth maneuverability of the devices avoiding possible instrument collision. In addition, it can provide improving cosmesis and theoretically reducing postoperative pain when compared with standard robotic surgery that usually needs at least six scars (Figs. 14.1 and 14.4a, b).

Here, we introduce our techniques for RARPTME with low colorectal anastomosis. Our approach makes it possible to standardize the procedure for robotic rectal surgery in a safe and a certain manner.

14.2 Indications and Contraindications

Indications for RARPTME are T1–T3 tumor, tumor diameter <4 cm, body mass index (BMI) <35 kg/m^2, and the American Society of Anesthesiologists class <2. Advanced T4 tumor, a huge or bulky tumor ≥4 cm, severe obesity, perforated tumor, stenosis with bowel distention, prior abdominal surgery, and any severe comorbidity are contraindications. Complete informed consent is imperative.

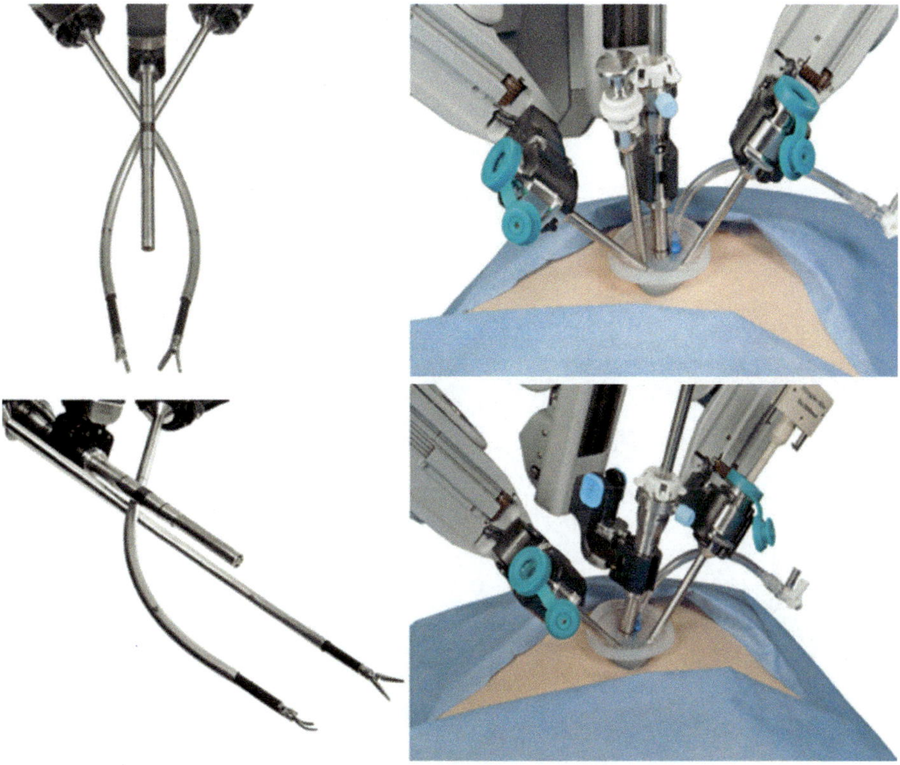

Fig. 14.3 da Vinci Single-Site Instrumentation platform (two-arm approach)

14.3 Technique

14.3.1 Patient Positioning and Operative Setup

The patient, under general anesthesia, is positioned on the operating table. The patient's feet are placed in boot-type leg holders with the legs spread apart and knees slightly flexed. The arms are tucked along the patient's sides. The operator, the assistant, and the scrub nurse stand on the right of the patient, and the robotic and laparoscopic monitor are situated between the patient's legs (Fig. 14.4b).

14.3.2 Access to the Abdominal Cavity

A 3-cm vertical skin incision and mini-laparotomy incision are made in the umbilicus. A multichannel access device such as GelPOINT devices (Applied Medical, Rancho Santa Margarita, CA, USA) with a previously installed a 12-mm trocar for the laparoscope, the first 8-mm robotic trocar which is for the operator's left hand and a 5-mm trocar for the assistant is fitted into the incision (Fig. 14.5). After

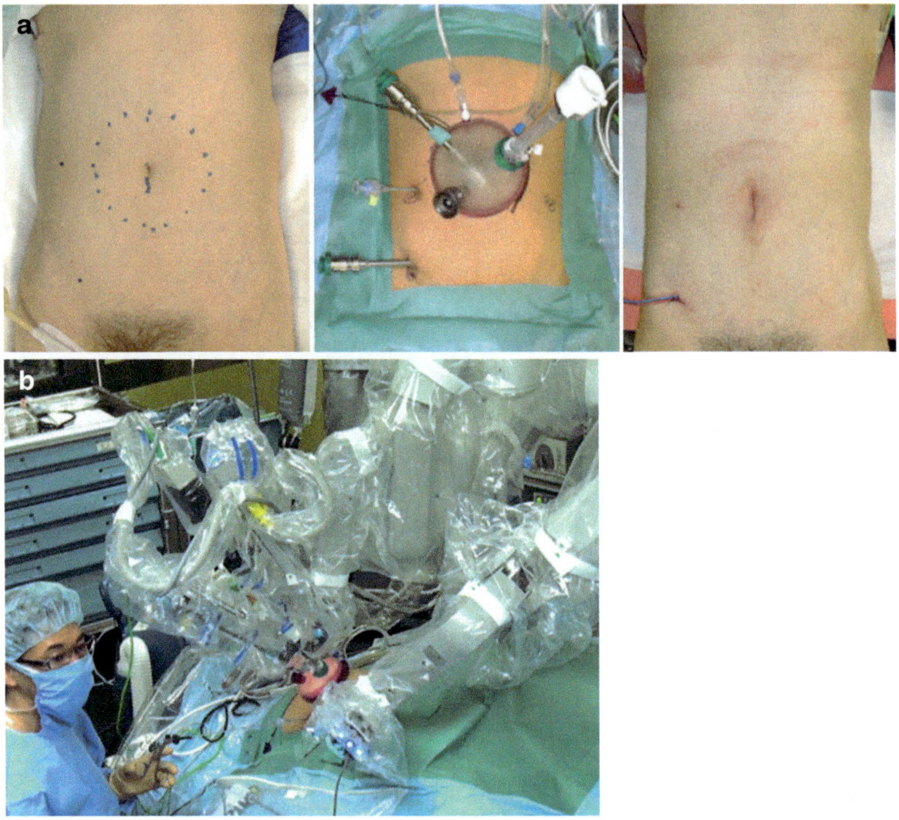

Fig. 14.4 (**a**) Trocar setting and an incision in a robotic reduced-port TME (two-arm approach) for rectal malignancies. (**b**) Robotic docking in a robotic reduced-port TME (two-arm approach) for rectal malignancies. The operator and the assistant stand on the right of the patient

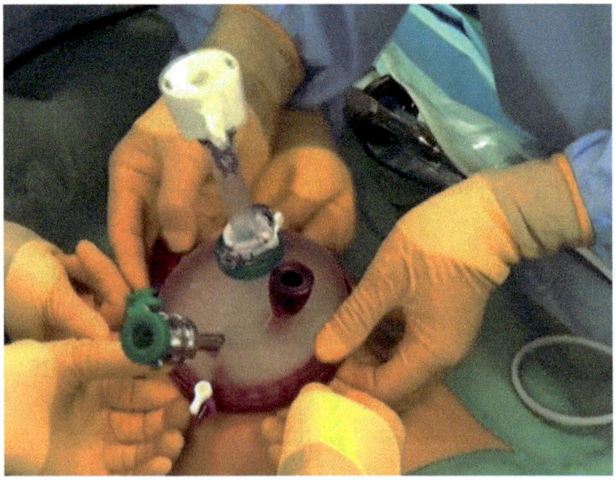

Fig. 14.5 A multichannel access device with a previously installed 12-mm trocar for the laparoscope; the first 8-mm robotic trocar and a 5-mm trocar for the assistant are fitted into a 3-cm vertical skin incision in the umbilicus

establishment of CO_2 pneumoperitoneum, the second 8-mm robotic trocar for the operator's right hand is inserted in the right lower quadrant. Finally, a 3-mm additional trocar for the assistant's right hand is placed in the right flank (Fig. 14.4a, b). We prefer to use atraumatic graspers or fine dissectors as the assistant's forceps. These two additional trocars should be placed at least 5 cm away from the GelPOINT devices for reducing the instruments collision. The assistant can facilitate in the suctioning of blood, retraction, or use of an energy device. Our procedure is a two-arm approach, and we do not use the third robotic arm (Fig. 14.4b).

Further additional incision or trocar port is made without hesitation if necessary to complete the procedure, and conversion to open laparotomy is kept as an option. The indication and timing of trocar insertion or conversion to open surgery depend on the surgeon's judgment.

14.3.3 Operative Exposure

CO_2 pneumoperitoneum is established and maintained at 10 mmHg. After complete exploration of the abdomen to identify any metastatic nodules or superficial hepatic metastases with a robotic laparoscope, the patient is tilted into a deep Trendelenburg position and inclined to the right. The small intestine is moved into the right upper quadrant, exposing the root of the left colonic mesentery with standard laparoscopic devices (Fig. 14.6). The greater omentum is then flipped to expose the transverse colon and the splenic flexure.

14.3.4 Robotic Docking

Our method is performed in a single docking to avoid undocking–redocking of the robotic cart and to save time. The da Vinci S or Si system in a two-arm approach is docked to the left hip of the patient at a slight angle aiming at the umbilicus, like

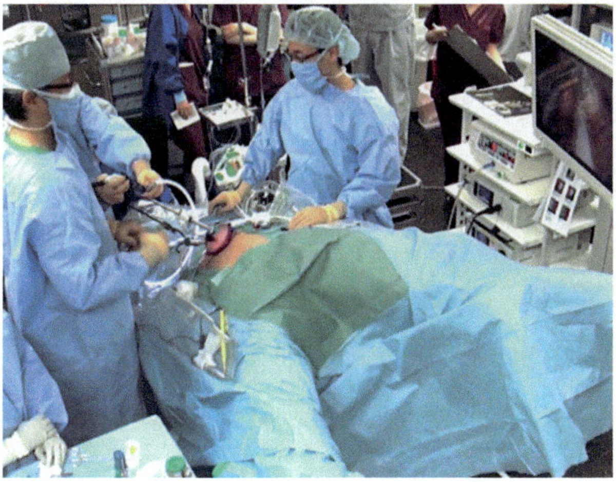

Fig. 14.6 Standard laparoscopic procedure for exposing good operative view at the beginning of the procedure before robotic docking

standard robotic procedure for rectal diseases (Fig. 14.4b). Precise adjustments of port placement and docking of the robotic system for the correct location are needed.

14.3.5 Dissection of the Left Colonic Mesentery and the Mesorectum

By tenting the left colonic mesentery with cooperation of the first robotic grasper and a 3-mm atraumatic grasper held in the assistant's right hand, the root of the left colonic mesentery is incised with the second robotic device, starting at the sacral promontory, in a medial to lateral approach (Fig. 14.7a). The appropriate plane is dissected, preserving the right hypogastric nerve (Fig. 14.7b). Continuous dissection below the inferior mesenteric artery (IMA) is performed by sweeping down the retroperitoneal fascia to preserve the left ureter and the gonadal vessels in the posterior plane (Fig. 14.8). The mesorectum is dissected posteriorly in the plane of total mesorectal excision, in front of the hypogastric plexus nerves. The medial dissection is continued until the inferior border of the pancreas on Gerota's fascia is reached.

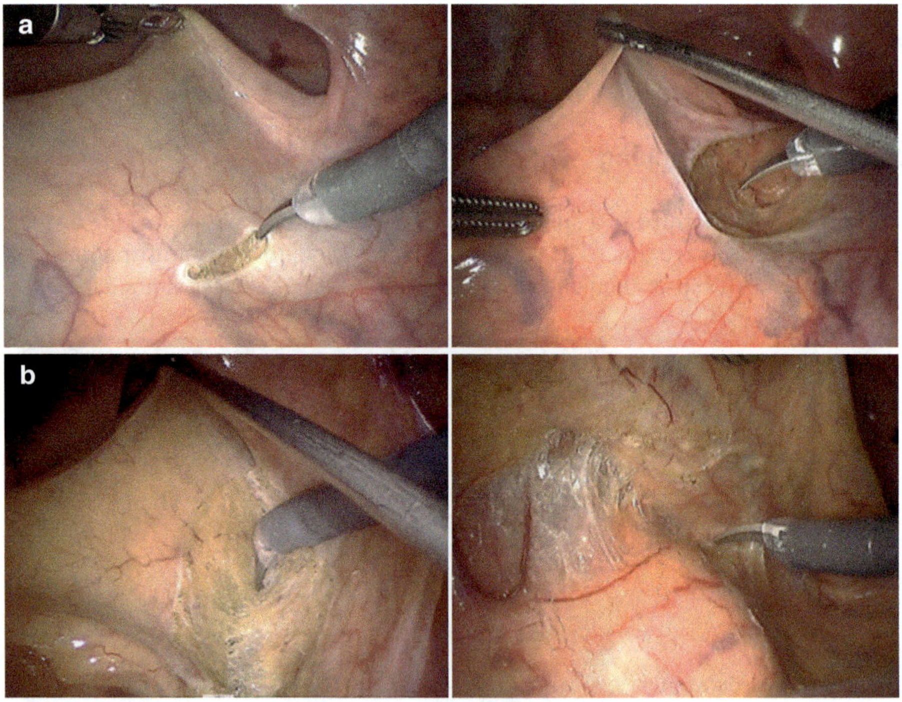

Fig. 14.7 (**a**) Initial incision on the root of the left colonic mesentery with a good operative view. (**b**) Medial-to-lateral approach for dissection of the left colonic mesentery and the mesorectum, preserving the right hypogastric nerve

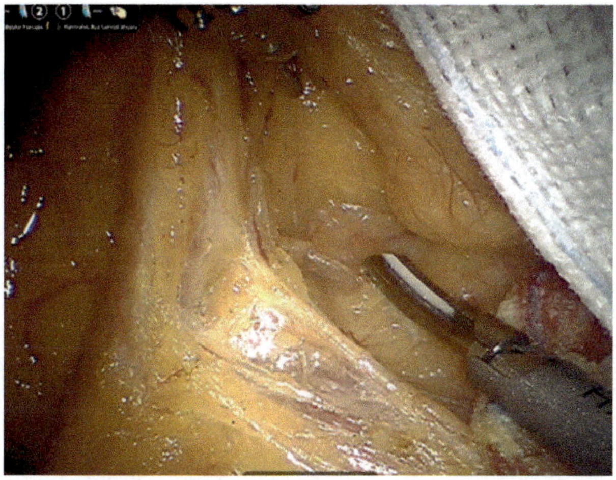

Fig. 14.8 Dissection below the inferior mesenteric artery by sweeping down the retroperitoneal fascia to preserve the left ureter and gonadal vessels

14.3.6 Ligation of the Inferior Mesenteric Vessels

The inferior mesenteric vessels are ligated. When there is a need to ligate the IMA at its origin, the IMA is dissected between clips 0.5 cm away from its aortic origin so as not to injure the lumbar splanchnic nerves (Fig. 14.9a). When possible, to preserve blood flow to the left colic artery (LCA), the superior rectal artery (SRA) is dissected between clips with or without D3 lymphadenectomy around the origin of the IMA (Fig. 14.9a). The inferior mesenteric vein is exposed and dissected at the same level of the IMA ligation between two clips (Fig. 14.9b).

14.3.7 Mobilization of the Left Colon and Rectum

The lateral attachment of the left colon and rectum is dissected from bottom to top and is freed up to near the splenic flexure (Fig. 14.10). The greater omentum is lifted cephalad in some cases with a retracting device such as the EndoGrab Retractor (Virtual Ports, Israel). In the case that needs complete mobilization of the splenic flexure, it is easier to do this procedure with standard laparoscopic devices in a laparoscopic-robotic hybrid technique. Precise partial or complete mesorectal dissection in the TME plane according to the location of the tumor is indispensable (Fig. 14.11a–c).

14.3.8 Transection of the Rectum

The fat surrounding the rectum at the transection line is removed, and the superior rectal vessels are dissected. In preparation for transection of the rectum, the second 8-mm robotic trocar in the right lower quadrant is changed to a 12-mm trocar for the introduction of a linear stapler. The rectum is clamped and transected by one firing

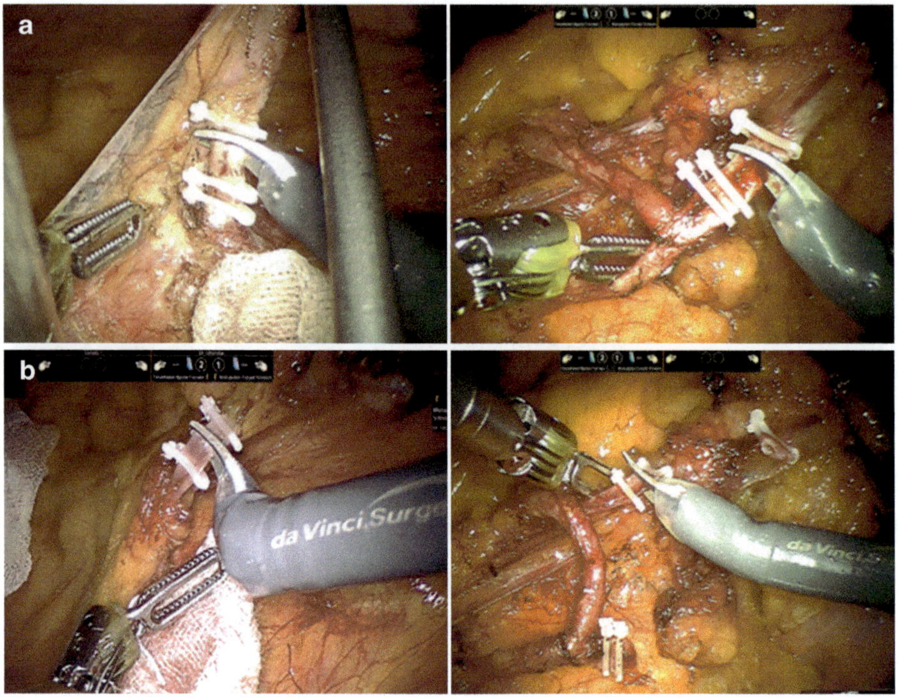

Fig. 14.9 (**a**) *Left*: Dissection of IMA between clips 0.5 cm away from its aortic origin so as not to injure the lumbar splanchnic nerves (high tie D3 lymphadenectomy). *Right*: Skeletonization of the IMA and its branches with D3 lymphadenectomy around the origin of the IMA to preserve the left colic artery (LCA preserving D3 lymphadenectomy). (**b**) Ligation of the IMV between two clips at the same level of the IMA ligation in high tie D3 lymphadenectomy (*left*) and LCA preserving D3 lymphadenectomy (*right*)

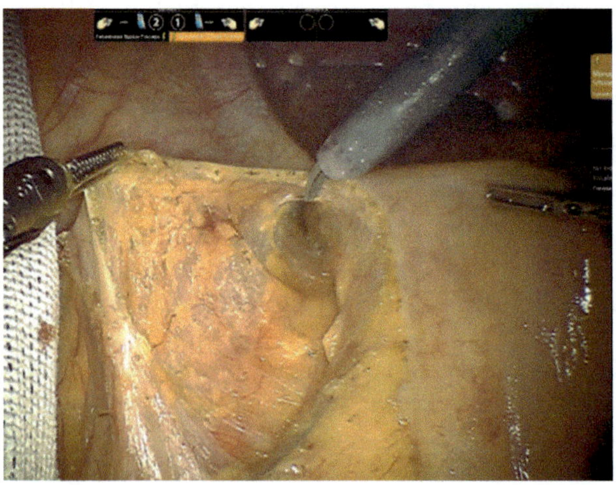

Fig. 14.10 Dissection of the left side of the rectum

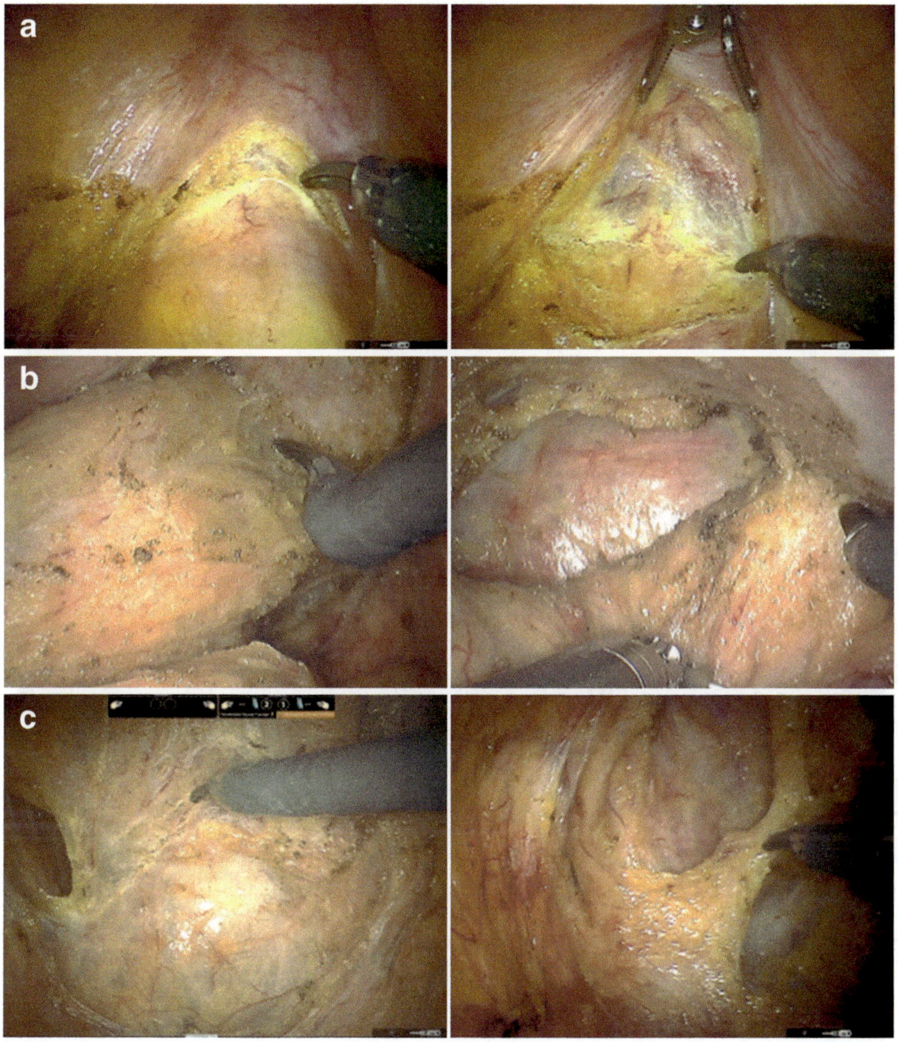

Fig. 14.11 (**a**) Open the peritoneal reflection. (**b**) Dissection of the mesorectum anteriorly in the plane of TME. (**c**) Dissection of the mesorectum posteriorly in the plane of TME

of an articulated linear stapler with a 60-mm cartridge or two firing with two 45-mm one (Fig. 14.12). The rectum is drawn cephalad so that the staple line is perpendicular to the axis of the rectum.

14.3.9 Extraction of the Specimen

After removal of the top of the GelPOINT device with the lap protector remaining in place, the left colon and rectum are extracted through the mini-laparotomy

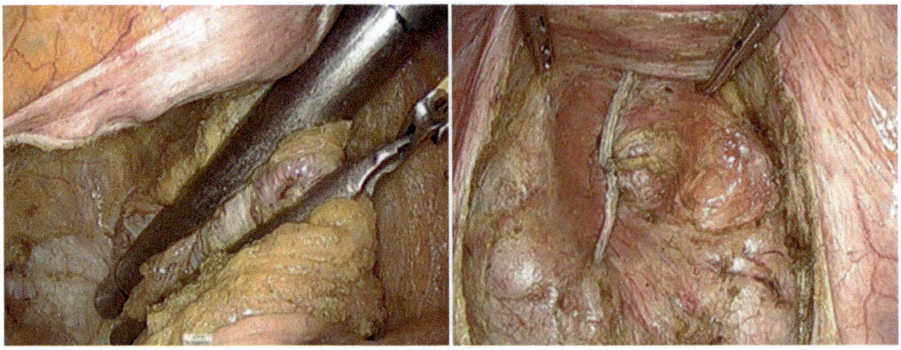

Fig. 14.12 Transection of the rectum by one firing of an articulated linear stapler with a 60-mm cartridge

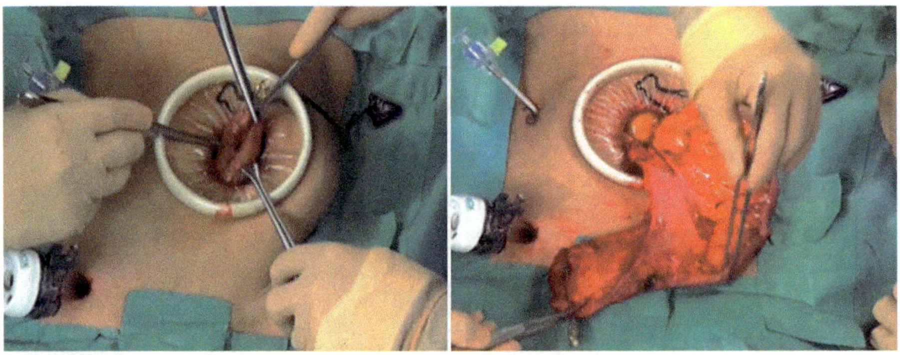

Fig. 14.13 Extraction of the specimen through the mini-laparotomy incision in the umbilicus

incision in the umbilicus (Fig. 14.13). The sigmoid colon and its mesentery are divided at least 10 cm proximal to the lesion after ligation of the mesentery vessels and the adjacent vascular arcade.

14.3.10 Colorectal Anastomosis

After undocking the robotic cart completely, the anvil of the circular stapling device is introduced into the stump of the proximal colon for anastomosis. The colon, with the anvil, is replaced in the abdomen, and the GelPOINT device is reapplied for reestablishment of the pneumoperitoneum. After confirming that the descending colon and the mesentery are not twisted, colorectal anastomosis is performed intracorporeally by the double-stapling technique with a standard laparoscopic manner (Fig. 14.14). Airtightness is tested by transanal injection of air while the anastomosis is checked endoscopically, and the intestinal rings are examined for secure placement. The small intestines are repositioned in front of the left mesocolon. An intracorporeal drainage tube is placed through a 12-mm trocar site (Fig. 14.4a).

Fig. 14.14 Colorectal anastomosis performed intracorporeally by the double-stapling technique

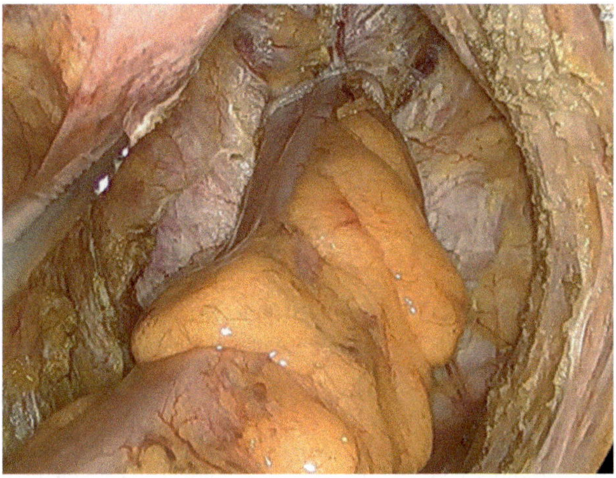

14.3.11 Wound Closure

The fascia is closed with interrupted absorbable sutures. The peritoneum is not closed separately. After the fascia is closed, the wound is rinsed free of blood and cell debris with Ringer's lactate solution. An anchoring suture is tied to the rectus sheath at the bottom of the umbilicus, and subcutaneous absorbable sutures are placed (Fig. 14.4a). Finally, the incision is re-measured.

References

1. Curcillo PG 2nd, Podolsky ER, King SA. The road to reduced port surgery: from single big incisions to single small incisions, and beyond. World J Surg. 2011;35:1526–31.
2. Takemasa I, Sekimoto M, Ikeda M, Mizushima T, Yamamoto H, Doki Y, Mori M. Video. Transumbilical single-incision laparoscopic surgery for sigmoid colon cancer. Surg Endosc. 2010;24:2321.
3. Papaconstantinou HT, Thomas JS. Single-incision laparoscopic colectomy for cancer: assessment of oncologic resection and short-term outcomes in a case-matched comparison with standard laparoscopy. Surgery. 2011;50:820–7.
4. Ramos-Valadez DI, Ragupathi M, Nieto J, Patel CB, Miller S, Pickron TB, Haas EM. Single-incision versus conventional laparoscopic sigmoid colectomy: a case-matched series. Surg Endosc. 2012;26:96–102.
5. Kim SJ, Ryu GO, Choi BJ, Kim JG, Lee KJ, Lee SC, Oh ST. The short-term outcomes of conventional and single-port laparoscopic surgery for colorectal cancer. Ann Surg. 2011;254:933–40.
6. Champagne BJ, Papaconstantinou HT, Parmar SS, Nagle DA, Young-Fadok TM, Lee EC, Delaney CP. Single-incision versus standard multiport laparoscopic colectomy: a multicenter, case-controlled comparison. Ann Surg. 2012;255:66–9.
7. Takemasa I, Uemura M, Nishimura J, Mizushima T, Yamamoto H, Ikeda M, Sekimoto M, Doki Y, Mori M. Feasibility of single-site laparoscopic colectomy with complete mesocolic excision for colon cancer: a prospective case-control comparison. Surg Endosc. 2014;28:1110–8.
8. Hiraki M, Takemasa I, Uemura M, Haraguchi N, Nishimura J, Hata T, Mizushima T, Yamamoto H, Doki Y, Mori M. Evaluation of invasiveness in single-site laparoscopic colectomy, using "the PainVision system" for quantitative analysis of pain sensation. Surg Endosc. 2014;28:3216–23.

9. Yun JA, Yun SH, Park YA, Huh JW, Cho YB, Kim HC, Lee WY. Oncologic outcomes of single-incision laparoscopic surgery compared with conventional laparoscopy for colon cancer. Ann Surg. 2016;263(5):973–8.
10. Katsuno G, Fukunaga M, Nagakari K, Yoshikawa S, Azuma D, Kohama S. Short-term and long-term outcomes of single-incision versus multi-incision laparoscopic resection for colorectal cancer: a propensity-score-matched analysis of 214 cases. Surg Endosc. 2015;30(4):1317–25.
11. Hamabe A, Takemasa I, Uemura M, Nishimura J, Mizushima T, Ikeda M, Yamamoto H, Sekimoto M, Doki Y, Mori M. Feasibility of single-port laparoscopic surgery for sigmoid colon and rectal cancers and preoperative assessment of operative difficulty. J Gastrointest Surg. 2014;18:977–85.
12. Haber GP, Autorino R, Laydner H, Yang B, White MA, Hillyer S, Altunrende F, Khanna R, Spana G, Wahib I, Fareed K, Stein RJ, Kaouk JH. SPIDER surgical system for urologic procedures with laparoendoscopic single-site surgery: from initial laboratory experience to first clinical application. Eur Urol. 2012;61:415–22.
13. Lanfranco AR, Castellanos AE, Desai JP, Meyers WC. Robotic surgery: a current perspective. Ann Surg. 2004;239:14–21.
14. Maeso S, Reza M, Mayol JA, Blasco JA, Guerra M, Andradas E, Plana MN. Efficacy of the Da Vinci surgical system in abdominal surgery compared with that of laparoscopy: a systematic review and meta-analysis. Ann Surg. 2010;252:254–62.
15. Park JS, Choi GS, Lim KH, Jang YS, Jun SH. Robotic-assisted versus laparoscopic surgery for low rectal cancer: case-matched analysis of short-term outcomes. Ann Surg Oncol. 2010;17:3195–202.
16. Pigazzi A, Luca F, Patriti A, Valvo M, Ceccarelli G, Casciola L, Biffi R, Garcia-Aguilar J, Baek JH. Multicentric study on robotic tumorspecific mesorectal excision for the treatment of rectal cancer. Ann Surg Oncol. 2010;17:1614–20.
17. White MA, Haber GP, Autorino R, Khanna R, Altunrende F, Yang B, Stein RJ, Kaouk JH. Robotic laparoendoscopic single-site surgery. BJU Int. 2010;106:923–7.
18. Rane A, Autorino R. Robotic natural orifice translumenal endoscopic surgery and laparoendoscopic single-site surgery: current status. Curr Opin Urol. 2011;21:71–7.
19. Kaouk JH, Goel RK, Haber GP, Crouzet S, Stein RJ. Robotic single-port transumbilical surgery in humans: initial report. BJU Int. 2009;103:366–9.
20. Ragupathi M, Ramos-Valadez DI, Pedraza R, Haas EM. Roboticassisted single-incision laparoscopic partial cecectomy. Int J Med Robot. 2010;6:362–7.
21. Ostrowitz MB, Eschete D, Zemon H, DeNoto G. Robotic-assisted single-incision right colectomy: early experience. Int J Med Robot. 2009;5:465–70.
22. Joseph RA, Goh AC, Cuevas SP, Donovan MA, Kauffman MG, Salas NA, Miles B, Bass BL, Dunkin BJ. "Chopstick" surgery: a novel technique improves surgeon performance and eliminates arm collision in robotic single-incision laparoscopic surgery. Surg Endosc. 2010;24:1331–5.
23. Heald RJ. The 'Holy Plane' of rectal surgery. J R Soc Med. 1988;81:503–8.
24. Quirke P, Durdey P, Dixon MF, Williams NS. Local recurrence of rectal adenocarcinoma due to inadequate surgical resection. Histopathological study of lateral tumour spread and surgical excision. Lancet. 1986;2:996–9.

Multiport Laparoscopic TME with Coloanal Anastomosis

15

Bart van Geluwe, Quentin Denost, and Eric Rullier

Abstract

Total mesorectal excision (TME) is the gold standard technique for the surgical treatment of rectal cancer. Despite the benefits of minimally invasive surgery, laparoscopic TME is a technically challenging procedure with a long learning curve. Quality of surgery is evaluated by completeness of the mesorectal envelope and resection margins. Other objectives are sphincter preservation and functional outcome. The concept for sphincter-saving resection is related to the distance between the tumor and the anal sphincter. It is now generally accepted that involvement of circumferential resection margin (CRM) is an important risk factor of local recurrence, and considerably circumferential resection margin is more relevant than the distal resection margin. The technique of intersphincteric resection has been developed to move to a more conservative (sphincter salvage) concept in lower rectal cancer. In this chapter we describe step-by-step our standardized technique of multiport laparoscopic TME, with or without an intersphincteric resection for low rectal cancer.

Keywords

Coloanal anastomosis • Intersphincteric • Low rectal cancer • Sphincter saving

B. van Geluwe (✉) • Q. Denost • E. Rullier
Department of Digestive Surgery, Saint-André Hospital, CHU Bordeaux, University of Bordeaux, 1 rue Jean Burguet, 33075 Bordeaux, France
e-mail: bartvangeluwe@hotmail.com

G. Dapri, J.H. Marks (eds.), *Surgical Techniques in Rectal Cancer*,
https://doi.org/10.1007/978-4-431-55579-7_15

15.1 Introduction

Surgery for rectal cancer has evolved immensely during the last decades, with improved pelvic imaging, optimizing neoadjuvant therapy and the minimally invasive "revolution" of laparoscopic surgery. The surgical quality is evaluated by completeness of the mesorectal envelope and resection margins. Other objectives are sphincter reservation and functional outcome. Regardless of whether an open or a laparoscopic procedure is used, the most pressing challenges relate to achieving these quality indicators in low rectal cancer (tumors located within 6 cm from the anal verge). The concept for sphincter-saving resection is related to the distance between the tumor and the anal sphincter. It is now generally accepted that involvement of circumferential resection margin (CRM) is an important risk factor of local recurrence, and considerably circumferential resection margin is more relevant than the distal resection margin [1]. A better understanding of rectal cancer disease allowed decreasing the distal surgical margin from 5 to 2 cm and more recently to 1 cm [2–4]. The surgical guidelines therefore recommend sphincter preservation in patients with a tumor more than 1 cm and abdominoperineal resection (APR) for tumors <1 cm from the anal ring [5]. Furthermore the perception that the lymphatic spread of these tumors occurs only in a cranial direction within the mesorectum and the local spread is only few millimeters in distal direction opened the challenge of sphincter preservation in very low rectal tumors. The internal anal sphincter consists of smooth muscle fibers which are continuous with the muscular layer of the rectal wall (visceral structures), whereas the external sphincter is a complex of striated muscle fibers, forming a functional entity with the pelvic floor (skeletal structures). There is an embryological plane of fusion between both. As long as the external sphincter apparatus is not infiltrated by the tumor, there is no reason to remove the sphincter. This new concept transforms a 1 cm discussion to a 1 mm one [6]. The technique of intersphincteric resection has been developed to move to a more conservative (sphincter salvage) concept in lower rectal cancer [7]. We therefore introduced a new surgical classification of low rectal cancer, separating patients with low rectal cancer in four groups, according to the location of the tumor from the anal sphincter (Table 15.1) [8]. Standardization of surgery defines

Table 15.1 The surgical classification of low rectal cancer separates patients in four groups according to the location of the tumor from the anal sphincter

Classification of low rectal cancer		Location of lesion	Surgical procedure
Type I	Supra-anal tumor	>1 cm from the anal ring (top anal canal) Or >2 cm from the dentate line	Coloanal anastomosis
Type II	Juxta-anal tumor	<1 cm from the anal ring (top anal canal) Or <2 cm from the dentate line	Partial intersphincteric resection (pISR)
Type III	Intra-anal tumor	Infiltration of the internal anal sphincter	Total intersphincteric resection (tISR)
Type IV	Transanal tumor	Infiltration of the external anal sphincter or levator ani muscles	Abdominoperineal excision (APR)

The standardization of surgery defines four surgical procedures, each dedicated to the four types of low rectal cancer [8]

four surgical procedures, each dedicated to the four types of low rectal cancer. Type I is treated by conventional (manual or mechanic) coloanal anastomosis, whereas abdominoperineal excision (APR) is indicated for type IV tumors. Abdominoperineal intersphincteric resection is proposed for tumors type II or III, lesions located <1 cm from the anal sphincter or lesions infiltrating the internal anal sphincter, respectively. The goal of this approach is to perform a dissection between the internal sphincter and the external sphincter by beginning the dissection either at the dentate line or underneath the dentate line to remove part (type II) or the whole of the internal anal sphincter (type III), respectively, in order to obtain an adequate distal resection margin and to avoid permanent colostomy. The purpose of this chapter is to describe step-by-step our standardized laparoscopic technique of intersphincteric rectum resection.

15.2 Preparation of the Operation

15.2.1 Installation

The positioning of the patient should be facilitated on a modern operating table, where lifting and lowering of the leg supports are possible by a remote control (Fig. 15.1). The patient is positioned in Lloyd-Davies position with the perineum slightly projecting from the end of the operating table. The patient's arms are fixed alongside the body. We use the system of padded shoulder straps in an X

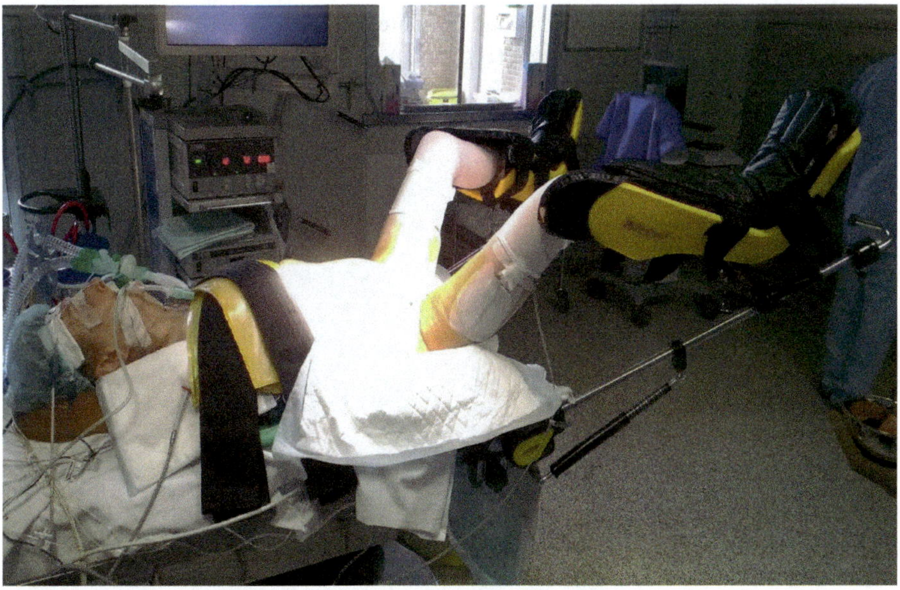

Fig. 15.1 Operating table with special leg support

fashion to secure the upper torso in order to achieve a stable fixation of the patient during steep Trendelenburg. Care has to be taken that movements of the table or leg supports do not cause unphysiological pressures on the nerves, skin, etc. Therefore, the movements and their effect on the patient should be checked before the patient is completely covered with sterile surgical drapes. During the abdominal part, a flexion of the hip joint of 20° is sufficient. As soon as the perineal part starts, the flexion should be changed to 80–90°. During the perianal part, it is helpful to move the table to a 10° head-down (Trendelenburg) position.

15.2.2 Instruments

In general we need two sets of instruments: one set for the abdominal part of the operation and one for the perineal part.

For the abdominal part, we need a typical set which can be used for all kinds of laparoscopic surgery. The dissection can be undertaken with monopolar laparoscopic instrumentation (graspers, scissors), harmonic scalpel (Ultracision™, Ethicon Endo-Surgery, Cincinnati, Ohio, USA), or thermal fusion (LigaSure™, Covidien, Mansfield, Massachusetts, USA). The optimal video-laparoscopic equipment may be a high-definition (HD) video tower, with one or two monitors, automatic insufflation with warmed CO_2 gas supply, and possibility for video documentation. A 10-mm, 0-degree optic lens is generally used.

For the perineal part we need a smaller set of conventional instruments. An important tool for exposure of the anal canal is the Lone Star retractor with eight hooks (CooperSurgical, Trumbull, Connecticut, USA). This disposable set allows an atraumatic exposure of the anal canal. For entering the intersphincteric space, we use two small Langenbeck retractors (Fig. 15.2).

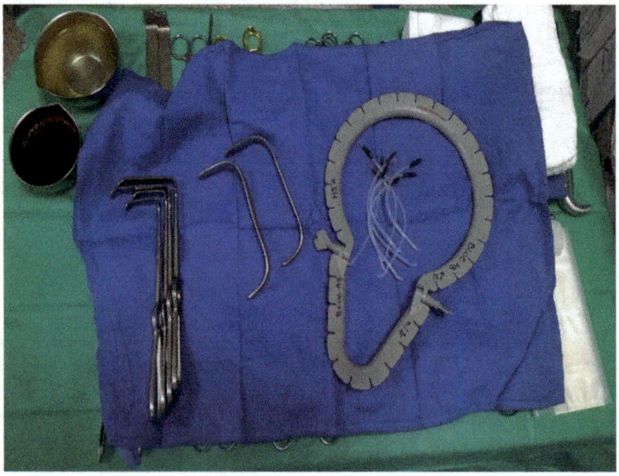

Fig. 15.2 Instruments for the perineal part of the dissection

15.2.3 Positioning of the Surgical Team

The surgeon stands to the right of the patient, and the monitor is located in his line of vision at the left of the patient. The camera assistant and the scrub nurse stand ipsilaterally, respectively, at the left and at the right of the surgeon. A second assistant stands between the legs of the patient. The operative technique is achieved by a five-port procedure.

15.3 Standardized Surgical Technique

15.3.1 Step 1: Pneumoperitoneum and Positioning of the Trocars

Before the first incision, the entire team takes a "time out" to complete the surgical safety checklist. Prophylactic antibiotics should be initiated within 1 h before surgical incision. We use an open access of the first 12-mm port through a longitudinal supraumbilical incision. The intra-abdominal pressure is maintained at 12 mmHg. After the initial diagnostic laparoscopic evaluation, the first 5-mm port (right lower quadrant) is placed on the midclavicular line under continuous optical control. The second 5-mm port is inserted in the right subcostal area. The third 5-mm trocar is placed in the left midclavicular line, at the level of the umbilicus. The fourth port is inserted at the midline, 1 cm above the pubic symphysis. This port can be changed for a 12-mm trocar in case of a distal stapling (Fig. 15.3).

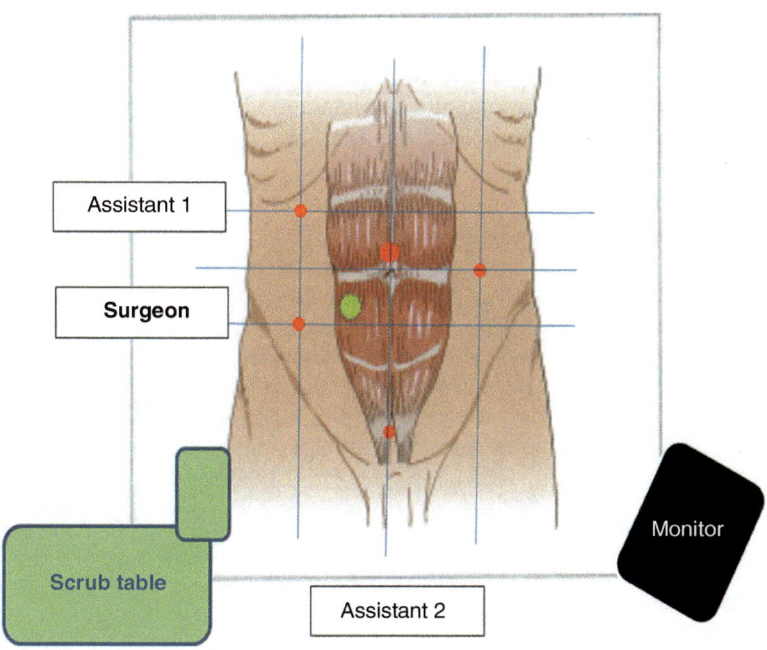

Fig. 15.3 Port placement and positions of the surgical team during the abdominal

15.3.2 Step 2: Laparoscopic Exposure

We start with a medial to lateral splenic flexure mobilization. The first step in the laparoscopic procedure consists in exposing the inferior mesenteric vein, which corresponds to the first anatomical landmark (Fig. 15.4). Therefore the patient is placed in a steep Trendelenburg position and is tilted right-side down, so the small intestine falls out of the pelvis into the upper right quadrant. The small bowel loops are retracted upon the liver, and the omentum is flipped over the transverse colon. If the stomach is distended, the anesthesiologist should aspirate the stomach with a well-positioned nasogastric tube for optimal exposure.

15.3.3 Step 3: Mobilization of the Splenic Flexure

The inferior mesenteric vein (IMV) is grasped, and the adhesions between the proximal jejunum and the vein are dissected (ligament of Treitz). The IMV is now elevated and the peritoneum just under the vein is incised. The mesocolon is gently elevated by both the surgeon and assistant ("as under a tent"), and a meticulous medial to lateral dissection is carried out to identify the embryological plane separating the mesocolon from Toldt's fascia and the retroperitoneal structures (Fig. 15.5). The risk is to dissect too deep and to open Gerota's fascia (perirenal); with some experience one learns to find easily the good plane of dissection, which is in fact an avascular one. Dissection is continued up along the white line of Toldt as lateral as possible. The landmarks of this dissection are the birth of the left colic artery caudally and the pancreas cranially (Fig. 15.6). The plane between the mesocolon and the anterior surface of the pancreas is developed. During this step, the IMV is preserved and served as potential landmark to identify the pancreas. By dissecting from the posterior approach, the incision of the transverse mesentery

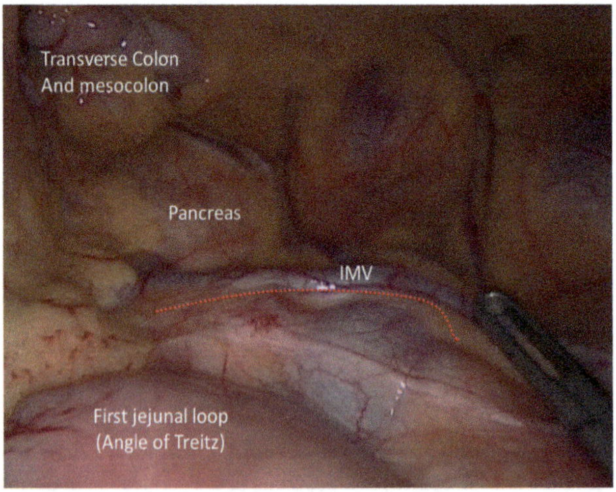

Fig. 15.4 Splenic flexure mobilization. Exposure of the first anatomical landmark: the inferior mesenteric vein (IMV). *Red dotted line*: line of peritoneal incision

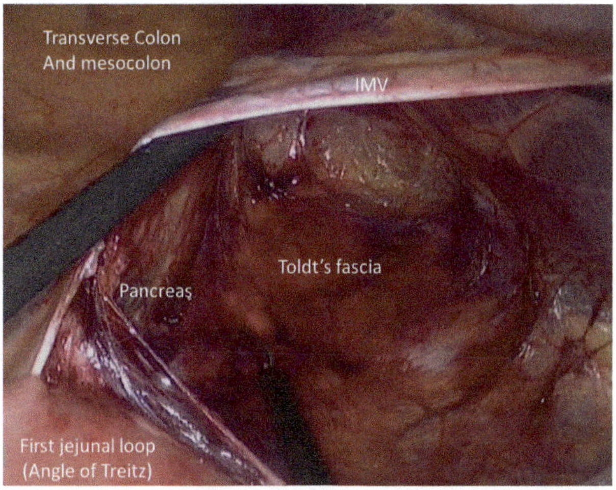

Fig. 15.5 The mesocolon is gently elevated by both the surgeon and assistant ("as under a tent"), and a meticulous medial to lateral dissection is carried out to identify the embryological plane separating the mesocolon from Toldt's fascia and the retroperitoneal structures

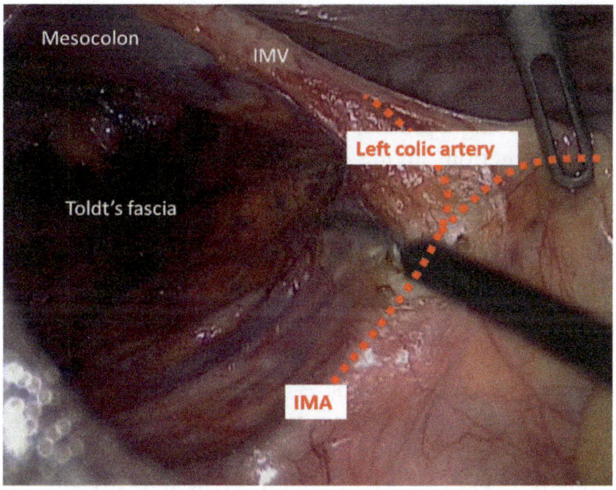

Fig. 15.6 The landmarks of the medial to lateral dissection are the pancreas cranially and the birth of the left colic artery caudally

permits to identify the pancreas and to enter in the lesser sac. The loose attachments between these two structures can be taken down with gentle blunt or monopolar dissection. Although this is an avascular plane, care must be taken not to injure the pancreas. The lesser sac is therefore entered from the medial side, and the stomach comes into view.

The complete anterior dissection of the pancreas makes the transverse mesentery totally free and finishes the medial approach (Fig. 15.7).

In some difficult cases, the complete dissection of the terminal part of the IMV improves the view of the pancreas giving the plane to open the lesser sac.

Once this plane is sufficiently opened laterally and caudally, we turn our attention to the inferior mesenteric artery (IMA) ligation. The presacral area is the second anatomical landmark in order to facilitate this vascular ligation.

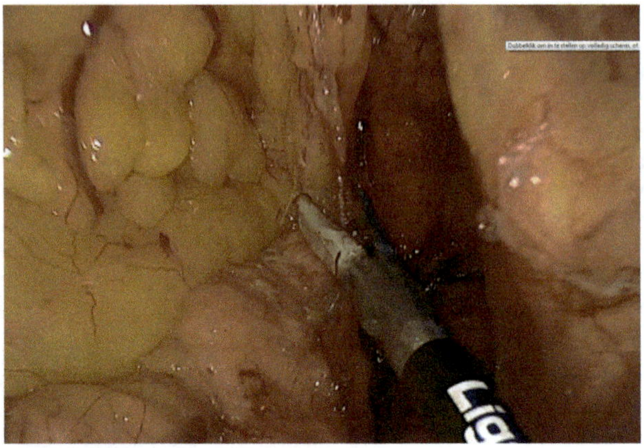

Fig. 15.7 The complete anterior dissection of the pancreas makes the transverse mesentery totally free and finishes the medial approach

15.3.4 Step 4: Arterial Ligation

Before starting pelvic dissection, it is important to locate, at the level of the sacral promontory, the cleavage between the parietal layer (presacral fascia) of the pelvic fascia and the visceral layer that underlines the mesorectum. We expose this presacral area using a grasper holding the sigmoid mesentery under traction in a ventrolateral direction, giving an optimal view of the promontory. This is an avascular plane, and by adequate ventral traction, we can demonstrate the shiny posterior surface of the mesorectum. An incision of the peritoneum is performed exactly 2 cm in front of the promontory allowing the beginning of the dissection of the upper part of the mesorectum, which is also the distal part of the IMA (Fig. 15.8). With some "help" of the pneumoperitoneum ("pneumodissection"), the "angel hairs" of the mesorectal space can be opened, and the proximal mesorectum is dissected posteriorly on a few centimeters. A medial to lateral plane is developed to separate the mesocolon and mesorectum from the retroperitoneum. Under continuous traction, the peritoneum is incised cephalad toward the direction of the origin of the IMA and caudally toward the right lateral rectal stalks. Using blunt dissection, the IMA is swept ventrally away from the preaortic hypogastric neural plexus, which is swept dorsally to prevent injury to it. Dissection is continued beneath the inferior mesenteric artery and vein; the left ureter and gonadal vessels are identified. The dissection is continued cranially. The objective is to connect the area of the proximal part of the mesorectum with the previously completed dissection under the IMV/left colic artery complex.

In this way, the origin of the IMA is isolated, and a characteristic T-shaped structure is identified comprising the origin of the IMA, the left colic/IMV complex, and the superior rectal artery (Fig. 15.9). This step allows identifying the artery exactly 2 cm from the aorta in order to preserve the sympathetic nerves and facilitate the end of the dissection of the IMA by using an accurate instrument. The IMA must be completely free before performing ligation or transection. Various kinds of ligation can be used, such as clips, suture, or vascular stapling devices. Thermal fusion by

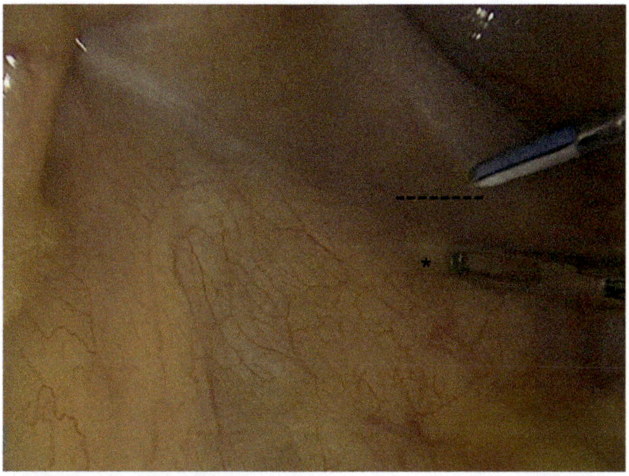

Fig. 15.8 An incision of the peritoneum is performed exactly 2 cm in front of the promontory allowing the beginning of the dissection of the upper part of the mesorectum (*, promontory. *dotted line*, incision line)

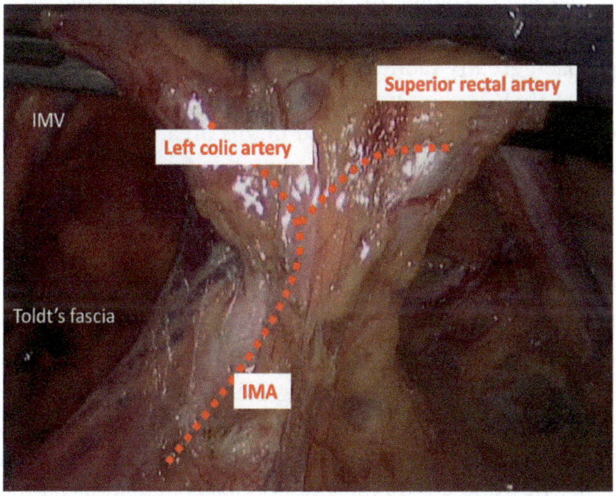

Fig. 15.9 A characteristic T-shaped structure is identified comprising the origin of the IMA, the left colic/IMV complex, and the superior rectal artery

LigaSure can be used in vessels no more than 7 mm without calcification but requires declining the tension on the artery before transecting to avoid incomplete sealing. After IMA ligation, the next step is to continue left colonic mobilization (Fig. 15.10).

15.3.5 Step 5: Lateral Mobilization of the Left Colon

The last part of colonic mobilization is the lateral mobilization. By pushing the sigmoid to the right, a peritoneal incision is performed along the white line of Toldt. The division of the lateral peritoneum continues along the descending colon and

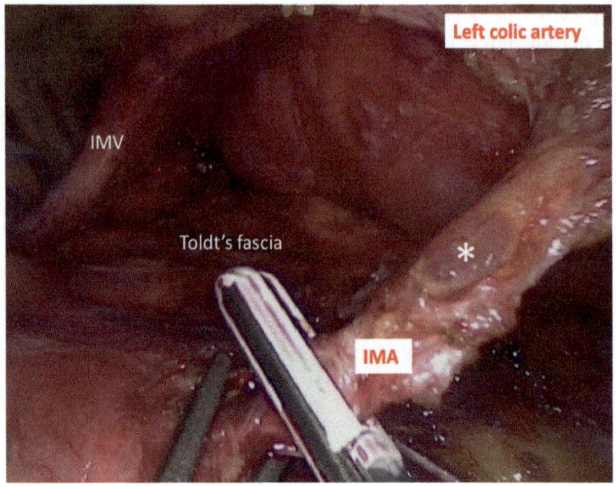

Fig. 15.10 The artery is cut exactly 2 cm from the aorta in order to preserve the sympathetic nerves

finishes at the splenic flexure. In order to avoid splenic decapsulation, adhesions of the greater omentum and the splenocolic ligament must be dissected. The medial approach greatly facilitates this last step of mobilization.

The IMV is then transected close to the pancreas, or 5 cm below if a left transverse colic artery is visualized in this area, to avoid colonic ischemia.

The colonic part of the dissection is finished; we can start with the TME.

15.3.6 Step 6: Dissection of the Mesorectum

The rectum has been described as "a cylinder within a box." The rectum and mesorectum form the cylinder, whereas the pelvis and levator ani form the box. We propose six different steps, dividing the dissection of the cylinder within the pelvic box.

The first step of the dissection of the mesorectum is the *high posterior dissection* (Fig. 15.11). This extrafascial anatomical dissection of the mesorectum can be performed by using scissors and monopolar coagulation, harmonic scalpel (Ultracision™), or thermal fusion (LigaSure™). We prefer using scissors with monopolar coagulation. The rectal exposure is achieved by stretching up the rectum out of the pelvis using a suprapubic grasper, while the assistant surgeon elevates the rectum vertically with a non-traumatic instrument via the left 5-mm port. The anatomical landmarks are the retrorectal space medially and the hypogastric nerves laterally. The dissection begins medially 2 cm in front of the sacral promontory and continues caudally and posteriorly along the presacral area. The key to successful dissection around the mesorectum is visualization of the loose areolar tissue of the presacral fascia (white tissue) surrounding the yellow mesorectal edge. Dissection on the "yellow side of the white" is the key to perfect perirectal/perimesorectal dissection. The medial dissection must be stopped 10 cm below the promontory at the level of the rectosacral ligament corresponding to the fusion between the presacral and the mesorectal fascias. Adequate tension to the tissues facilitates dissection. Non-traumatic instruments are used

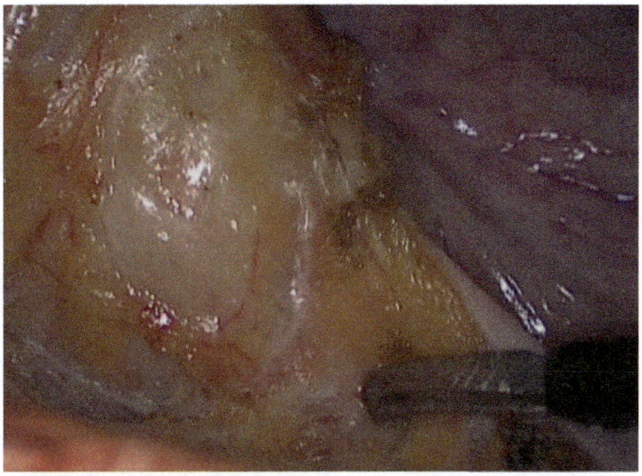

Fig. 15.11 High posterior rectal dissection, the dissection should be performed at the "yellow site of the white"

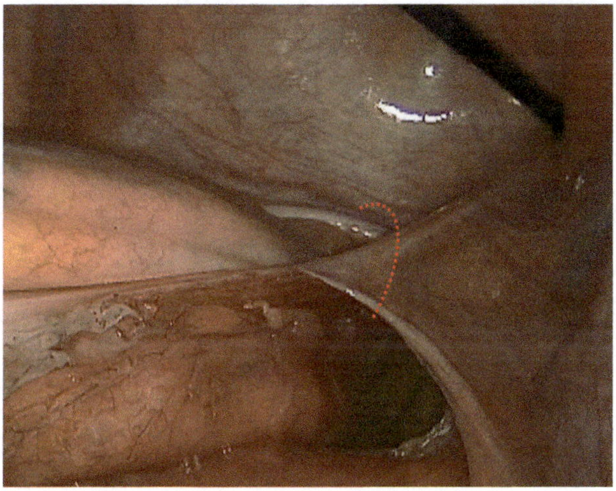

Fig. 15.12 High lateral dissection: an incision of the peritoneum along both sides of the rectum is performed down to the anterior reflection

without grasping the mesorectum to preserve its integrity. In cases of difficult dissection, elevating the mesorectum with a gauze on a graper can be helpful to create a better traction and countertraction. This medial posterior dissection avoids injuries of both superior hypogastric plexus and hypogastric nerves.

The second step is the *high lateral dissection* after identification of the hypogastric nerves (Fig. 15.12). A cephalic traction of the superior hypogastric plexus at the sacral promontory level induces tension of the hypogastric nerves, which can be visualized as a "white fiber" through the soft pelvic tissues or below the peritoneum (Fig. 15.13). An incision of the peritoneum along the right side of the rectum is performed down to the anterior reflection. The lateral avascular plane between the mesorectum and the right lateral pelvic fascia can be opened, connecting the previous medial (high posterior) dissection. After full right lateral mesorectum mobilization, the same dissection is performed on the left side.

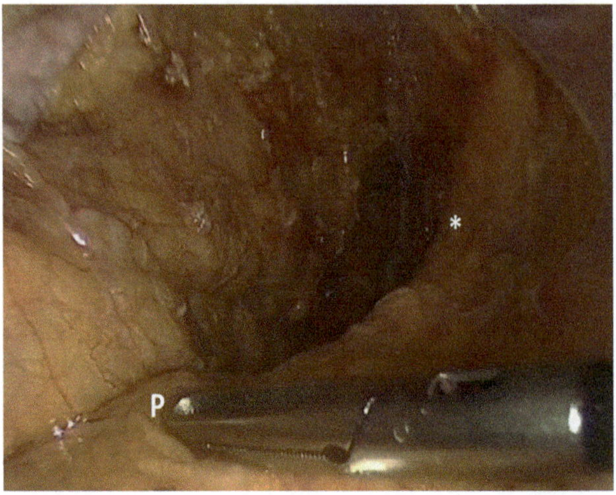

Fig. 15.13 A cephalic traction of the superior hypogastric plexus at the sacral promontory (**P**) level induces tension of the hypogastric nerves (*), which can be visualized as a "white fiber" through the soft pelvic tissues or below the peritoneum

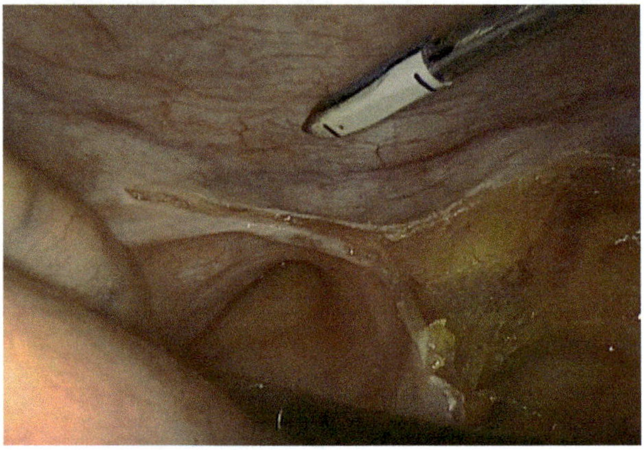

Fig. 15.14 High anterior dissection: a peritoneal incision is performed anteriorly 2 cm above the Douglas' pouch and connects the lateral right incision performed during the previous step. Seminal vesicles in men and cervix in female are the landmarks, which need to be identified

The third step consists in the *high anterior dissection*. Seminal vesicles in men and cervix in female are the landmarks, which need to be identified (Fig. 15.14). The upper rectum is grasped with a cephalic and left lateral traction giving a tension to the opposite anterior and right sides of the rectum. A peritoneal incision is performed anteriorly 2 cm above the Douglas' pouch and connects the lateral right incision performed during the previous step. Distal dissection from 1 to 2 cm of right anterior peritoneum allows discovering the right seminal vesicle, which must be completely isolated. In order to preserve both small efferent nerves along the vesicles and the mesorectum which is very thin and fragile at this level, the dissection must be led close to the seminal vesicles. In female patients, pelvic exposure is facilitated by uterus fixation to the anterior abdominal wall using a suprapubic stitch. The anterior incision of the peritoneum permits one to identify the cervix and then to connect the high lateral dissection.

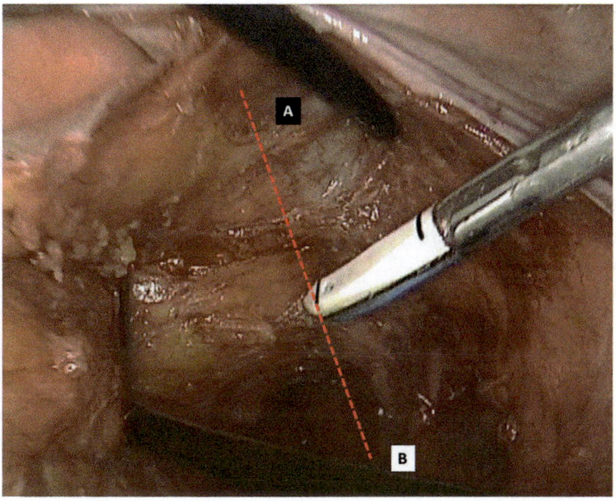

Fig. 15.15 The inferior hypogastric plexus is used as anatomical landmark in the low lateral dissection. The objective is to transect the lateral ligament of the rectum. Dissection is performed along a virtual line between the seminal vesicle and the hypogastric nerve; the pelvic plexus appears as a 2–3-cm triangle located along the lateral sidewall of the pelvis

The fourth step is *low lateral dissection* using the inferior hypogastric plexus as anatomical landmark. The objective is to transect the lateral ligament of the rectum. Great care is to preserve the neurovascular bundle during this dissection. By following dissection along a virtual line between the seminal vesicle and the hypogastric nerve, the pelvic plexus appears as a 2–3-cm triangle located along the lateral sidewall of the pelvis (Fig. 15.15). To free the mesorectum from the pelvic plexus, some attachments due to vessels and nerves coming from the plexus to the mesorectum have to be cut. To prevent plexus injury, perfect hemostasis and adequate traction of the tissue are essential.

Then, the rectum is pulled up for optimal visualization of the low pelvis. After incision of the rectosacral ligament, *low posterior dissection* is continued along the levator ani muscle. Presacral nerves (S2–S4) are identified at the midpart of the sacrum and preserved by dissecting close to the mesorectum.

Denonvilliers' fascia can be considered as the anterior part of the mesorectum. The oncologic *low anterior dissection* must be performed in front of the Denonvilliers' fascia, except in case of posterior tumors. So care is taken to do an anatomical dissection which preserves both the Denonvilliers' fascia and the anterior mesorectum, which need to be removed together to achieve a radical oncologic laparoscopic TME (Fig. 15.16).

The laparoscopic dissection continued along the pelvic floor toward the top of the anal canal anteriorly and the puborectal sling posteriorly. The distal level of the laparoscopic dissection is confirmed by digital rectal examination. For a sphincter-saving procedure, the dissection is performed until the top of the anal canal. The aponeurosis of the levator ani muscles (sheath of the pelvic floor) can be incised to enter into the intersphincteric plane. This step is enhanced by the optimal view of the laparoscopic approach and facilitates the connection with the perineal dissection.

In case of a stapled coloanal anastomosis (type I low rectal cancer, supra-anal tumors, lesions located >1 cm from the anal ring), the suprapubic 5-mm trocar is

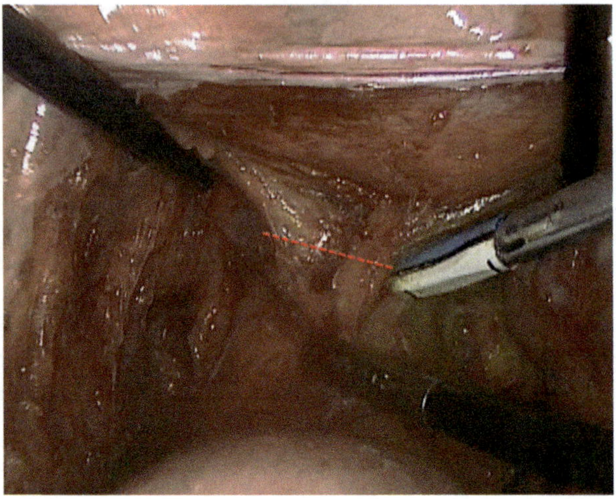

Fig. 15.16 The oncologic low anterior dissection must be performed in front of the Denonvilliers' fascia, except in case of posterior tumors. So care is taken to do an anatomical dissection which preserves both the Denonvilliers' fascia and the anterior mesorectum

changed for a 10-mm port, and a stapler is introduced to perform a vertical stapling with a linear stapler (Endo GIA™, Covidien, Mansfield, Massachusetts, USA). Pushing on the perineum facilitates rectal division. The specimen is then removed from a suprapubic 6-cm incision. A wound protector is necessary to decrease risks of port-site and local recurrences. Reconstruction with a colonic pouch or a latero-terminal anastomosis is performed laparoscopically.

For an APR (type IV low rectal cancer, transanal tumors, lesions with infiltration of the external anal sphincter or levator ani muscles), dissection is stopped earlier at the level of the seminal vesicles anteriorly and the coccyx posteriorly to avoid disconnection between tumor adhesion and levator ani muscles.

Nevertheless the scope of this chapter was to describe the surgical technique of the abdominoperineal intersphincteric dissection (for types II and III low rectal cancers, juxta-anal and intra-anal tumors, respectively). In these cases the pneumoperitoneum is released, and the transanal portion of the procedure begun.

15.3.7 Step 7: Perineal Part

This part is very dependent on good positioning of the patient. The legs have to be lifted from a Lloyd-Davies position to almost lithotomy position.

When the anal region is well exposed, the Lone Star retractor is inserted. We always use eight hooks in order to have a good approach to the anal canal and lower rectum. Low tumors are now visible, and their effective distance to the sphincter apparatus can be determined. A gauze is introduced into the rectum to avoid rectal and tumor spillage.

A circular incision of the anal canal is performed 1 cm below the tumor with the electric scalpel. If the mucosa is incised below the dentate line, the whole of the internal sphincter will be removed (total or low intersphincteric resection (ISR))

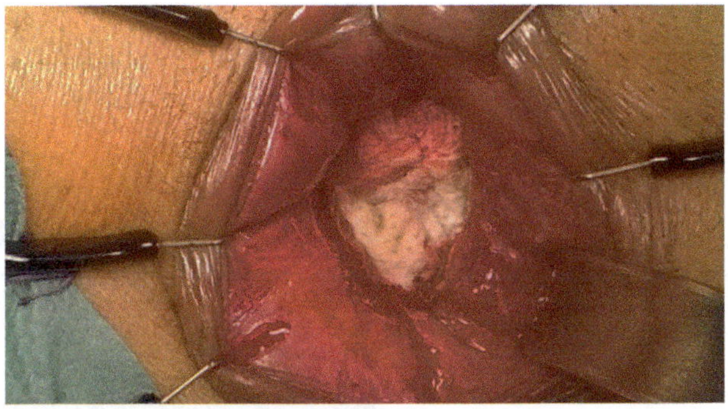

Fig. 15.17 A circular incision of the anal canal is performed 1 cm below the tumor with the electric scalpel. In this case the mucosa is incised below the dentate line; the whole of the internal sphincter will be removed (total or low ISR). A gauze is introduced into the rectum to avoid rectal and tumor spillage

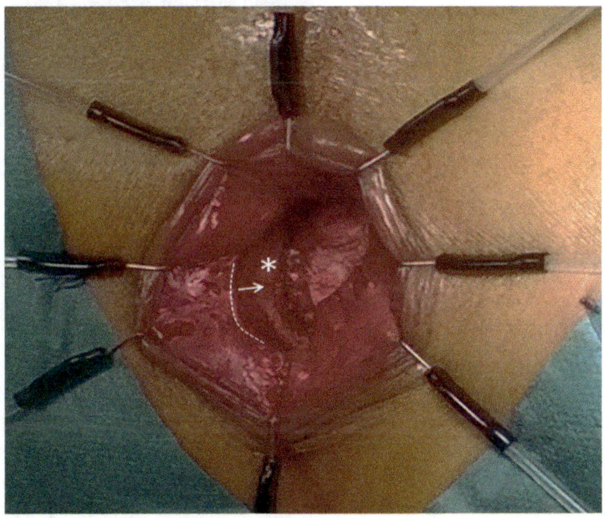

Fig. 15.18 Both the mucosa and the muscular layer are incised (*dotted white line*) to transect the underlying internal anal sphincter (which is identified as a *white band, asterisk*) to enter the intersphincteric groove. This dissection should begin posteriorly. When the correct intersphincteric plane has been reached, a spontaneous retraction of the rectal wall cranialward can be observed (*white arrow*)

(Fig. 15.17). If the ISR is started at the dentate line, the upper half of the internal sphincter (partial or high ISR) will be removed. Both the mucosa and the muscular layer are incised to transect the underlying internal anal sphincter (which is identified as a white band) to enter the intersphincteric groove. This dissection should begin posteriorly where the external sphincter is easier to identify. When the correct intersphincteric plane has been reached, a spontaneous retraction of the rectal wall cranialward can be observed. This is not possible anteriorly due to intermuscular connections and adhesions. We lift the muscle fibers with a forceps, and with gentle dissection, the external sphincter, which has a reddish appearance, can be separated (Fig. 15.18).

As soon as a good intersphincteric dissecting plane is achieved, the internal sphincter is mobilized in the entire circumstance (Fig. 15.19). Again, it is better, if possible, to get the posterior and lateral part of the dissection well started before moving to the anterior part. The rectum is then closed by continuous

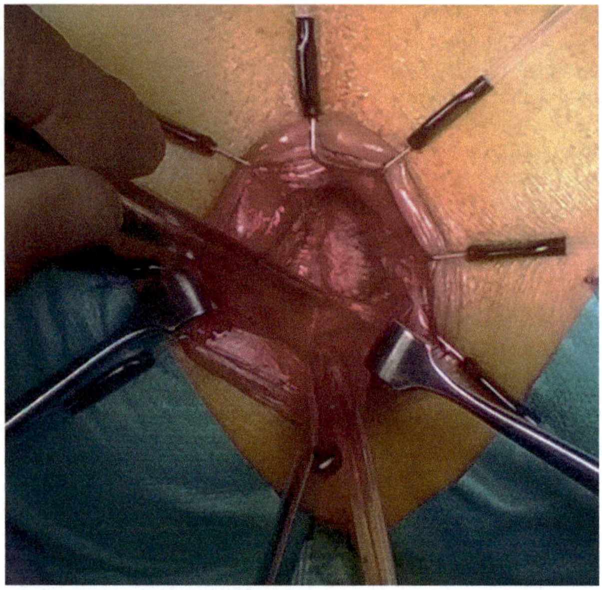

Fig. 15.19 As soon as a good intersphincteric dissecting plane is achieved, the internal sphincter is mobilized in the entire circumstance. The dissection between the internal and the external sphincter is continued by using scissors in a bloodless plane

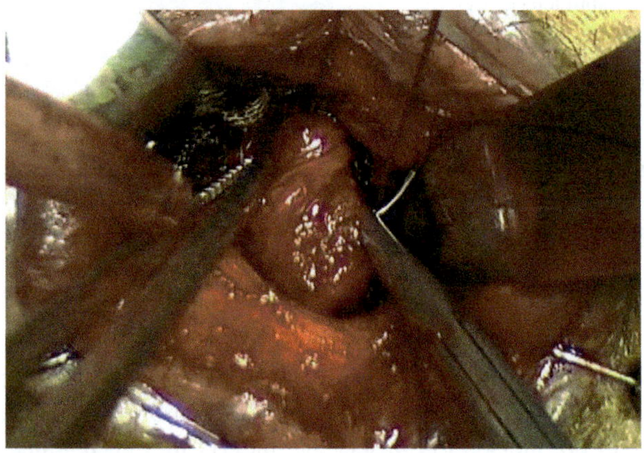

Fig. 15.20 The rectum is closed by continuous vicryl sutures (ends kept long) to prevent spillage

vicryl sutures (ends kept long) to prevent spillage, and the dissection between the internal and the external sphincter is continued by using scissors in a bloodless plane (Fig. 15.20).

The critical issue during the dissection in this space is whether the external sphincter is free of tumor or not. If the intersphincteric plane and the external sphincter muscle are infiltrated with tumorous tissue, the attempt of sphincter preservation should be aborted. A minimal infiltration can be treated by segmental resection and immediate reconstruction of the external sphincter.

The plane of intersphincteric dissection is continued posteriorly to the sheath of the pelvic floor for at least 5 cm (Fig. 15.21). The sheath of the levator ani muscles,

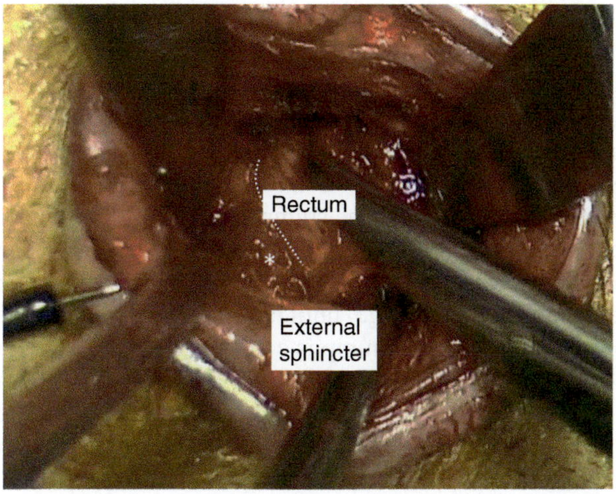

Fig. 15.21 The plane of intersphincteric dissection (*dotted line*) is continued posteriorly to the sheath of the pelvic floor (*) for at least 5 cm

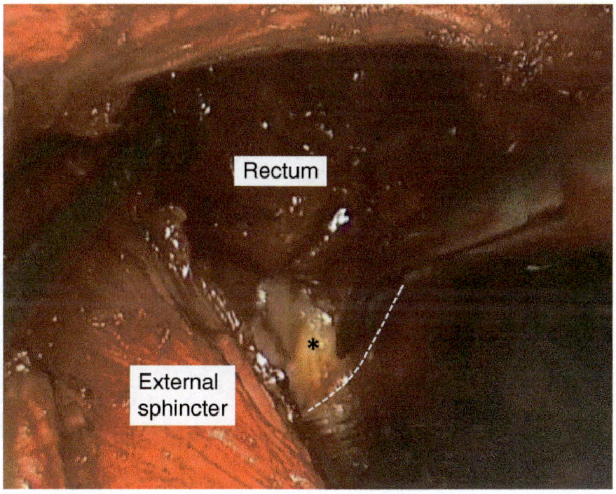

Fig. 15.22 The sheath of the levator ani muscles (*), which was usually thickened due to irradiation, was then transected to join the plane of the abdominal dissection

which is usually thickened due to irradiation, is then transected to join the plane of the abdominal dissection (Fig. 15.22).

The most difficult part of the dissection is the anterior circumference between the rectum and the prostate or vagina. In males, it is important not to proceed beyond the intersphincteric plane, as it is possible to damage the urethra. This plane can be followed up well to the seminal vesicles or cervix uteri. This is the juncture at which a "rendezvous" with the abdominal dissection is appropriate. The plane of dissection, especially the neurovascular bundle on both sides, is inspected, and additional hemostasis is performed if necessary. Vessels that are not easily coagulated should be individually secured with interrupted stitches. The pelvic cavity is now irrigated with saline solution.

15.3.8 Step 8: Rectal Transection and Reconstruction

The final step is the reconstruction of the bowel continuity. The upper end of the rectum is gently grasped with a long Babcock forceps and delivered through the anal canal ("pull through"), except for thick mesentery or anal stricture, and the colon is dissected with a linear stapler (Endo GIA™, Covidien, Mansfield, Massachusetts, USA). The stump of the colon must come up without angulation or tension (Fig. 15.23). The bowel is freed of all fatty attachments. If the colonic stump color indicates an inadequate blood supply, the surgeon should not hesitate to remove a sufficient length until its viability is unquestionable. When adequate blood supply of the colonic stump is confirmed, the decision has to be made as whether a pouch (a 5–6-cm colonic J-pouch or a latero-terminal anastomosis) is performed or not (Fig. 15.24). This will depend on the available length of the colon and the volume of the mesenteric fat in relation to the capacity of the pelvis. Obesity makes it impossible to perform an anal pouch anastomosis. In these cases a straight

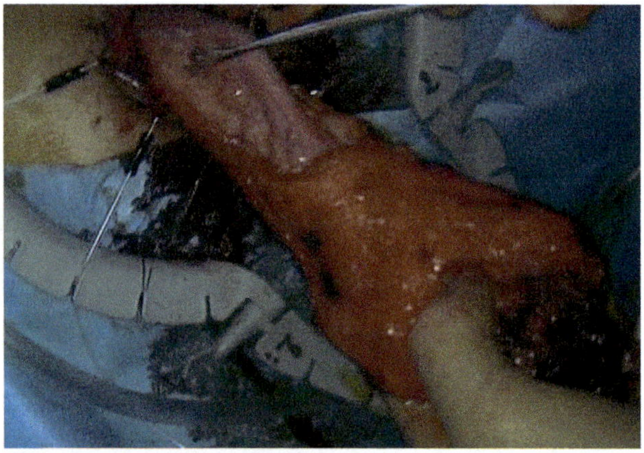

Fig. 15.23 The upper end of the rectum is gently grasped with a long Babcock forceps and delivered through the anal canal ("pull through"), and the colon is dissected with a linear stapler

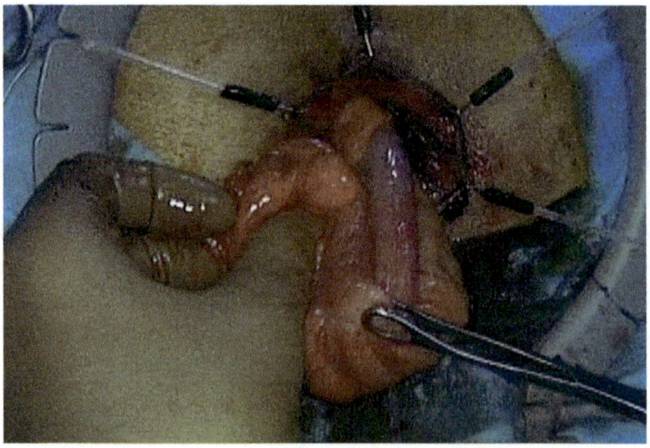

Fig. 15.24 The decision has to be made as whether a pouch (a 5–6-cm colonic J-pouch or a latero-terminal anastomosis) is made or not

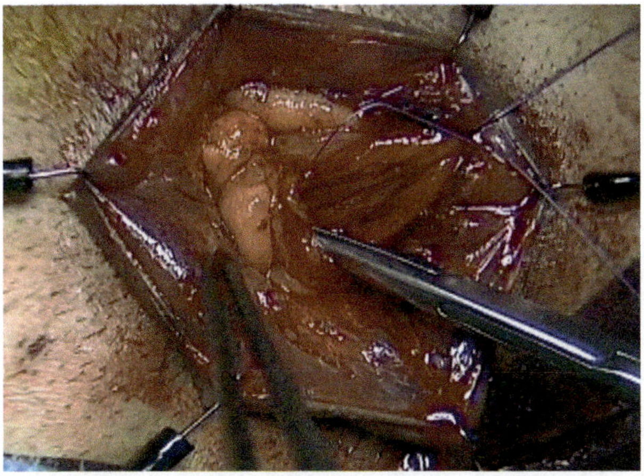

Fig. 15.25 The anastomotic single sutures Vicryl 2.0 must be placed carefully to include the anoderm as well as the remaining sphincter complex with the full intestinal wall

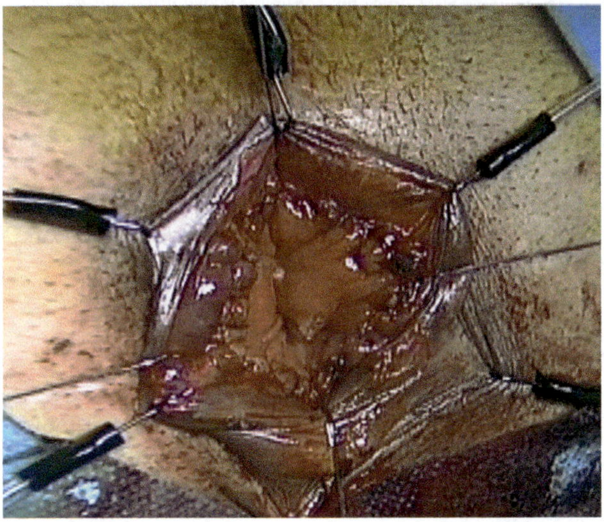

Fig. 15.26 Four stitches at each hour of the clock should be placed to anchor the pulled-down colon and to ensure accurate and secure approximation. Several additional sutures, totaling approximately 2 or 3 in every quadrant, may be placed to reinforce the anastomosis

termino-terminal anastomosis should be performed. When possible, we perform a latero-terminal anastomosis. The stump of the colon is brought at the right site of the pelvis with a grasper, while the anti-mesocolic side (at 4 cm of the stapler line) is exposed through the anal orifice. A small horizontal incision of 2 cm is made while preventing gross contamination. The manual coloanal anastomosis is constructed at the dentate line or below according to the primary incision of the anoderm. Four stitches at each hour of the clock should be placed to anchor the pulled-down colon and to ensure accurate and secure approximation. The anastomotic single sutures Vicryl 2.0 must be placed carefully to include the anoderm as well as the remaining sphincter complex with the full intestinal wall (Fig. 15.25). Several additional sutures, totaling approximately 2 or 3 in every quadrant, may be placed to reinforce the anastomosis (Fig. 15.26). A release of the hooks of the Lone

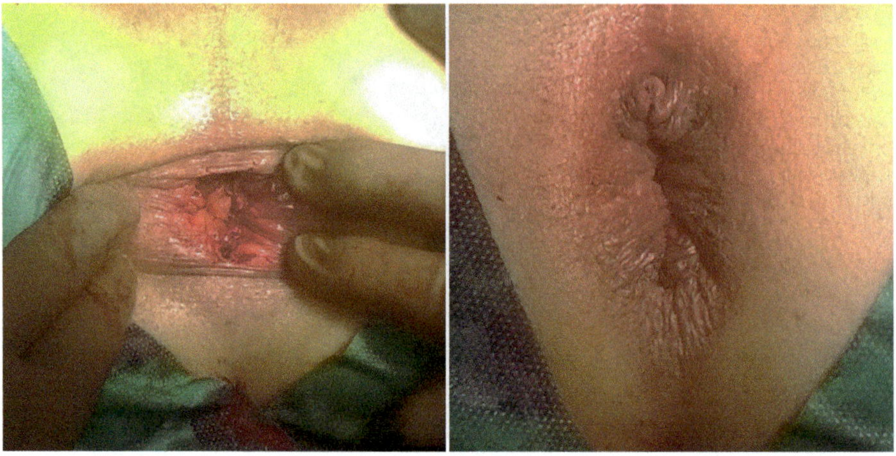

Fig. 15.27 Contraction of the sphincter is usually observed after removal of the Lone Star retractor and the anastomosis disappears into the anal canal

Star retractor is helpful to lessen possible traction. All stitches are finally cut while rechecking each stitch interval. Finally, adequacy of the blood supply to the site of the anastomosis should be carefully inspected again. The anastomosis is irrigated with saline, and the residual hooks of the Lone Star are removed. Contraction of the sphincter is usually observed after removal of the Lone Star retractor, and the anastomosis disappears into the anal canal (Fig. 15.27).

15.3.9 Step 9: End of the Procedure

The final step of the operation is a protective ileostomy. This is closed after 6 weeks provided that an anastomotic fistula is excluded by a contrast enema examination. A drain may be inserted into the posterior side of the pelvis and brought out via the left 5-mm port.

At the end of the procedure, the TME resection specimen should be examined by the surgeon: the external surface should be carefully inspected, and the quality of the mesorectal excision should be assessed. The mesorectal surface of a good resection should be smooth with a good bulk of mesorectum. Defects at the surface should be <5-mm deep. In case of perforation of the resection specimen or in case the muscular layer is visible exteriorly, the resection is classified as incomplete. There should be no coning near the distal margin. The continuous vicryl suture, used to close the rectum during dissection, is resected, and the distance between the tumor and the distal margin, as well as the circumferential resection margin, can be evaluated by digital manipulation and meticulous inspection. Preferentially, the resection specimen should be delivered unopened to the pathologist, in a fresh, unfixed state.

15.4 Epilog

TME offers the lowest reported rates of local recurrence and the best survival results in patients with middle or low rectal cancer. However, the laparoscopic approach to perform resections for rectal cancer remains controversial due to fears that oncologic principles will be compromised. The CLASICC trial, published in 2005, was the first randomized controlled trial to report results of laparoscopic TME for cancer and initially suggested a high risk of conversion, associated with a high risk of postoperative morbidity and incomplete resection [9]. Since then, the COREAN trial and, more recently, the COLOR II studies have reported excellent results of laparoscopic TME with low risk of conversion and improved short-term results compared to the open approach. Moreover, the laparoscopic approach was associated with rates of locoregional recurrence and disease-free and overall survival similar to those for open surgery, indicating that laparoscopic TME can become the standard approach for TME [10, 11].

The ISR after neoadjuvant chemoradiation is helpful in the management of patients with low rectal cancer. With the advent of this technique, the need for performance of APR seems to have decreased in patients with very low rectal tumors [12]. After the intersphincteric dissection, the distal part of the TME can be performed transanally. It is mostly performed with conventional anal retractors under direct vision (as described above). The transanal approach, mostly performed with conventional retractors (as described above), appears to be the optimal way because the dissection is more anatomic and under direct vision and permits a more accurate evaluation of the lower edge of the ultralow rectal cancer. In addition, this enables to obtain optimal distal and circumferential margins respecting oncological principles and restore bowel continuity, even in a difficult narrow pelvis or in obese patients.

Furthermore the total transanal TME (taTME) has recently been introduced and must be considered as a new progress in the field of low rectal cancer surgery [13]. The total taTME (laparoscopic taTME) dissects the whole mesorectum with the aim to improve the oncologic quality of surgery and to avoid pelvic nerve injury. A GelPOINT Path platform (Applied Medical, Rancho Santa Margarita, CA, USA) can be introduced into the anal canal after intersphincteric dissection and distal rectal mobilization to free up 2–3 cm. The transanal view, in combination with CO_2 insufflation, offers a better visualization of the distal rectum. Although the same anatomic and embryological planes of dissection have to be recognized from above and beneath, the most distal part might be better visualized and approached from beneath. The fact that the rectum is pushed and not retracted improves the precision of the dissection [14].

Although the principles of the perineal dissection remain the same as a conventional TME, the results could be improved in all fields of the postoperative outcome: lower morbidity and conversion rate, shorter hospital stay, higher radicality of surgery, and sphincter preservation with improved autonomic pelvic nerve preservation. All these factors could contribute to an improved oncological survival and quality of life in patients treated for rectal cancer [15–17]. We recently conducted a pilot-randomized trial in patients treated by laparoscopic sphincter preservation for low rectal cancer (<6 cm from the anal verge) and demonstrated that perineal dissection of the low rectum reduces the rate of positive CRM with similar quality of mesorectal dissection, number of lymph nodes analyzed, and morbidity, as compared with the conventional abdominal dissection of the low rectum. Moreover, these results showed a trend to lower technical difficulties and conversion by using the perineal approach for low rectal dissection [18]. The further development of taTME may therefore change radically rectal cancer surgery.

Because of these potential oncologic and technical advantages of the perineal dissection, regardless of whether an open or a laparoscopic approach is performed, we recommend this approach instead of the conventional abdominal dissection, in laparoscopic sphincter-preserving resection for low rectal cancer.

References

1. Birbeck KF, Macklin CP, Tiffin N, Parsons W, Dixon MF, Mapstone NP, et al. Rates of circumferential resection margin involvement vary between surgeons and predict outcomes in rectal cancer surgery. Ann Surg. 2002;235:449–57.
2. Williams NS, Dixon MF, Johnston D. Reappraisal of the 5 centimeter rule of distal excision for carcinoma of the rectum: a study of distal intramural spread and patients survival. Br J Surg. 1983;70:150–4.
3. Pollett WG, Nicholls RJ. The relationship between the extent of distal clearance and survival and local recurrence rates after curative anterior resection for carcinoma of the rectum. Ann Surg. 1983;198:159–63.
4. Ueno H, Mochizuki H, Hashiguchi Y, Ishikawa K, Fujimoto H, Shinto E, Hase K. Preoperative parameters expanding the indication of sphincter preserving surgery in patients with advanced low rectal cancer. Ann Surg. 2004;239:34–42.
5. Rullier A, Laurent C. Recommendations for clinical practice. Therapeutic choices for rectal cancer. What quality criteria are important for surgical excision of rectal cancer? Gastroenterol Clin Biol. 2007;31:1S34–51.
6. Taylor FG, Quirke P, Heald RJ, Moran B, Blomgvist L, Swift I, et al. One millimeter is the safe cut-off for magnetic resonance imaging prediction of surgical margin status in rectal cancer. Br J Surg. 2011;98:872–9.
7. Schiessel R, Karner-Hanusch J, Herbst F, Teleky B, Wunderlich M. Intersphincteric resection for low rectal tumors. Br J Surg. 1994;81:1376–8.
8. Rullier E, Denost Q, Vendrely V, Rullier A, Laurent C. Low rectal cancer: classification and standardization of surgery. Dis Colon Rectum. 2013;56:560–7.
9. Guillou PJ, Quirke P, Thorpe H, et al. Short-term endpoints of conventional versus laparoscopic-assisted surgery in patients with colorectal cancer (MRC CLASICC trial): multicentre, randomised controlled trial. Lancet. 2005;365:1718–26.
10. Kang SB, Park JW, Jeong SY, et al. Open versus laparoscopic surgery for mid or low rectal cancer after neoadjuvant chemoradiotherapy (COREAN trial): short-term outcomes of an open-label randomised controlled trial. Lancet Oncol. 2010;11:637–45.
11. Bonjer HJ, Deijen CL, Abis GA, Cuesta MA, van der Pas MH, de Lange-de Klerk ES, et al. A randomized trial of laparoscopic versus open surgery for rectal cancer (COLOR II tial). N Engl J Med. 2015;372:1324–32.
12. Dowdall JF, Maguire D, McAnena OJ. Experience of surgery for rectal cancer with total mesorectal excision in a general surgical practice. Br J Surg. 2002;89:1014–9.

13. Sylla P, Rattner DW, Delgado S, et al. NOTES transanal rectal cancer resection using transanal endoscopic microsurgery and laparoscopic assistance. Surg Endosc. 2010;24:1205–10.
14. Knol J, Dhondt M, Souverijns G, Heald B, Vangertruyden G. Transanal endoscopic total mesorectal excision: technical aspects of approaching the mesorectal plane from below – a preliminary report. Tech Coloproctol. 2015;19(2):69–82.
15. Fernandez-Hevia M, Delgado S, Castells A, et al. Transanal total mesorectal excision in rectal cancer: short-term outcomes in comparison with laparoscopic surgery. Ann Surg. 2015;261:221–7.
16. Rouanet P, Mourregot A, Azar CC, et al. Transanal endoscopic proctectomy: an innovative procedure for difficult resection of rectal tumors in men with narrow pelvis. Dis Colon Rectum. 2013;56:408–15.
17. Velthuis S, Nieuwenhuis DH, Ruijter TEG, et al. Transanal versus traditional laparoscopic total mesorectal excision for rectal carcinoma. Surg Endosc. 2014;28:3494–9.
18. Denost Q, Adam JP, Rullier A, Buscail E, Vendrely V, Rullier E. Perineal transanal approach: a new standard for laparoscopic sphincter-saving resection in low rectal cancer, a randomized trial. Ann Surg. 2014;260:993–9.

Reduced Port Laparoscopic TME with Coloanal Anastomosis

16

Shigenori Homma, Futoshi Kawamata, Susumu Shibasaki, Takahisa Ishikawa, Tadashi Yoshida, Hideki Kawamura, Norihiko Takahashi, and Akinobu Taketomi

Abstract

We began performing a single-incision plus one additional port laparoscopy-assisted anterior resection of the rectum (SILS+1-AR) in August 2010. In recent years, intersphincteric resection (ISR) is proposed as a means of offering sphincter preservation in patients with very low rectal cancer and has become an accepted surgical procedure. Moreover, the procedure of ultralow anterior resection mainly includes an ISR for sphincter-saving operation. Therefore, we applied SILS+1 partial ISR in cases of rectal cancer located within 5 cm from the anal verge.

In the SILS+1-AR without ISR, a 3-cm trans-umbilical incision was made, and the SILS™ port was inserted, and an additional 12-mm trocar was placed in the right lower quadrant. In the SILS+1 partial ISR, a SILS™ port was placed in the right lower quadrant at the intended ileostomy site, and a 5-mm trocar was inserted at the umbilicus at the subsequent drain site. The surgical procedure of partial ISR included five stages: colonic mobilization, pelvic dissection with total mesorectal excision (TME), transabdominal dissection of the intersphincteric space, stapled coloanal anastomosis, and diverting stoma. All postoperative outcomes were satisfactory (data not shown).

Reduced port laparoscopic TME for rectal carcinoma with or without ISR can be performed safely, and its feasibility depends on proper selection of patients.

S. Homma (✉) • F. Kawamata • S. Shibasaki • T. Ishikawa • T. Yoshida • H. Kawamura
N. Takahashi • A. Taketomi
Department of Gastroenterological Surgery I, Hokkaido University Graduate School of Medicine, North 15, West 7, Kita-ku, Sapporo 060-8638, Japan
e-mail: homma.s@nifty.com

G. Dapri, J.H. Marks (eds.), *Surgical Techniques in Rectal Cancer*,
https://doi.org/10.1007/978-4-431-55579-7_16

Keywords
Reduced port surgery • Single-incision laparoscopic surgery • Total mesorectal excision • Intersphincteric resection • Rectal cancer

16.1 Introduction

Single-incision laparoscopic surgery (SILS) has been used in urologic, gynecologic, general, and colorectal surgery, and it has demonstrated even better cosmetic benefits than conventional multiport laparoscopic surgery (CLS) [1–3]. Regarding colorectal surgery specifically, SILS has been associated with improved cosmesis and enhanced recoveries because there is less postoperative pain [4]. However, SILS for the treatment of rectal cancer is challenging even in the hands of a colorectal surgeon who is skilled in laparoscopic techniques, because of the difficulties associated with creating triangulation and applying laparoscopic staples in a narrow pelvic cavity. Moreover, an incomplete total mesorectal excision (TME) may lead to local recurrence of the tumor. Current evidence regarding SILS is based on information about the outcomes from right-sided colectomies performed on selected patients by experienced surgeons; however, the evidence relating to SILS for rectal cancer is limited, and only a few reports have been published [5, 6]. Intersphincteric resection (ISR) has become an increasingly popular surgical option for the treatment of very low rectal cancer. To preserve the anus with ISR, the rectum is divided from the levator ani muscle using an abdominal approach, followed by dissection between the internal anal sphincter and the external anal sphincter using both abdominal and perianal approaches.

To resolve the technical difficulties associated with SILS for rectal surgery, we developed the single-incision plus one additional port (SILS+1) technique. Adding an additional port to SILS may bridge the gap between CLS and SILS, and it may be associated with a relatively shorter learning curve, while maintaining oncologic principles.

We began performing SILS+1 laparoscopy-assisted anterior resection of the rectum (SILS+1-AR) [5] and SILS+1 partial ISR in August 2010. We herein describe these novel techniques and present our experience with these procedures.

16.2 Materials and Methods

16.2.1 Patients and Methods

The patients who had preoperative clinical stage 0 to stage III rectal cancers that required anterior resection of the rectum and ultralow anterior resection with extensive lymph node dissections were included. We excluded T3 rectal cancers that were located within 2 mm of the endopelvic fascia or with positive circumferential margins, based on computed tomography (CT) or magnetic resonance imaging (MRI).

Table 16.1 Demographics and clinical characteristics of the SILS+1-AR

Parameter	SILS+1-AR (*n* = 20)
1. Age (year)	66.4 ± 6.6
2. Sex	
Male	14
Female	6
3. BMI (kg/m^2)	23.5 ± 2.9
4. Operation history (yes/no)	1/19
5. Tumor size (cm)	36.5 ± 21.2
6. Stage	
0–I	7
II–III	13
7. Tumor location	
Rs	8
Ra	10
Rb	2

Stage and tumor location were determined according to the Japanese Society for Cancer of the Colon and Rectum (JSCCR)
The localization of the tumor was categorized as rectosigmoid (Rs), rectum above the peritoneal reflection (Ra), and rectum below the peritoneal reflection (Rb)
BMI body mass index

We applied partial ISR (ultralow anterior resection) in cases of rectal cancer located within 5 cm from the anal verge. The selection of patients who may benefit from the ISR should be based on the results of MRI, CT, endoanal ultrasonography, rigid proctoscopy, and digital examination [7]. Particularly, digital examination under anesthesia is important for evaluating tumor mobility, tumor relation to the anal sphincter, and final decision-making. Absolute contraindications for the method are T4 tumors, invasion of external anal sphincter (EAS), fixed tumors on digital examination (indication that the tumor has broken through the intersphincteric plane), poorly differentiated tumor, poor preoperative sphincter function, distant metastases, and presence of mental disease. The staging of the tumors and the tumors' locations were determined using the Japanese Society for Cancer of the Colon and Rectum 2010 guidelines [8] (Table 16.1).

16.2.2 Operative Procedures

All of the procedures were performed by the same colorectal surgeon who had qualified within the Japanese endoscopic surgical skills qualification system [9] and whose experience encompassed more than 900 laparoscopic colorectal resections and more than 100 SILS for colorectal diseases. All of the patients were placed in a modified lithotomy-Trendelenburg position.

In the SILS+1-AR without ISR, a 3-cm trans-umbilical incision was made, and the SILS™ port (Covidien, New Haven, CT, US) with three built-in trocars was inserted into the single umbilical incision. An additional 12-mm trocar was placed in the right lower quadrant (Fig. 16.1a, b). A 5-mm standard definition flexible videoscope (LTF-VP; Olympus, Tokyo, Japan) was inserted into the 5-mm trocar at the extreme caudal end of the SILS™ port for the procedure's duration. After the trocars were positioned, the patient was placed in a 20° Trendelenburg position with a 10° right lateral tilt. The surgeon and his assistant were positioned on the patient's right side, and the videoscope operator was positioned on the patient's left side. Ultrasonic-activated scissors (Harmonic ACE™, Ethicon Endo-Surgery Inc., Cincinnati, OH, US) were used for the dissection. Straight and curved graspers (Roticulator™ Endo Grasp™; Covidien) were used to grasp the tissues, and the dissection was performed using a medial-to-lateral approach, while preserving the left ureter and gonadal vessels. The dissection continued superior to the level of the root of the inferior mesenteric artery, and a high ligation of the inferior mesenteric artery was achieved (Fig. 16.2a). Then, the root of the superior rectal artery and the inferior mesenteric vein was divided without damaging the hypogastric plexus. All of the procedures complied with the principles of TME, which requires the removal of the entire mesorectum down to the pelvic floor, while ensuring that the hypogastric and pelvic autonomic nerves are preserved (Fig. 16.2b). After sufficient intestinal irrigation with a saline solution, the transection of the rectum was performed through the additional port using a linear stapler with a 3.8-mm gold cartridge (Echelon-Flex™ 60; Ethicon Endo-Surgery), and the specimen was retrieved through the umbilical port. The anastomosis was performed intracorporeally using an EEA circular stapler (Ethicon Endo-Surgery) after the anvil was inserted extracorporeally. After lavage of the abdominal cavity, a 4.7-mm closed suction drain (Davol Reliavac Silicone Drain; CR Bard, Inc., Murray Hill, NJ, US) was inserted through the port incision in the right flank.

The procedure of ultralow anterior resection mainly includes an ISR for a sphincter-saving operation. We applied partial ISR (ultralow anterior resection with double stapling technique) in cases of rectal cancer such as those located

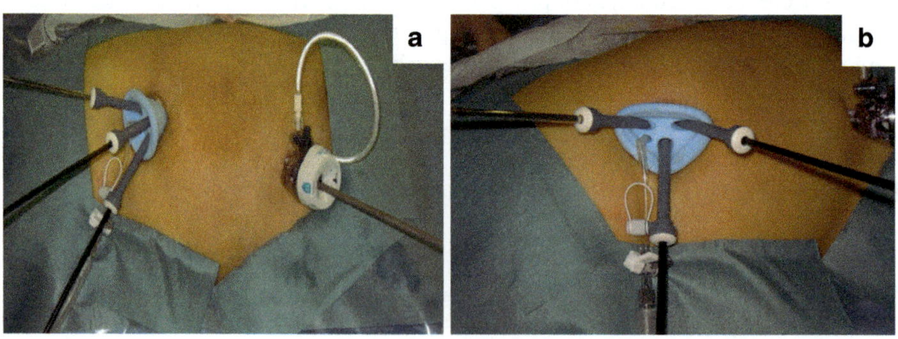

Fig. 16.1 (**a**) Port setting. In the SILS+1-AR, a 3-cm trans-umbilical incision was made and the SILS™ port (Covidien) was inserted into a single umbilical incision. A 12-mm port was inserted into the right lower quadrant of the abdomen. (**b**) Intraoperatively, the system allows for the instruments to be manipulated with greater freedom

5 cm from the anal verge. The surgical procedure of partial ISR included five stages: colonic mobilization, pelvic dissection with TME, transabdominal ISR, stapled coloanal anastomosis, and diverting stoma [10]. In this case, a SILS™ port was inserted through a 2.5-cm skin incision at the intended ileostomy site in the right lower quadrant (Fig. 16.3a). An additional 5-mm bladeless trocar was inserted at the umbilicus at the postoperative drain site (Fig. 16.3). The surgery was performed using a technique that was similar to that used in the patients in the SILS+1-AR. TME was performed from the right side to the posterior and left side, while ensuring that the hypogastric and pelvic autonomic nerves were preserved. For the pelvic dissection, the rectum was straightened to achieve the appropriate tension using the assistant's curved grasper. Using the Harmonic ACE™, a sharp dissection was performed along the presacral avascular plane down to the pelvic floor and to the top of the anal canal (Fig. 16.4). For the anterior dissection, the peritoneal reflections in men or the uteri in women were suspended using two 3-0 monofilament sutures that penetrated the left and right lower abdominal wall near the pubic bone (Fig. 16.5). After the rectum had been completely mobilized to the

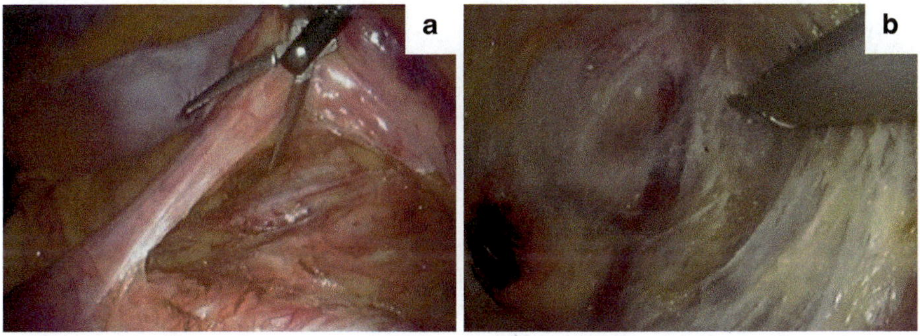

Fig. 16.2 (**a**) SILS+1-AR with lymph node dissection around the inferior mesenteric artery. (**b**) All procedures had to comply with the principles of total mesorectal excisions

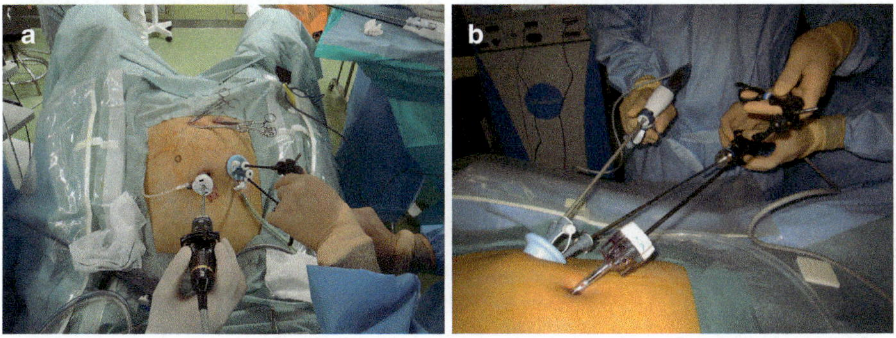

Fig. 16.3 The SILS™ port (Covidien) was placed at the ileostomy site through a 25-mm skin incision in the right quadrant. A 5-mm trocar for the operator's right hand was inserted at the umbilicus. The surgeon and his assistant were positioned on the patient's right side, and the videoscope operator was positioned on the patient's left side

level of the levator ani muscle, one of the 5-mm ports was changed to a 12-mm port, and the sigmoid colon was transected using an Echelon-Flex™ 60. The perineal approach began after the intracorporeal manipulations. The posterior adhesion line between the puborectalis muscle and rectal wall was exposed, and the intersphincteric space could be entered along the dissection plane at the dorsolateral side of the rectum (Fig. 16.6). The hiatal ligament was then dissected and transected at the posterior side. The distal bowel wall was mobilized for 3 cm from the lower edge of the tumor to obtain an adequate distal margin of 1 or 2 cm (Fig. 16.7). At this point, circular dissection of the intersphincteric space was completed.A digital rectal examination was required to determine the height of the tumor and the cutting line of the stapling device. A flexible linear stapler was used to cut the distal margin. A stapled end-to-end coloanal anastomosis was constructed as previously described [10]. A drain was placed through the umbilicus and into the bottom of the pelvis, and a diverting ileostomy was created at the site of the SILS™ port (Fig. 16.8a). The diverting ileostomy was closed 6 weeks after primary surgery (Fig. 16.8b).

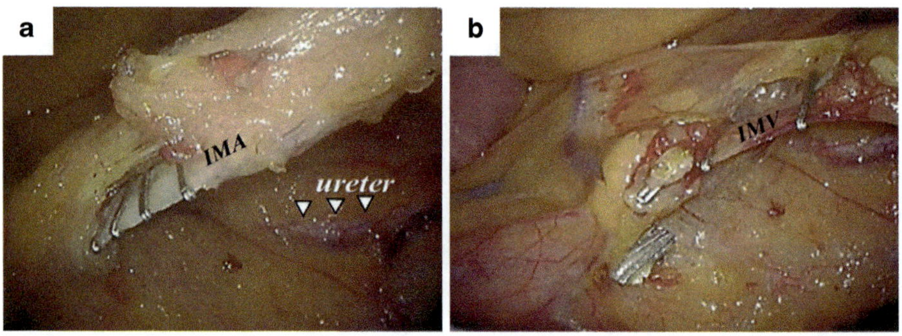

Fig. 16.4 (**a**, **b**) After identifying the left ureter, the inferior mesenteric artery was isolated and ligated 1 cm distal to the aorta

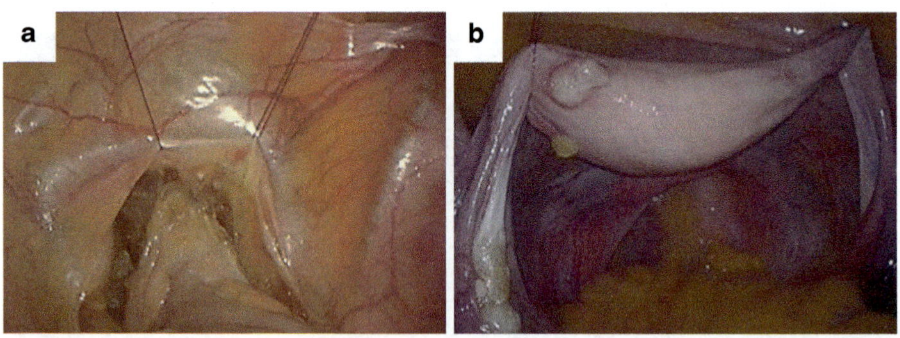

Fig. 16.5 (**a**, **b**) The peritoneal reflection in males or uterus in females was suspended using two 3-0 monofilament sutures that penetrated the left and right lower abdominal wall near the pubic bone

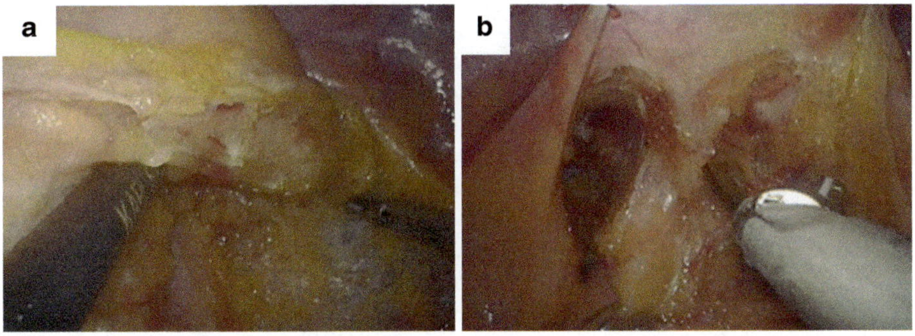

Fig. 16.6 (**a**, **b**) A total mesorectal excision was performed from the right side to the posterior and left side, while ensuring the hypogastric and pelvic autonomic nerves were preserved

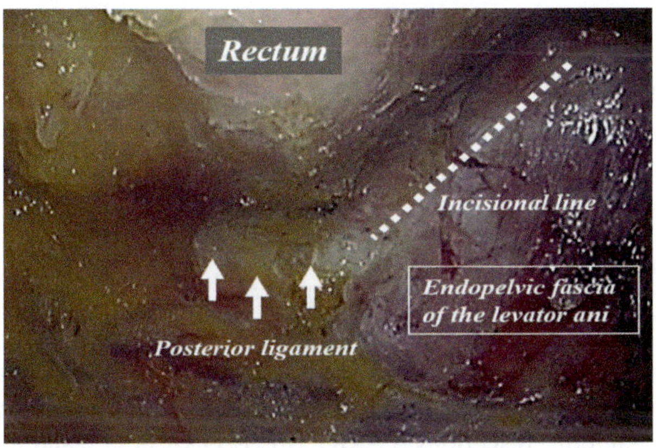

Fig. 16.7 (**a**, **b**) The pelvic dissection was performed along the presacral avascular plane down to the pelvic floor and the top of the anal canal. The rectum was completely mobilized to the level of the levator ani muscle. The broken lines represent the incisional line of the levator ani muscle from the perineal approach

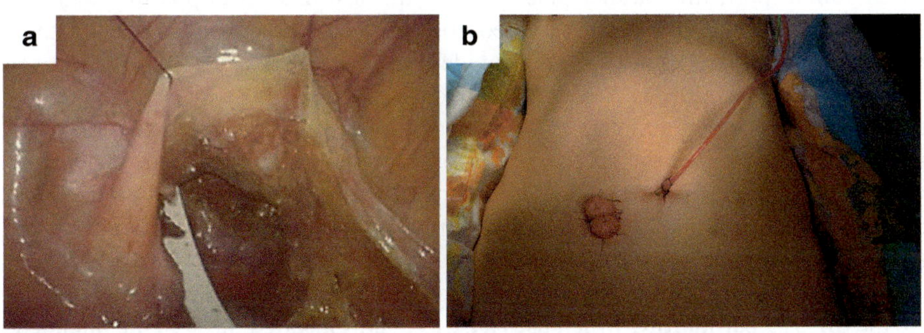

Fig. 16.8 (**a**) A 4.7-mm closed suction drain was inserted through the umbilicus into the bottom of the pelvis. (**b**) The diverting loop ileostomy was created at the right iliac fossa at the port site and the pelvic drain was brought out through the umbilical port site

Table 16.2 Operative variables in SILS+1-AR

Parameter	SILS+1-AR (*n* = 20)
1. Operation time (min)	187 (126–308)
2. Blood loss (ml)	22.5 (0–190)
3. The number of lymph node dissection	13.3 ± 7.3
4. Lymph node metastasis (%)	5 (25.0)
5. Distal resection margin (mm)	32.0 ± 14.4
6. Adding further port	0 (0.0)
7. Intraoperative complication	0 (0.0)
8. Conversion rate (%)	2 (10.0)
9. Complications	0 (0.0)
10. Hospital stay (days)	11.3 (7–18)

NA not available

16.3 Results

The results are presented in Tables 16.2 and 16.3.

16.4 Discussion

We were able to demonstrate that the reduced port laparoscopic TME for rectal cancer surgery was safe and feasible without severe intra- or postoperative complications. The results from our previous study indicated that compared with conventional multiport-anterior resections (C-AR), SILS+1-AR is safe and feasible, and it is not associated with longer operation times, postoperative complications, morbidity, or increased hospital stays [5]. Furthermore, there were no adverse effects with respect to cancer-specific outcomes, including blood losses, lymph node dissections, lymph node metastases, and the lengths of the resection margins [5]. By using an additional port, the parallel placement of the instruments is possible without causing interference between the videoscope and the surgeon's dominant hand; hence, all of the benefits of CLS are provided.

We applied partial ISR in cases of rectal cancer such as those located 5 cm from the anal verge. As an alternative to abdominoperineal resection, ISR offers the possibility of preserving anal continence in patients in whom the tumor is located within 5 cm from the anal verge. The goal of ISR is to dissect the rectum transabdominally and transanally and to remove part or the whole of the internal anal sphincter, to obtain adequate distal margin, and to restore bowel continence [11].

Based on our experience, we developed the SILS+1-AR technique further to create the SILS+1 partial ISR, which uses a SILS™ port inserted through the intended stoma site and a 5-mm umbilical port. In the perineal approach, a circumferential incision of the mucosa, submucosa, and the internal sphincter is performed 1–2 cm distal to the tumor (just on or very close to the dentate line), followed by a careful

Table 16.3 Summary of three patients with recurrence after SILS+1-AR

Case No.	Operation	Age	Sex	Location	Histological classification	Invasion depth	pN factor	pStage	Lymphatic permeation	Blood vessel permeation	Adjuvant chemotherapy	Site of recurrence (month)	Outcome (month)
1	SILS+1-AR	68	M	Ra	tub2	SM	0	I	negative (0)	positive (1)	XELOX	liver (25)	alive (39)
2	SILS+1-AR	75	M	Ra	tub2	SS	1	III	negative (0)	positive (1)	mFOLFOX6	liver (10)	alive (29)
											declined	lung (8)	alive (17)

Lymphatic and blood vessel permeation: (1): mild, (2) moderate, (3) severe dissection of the internal sphincter free of the external sphincter in a bloodless plane (intersphincteric plane). The rectum is removed en bloc with the internal sphincter. Finally, a stapled coloanal anastomosis is made [12].

A key requirement for the successful performance of our SILS+1 partial ISR that uses the intended stoma site is the addition of another port for the operator's right hand. With the exception of the SILS™ port inserted through the intended stoma site, the operator can use his right hand to freely manipulate the instruments and tissues precisely. The use of a curved grasper and flexible videoscope allows the operator to use his left hand freely. Therefore, the operator can maintain the triangular formation and reduce the stress that is imposed by laparoscopic instruments interfering with each other.

Our SILS+1 port procedure represents a major advance compared with conventional surgery with respect to cosmesis and a major advance compared with pure SILS with respect to its feasibility. Curative resections of rectal cancers require TME. Moreover, incomplete TME may lead to local recurrences [13, 14], and the circumferential margin is a major prognostic factor in rectal cancer [15]. Therefore, achieving negative circumferential resection margins through complete TME is essential for curative rectal cancer surgery, which includes anterior, ISR, and abdominoperineal resections. The results from our previous study indicated that SILS+1-AR provided a degree of oncological radicality that was similar to that observed with C-AR by achieving TME [5]. In addition, no local recurrences were noted during the follow-up period. Therefore, TME can be performed accurately. However, the current study only evaluated the short-term outcomes, and we will continue to monitor these patients to determine their long-term outcomes.

In the partial ISR, when an additional trocar is inserted into the umbilicus, it seems to be difficult to perform medial-to-lateral approach, ligate the inferior mesenteric artery, and dissect lymph nodes, compared with insertion into the right lower quadrant. However, there are two reasons for selecting the umbilicus for the insertion of a 5-mm trocar for use by the operator's right hand. First, there is the cosmetic benefit, because an umbilical scar becomes almost invisible after the operation, whereas a scar in the right lower quadrant remains visible. Consequently, our laparoscopic procedure produces only two barely perceptible scars, one behind the stoma and one at the umbilicus. Indeed, patients who underwent this procedure were extremely satisfied with their nearly invisible scars. The second reason for selecting the umbilicus for the insertion of a 5 mm trocar is that compared with an additional port placed at the right lower quadrant, the umbilical port enables the operator's right hand to perform the pelvic dissection relatively freely, especially that of the right rectal wall. As a result, we achieved curative R0 resections in all of the patients. Therefore, the additional port placed at the umbilicus seems to be advantageous when performing complete TME [16].

A recent paper by Hirano et al. [17] reported that SILS+1-AR is a promising alternative method for scarless abdominal surgery for the treatment of some patients with rectal disease. Moreover, Lim et al. [18] demonstrated that adding another port to SILS may bridge the gap between CLS and SILS. In addition, Adair et al. [19]

reported that adding another port to SILS is a more realistic representation of the technique used in clinical settings. Based on the results we achieved, we agree with the viewpoints of these investigators.

We compared changes in specific parameters over time with those obtained from C-AR to evaluate the less invasive nature of SILS+1-AR. The two groups of patients were similar with respect to the changes in the parameters that are associated with inflammation, including their body temperatures, white blood cell counts, and C-reactive protein levels. We hypothesized that the postoperative neutrophil counts might reflect the dynamic changes in the hosts' inflammatory responses. However, given that the postoperative neutrophil counts in patients in the SILS+1-AR group were substantially lower than those in patients in the C-AR group, less inflammation may have occurred in the SILS+1-AR group [5]. Moreover, the significant differences in the body temperatures that were observed on the first postoperative day in patients in the SILS+1-AR group may indicate earlier normalization [5].

In conclusion, reduced port laparoscopic TME with coloanal anastomosis with or without ISR for rectal cancer can be performed safely and feasibly when used in selected patients. Long-term follow-up assessments are necessary to determine the local recurrence and survival rates and to ascertain the oncological safety of reduced port laparoscopic TME with coloanal anastomosis with or without ISR.

References

1. Ahmed K, Wang TT, Patel VM, Nagpal K, Clark J, Ali M, et al. The role of single-incision laparoscopic surgery in abdominal and pelvic surgery: a systematic review. Surg Endosc. 2011;25(2):378–96. doi:10.1007/s00464-010-1208-6.
2. Fichera A, Zoccali M, Gullo R. Single incision ("scarless") laparoscopic total abdominal colectomy with end ileostomy for ulcerative colitis. J Gastrointest Surg. 2011;15(7):1247–51. doi:10.1007/s11605-011-1440-y.
3. Egi H, Hattori M, Hinoi T, Takakura Y, Kawaguchi Y, Shimomura M, et al. Single-port laparoscopic colectomy versus conventional laparoscopic colectomy for colon cancer: a comparison of surgical results. World J Surg Oncol. 2012;10:61. doi:10.1186/1477-7819-10-61.
4. Chambers WM, Bicsak M, Lamparelli M, Dixon AR. Single-incision laparoscopic surgery (SILS) in complex colorectal surgery: a technique offering potential and not just cosmesis. Colorectal Dis. 2011;13(4):393–8. doi:10.1111/j.1463-1318.2009.02158.x.
5. Kawamata F, Homma S, Minagawa N, Kawamura H, Takahashi N, Taketomi A. Comparison of single-incision plus one additional port laparoscopy-assisted anterior resection with conventional laparoscopy-assisted anterior resection for rectal cancer. World J Surg. 2014;38(10):2716–23. doi:10.1007/s00268-014-2642-8.
6. Osborne AJ, Lim J, Gash KJ, Chaudhary B, Dixon AR. Comparison of single-incision laparoscopic high anterior resection with standard laparoscopic high anterior resection. Colorectal Dis. 2013;15(3):329–33. doi:10.1111/j.1463-1318.2012.03178.x.
7. Dimitriou N, Michail O, Moris D, Griniatsos J. Low rectal cancer: sphincter preserving techniques-selection of patients, techniques and outcomes. World J Gastrointest Oncol. 2015;7(7):55–70. doi:10.4251/wjgo.v7.i7.55.
8. Watanabe T, Itabashi M, Shimada Y, Tanaka S, Ito Y, Ajioka Y, et al. Japanese Society for Cancer of the Colon and Rectum (JSCCR) guidelines 2010 for the treatment of colorectal cancer. Int J Clin Oncol. 2012;17(1):1–29. doi:10.1007/s10147-011-0315-2.

9. Mori T, Kimura T, Kitajima M. Skill accreditation system for laparoscopic gastroenterologic surgeons in Japan. Minim Invasive Ther Allied Technol. 2010;19(1):18–23. doi:10.3109/13645700903492969.
10. Chi P, Huang SH, Lin HM, Lu XR, Huang Y, Jiang WZ, et al. Laparoscopic transabdominal approach partial intersphincteric resection for low rectal cancer: surgical feasibility and intermediate-term outcome. Ann Surg Oncol. 2015;22(3):944–51. doi:10.1245/s10434-014-4085-8.
11. Saito N, Ito M, Kobayashi A, Nishizawa Y, Sugito M. Sphincter-saving resection for low rectal cancer. Nihon Geka Gakkai Zasshi. 2011;112(5):318–24.
12. Saito N, Ito M, Kobayashi A, Nishizawa Y, Kojima M, Nishizawa Y, et al. Long-term outcomes after intersphincteric resection for low-lying rectal cancer. Ann Surg Oncol. 2014;21(11): 3608–15. doi:10.1245/s10434-014-3762-y.
13. Heald RJ, Husband EM, Ryall RD. The mesorectum in rectal cancer surgery--the clue to pelvic recurrence? Br J Surg. 1982;69(10):613–6.
14. Martling A, Holm T, Rutqvist LE, Johansson H, Moran BJ, Heald RJ, et al. Impact of a surgical training programme on rectal cancer outcomes in Stockholm. Br J Surg. 2005;92(2):225–9. doi:10.1002/bjs.4834.
15. Tilney HS, Rasheed S, Northover JM, Tekkis PP. The influence of circumferential resection margins on long-term outcomes following rectal cancer surgery. Dis Colon Rectum. 2009;52(10):1723–9. doi:10.1007/DCR.0b013e3181b54fbd.
16. Ishikawa T, Homma S, Shibasaki S, Yoshida T, Minagawa N, Kawamura H, et al. Dual-port laparoscopic abdominoperineal resection using the intended stoma site as the multichannel port. Surg Today. 2015;45(12):1583–7. doi:10.1007/s00595-015-1224-1.
17. Hirano Y, Hattori M, Douden K, Shimizu S, Sato Y, Maeda K, et al. Single-incision plus one port laparoscopic anterior resection for rectal cancer as a reduced port surgery. Scand J Surg. 2012;101(4):283–6.
18. Lim SW, Kim HJ, Kim CH, Huh JW, Kim YJ, Kim HR. Umbilical incision laparoscopic colectomy with one additional port for colorectal cancer. Tech Coloproctol. 2013;17(2):193–9. doi:10.1007/s10151-012-0900-z.
19. Adair J, Gromski MA, Lim RB, Nagle D. Single-incision laparoscopic right colectomy: experience with 17 consecutive cases and comparison with multiport laparoscopic right colectomy. Dis Colon Rectum. 2010;53(11):1549–54. doi:10.1007/DCR.0b013e3181e85875.

Single-Port Laparoscopic TME with Coloanal Anastomosis

17

Armando Geraldo Franchini Melani, Luis Gustavo Capochin Romagnolo, and Frédéric Bretagnol

Abstract

Minimally invasive surgery is one of the major technical advances of the past 20 years. Interest in laparoscopy has led to the development of more minimally invasive surgeries such as natural orifice transluminal endoscopic surgery (NOTES) and laparoendoscopic single-site surgery (LESS).

The laparoendoscopic single-site surgery (LESS) emerged with the potential benefit of a single incision associated with the advantages of the laparoscopy to perform colorectal procedures. LESS is an emerging technique that meets enthusiastic surgical community, as stated by the large and increasing number of publications within the last years. The challenge to perform LESS is the triangulation needed among the instruments using a single-incision access. Compared with conventional laparoscopy using multiport access, the LESS approach may be more difficult to provide a good exposure of the surgical field. But in addition to the benefits of laparoscopy, LESS may offer a reduction in port-related complications such as pain, faster postoperative recovery, and improved cosmesis. The aim of this chapter is to describe the single-port technique to do total mesorectal excision (TME) resection with coloanal anastomoses.

A.G.F. Melani, M.D. (✉)
Colorectal Oncology Surgery, Americas Medical City,
Av. Jorge Curi 550, Barra da Tijuca, Rio de Janeiro 22793-334, Brazil

IRCAD, Rio de Janeiro, Brazil
e-mail: armandomelani@icloud.com

L.G.C. Romagnolo, M.D.
Department of Colorectal Surgery, Barretos Câncer Hospital, Barretos, Brazil

F. Bretagnol, M.D.
Department of Digestive Surgery, Hôpital Louis Mourier (APHP), Colombes, France

G. Dapri, J.H. Marks (eds.), *Surgical Techniques in Rectal Cancer*,
https://doi.org/10.1007/978-4-431-55579-7_17

Keywords
Laparoscopy • Laparoendoscopy • Rectal cancer

17.1 Introduction

The use of laparoscopy has increased in the management of malignant colorectal diseases, especially in oncologic procedures. However other minimally invasive techniques are also growing. The advantages of faster recovery, reduced hospital stay, and better cosmetics are associated with similar oncological outcomes to standard open surgery. Although conventional laparoscopy is less traumatic than open surgery, the trauma associated with multiport surgery could be reduced using a single incision. Each incision carries the potential risk of bleeding, incisional hernia, pain, and hematoma in the abdominal wound. Laparoendoscopic single-site surgery (LESS) emerged with the potential benefit of a single incision associated with the advantages of the laparoscopy to perform colorectal procedures. The challenge to perform LESS is the triangulation needed among the instruments using a single-incision access. Comparing with conventional laparoscopy using multiport access, LESS approach may be more difficult to provide good exposure of the surgical field. There is an increased frequency of clashing the instruments, and the learning curve is greater [1].

In the treatment of rectal cancer, the total mesorectal excision (TME) decreases the risk of local recurrence. Nowadays, standard surgical treatment for low rectal cancers should be performed with TME and coloanal anastomosis (CAA) for those tumors close to dentate line. The feasibility, safety, and long-term outcome of laparoscopic rectal cancer resections can be performed following the principles of TME. LESS is recognized to offer excellent cosmetic results compared with conventional multiport laparoscopic surgery [2]. We assessed the safety and feasibility of single-incision laparoscopic TME for rectal cancer [3]. LESS represents the latest advance in laparoscopic surgery, and the feasibility and safety of this procedure has been previously described [4].

The aim of this chapter is to describe the technique of single-port TME resection with coloanal anastomoses.

17.2 Surgical Technique

17.2.1 Abdominal Step

After the induction of the general anesthesia, the patient is placed in Lloyd–Davis position; the surgeon and the assistant are located to the right side of the patient. Pneumoperitoneum is achieved with CO_2 at a pressure of 12 mmHg at Palmer's point (under the ribs on the left side, medium clavicle line.) At the previously demarcated ileostomy site (right lower quadrant), we perform a single incision

(2.5–3.0 cm of diameter—depending on the device to be used), and under direct vision, the single-port device is placed in the abdominal wall (Fig. 17.1). We choose to use a 10 mm straight 30° optic. Nowadays it is possible to use a flexible or rigid 5 mm scope. A 5 mm energy device and a 5 mm grasper are used in the two other 5 mm ports, for dissection and hemostasis. It is important to choose an energy device with the capability to grasp, seal vessels, and cut with or without energy. To improve the exposure without the need of extra instruments, the patient is then placed in a Trendelenburg position (35–40°) and right-side tilt (20–25°). To achieve maximum exposure, it is important to fix the patient on the surgical table. We try to avoid shoulder fixation to prevent brachial plexus injury. To facilitate the manipulation of the sigmoid colon, the upper rectum is mobilized posteriorly, and the sigmoid colon is suspended toward the abdominal wall with the transparietal suture at the beginning of the rectal dissection and is mobilized medial to lateral. These maneuvers facilitate and increase the exposure of the rectum, providing a good surgical field to proceed with TME.

We start by preparing the abdominal cavity; the first movement is to place the omentum over to the stomach and expose the distal transverse mesocolon (Fig. 17.2). We keep the transverse mesocolon positioned and then ask for Trendelenburg position. The second step is to expose the inferior mesenteric vein. We enter with the shaft of our forceps at the base of the small bowel mesentery, and we move as a handspike from the left toward the right side of the abdomen (Fig. 17.3). Then we ask for right tilt. We expose the inferior mesenteric vein (IMV), distal transverse mesocolon, and descending colon (Fig. 17.4). We grab the vein with our left hand forceps and start our dissection opening the visceral peritoneum below the vein (Fig. 17.5). We detach the descending mesocolon from the retroperitoneum with a medial to lateral dissection following the embryological plane (Fig. 17.6). Our movements are facilitated using vertical dissection.

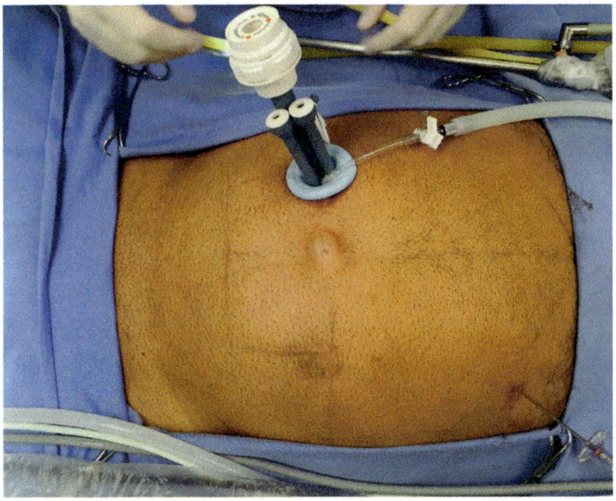

Fig 17.1 Ileostomy site and single port site

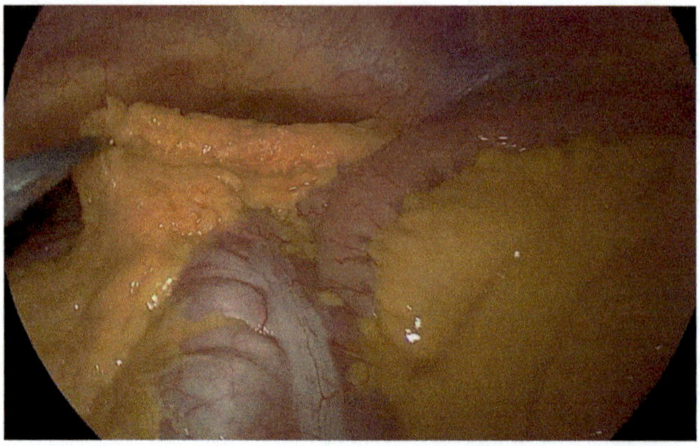

Fig 17.2 First movement: omentum over the stomach

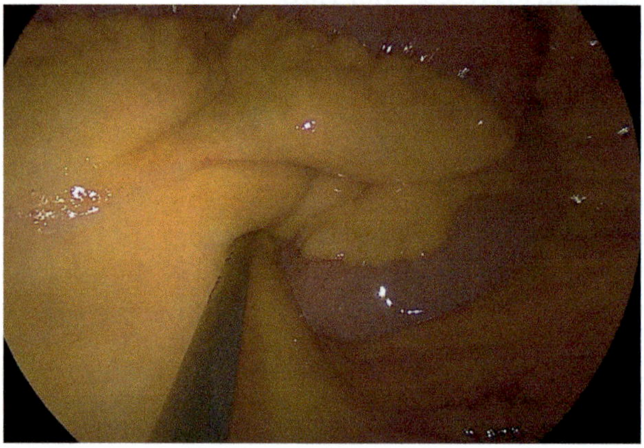

Fig 17.3 Maneuver to put small bowel to the right side

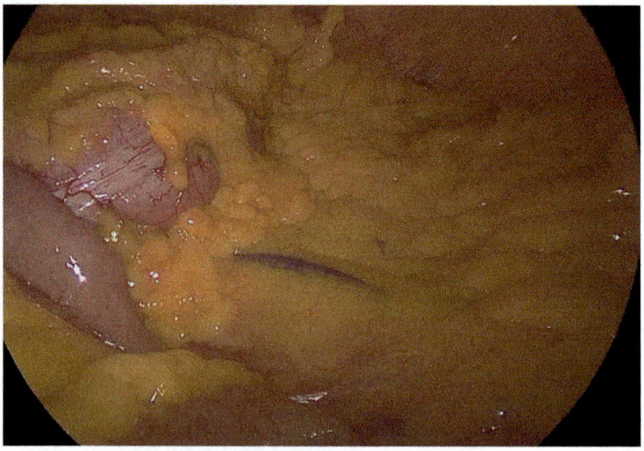

Fig 17.4 Inferior mesenteric vein (IMV)

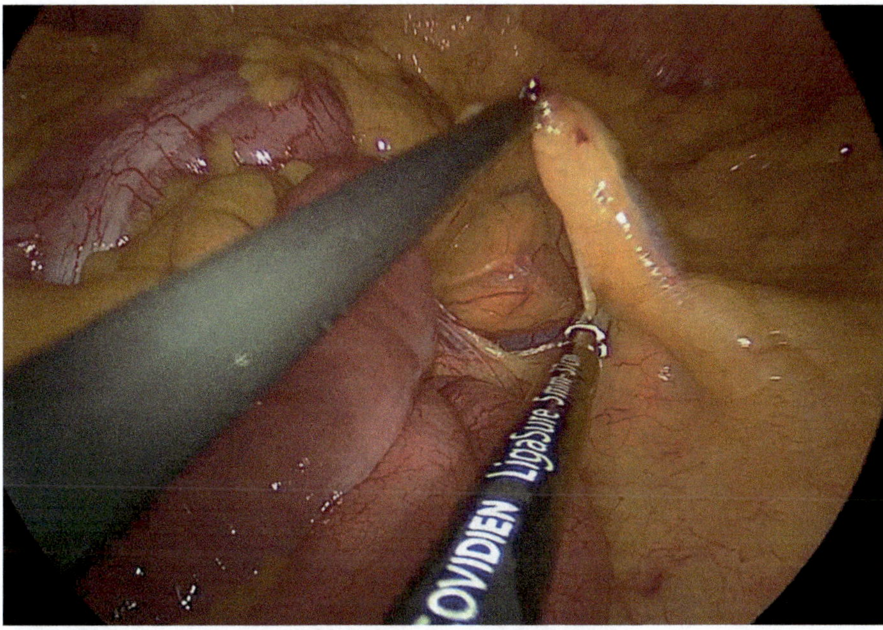

Fig 17.5 Opening the visceral peritoneum below the IMV

Fig 17.6 Dissection following the embryological plane: below the IMV

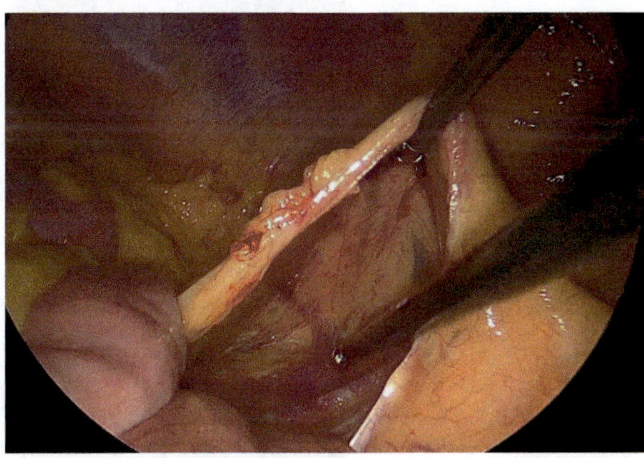

To enter into the lesser sac, we grab the distal transverse mesocolon. We try to recognize the shadow of the pancreas body, insertion of IMV, and Treitz angle to determine the correct place to open the transverse mesocolon (Fig. 17.7). We use a simple rule to achieve a good position to make this window—1.5 in. up to the IMV and 1.5 in. to the left of the IMV (Fig. 17.7).

After that we ligate the IMV. It can be done with surgical clips or energy (Figs. 17.8 and 17.9).

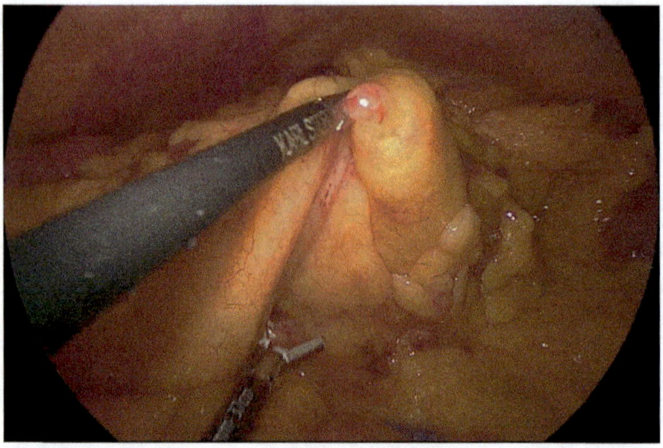

Fig 17.7 Maneuver to enter into the lesser sac

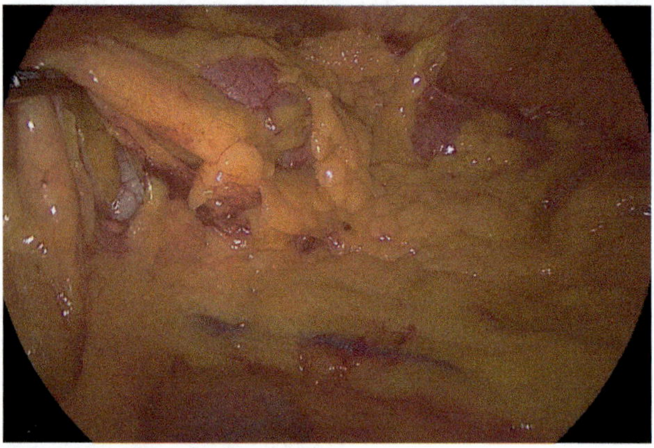

Fig 17.8 Correct plane after entering into the lesser sac

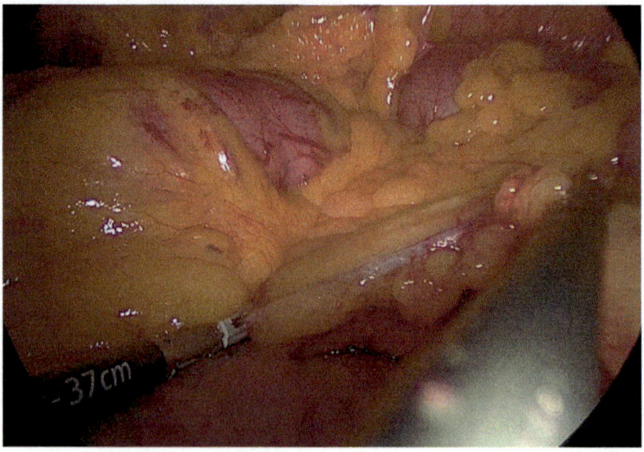

Fig 17.9 Using an energy device to ligate the IMV

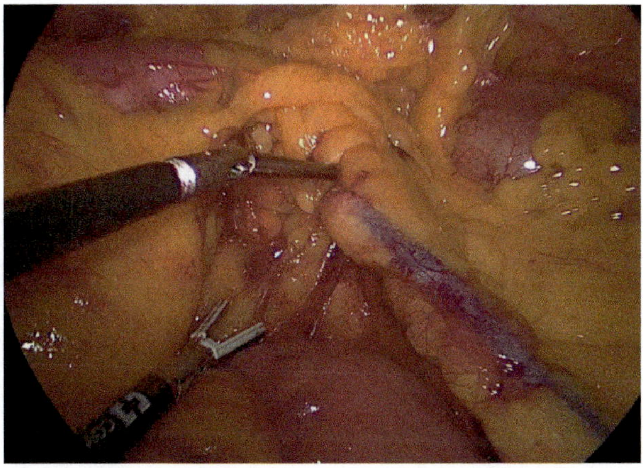

Fig 17.10 Detaching the distal transverse mesocolon to the pancreas

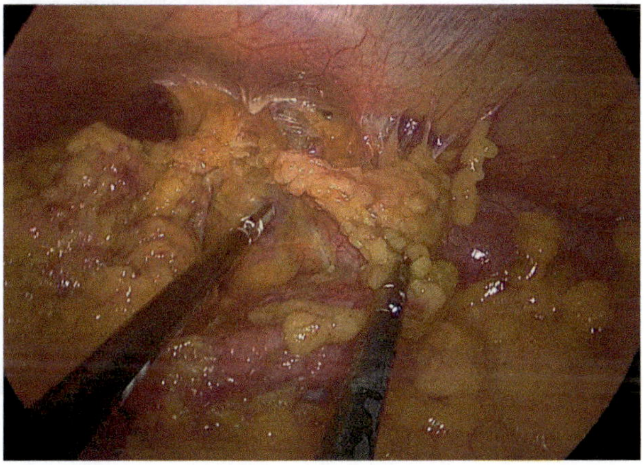

Fig 17.11 Detaching the transverse mesocolon from the epiploon

The next step is to detach the distal transverse mesocolon from the pancreas. We use our right hand to lift the transverse mesocolon. In this procedure it is important to use a forceps with a big jaw. To lift we open the jaw of the forceps to avoid damage to the marginal arcade. Opening the jaw increases the contact area between the instrument and the mesocolon decreasing the pressure of the forceps (Fig. 17.10). We finish our medial to lateral exposure dissecting the pancreas until the tail.

Next move is to detach the transverse mesocolon from the epiploon. We grab the omentum close to the medial transverse mesocolon, with the aim to reach the lesser sac and our previous dissection (Fig. 17.11). During these maneuvers sometimes to achieve more comfortable exposition, we could ask for a reverse Trendelenburg. We detach all the adhesions between the posterior wall of the stomach, omentum, and distal transverse mesocolon until the splenic flexure (Fig. 17.12).

With these strategies we finish the upper abdominal dissection of the left side detaching the splenic flexure and ligating the IMV.

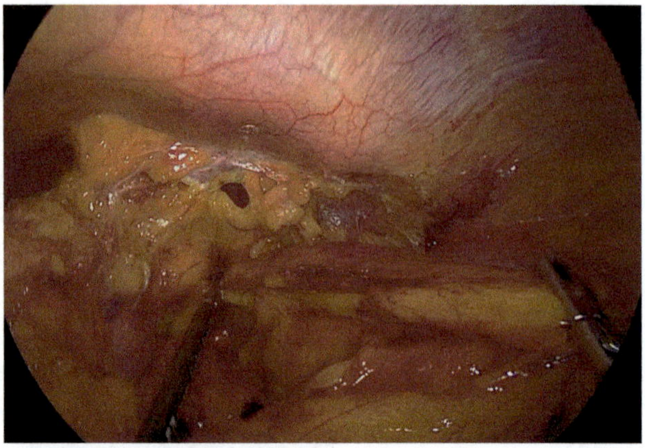

Fig 17.12 Splenic flexure

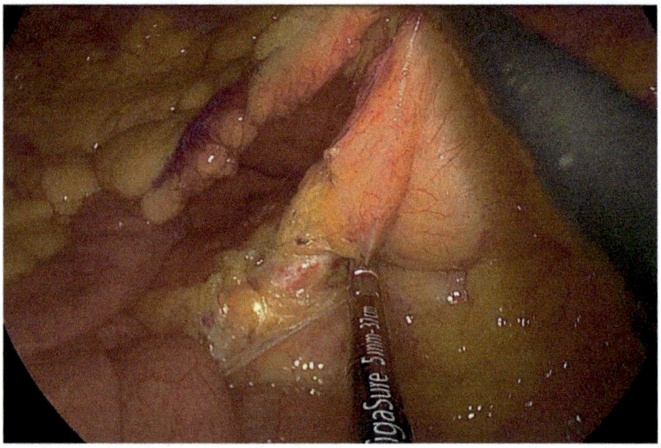

Fig 17.13 Dissecting the inferior mesenteric artery (IMA)

Our next challenge is to dissect and ligate the inferior mesenteric artery and detach the distal descending and sigmoid colon. Now it is important to return to the previous Trendelenburg position.

We grab the mesentery over the inferior mesenteric artery (IMA) (Fig. 17.13). The artery is dissected and ligated using the energy device (Fig. 17.14). It is important that the left ureter should be recognized before the ligation of the IMA. We release the descending and sigmoid mesocolon from the retroperitoneum, so we can see the left ureter and left gonadal vessels (Fig. 17.15). Next step is to release the left Toldt's fascia for the descending and sigmoid colon (Figs. 17.16 and 17.17).

To start the dissection of the rectum, it is important to have traction on the sigmoid colon. We use transfacial sutures for it (Fig. 17.18). We start dissecting the posterior rectal space through the promontory (Fig. 17.19). A careful dissection should be performed at this point to avoid injuries to the hypogastric nerves and also dissecting through the presacral avascular plane toward the pelvic floor. The dissection of the lateral rectal space is performed first on the right side, because it is

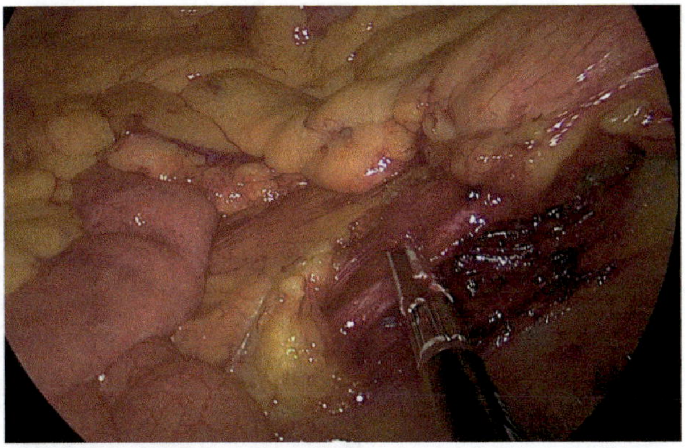

Fig 17.14 Energy device to take the IMA

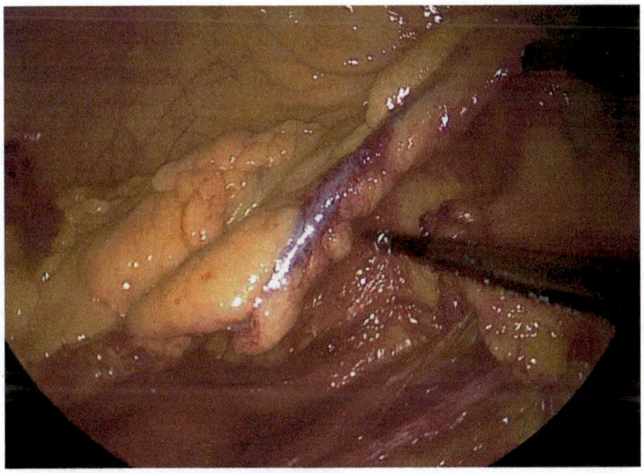

Fig 17.15 Dissecting below the IMA (detail: the ureter and gonadal vein)

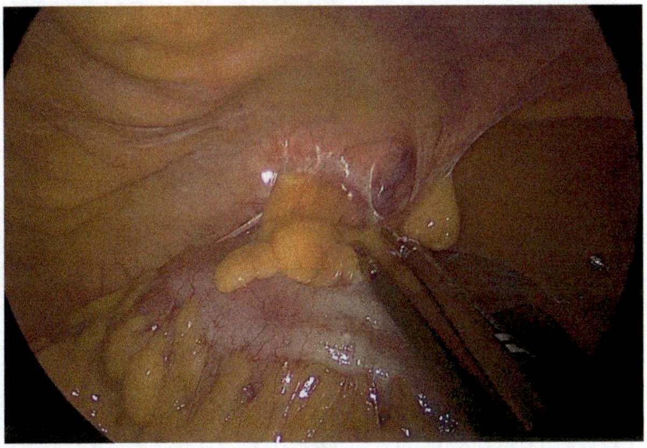

Fig 17.16 Toldt's fascia

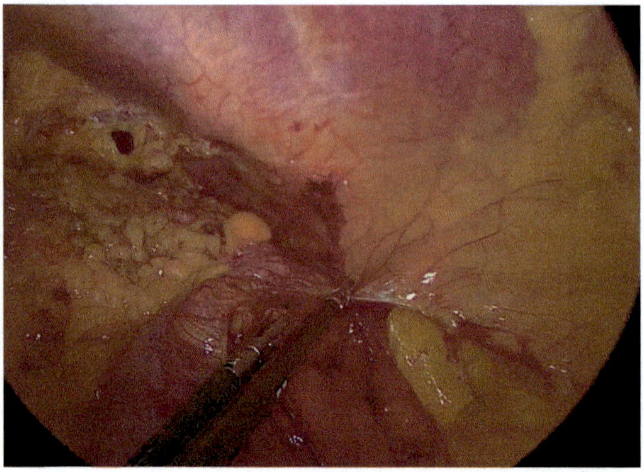

Fig 17.17 Toldt's fascia next to the splenic flexure

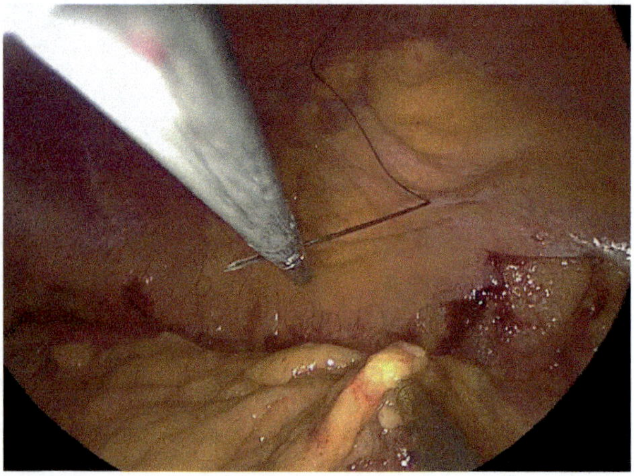

Fig 17.18 Rectum dissection: transfacial suture to have traction

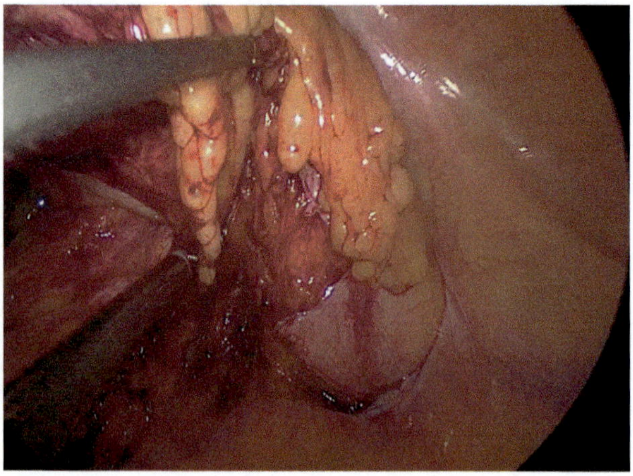

Fig 17.19 Posterior rectal dissection

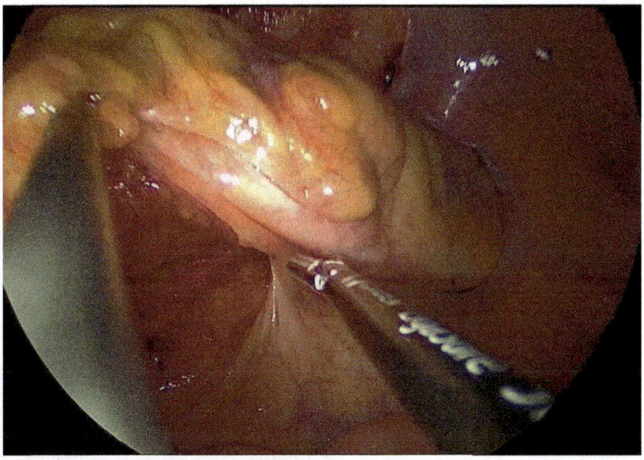

Fig 17.20 Lateral rectal space: right side first

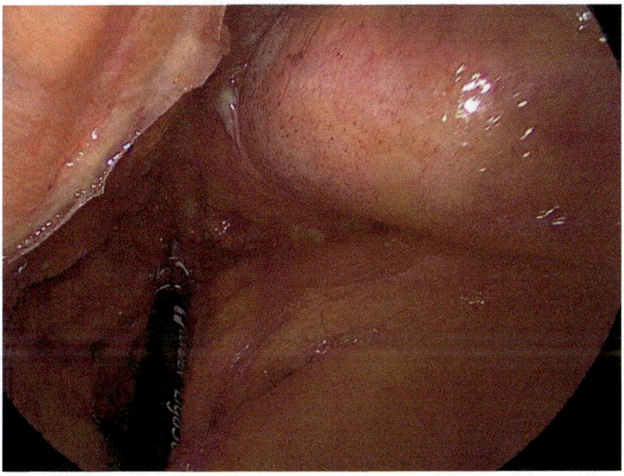

Fig 17.21 Left side of the rectal space

already partially exposed by the initial dissection (Fig. 17.20). The left side is then dissected as far as possible, to reach the levator muscles (Figs. 17.21 and 17.22). Before we start the anterior rectal wall dissection, we use transfacial sutures to lift the bladder in male patients (Fig. 17.23). In female patients, to facilitate the exposure, an additional suture can be placed at the uterus fixing it at the abdominal wall.

Now, the dissection continues toward the anterior rectum opening the posterior peritoneal fold and in a plane between the rectum and the posterior vagina or the seminal vesicles and the prostate (Fig. 17.24). If tumor is located at the anterior wall, we include the Denonvelliers' fascia. We complete the deep right-side dissection toward the levator muscles (Figs. 17.25 and 17.26).

A digital rectal exam is performed after the anterior dissection is complete to identify the distal margin of tumor and before starting the intersphincteric dissection.

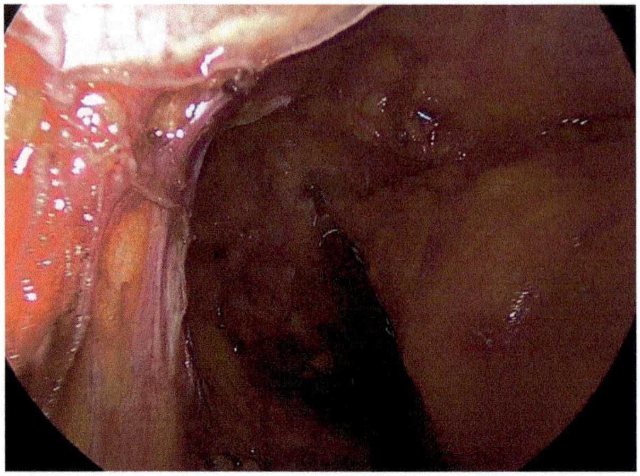

Fig 17.22 Levator muscles

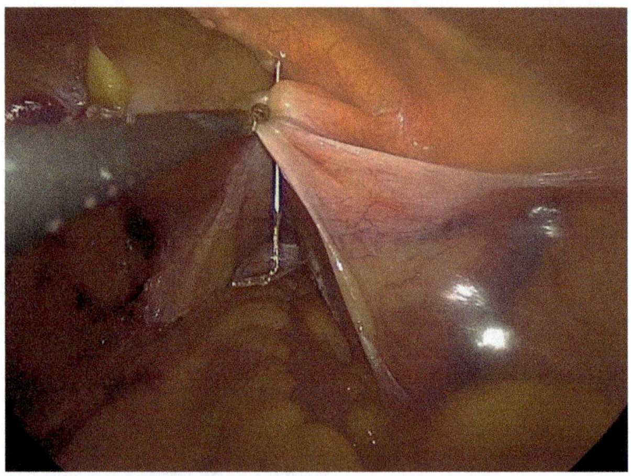

Fig 17.23 Anterior rectal dissection: transfacial suture to lift the bladder

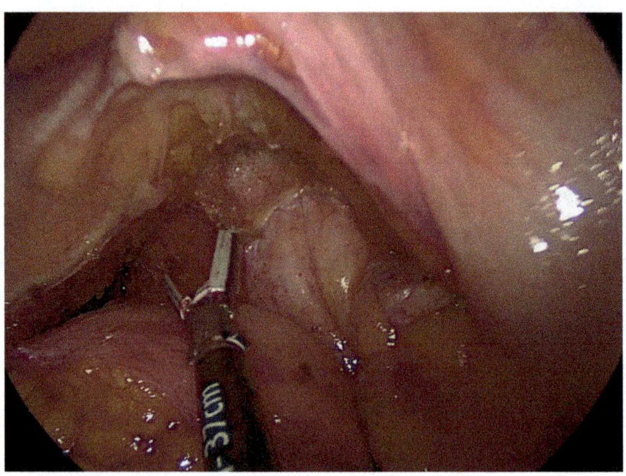

Fig 17.24 Anterior rectal plane

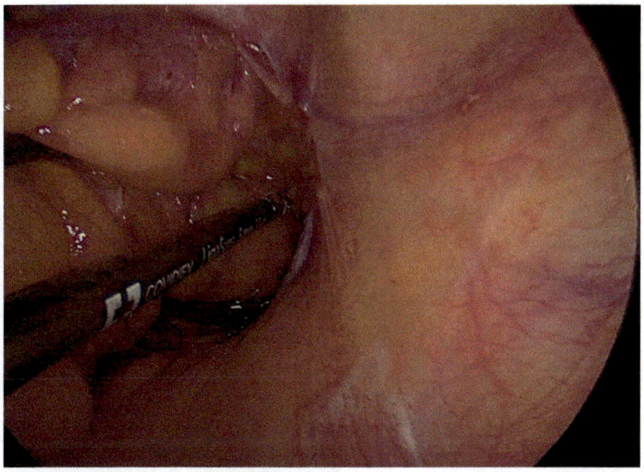

Fig 17.25 Deep right-side dissection

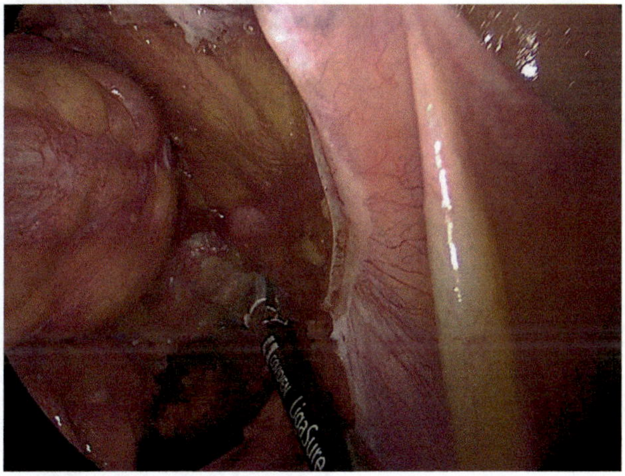

Fig 17.26 Levator muscles on the right side

17.2.2 Perianal Step

After exposure of the anus, a circular incision at the dentate line is performed, and the dissection through the internal anal sphincter muscle is performed to meet the level of the dissection performed laparoscopically (Figs. 17.27 and 17.28).

The specimen is removed through the anus until the recognition of the transition of ischemic area caused by the ligation of IMA and the vascularized remaining colon (Fig. 17.29). The colon is then resected, and a hand-sewn anastomosis with Vicryl 3–0 is performed.

We perform at the site of SILS single port, the loop ileostomy (Fig. 17.30).

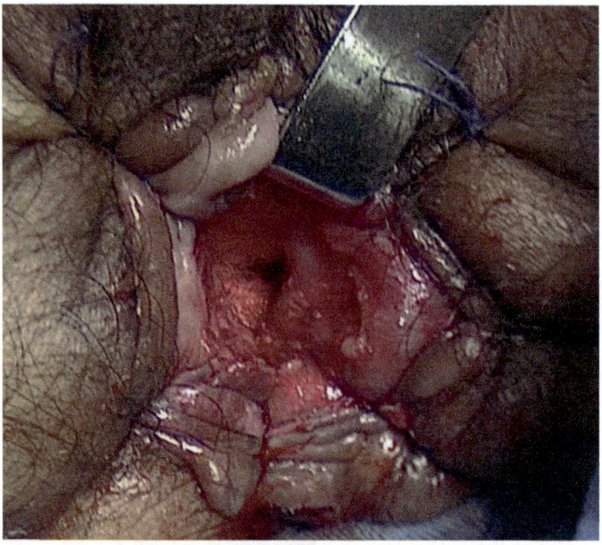

Fig 17.27 Perineal step: internal anal sphincter muscle

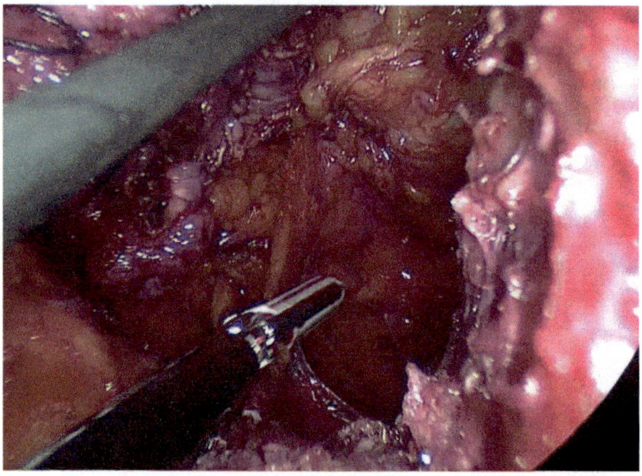

Fig 17.28 Finding laparoscopy and perineal plane

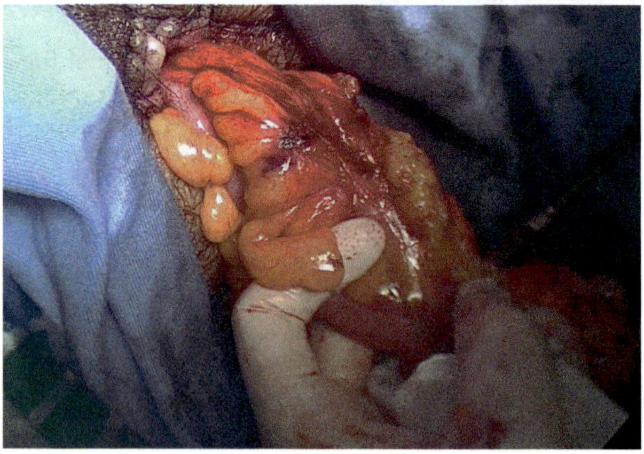

Fig 17.29 Extracting the specimen through the anus

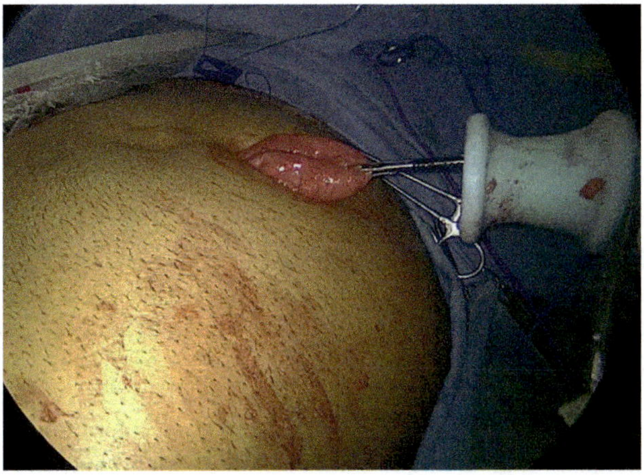

Fig 17.30 Loop ileostomy at the site of single port

17.3 Tips and Tricks

In colorectal surgery the majority of the movements in LESS are vertical, which enables the surgeon to have more amplitude and to be more effective.

The position of the scope and the forceps are very important, and to understand this it is necessary to imagine a triangle: the base is always turned to the surgical field and the vertex apex in the opposite site. The scope is positioned in the vertex of the triangle, and the forceps are always located at the base. It is easier to understand it if you imagine Mickey Mouse's face. The optic is always in the mouth, and the forceps and the energy device are in the ears. The mouth is the opposite to the target area.

The surgical table setting: the proper position of the patient, the lateral tilt, and the lateral Trendelenburg position can be considered the first assistant because if performed accordantly, they can provide a safe exposure without the need of extra ports. Gravity is the best ally.

Energy dissectors should be chosen carefully. This device must have some important capabilities, because if it does not, the surgeon will be forced to interchange his/her dissector with any hemostasis instrument in the right hand multiple times during the operation. In our opinion, the dissector used in the right hand should have the capabilities to grab, dissect, cut without energy, cut with energy, coagulate, and seal the vessel. On the other hand, the temperature of the device cannot reach more than 100 °C, and it must decrease quickly [5]. Considering for these features, we do not recommend ultrasonic device for colon resection, because it goes to 263 °C and it needs 40 s to be cold enough to touch the tissue around.

Laparoscopy set: for the majority of the procedure, the main area of interest will be on the peripheral area of the screen; it means that the use of a real high-definition camera could increase the vision up to 30%. So it is necessary to work with a 16:9 instead of a 4:3 screen. Also, we prefer to use a 10 mm instead of 5 mm scope for the reasons of durability and capability to improve brightness of the light by 300% and because we do not need to buy a new one. However, it is important that the connection between the light cable and the scope must be in 90° to avoid clashing among the instruments in a small space and also to avoid interference between the camera driver and the surgeon.

17.4 Discussion

Minimally invasive surgery is one of the major technical advances of the past 20 years. Interest in laparoscopy has led to the development of more minimally invasive surgery such as natural orifice transluminal endoscopic surgery (NOTES) and LESS.

Indeed, one of the last innovations has been the development of a new generation of multi-instrument ports allowing the introduction of a camera and several instruments through a unique skin incision of 25–50 mm and to perform various surgical procedures. In addition to the benefits of laparoscopy, LESS offers a reduction in port-related complications such as pain, faster postoperative recovery, and improved cosmesis.

LESS is an emerging technique that meets an enthusiastic surgical community, as stated by the large and increasing number of publications within the last years. Indeed, case reports and small series [6–12] have rapidly grown and demonstrated the technical feasibility of LESS for various colorectal procedures including complex ones such as subtotal colectomies or rectal resections. But, for these latter complex procedures, specific challenges of the handling of straight tools in parallel with the optic through a small single incision decreasing the range of movement for the surgeon and the assistant holding the camera were more evident and crucial. Problems of triangulation, tissue retraction, internal and external instrument collision, and in-line vision are the main challenges limiting the procedure. In our experience, for rectal resection, the best approach might be to insert the port at the site of the planned ileostomy in the right iliac fossa to be far enough from the surgical site and to leave the patient just one scar.

In fact, the main limit to a larger development of this technique was the lack of evidence of its equivalence or superiority to conventional laparoscopy. Indeed, the expected benefit of LESS over conventional laparoscopy would mainly be cosmetic or a moderate decrease in parietal trauma. These expected limited benefits must be balanced with possible increased morbidity due to the technical challenge of the procedure.

Some comparative studies have already been published regarding cholecystectomy [13], appendicectomy [14], or nephrectomy [15] showing encouraging results. Its technical feasibility in experienced hand is now widely established, but safety and benefits compared to standard laparoscopy procedure just start to be assessed as for cholecystectomy by randomized control trials [13]. LESS remains a controversial procedure. Some authors argue better patient satisfaction due to faster recovery and better cosmetic result, but on the other hand, others claim that reduction of only a few small abdominal incisions offers no objective benefit to patients and the surgical quality could be jeopardized leading to bad long-term oncological results.

This was the reason the first systematic review and meta-analysis, including more than 1000 procedures, was published [16]. We have seen, compared to conventional laparoscopy, LESS was associated with a similar postoperative morbidity, a significantly shorter length of skin incision and a significantly shorter length of stay. During the same year, Fung et al. published a very interesting review [17] where colonic LESS data were compared with those from a Cochrane review on the short-term outcomes of laparoscopic colonic surgery and four main randomized trials. The authors showed that operating times and time to first bowel motion for LESS were comparable with those for laparoscopic surgery. The median lymph nodes' retrieval for cancer with LESS were acceptable (17 vs. 14.8). Evidence for a reduction in postoperative pain with LESS was conflicting, and there was no significant reduction in the length of hospital stay. Most patients in the LESS group had a low body mass index and non-bulky tumors and were operated on by experienced colorectal surgeons. The authors concluded that LESS should be restricted to highly selected patients, and operations should be performed by experienced laparoscopic surgeons.

Potential advantages of LESS compared with multiport laparoscopy are well identified in the literature including decreased postoperative pain, faster recovery, shorter length of hospital stay, and improved cosmesis. But, one of the major disadvantages in LESS cholecystectomy, the need for an incision 3–5 cm in length, which might lead to a greater tendency for wound herniation, is not an issue with LESS colon surgery. In LESS colon surgery, this size incision is needed to extract the specimen, or for low anastomosis the site is used as a stoma site. No study to date has reported the long-term results including function and late wound herniation. Another point is the need for additional equipment and a consequent increase in cost. Specific articulated instruments have now been designed to facilitate the operation, but these developments have led to a rise in the cost. Some authors have reported the use of extracorporeal magnetic retraction which is also expensive. In our experience, LESS is possible using conventional laparoscopic instrumentation. The technical feasibility might also be related to the port itself. Several designs of ports are now available, but to date there are no studies comparing different ports. It was therefore not possible to analyze this potential effect. Furthermore, the heterogeneity of design of the LESS ports used in the various studies would create bias.

But, published reviews [16, 17] raise the question of an oncological outcome following LESS. In a consensus statement of a consortium for LESS [18], the authors stated that for patients undergoing cancer surgery, given the gravity of oncologic issues vis-a-vis procedural morbidity, the bar for considering LESS oncologic procedures should be higher than for non-cancer applications. Questions remain about the safety of LESS for colorectal cancer resection. From an oncological point of view, in all published cases, margins were negative, and the number of harvested lymph nodes was equal to that reported in randomized studies of multiport laparoscopic surgery. So while these are theoretical concerns, there is no data to support an inferior oncological outcome compared to standard laparoscopic colorectal surgery. There are, however, no data on the long-term outcomes.

To date, two randomized studies are available comparing LESS and conventional multiport laparoscopy [19, 20]. In a study of 50 patients, Poon et al. [19] demonstrated that LESS for cancer colectomy reduced postoperative pain and was associated with shorter hospital stay in good-risk patients with small colon cancer. The authors concluded that further studies including a larger scale for broader application were required. Huscher et al. [20], including 16 patients in each group, showed no significant differences in terms of mortality and morbidity between LESS and conventional laparoscopy. Pathological data were similar in terms of margins, number of resected lymph nodes.

In conclusion, LESS represents a logical next step in minimally invasive surgery, but its place is not yet well defined in colorectal surgery. Clinical advantages after LESS are well identified including decreased pain score, shorter hospital stay, and better cosmetic results. By contrast, disadvantages are related to the perceived complexity of the procedure. Regarding colorectal cancer, LESS is feasible and safe in experienced surgical hands. As technology advances and new techniques evolve, we must ensure that oncologic principles are maintained.

References

1. Leroy J, Jamali F, Forbes L, Smith M, Rubino F, Mutter D, et al. Laparoscopic total mesorectal excision (TME) for rectal cancer surgery: long-term outcomes. Surg Endosc. 2004;18(2):281–9.
2. Maeda K, Noda E, Nagahara H, Inoe T, Takii M, Watanabe K, et al. A comparative study of single-incision versus conventional multiport laparoscopic ileocecal resection for Crohn's disease with strictures. Asian J Endosc Surg. 2012;5(3):118–22.
3. Choi B, Lee S, Kang W. Single-port laparoscopic total mesorectal excision with transanal resection (transabdominal transanal resection) for low rectal cancer: initial experience with 22 cases. Int J Surg. 2013;11(9):858–63.
4. Tokuoka M, Ide Y, Taleda M, Hashimoto Y, Matsuyama J, Yokoyama S, et al. Single-incision plus one port laparoscopic total mesorectal excision and bilateral pelvic node dissection for advanced rectal cancer - a medial umbilical ligament approach. Int Surg. 2015;100(3):417–22.
5. Kim F, Chammas M, Gewehr E, Morihisa M, Caldas F, Hayacibara E. Temperature safety profile of laparoscopic devices: harmonic ACE (ACE), Ligasure V (LV), and plasma trisector (PT). Surg Endosc. 2008;22(6):1464–9.
6. Remzi FH, Kirat HT, Kaouk JH, Geisler DP. Single-port laparoscopy in colorectal surgery. Color Dis. 2008;10(8):823–6.
7. Leroy J, Cahill RA, Asakuma M, Dallemagne B, Marescaux J. Single-access laparoscopic sigmoidectomy as definitive surgical management of prior diverticulitis in a human patient. Arch Surg. 2009;144(2):173–9. discussion 9
8. Merchant AM, Lin E. Single-incision laparoscopic right hemicolectomy for a colon mass. Dis *Colon rectum*. 2009;52(5):1021–4.
9. Bucher P, Pugin F, Morel P. Transumbilical single incision laparoscopic sigmoidectomy for benign disease. Color Dis. 2010;12(1):61–5.
10. Geisler DP, Condon ET, Remzi FH. Single incision laparoscopic total proctocolectomy with ileopouch anal anastomosis. Color Dis. 2010;12(9):941–3.
11. Law WL, Fan JK, Poon JT. Single incision laparoscopic left colectomy for carcinoma of distal transverse colon. Color Dis. 2010;12(7):698–701.
12. Rieger NA, Lam FF. Single-incision laparoscopically assisted colectomy using standard laparoscopic instrumentation. Surg Endosc. 2010;24(4):888–90.

13. Lee PC, Lo C, Lai PS, Chang JJ, Huang SJ, Lin MT, et al. Randomized clinical trial of single-incision laparoscopic cholecystectomy versus minilaparoscopic cholecystectomy. Br J Surg. 2010;97(7):1007–12.
14. Chow A, Purkayastha S, Nehme J, Darzi LA, Paraskeva P. Single incision laparoscopic surgery for appendicectomy: a retrospective comparative analysis. Surg Endosc. 2010;24(10):2567–74.
15. Raman JD, Bagrodia A, Cadeddu JA. Single-incision, umbilical laparoscopic versus conventional laparoscopic nephrectomy: a comparison of perioperative outcomes and short-term measures of convalescence. Eur Urol. 2009;55(5):1198–204.
16. Maggiori L, Gaujoux S, Tribillon E, Bretagnol F, Panis Y. Single-incision laparoscopy for colorectal resection: a systematic review and meta-analysis of more than a thousand procedures. Color Dis. 2012;14(10):e643–54.
17. Fung AK, Aly EH. Systematic review of single-incision laparoscopic colonic surgery. Br J Surg. 2012;99(10):1353–64.
18. Gill IS, Advincula AP, Aron M, Caddedu J, Canes D, Curcillo PG 2nd, et al. Consensus statement of the consortium for laparoendoscopic single-site surgery. Surg Endosc. 2010;24(4):762–8.
19. Poon JT, Cheung CW, Fan JK, Lo OS, Law WL. Single-incision versus conventional laparoscopic colectomy for colonic neoplasm: a randomized, controlled trial. Surg Endosc. 2012;26(10):2729–34.
20. Huscher CG, Mingoli A, Sgarzini G, Mereu A, Binda B, Brachini G, et al. Standard laparoscopic versus single-incision laparoscopic colectomy for cancer: early results of a randomized prospective study. Am J Surg. 2012;204(1):115–20.

Robot-Assisted TME with Coloanal Anastomosis

18

Han Deok Kwak and Seon-Hahn Kim

Abstract

Since total mesorectal excision (TME) was introduced in 1982 [1], it has become a standard procedure for the treatment of rectal cancer. For low rectal cancer, coloanal anastomosis (CAA) [2] after ultralow anterior resection (uLAR) or intersphincteric resection (ISR) [3] along with TME has provided positive functional, psychological, and oncological outcomes. These outcomes of surgical techniques are also owed to the development of anatomical knowledge and perioperative treatment [4]. Robotic systems offer surgeons several benefits, though there have been controversial issues. Recent reports have indicated that robotic surgery is feasible and safe compared to laparoscopic surgery [5–7]. Robotic surgery enables easier performance of intersphincteric dissection for very low-lying rectal cancer, especially when accompanied with unfavorable factors such as high body mass index or preoperative radiation, leading to satisfactory surgical, functional, and oncological outcomes compared to conventional laparoscopy [8]. It also provides earlier recovery of sexual and bladder functions [6], lower conversion rate, and shorter hospital stay [9]. Although multicenter, randomized prospective trials are needed, robot-assisted TME with CAA with or without ISR has potential benefits for low rectal cancer.

In this chapter, the authors introduce the robotic approach of TME with CAA, which is performed with or without ISR. The procedures include patient

H.D. Kwak, M.D. (✉)
Department of Surgery, Chonnam National University Hospital,
Gwangju, Republic of Korea

S.-H. Kim, M.D., Ph.D.
Department of Surgery, Korea University Anam Hospital,
73 Inchon-ro, Seoul 02841, Republic of Korea
e-mail: drkimsh@korea.ac.kr

G. Dapri, J.H. Marks (eds.), *Surgical Techniques in Rectal Cancer*,
https://doi.org/10.1007/978-4-431-55579-7_18

positioning, trocar placement, docking, abdominal/pelvic phases, and useful technical tips as well as CAA and ISR.

Keywords
Robotic • Total mesorectal excision • Coloanal anastomosis • Intersphincteric resection • Rectal cancer

18.1 Procedure Overview

18.1.1 Patient Positioning

Proper positioning of the patient is an essential first step for patient safety, docking of the robot, and good exposure of the surgical field. After the induction of general anesthesia, the patient is placed in a modified lithotomy position with a beanbag mattress to prevent sliding. Legs are placed in adjustable stirrups with the knees flexed. The legs are lowered, so the thigh is at the same level as the torso, so that the legs do not interfere with the approach of the robotic system. After positioning, the angles of the Trendelenburg position and the right-sided downward tilt can be adjusted during the initial exposure step.

18.1.2 Trocar Placement

Proper port placement is crucial, since the da Vinci® system (Intuitive Surgical Inc., Sunnyvale, CA, USA) requires sufficient room between arms to avoid external collision and maximize internal movement. Our standard robotic setup includes six instrument ports, including a 12 mm camera port.

Pneumoperitoneum is established via direct cutdown around the umbilicus. The camera port can be shifted a few centimeters up or down relative to the umbilicus, based on the distance from the target anatomy. The first 8 mm right lower quadrant (RLQ) port is usually placed at McBurney's point. It is important to avoid bony structures such as the iliac crest to allow the maximum range of motion for the robotic arm. This port will be used for an ileostomy, if required. Then, the right upper quadrant (RUQ) port is placed 2 cm from the costal margin and just medial to midclavicular line (MCL). Left-sided ports are placed along the left MCL. The left upper quadrant (LUQ) port is placed approximately 1–2 cm above the camera port at the crossing of the MCL; this placement is lower than the RUQ port to avoid clashing during colonic dissection. The left lower quadrant (LLQ) port is inserted approximately 1–2 cm lateral to the MCL. The assistant port is placed in the right flank position between the RUQ and camera port near the anterior axillary line at the umbilicus level to allow the assistant access. This is used for suction or irrigation, clipping of vessels, and retraction of tissues (Figs. 18.1 and 18.2).

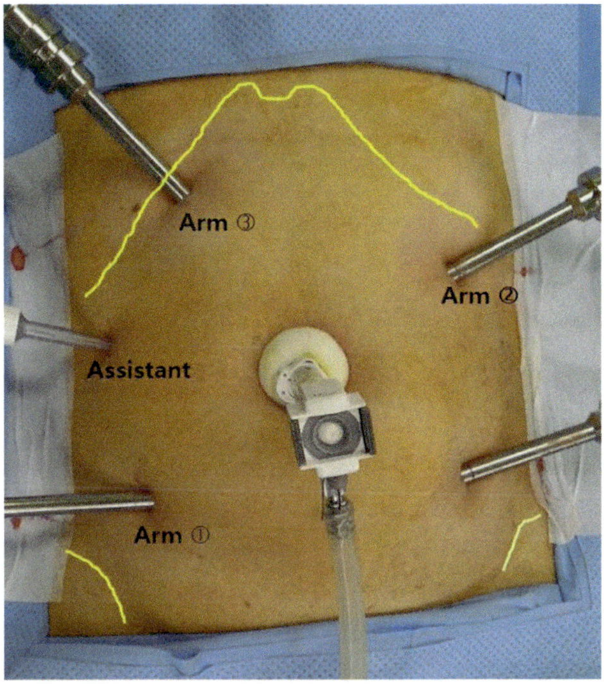

Fig. 18.1 Port placement, initial abdominal phase

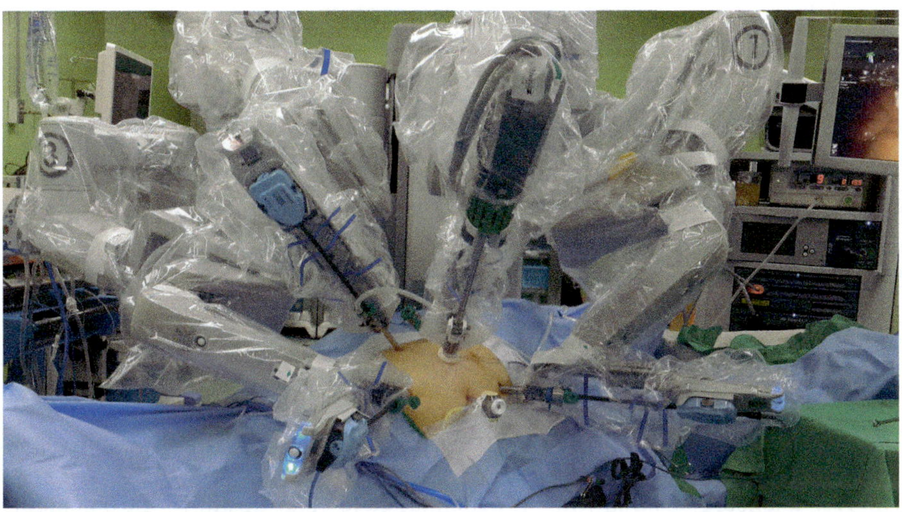

Fig. 18.2 Initial robotic setup

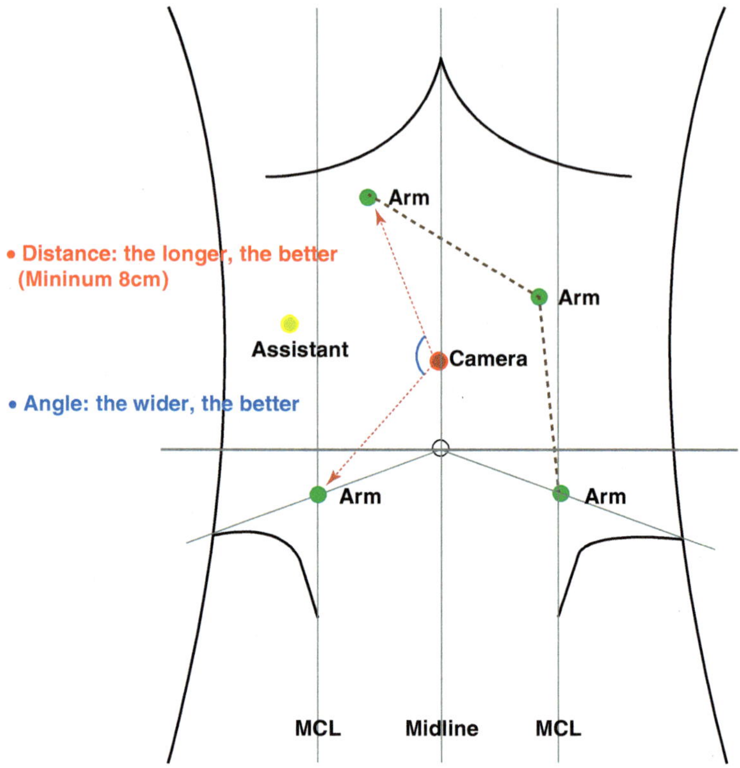

Fig. 18.3 Diagram showing the angle between the robotic ports in the RUQ and RLQ, which should be as wide and long as possible

Trocar placement is important to prevent ongoing problems during the operation. The distance between the camera or instrument and the target anatomy as well as the distance between the instrument ports is important. The camera port should be at least 15 cm from the target anatomy. The distance between the instrument ports on the same side of the patient should be at least 8 cm apart. The angle between the two right-sided instrument ports should be as wide as possible (Fig. 18.3). Correct trocar placement will prevent clashing of the instrument arms during the operation.

18.1.3 Patient Repositioning

The Trendelenburg position with the patient tilted left side up allows the omentum and the small bowel loops to fall away from the operative field due to gravity. Often, the patient needs to be positioned 15–20° head-down and 15–20° right side-down. The right side of the greater omentum should also be positioned over the liver (Fig. 18.4). The patient cart is positioned and docked obliquely at the

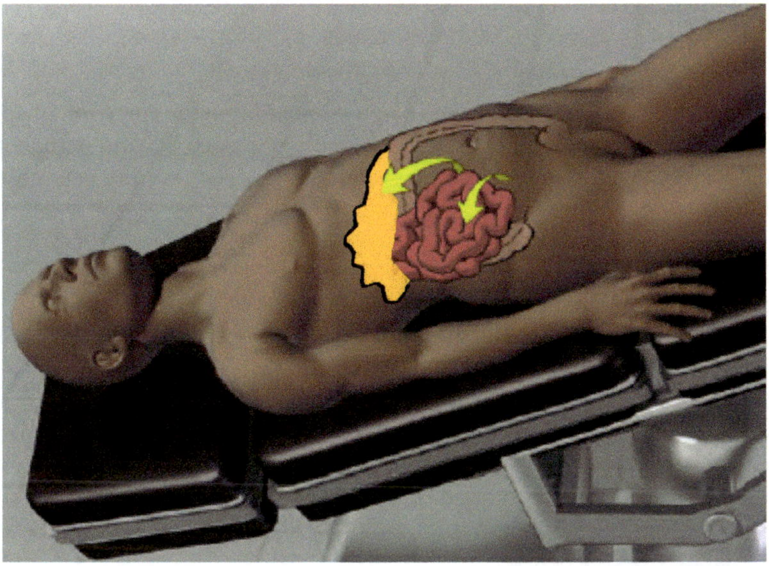

Fig. 18.4 Patient positioning for robotic LAR or ISR

patient's left side. The robotic arms are well fanned out to minimize external collision. During the operation, both the assistant and the scrub nurse should stand on the patient's right side, allowing them access to the robotic instruments. The video cart is placed toward the patient's right foot to allow visualization of the video screen.

18.1.4 Initial Laparoscopic Exposure

The aim of exposure in the left colon is to identify the base of the mesentery and the inferior mesenteric artery (IMA) and inferior mesenteric vein (IMV). The intra-abdominal pressure is maintained at 8 mmHg (12 mmHg, when needed). Just after manual introduction of the robotic camera, full initial diagnostic exploration is performed for evidence of peritoneal or metastatic disease. If adhesions limit mobilization and exposure, they should be divided. The omentum is retracted above the stomach and the liver along with the transverse colon. The weight of the omentum, along with the Trendelenburg position, helps keep the transverse colon away from the operative field. To expose the base of the mesentery, small bowel loops should be retracted medially and toward the RUQ. The surgeon should assess the left colon and sigmoid, as mobilization of the splenic flexure may not be necessary if there is redundant sigmoid colon. Then, one or two pieces of small gauze may be placed intraperitoneally to help retract the small bowel and to wipe up blood from the tissues. This step is achieved with conventional laparoscopic instruments, except using the robotic camera.

18.1.5 Docking

18.1.5.1 Double Docking

Two separate dockings are performed: an initial docking for mobilization of splenic flexure and a second docking for sigmoid and pelvic dissection. An alternate technique undocks the patient cart and moves the patient's bed into the new position, rather than moving the patient cart.

18.1.5.2 Single Docking

The patient cart is obliquely placed on the patient's left. The central column of the patient cart should line up along an imaginary line between the camera port and the left anterior superior iliac spine. Moving the robotic arms into different ports allows dissection of the left colon/splenic flexure as well as pelvic dissection. Docking on the patient's left also allows access to patient's perineum, enabling the surgeon to check his/her dissection by digital examination without undocking the patient cart.

18.2 Abdominal Phase

18.2.1 Ports Placement (Fig. 18.1)

- Instrument arm ① Monopolar curved scissors at the RLQ port.
- Instrument arm ② Maryland bipolar forceps at the LUQ port.
- Instrument arm ③ Cadiere forceps through at the RUQ port.
- Assistant uses an instrument: a non-toothed bowel grasper or a suction device at the right flank port.

18.2.2 Medial-to-Lateral Approach

The sigmoid colon mesentery is lifted up by instrument arm ② to reveal the base of the mesentery and the IMA (Fig. 18.5). The assistant uses a non-toothed bowel grasper to retract the small bowel away from the operative field. The base of the mesentery above the sacral promontory is incised and dissected using instrument arms ① and ③. The IMA is identified and skeletonized. The aorta is used as a landmark for dissection of the IMA. We keep the aorta horizontal while visualizing the IMA. D3 dissection is performed by dissecting a cuff of the mesentery at least 1 cm around the origin of the IMA and included in the specimen, while the periaortic sympathetic nerve plexus is preserved (Fig. 18.6). Once skeletonized, the IMA is ligated at its origin with Hem-o-lok® clips. This can be performed either by the assistant or via robotic arm ①. When the robotic arm is used, exchange of instrument arm ① has the advantage of rotation and angulation provided by the robotic wrist.

We have modified the procedure for patients with cardiovascular diseases, in which the IMA is ligated at a low level while preserving the left colic vessels.

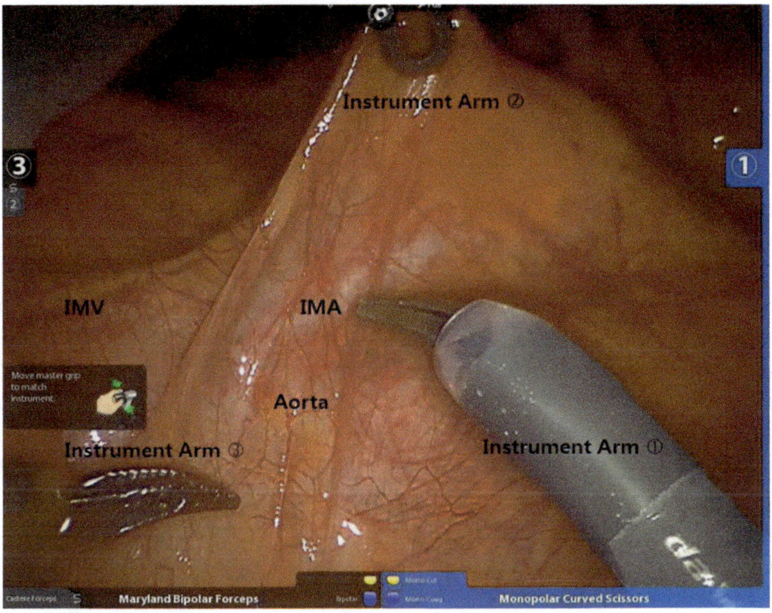

Fig. 18.5 Exposure of the IMA. The instrument arm ② retracts the sigmoid mesentery toward the anterior abdominal wall, leaving instrument arms ① and ③ for dissection

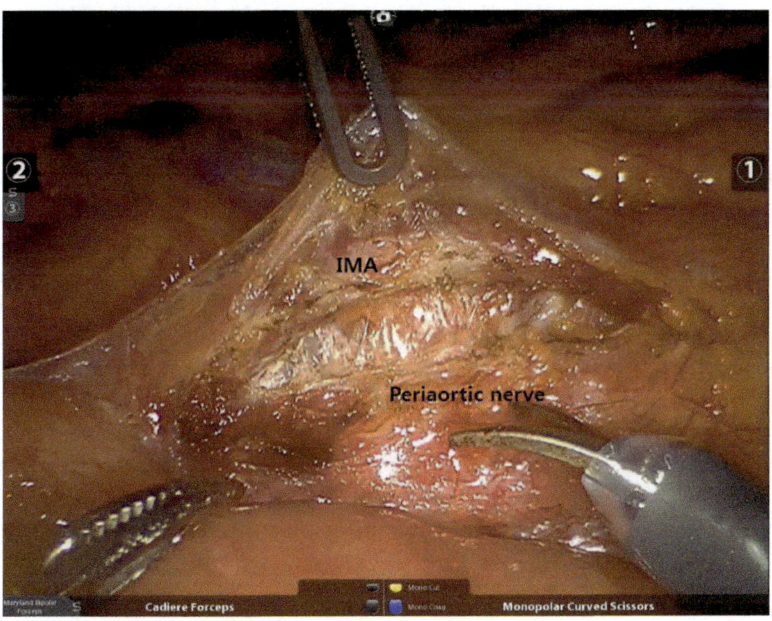

Fig. 18.6 The IMA is skeletonized and the periaortic sympathetic nerves are preserved

However, oncological resection is not compromised because the lymph nodes included are the same mesenteric tissue as the final specimen, as compared with high ligation. This should be done carefully when skeletonizing the IMA; dissecting mesenteric tissue from the IMA until the left colic artery is identified. Mesenteric tissue is dissected off the left colic pedicle to allow the IMA to be ligated above the left colic branch.

It is important to identify and to preserve nerves. The three-dimensional view is very helpful in identifying the nerves. The assistant may assist by retracting them with a grasper.

The IMA is then lifted toward the anterior abdominal wall, and the descending colon and sigmoid mesentery are dissected from the retroperitoneum. Sharp dissection technique is used. The plane between the mesentery and Gerota's fascia can be identified using both traction and countertraction with instrument arms ② and ③. Sometimes, the plane can be better identified by gentle pushing of the instrument arms. It is important to reposition instrument arm ② with retraction. Instrument arm ② should retract the mesentery up toward the anterior abdominal wall. This allows instrument arm ③ to be used for countertraction. Any bleeding can be controlled by bipolar of instrument arm ③ with Maryland bipolar forcep and instrument arm ① with monopolar curved scissor.

Dissection of the colonic mesentery of the retroperitoneum is continued proximally toward the splenic flexure. The IMV is identified on the lateral side of the duodenum and dissected. Before ligation of the IMV, the arc of Riolan (otherwise known as the meandering artery) needs to be identified. The arc of Riolan, when present, may be significant in affecting the blood supply provided by the marginal artery. If required, the IMV should be ligated to ensure that the arc of Riolan remains intact (Fig. 18.7a, b). Ligation of the IMV does not affect oncological outcome but provides colonic mobilization to reach the pelvis during anastomosis.

The boundaries of medial dissection are the inferior border of the pancreas proximally and the aorta medially. Laterally, dissection is carried out as far as possible until the psoas muscle can be visualized. The left ureter should be visualized crossing the left iliac vessels and preserved.

After the splenic flexure is mobilized, proximal dissection is extended above the pancreas and lesser sac, which is entered inferiorly during medial dissection. This is done by incision of the peritoneum overlying the transverse colon mesentery at the level of the pancreas. Mesenteric dissection of the superior aspect of the pancreas leads to the lesser sac. Once inside the lesser sac, the mesentery of the transverse colon can be dissected off its attachment to the anterior aspect of the pancreas (Fig. 18.8). The assistant places the grasper into the lesser sac and lifts the transverse colon mesentery upward. This dissection is carried laterally toward the splenic flexure. This is identified by the omentum that attaches to the tail of the pancreas.

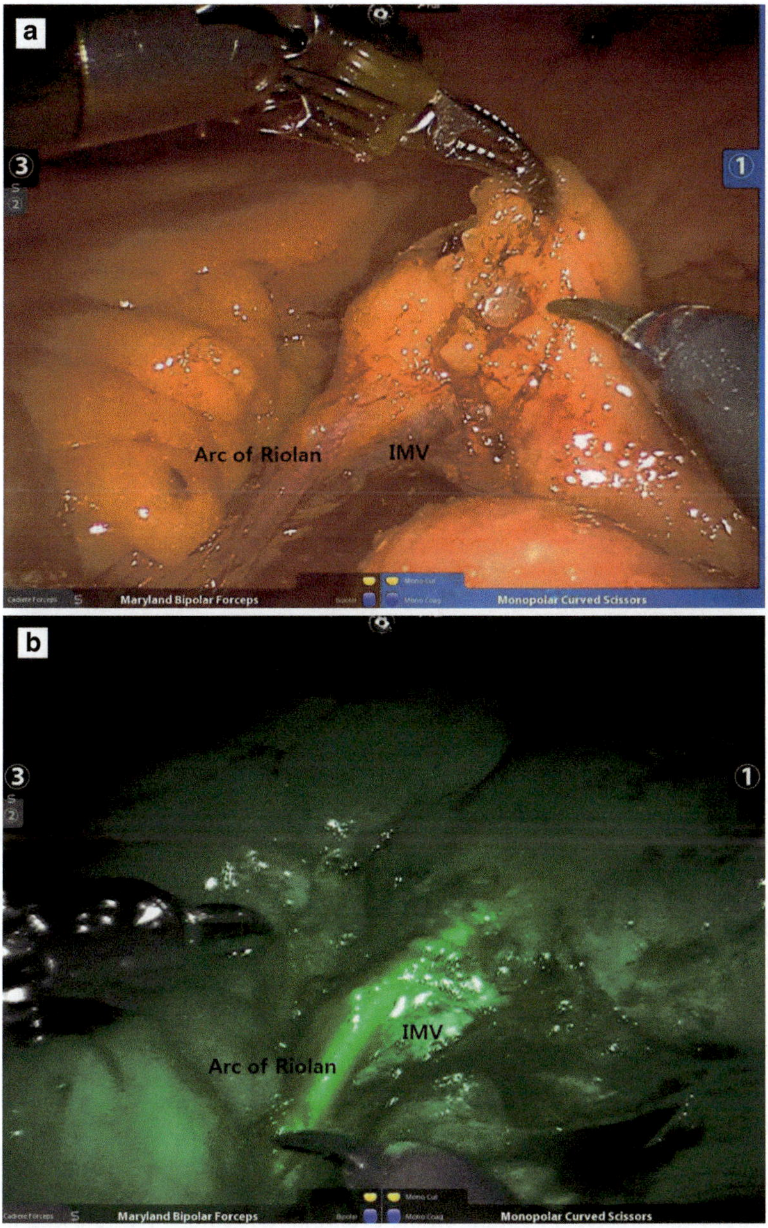

Fig. 18.7 (**a** and **b**) Preservation of the arc of Riolan

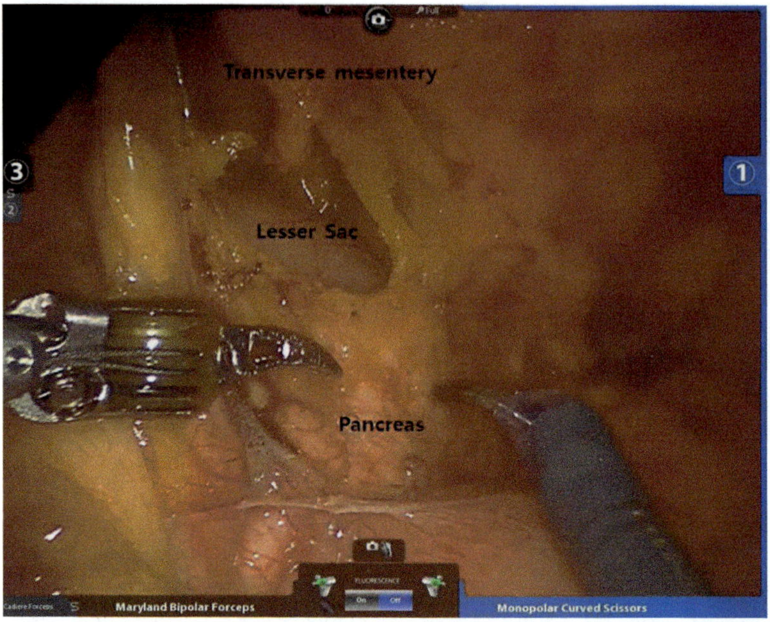

Fig. 18.8 Medial dissection above the pancreas to enter the lesser sac and dissection of the transverse colon mesentery off the pancreas. The black-colored instrument is the assistant's grasper

Once medial dissection is completed, lateral dissection should be performed. The sigmoid colon is separated from its peritoneal attachment commencing at the sigmoid notch by dissecting along the white line of Toldt. The colon is retracted medially and inferiorly (i.e., toward the RLQ) by the assistant, leaving the surgeon's left robotic arm to be used for countertraction (Fig. 18.9). If the medial dissection is adequate, lateral dissection will be joined with the medial portion that was done previously.

18.2.3 Splenic Flexure Mobilization

The splenic flexure is mobilized by lateral dissection of the left colon toward the spleen. It is important to reposition constantly, and the assistant should provide adequate traction on the left colon during dissection. One will then encounter the attachment of the greater omentum on the proximal left colon. While using instrument arm ② to lift the greater omentum toward the anterior abdominal wall, the greater omentum is dissected off the splenic flexure using instrument arms ② and ③. Once the omentum is dissected off the colon, the lateral attachments of the splenic flexure may be divided to fully mobilize the splenic flexure. The greater omentum is then further dissected off the transverse colon toward the midline. This is best performed by lifting the omentum using instrument arm ② and utilizing the countertraction provided by the assistant.

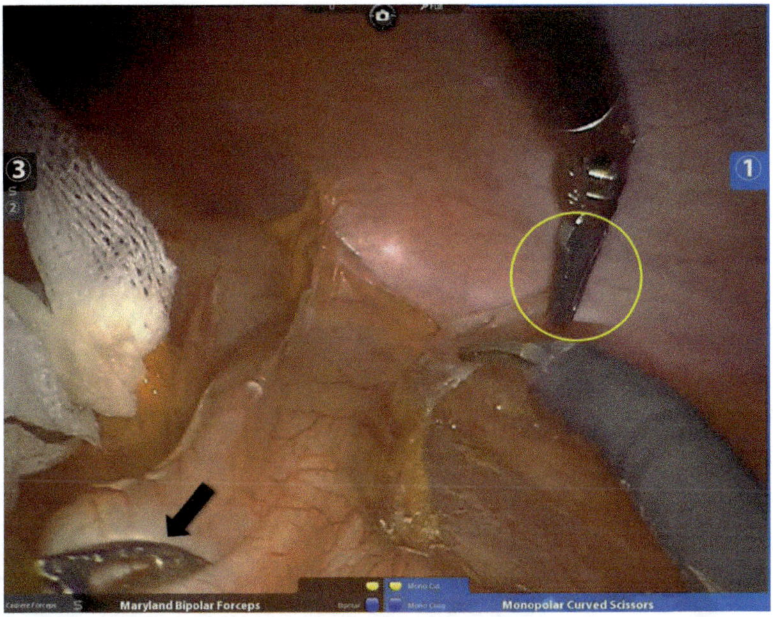

Fig. 18.9 The descending colon is retracted medially and inferiorly by the assistant (*arrow*), and the surgeon's left robotic arm is used for countertraction (*yellow ellipse*) during lateral dissection

Most of the dissection of the greater omentum off the transverse colon requires only instrument arms ① and ③. There may be excessive clashing, especially toward the middle of the transverse colon. If there is excessive clashing between instrument arms ② and ③, arm ② can be removed.

18.3 Pelvic Phase

18.3.1 Port Placement (Fig. 18.10)

- Instrument arm ① Monopolar curved scissors at the RLQ port.
- Instrument arm ② Maryland bipolar forceps at the LLQ port.
- Instrument arm ③ Cadiere forceps through at the LUQ port.
- Assistant uses two instruments: a non-toothed bowel grasper at the RUQ and a suction device at the right flank port

18.3.2 Total Mesorectal Excision (TME)

The instrument arms are swapped to their new positions by repositioning them without completely undocking the patient cart. The robotic instruments in the RUQ and LUQ ports are de-docked and re-docked to the LUQ and LLQ ports, respectively (Figs. 18.2 and 18.11).

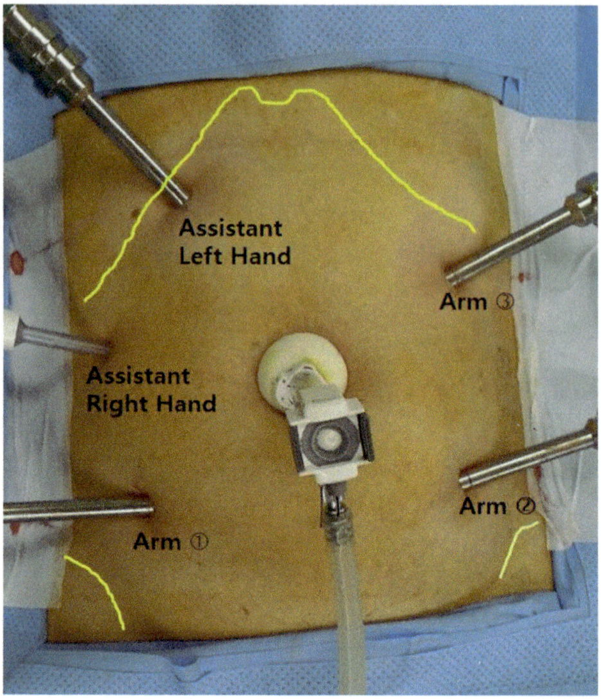

Fig. 18.10 Port placement, pelvic phase

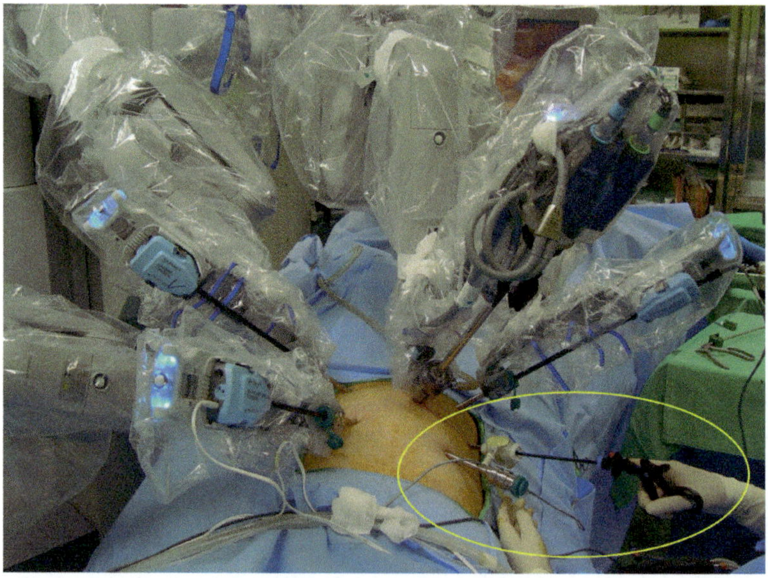

Fig. 18.11 An overview from the patient's head after repositioning the robotic arms for the pelvic dissection. Note the two trocars available for the assistant on the right side of the patient (*yellow ellipse*). Also note that the robotic arms are well fanned out to minimize external collision

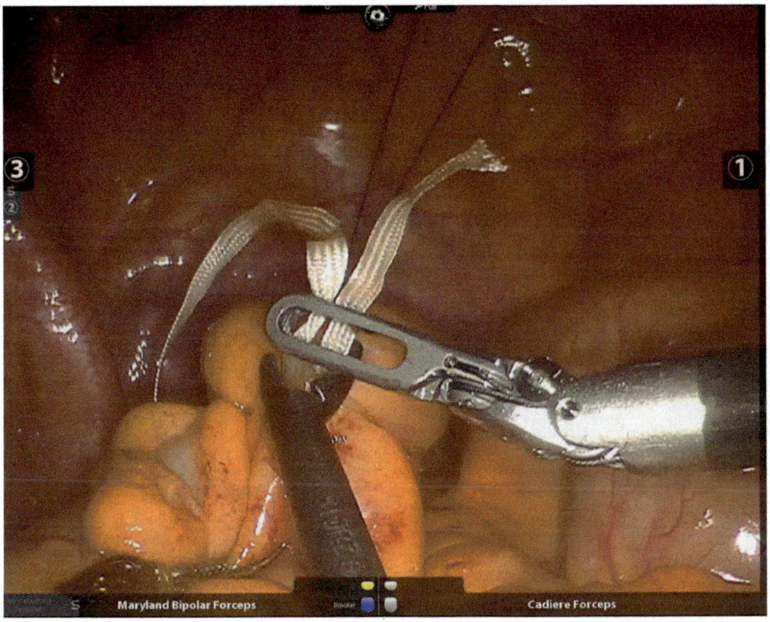

Fig. 18.12 A nylon tape around the rectosigmoid colon to assist with retraction of the rectum out of the pelvis using the RUQ port. Also note the stitch in the anterior peritoneal reflection to assist with exposure in the narrow male pelvis

The rectum is lifted out of the pelvis by upward retraction of the sigmoid colon by the assistant toward the spleen. This can be done with a grasper or by using nylon tape to wrap around the rectosigmoid junction (Fig. 18.12). This frees the surgeon to use instrument arms ② and ③ for retraction, with one arm retracting and the other providing countertraction (we call this the "two-hand free technique"). The assistant has access to two instrument ports to provide retraction of the colon and suction of any fluid or smoke from the diathermy. Usually, the assistant would have a grasper in the left hand and a suction device in the right hand.

When the total mesorectal excision (TME) plane is identified with adequate traction, there should be a relatively bloodless plane. Posterior dissection along the sacrum is followed by lateral dissection with division of the lateral peritoneal folds. Anterior dissection, which is usually considered the most difficult part, is performed last.

Instrument arm ② is used to retract the rectum upward toward the anterior abdominal wall. Instrument arm ③ may be used to provide further retraction or countertraction. Note that retraction can be done either by opening the instrument or using the wrist of the instrument to push the tissue away. A layer of alveolar tissue can demonstrate the avascular plane of TME when adequate retraction is achieved. It is important to keep the dissection close to the mesorectal fascia. The hypogastric nerves should be identified and preserved during posterior dissection. The key is adequate retraction and sticking close to the TME plane on the rectal side.

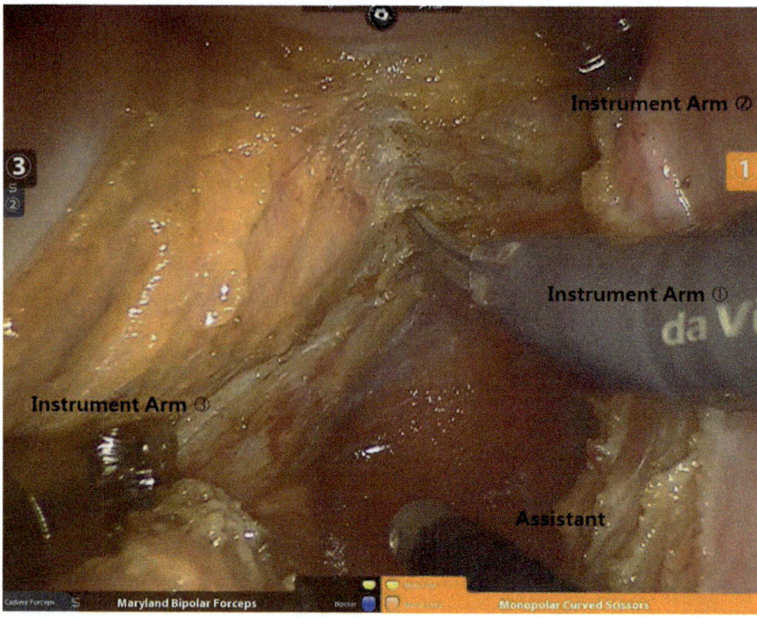

Fig. 18.13 Lateral pelvic dissection demonstrating positions of each instrument arm

During lateral dissection, instrument arm ② is usually used to provide lateral traction on the pelvic side wall, while the assistant uses the suction device to retract the rectum medially (Fig. 18.13). Adequate traction is vital to provide good exposure because this is the key to correct identification of the lateral TME plane.

When assisting in anterior exposure, the peritoneum overlying the bladder near the peritoneal reflection can be hitched up toward the anterior abdominal wall using a straight needle. This method also can be applied to postmenopausal women for suspension of the uterus from the abdominal wall.

Instrument arm ② can assist with further retraction of the peritoneum overlying the bladder, while instrument arm ③ pushes down on the rectum to provide countertraction. Seminal vesicles are identified, and dissection is continued along Denonvilliers' fascia. When the fascia cannot be resected en bloc for oncological reasons (i.e., anterior rectal cancer), the resection plane should be behind Denonvilliers' fascia to preserve the neurovascular bundle that lies immediately anterior to the fascia (Fig. 18.14). It is also important to note that there are usually vessels that cross the fascia anteriorly from the prostate toward the mesorectum. These can be a source of bleeding if not adequately controlled. When tumor involves the anterior rectum, the dissection plane should be anterior to Denonvilliers' fascia to achieve a negative circumferential margin (Fig. 18.14b).

Instruments in arms ② and ③ can be swapped at any time to provide better retraction. As the da Vinci® system eliminates any physiological tremor, dissection with the left hand can be utilized. Hot shear can be swapped to instrument arm ③ for dissection, especially on the left side.

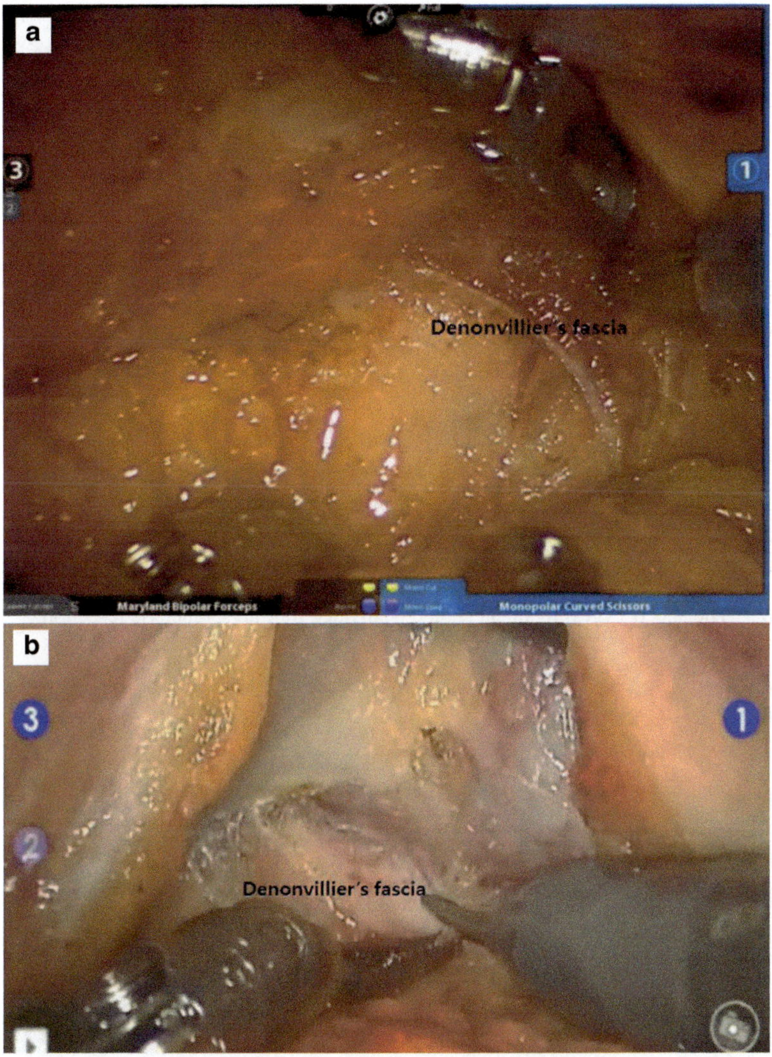

Fig. 18.14 (**a**) The dissection plane is behind the Denonvilliers' fascia to preserve the neurovascular bundle that lies immediately anterior to the fascia. (**b**) The dissection plane is anterior to the Denonvilliers' fascia to achieve a negative circumferential margin when the tumor involves the anterior rectum

Dissection is continued until identification of the pelvic floor. Laterally, the puborectalis muscle sling is noted, and posteriorly, the anococcygeal ligament should be found. These can be easily identified, as the muscle fibers of the pelvic floor will contract when touched with diathermy. The extent of the dissection can be confirmed by digital examination.

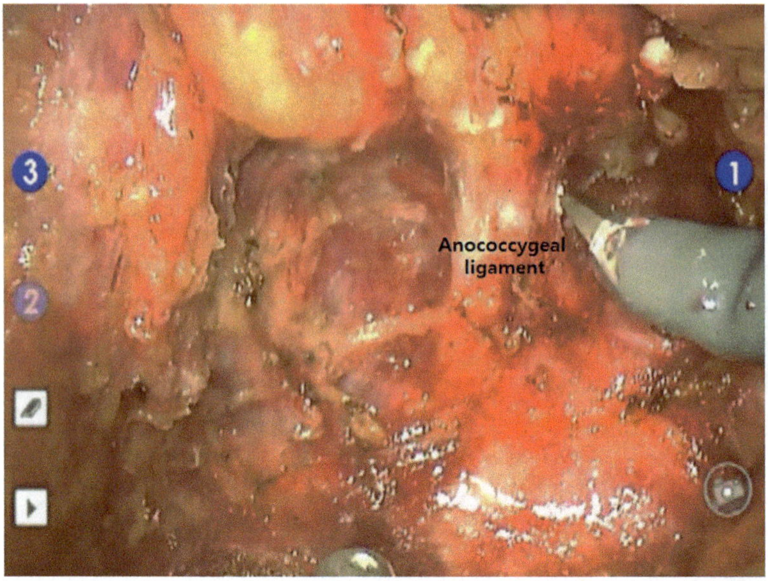

Fig. 18.15 The anococcygeal ligament should be divided for intersphincteric resection

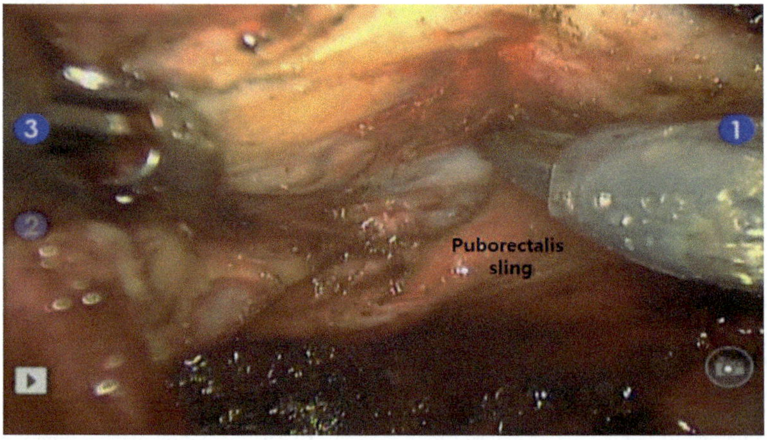

Fig. 18.16 The puborectalis sling is identified and dissected off

For intersphincteric dissection, the anococcygeal ligament (Fig. 18.15) posteriorly and the puborectalis slings bilaterally are identified (Fig. 18.16). The anococcygeal ligament has to be divided to enter the intersphincteric plane. Dissection is continued as low as possible and then completed from below.

During pelvic dissection, it can be easy to develop "tunnel vision" in the narrow pelvis. It is easy to become disoriented as the camera can rotate, especially early in the learning curve. It is advisable to frequently bring the camera back to gain an overview of the pelvis and reorientate. Another tip is to look at the camera icon in the surgeon's console, located in the middle of the top part of the screen. It shows the level and orientation of the camera.

18.4 Coloanal Anastomosis (CAA) Without Intersphincteric Resection (ISR)

18.4.1 Rectal Division

Once pelvic dissection is completed and rectum is mobilized to the pelvic floor, the distal rectum is divided within 1 cm from the dentate line, which is around 3–3.5 cm from the anal verge, with a double stapling technique. The da Vinci® system has recently added a stapling device to an instrument arm. We use this robotic stapling device on instrument arm ① after swapping to a 12 mm port at the RLQ (Fig. 18.17). If this robotic system is unavailable, the patient cart is undocked and moved away from the patient at this stage. The RLQ port is swapped to a 12 mm port, and a laparoscopic stapler is used for resection of the distal rectum. The rectum is resected in a conventional laparoscopic manner (Fig. 18.18). In patients with a narrow pelvis, the patient cart can be partially undocked. The camera is left in situ to provide stable view of the distal rectum. Instrument arm ② is also left in situ to provide anterior retraction of the pelvis. Instrument arms ① and ③ are undocked.

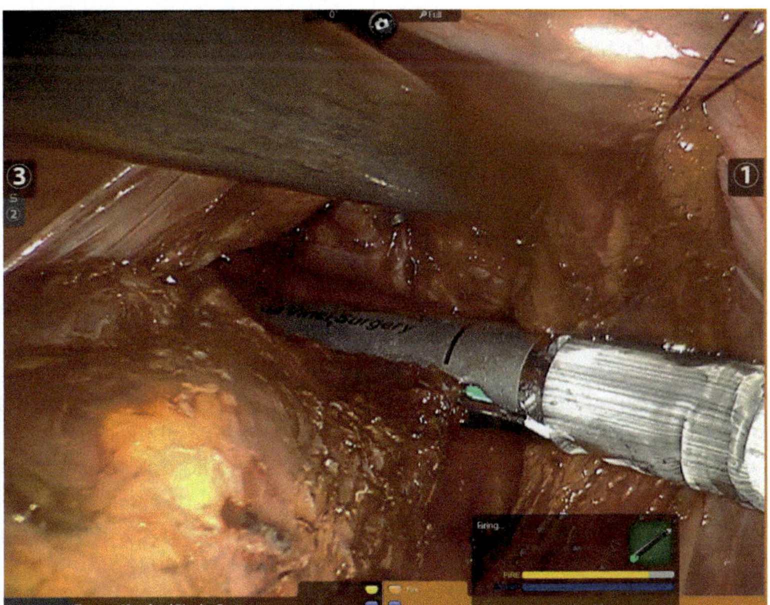

Fig. 18.17 Robotic stapling during the rectal transection

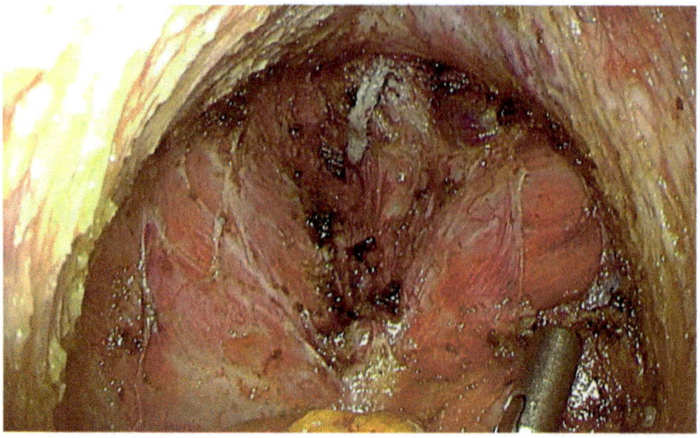

Fig. 18.18 Pelvic cavity after rectal division

18.4.2 Specimen Extraction

Wound extraction may be performed either through the left iliac fossa or the umbilical incision. Usually, the left lower quadrant port site is preferred due to the lower rate of incisional hernia in the published literature. A wound protector (Endo Keeper, NELIS, Bucheon-si, Gyeonggi-do, Korea) is used and the specimen is externalized. This protector is used for a working or a camera port using its cover. The surgeon makes a decision regarding the length of resection. This is usually determined by the location of the IMA, as the resection is usually performed in line with the IMA. The mesenteric vessels are ligated. The marginal artery is identified and cut to check for adequate blood flow before ligation. Proximal colonic resection is then performed using a hard bowel clamp and a knife in the usual fashion.

18.4.3 Anastomosis

A standard double stapling technique is used. A purse string is placed using nonabsorbable sutures in the proximal colon. The anvil of the circular stapling device is placed in the proximal colon and secured with the purse string. The colon is placed back into the peritoneal cavity, and pneumoperitoneum is reestablished. This can be done by placing a cover over the wound protector.

Bowel is retracted from the pelvis to obtain a good view of the staple line. We often consider using a 25 mm circular stapler instead of the 29 mm stapler because of the short and shallow rectal stump. A stapler is introduced into the rectum via the anus by the assistant under direct vision and direction of the surgeon. Once the stapler is properly positioned, it is opened to enable the spike of the stapler to come through the rectal stump. The anvil is placed over the spike, and a click should be audible. One should also feel the anvil click into place. The spike is then retracted into the stapler, which is closed until the green zone is reached on the indicator. Before firing, it is important to check the orientation of the colon and to ensure that the mesentery is not twisted. This is done easily by making sure the tinea of the colon is facing up and not rotated. It is our practice to hold that position for at least 15 s before the safety is removed and the stapler fired. The stapler is then opened slightly before being removed from the patient. Often, the stapler needs to be rotated slightly clockwise and anticlockwise to disengage the bowel before withdrawal. The donuts are then checked for completeness and a leak test is performed. This is done by filling the pelvis with saline and compressing the proximal colon with a grasper, while the assistant blows air into the rectum with an empty syringe. Leakage of air detected by bubbles would be an indicative of a positive test and suggests some compromise of the anastomosis.

When performing a coloanal approach, the distal rectum is transected around the dentate line. Then, we use a "pulled through" approach for specimen extraction and a hand-sewn anastomosis. In this method, resection of the colon or rectum is not performed during robotic dissection, but the left colic artery should be divided robotically to reach the specimen out through the anus. A direct coloanal side-to-end anastomosis, colonic J-pouch, or transverse coloplasty pouch can be performed according to the surgeons' preference. After the specimen is extracted through the anus, the anastomosis will be performed less than 1 cm from the dentate line.

18.5 Coloanal Anastomosis (CAA) with Intersphincteric Resection (ISR)

In a high lithotomy position, the anus is exposed with interrupted everting sutures (Fig. 18.19). Epinephrine solution (1:200,000) is administered into the intersphincteric space. Dissection of anal canal starts at the level of the intersphincteric groove. Once dissection from the perineal side is completed, the distal end is closed with sutures. Then, the rectum and proximal colon are delivered through the anus.

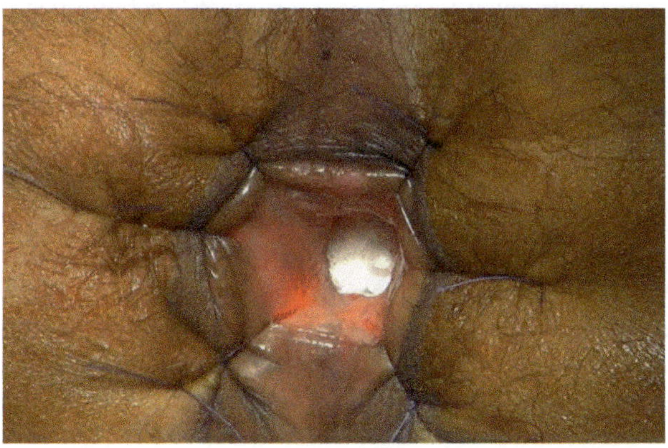

Fig. 18.19 Preparation of the anus with interrupted sutures for a perineal approach

Proximal resection of the colon is then performed after ligation of the mesenteric vessels. This is done with a linear stapling device. A side-to-end anastomosis is preferable for securing the staple line with interrupted absorbable sutures. An enterotomy is made on the anti-mesenteric border of the colon 3 cm away from the distal end, and the full thickness of the colon is anastomosed to the sphincter muscles and anal mucosa using 3-0 absorbable sutures.

18.6 Other Techniques

18.6.1 Covering Ileostomy

Covering ileostomy is not routinely used in anterior resection at our institution.

Indications for covering ileostomy include neoadjuvant radiotherapy, intersphincteric resection and hand-sewn coloanal anastomosis, an ultralow anterior resection (double-stapled anastomosis within 1 cm from the dentate line), or technical difficulty during the case, including incomplete doughnuts or a positive air leak test.

If required, the right lower quadrant port site is used for ileostomy. An incision is made with a trephine over the port site and dissected down to the fascia, which is then incised vertically, while the muscle is retracted and split transversely. The peritoneum is then incised, and a loop of terminal ileum is brought out through the trephine. Orientation of the terminal ileum is confirmed on laparoscopy. Loop ileostomy is matured after the closure of all abdominal wounds, and a dressing is applied.

18.6.2 "Hand-on-Hand" Technique

During instrument repositioning, communication between the surgeon and assistant is important. We called this a "hand-on-hand" technique. The surgeon retracts the colon or mesentery into the desired position, and then the assistant comes in with his or her instrument to replace the surgeon's robotic instrument arms. It is important that only one person moves at a time to avoid losing the established retraction, i.e., the surgeon moves, and then the assistant moves. This also reduces unnecessary movement and the risk of inadvertent injury.

18.6.3 Interference Among Robotic Arms

When a robotic operation is in progress, there may be a collision among the robotic arms. Especially, instruments arm ② and ③ tend to collide to be stuck on their position. It is helpful to shift the location of the arms after pulling the arms out of the operative field (Fig. 18.20).

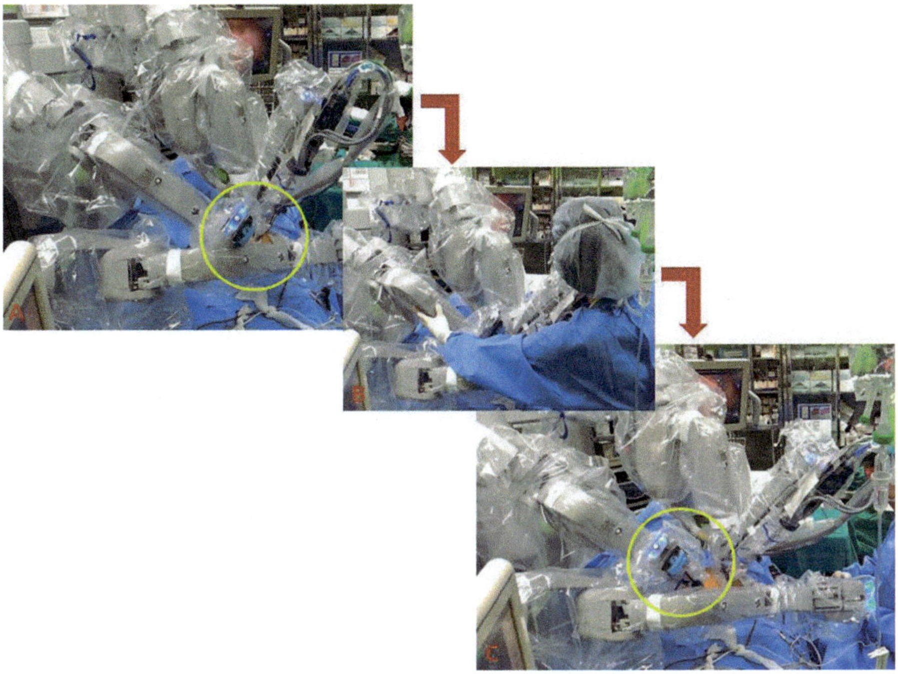

Fig. 18.20 Adjusting the location of robotic arms when colliding

18.6.4 Wound Closure

The wound is closed in the usual manner. For the specimen extraction site, we prefer a layered closure using interrupted absorbable sutures. The fascia is closed over the 12 mm trocar site.

References

1. Heald RJ, Husband EM, Ryall RD. The mesorectum in rectal cancer surgery--the clue to pelvic recurrence? Br J Surg. 1982;69(10):613–6.
2. Parks AG, Percy JP. Resection and sutured colo-anal anastomosis for rectal carcinoma. Br J Surg. 1982;69(6):301–4.
3. Schiessel R, Karner-Hanusch J, Herbst F, Teleky B, Wunderlich M. Intersphincteric resection for low rectal tumours. Br J Surg. 1994;81(9):1376–8.
4. Rullier E, Goffre B, Bonnel C, Zerbib F, Caudry M, Saric J. Preoperative radiochemotherapy and sphincter-saving resection for T3 carcinomas of the lower third of the rectum. Ann Surg. 2001;234(5):633.
5. Leong QM, Son DN, Cho JS, Baek SJ, Kwak JM, Amar AH, et al. Robot-assisted intersphincteric resection for low rectal cancer: technique and short-term outcome for 29 consecutive patients. Surg Endosc. 2011;25(9):2987–92.

6. Park SY, Choi GS, Park JS, Kim HJ, Ryuk JP. Short-term clinical outcome of robot-assisted intersphincteric resection for low rectal cancer: a retrospective comparison with conventional laparoscopy. Surg Endosc. 2013;27(1):48–55.
7. Kuo LJ, Lin YK, Chang CC, Tai CJ, Chiou JF, Chang YJ. Clinical outcomes of robot-assisted intersphincteric resection for low rectal cancer: comparison with conventional laparoscopy and multifactorial analysis of the learning curve for robotic surgery. Int J Colorectal Dis. 2014;29(5):555–62.
8. Yoo B-E, Cho J-S, Shin J-W, Lee D-W, Kwak J-M, Kim J, et al. Robotic versus laparoscopic intersphincteric resection for low rectal cancer: comparison of the operative, oncological, and functional outcomes. Ann Surg Oncol. 2015;22(4):1219–25.
9. Baek SJ, Sami A-A, Jeong DH, Hur H, Min BS, Baik SH, et al. Robotic versus laparoscopic coloanal anastomosis with or without intersphincteric resection for rectal cancer. Surg Endosc. 2013;27(11):4157–63.

Multiport Laparoscopic Abdominoperineal Resection

19

W. Conan Mustain and Conor P. Delaney

Abstract

Despite advances in surgical techniques allowing for the preservation of the sphincter complex in the majority of patients with rectal cancer, en bloc resection of the rectum and anus using a combined abdominal and perineal approach is still required in some circumstances. Abdominoperineal resection (APR) can be performed through an open or laparoscopic approach, though the laparoscopic approach is associated with less blood loss, decreased postoperative pain and narcotic use, and shorter hospital stay. Multiport laparoscopic APR is performed in much the same manner as laparoscopic lower anterior resection for rectal cancer, adhering to the oncologic principles of high ligation on the inferior mesenteric artery and total mesorectal excision (TME). Key differences include the omission of splenic flexure mobilization and the conscious avoidance of distal mesorectal dissection off of the levator ani muscles to preserve the cylindrical nature of the specimen and avoid "wasting" at the proximal anal canal. Performance of the perineal dissection in lithotomy allows for excellent visualization in most circumstances, without the need for prone positioning. Postoperative recovery is managed according to established enhanced recovery pathways.

Keywords

Abdominoperineal resection • Laparoscopic • Rectal cancer • Enhanced recovery

W. Conan Mustain, M.D.
Division of Colon and Rectal Surgery, University of Arkansas for Medical Sciences, Little Rock, AR, USA

C.P. Delaney, M.D., Ph.D. (✉)
Digestive Disease and Surgery Institute, Cleveland Clinic, 9500 Euclid Avenue, Cleveland, OH 44195, USA
e-mail: delanec@ccf.org

G. Dapri, J.H. Marks (eds.), *Surgical Techniques in Rectal Cancer*,
https://doi.org/10.1007/978-4-431-55579-7_19

19.1 Introduction

In his landmark 1908 publication in *The Lancet*, William Ernest Miles introduced the concept of a combined abdominal and perineal approach for the removal of the rectum [1]. Having appreciated a high rate of mesorectal and pelvic nodal recurrences in the postmortem examination of over 50 patients treated by perineal resection alone, Miles recognized the importance of en bloc removal of the rectum and its associated lymphatics [2]. With the demonstrated success of sphincter-sparing anterior resection by Claude Dixon and others in the 1940s, the use of Miles' abdominoperineal resection (APR) became reserved primarily for cancers in the distal third of the rectum in which a 5 cm distal margin could not be obtained. As our understanding of the pathophysiology and mechanisms of lymphatic spread has increased and the concept of total mesorectal excision (TME) has clarified the importance of circumferential rather than distal margins, the use of APR for rectal cancer has been further restricted to only the most distal tumors, often those with direct sphincter involvement, or to patients with impaired preoperative continence [3]. Malignancies of the anal canal and perianal skin, specifically squamous cell carcinoma refractory to chemoradiation and anal melanoma, are still treated by APR. Rarely, cases of inflammatory bowel disease (IBD) and severe perianal disease require APR.

Laparoscopic APR was first described in the early 1990s [4, 5] though its applicability to rectal cancer remained unclear. Early randomized clinical trials to assess the oncologic equivalency of laparoscopy to open surgery for colon cancer specifically excluded rectal cancer and APR [6, 7]. Since then, multiple randomized clinical trials have demonstrated the benefits of decreased blood loss and faster recovery with laparoscopic surgery for rectal cancer, with equivalent oncologic outcomes to open surgery [8–10]. While these studies included both anterior resection and APR, it is understood that APR carries different risks related to the perineal wound that may influence the potential benefit of laparoscopy on short-term outcomes. However, a recent analysis of data from the Nationwide Inpatient Sample (NIS) found that patients undergoing laparoscopic APR experienced decreased postoperative complications and shorter length of stay and were less likely to require post-hospitalization care compared to open APR [11].

19.2 Anatomical Considerations for APR

The goal of APR for rectal cancer is to remove the entire rectum and anus along with its associated lymphatic drainage, consisting of the mesorectum and the mesentery of the sigmoid colon, while obtaining negative oncologic margins and avoiding injury to adjacent structures. A permanent colostomy is created, and the perineum is closed primarily unless extenuating circumstances require autologous tissue transfer. With these goals in mind, some important anatomical considerations merit review, especially insofar as the approach differs from that of anterior resection with anastomosis.

High ligation of the inferior mesenteric artery (IMA) is desired for purposes of adequate lymph node staging. However, because a permanent colostomy rather than a coloanal anastomosis is being created, high ligation of the inferior mesenteric vein (IMV) near the pancreas and mobilization of the splenic flexure are unnecessary and may predispose to the development of parastomal hernia. The lateral attachments of the descending colon are divided only as far as is necessary for the colostomy to reach the skin. After division of the IMA at its origin, the left colic artery and IMV are divided just cephalad to the bifurcation with the superior rectal artery, thus preserving all branches of the arcade arising from the left colic artery. The mesentery is then transected perpendicularly to the level of the marginal artery just proximal to the first sigmoid branch. The sigmoid mesentery is mobilized in the proper plane to preserve Toldt's fascia, thereby ensuring that retroperitoneal structures such as the left ureter, left gonadal vessels, and the para-aortic autonomic nerves are protected. Complete TME is performed with attention paid to the preservation of the presacral autonomic nerves which affect ejaculation and anterolateral cavernous nerves which control tumescence.

The mesorectum ends at the levator ani and naturally tapers toward the anorectal ring where only the narrow muscular tube of the rectum enters the anal canal. Unlike in ultralow resections in which coloanal anastomosis is planned, surgeons performing APR must consciously avoid continuing the dissection toward the anal canal once the levator ani muscles are reached. The potential consequence is a specimen with a narrow "waist" of tissue at the anorectal ring and the risk of a positive circumferential resection margin at the level of the tumor. A so-called "cylindrical" APR specimen is associated with a lower risk of specimen perforation and margin positivity and is achieved by limiting the extent of abdominal dissection once the levators are reached [12, 13].

19.3 Preoperative Evaluation

Patients should be evaluated with a complete history and physical exam. Digital rectal exam and proctoscopy are performed to assess the size, extent, and location of the tumor as well as baseline sphincter function. In female patients, digital vaginal exam and vaginoscopy to assess for tumor invasion should be performed. The depth of tumor invasion and the status of mesorectal lymph nodes are assessed by endorectal ultrasound or pelvic MRI. MRI carries the additional advantage of defining relationships to other potentially involved organs including the cervix, vagina, bladder, prostate, or seminal vesicles. A complete colonoscopy is required to screen the remaining colon. Staging CT scans of the chest, abdomen, and pelvis are performed to assess for metastatic disease. Patients with stage II and stage III disease are typically referred for neoadjuvant chemoradiation, to decrease the risk of local recurrence and potentially improve the chance for sphincter preservation in patients with distal tumors. The exception to this may be in elderly patients with small T3 tumors who are not candidates for sphincter preservation based on poor continence or functional impairment, in whom chemoradiation may be poorly tolerated and the risk of a positive circumferential margin is deemed low in the setting of an APR. In patients with T4 tumors in whom en bloc resection of the posterior vagina, prostate, or bladder may be required, preoperative consultation with gynecology and/or urology may be necessary. Likewise, patients in whom primary closure of the perineal wound may be difficult due to extensive radiation, poor nutrition, or the need for wide resection of a bulky tumor are referred to a plastic surgeon to discuss myocutaneous flap reconstruction of the perineum.

Baseline carcinoembryonic antigen (CEA) level should be checked for surveillance purposes. Routine labs, including complete blood count (CBC), metabolic and coagulation panels, blood type and screen, and an assessment of nutritional status with albumin or prealbumin, should be performed. Patients with significant medical comorbidities should be referred for preoperative medical and/or cardiology clearance and preanesthesia testing.

Standardized preoperative measures are implemented according to established enhanced recovery pathways [14, 15]. Time is spent in the office preparing the patient for what to expect on the day of surgery and during the postoperative period. Patients meet with a trained enterostomal therapy nurse to discuss stoma care and select a site for a permanent left-sided colostomy. In patients who are not obstructed, we routinely order mechanical bowel prep and preoperative oral antibiotics prior to laparoscopic APR to facilitate manipulation of the colon and rectum laparoscopically, although some prefer an enema alone. In the preoperative holding area, patients receive 5000 units of unfractionated heparin subcutaneously and 12 mg alvimopan by the mouth when the surgery is being performed open. Intravenous antibiotics are given at induction according to hospital protocol.

19.4 Operative Technique

19.4.1 Positioning and Trocar Placement

The room is configured with the bed in the center of the room and the laparoscopic tower at the patient's right. A second monitor is positioned on the patient's left side just inferior to the left hip (Fig. 19.1). During the operation, the primary operator will be on the patient's right with the assistant/camera operator standing to his left. It is important to ensure that the anesthesia machine and ether curtain are positioned to leave enough space for both parties to stand on the right side. The patient is placed on the bed in the supine position with the arms tucked and a beanbag or gel pad to prevent slipping during periods of steep Trendelenburg. The legs are placed in Allen stirrups, and the foot of the bed is removed (Fig. 19.2). The edge of the bed should rest between the top of the gluteal cleft and the anus so that the perineum can be prepped posterior to the tip of the coccyx. A digital rectal exam is performed, and the rectum is irrigated with a dilute betadine solution. The anus is then sutured closed with a purse string of 2-0 polypropylene to minimize contamination. The

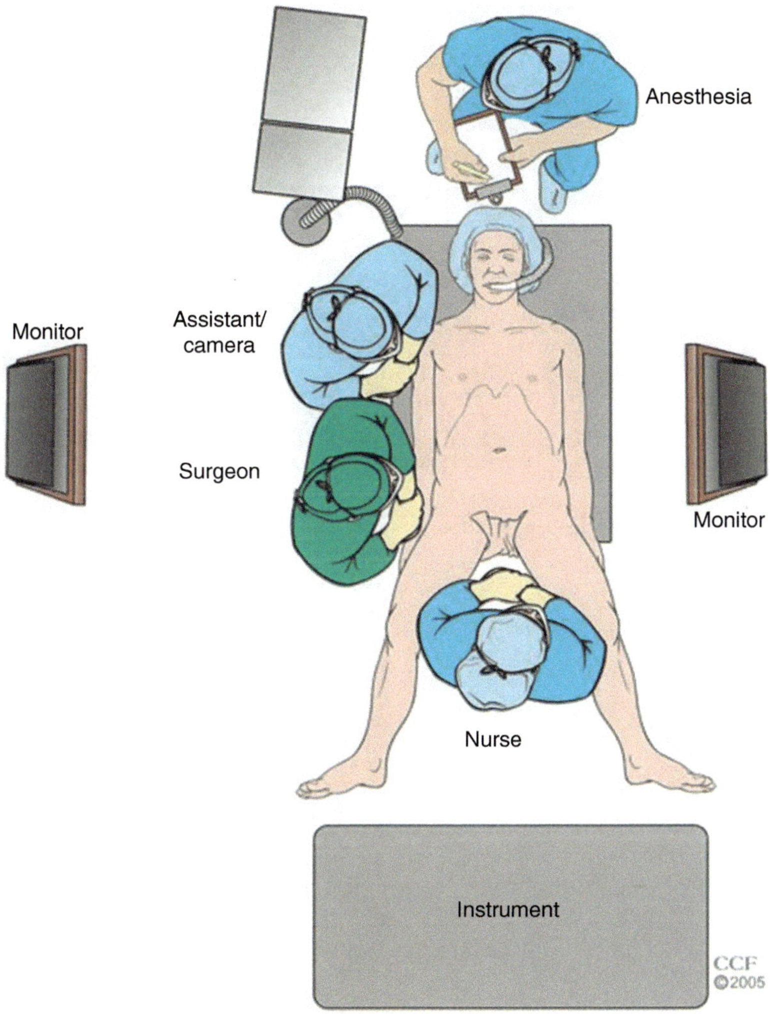

Fig. 19.1 Equipment positioning in operating room

perineum is prepped and draped, and a sterile Foley catheter is placed prior to prepping the abdomen.

The abdominal portion of a laparoscopic APR can be performed through a variety of configurations. The authors' preference is to enter the abdomen under direct visualization through an infraumbilical cutdown followed by placement of a U-stitch of O-polyglactin suture and a 10 mm trocar. After the establishment of pneumoperitoneum, two right-sided trocars are placed; the first is placed approximately three fingerbreadths medial and three fingerbreadths cephalad to the anterior superior iliac spine and a 5 mm trocar one handbreadth cephalad and parallel to the first. A 12 mm trocar is placed on the left side through the planned colostomy site (Fig. 19.3).

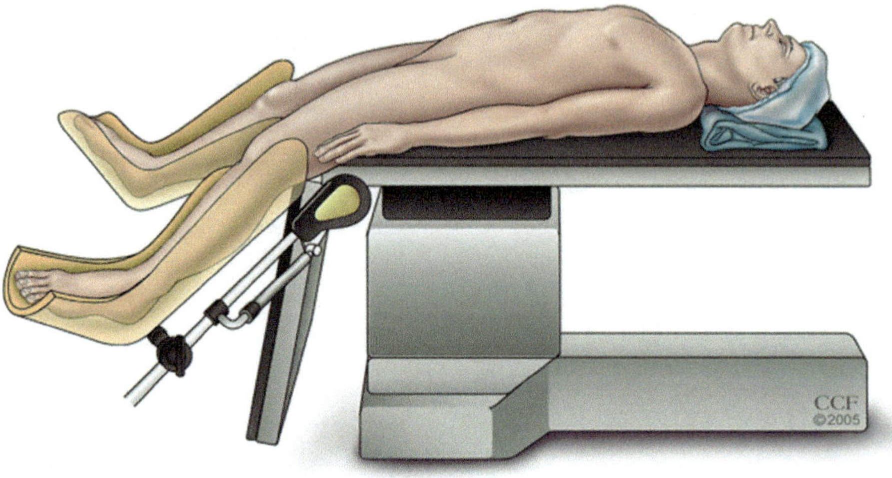

Fig. 19.2 Patient in Trendelenberg position

Fig. 19.3 Port positions

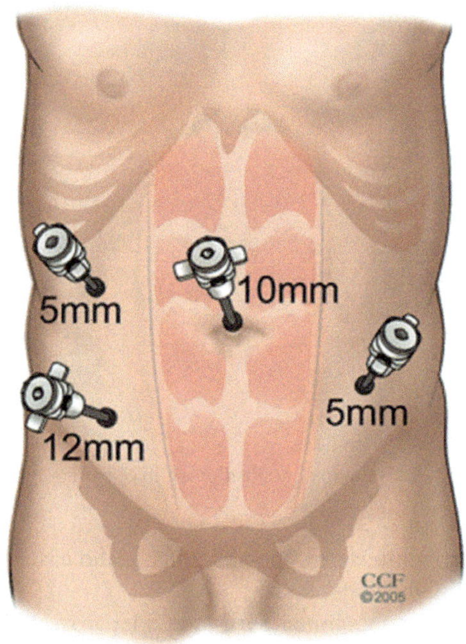

19.4.2 Initial Survey and Restoring Normal Anatomy

After the necessary trocars are in place, a survey of the abdomen and pelvis, including the peritoneal surfaces and especially the liver, is performed to rule out undetected metastatic disease. In patients with prior surgery or pelvic radiation, there may be significant adhesions involving the omentum, small bowel, and sigmoid colon. These should be addressed sequentially to restore normal anatomy and provide adequate working space. The omentum is retracted out of the pelvis and positioned above the transverse colon, creating the necessary space to reposition the small bowel. The patient is positioned in Trendelenberg with the right side down. The small bowel is swept out of the pelvis, exposing the sacral promontory and the medial aspect of the sigmoid mesentery. Frequently in patients with prior radiation, the terminal ileum may be adherent to pelvic structures requiring partial mobilization of the root of the small-bowel mesentery and cecum. Lateral adhesions to the mid- or distal sigmoid colon may be beneficial if they help to hold the colon in place during dissection of the IMA. Adhesions that tether a redundant sigmoid in the pelvis, however, will narrow the angle of the IMA off the aorta and should be divided early to allow the sigmoid to be retracted out of the pelvis. The medial aspect of the rectosigmoid mesentery is grasped by the assistant through the left-sided trocar and retracted anteriorly and laterally.

19.4.3 Identification of the IMA and Left Ureter

The medial aspect of the sigmoid mesentery is incised with cautery over the sacral promontory and extending cephalad to allow air to enter the retromesenteric plane. The proper location for this incision can be identified by lifting the sigmoid several times to visualize the mesorectum sliding beneath the peritoneum adjacent to the fixed retroperitoneum. The line of peritoneal transection is extended cephalad along the medial side of the mesentery adjacent to the aorta. Once cephalad to the origin of the IMA, the line is extended laterally to score the peritoneum overlying the vessel. Returning to the rectosigmoid junction, the posterior surface of the IMA and adjacent mesocolon is carefully dissected free from the retroperitoneum, taking care to preserve Toldt's fascia and keeping the para-aortic autonomic nerve fibers posterior and away from harm. A bowel grasper in the left hand is positioned beneath the IMA, and the mesocolon is retracted first anteriorly and then cephalad. The left ureter is identified by vermiculation along the left pelvic sidewall lateral to the vessel.

19.4.4 High Ligation of the IMA

With the left ureter in view, a window is created behind the origin of the IMA through the previously scored area on the anterior surface of the mesentery. The IMA is then ligated about its origin using a 5 mm laparoscopic vessel-sealing device through the right lower quadrant port. The left colic artery is identified running cephalad with the IMV. An avascular window lateral to the IMV is identified and scored with electrocautery. Both the left colic artery and IMV are divided with the vessel-sealing device near the bifurcation with the superior rectal artery. In elderly patients, the inferior mesenteric artery may be taken distal to the left colic artery to maximize perfusion of the descending colon.

19.4.5 Left Colon Mobilization and Transection

Because a permanent colostomy rather than a coloanal anastomosis is to be created, complete mobilization of the left colon and splenic flexure is unnecessary. However, in order for the colostomy to reach the anterior abdominal wall, some degree of mobilization of the descending colon mesentery and its lateral attachments is required. Working from medial to lateral, the left mesocolon is dissected free from the retroperitoneum as far as the lateral abdominal wall. With the colon then reflected medially, the dissection plane can be visualized as ecchymosis behind the white line of Toldt's fascia. These lateral attachments are then divided with electrocautery through the left lower quadrant port. Mobilization is continued cephalad as far as necessary for the colostomy to reach skin level. The mesentery of the sigmoid colon is then divided perpendicularly, beginning at the site of IMV transection and proceeding laterally toward the marginal vessels. With careful blunt dissection on the posterior wall of the colon, a clear window is created between the marginal vessels and the bowel wall. This allows for safe ligation of the vessels with the vessel-sealing device without injuring the colon. The colon is then divided with a single 60 mm fire of a 3.5 mm staple height endoscopic stapler passed through the 12 mm colostomy site port. Confirmation is made that the proximal segment will reach the anterior abdominal wall, with additional mobilization performed if necessary.

19.4.6 Total Mesorectal Excision

Attention is then turned to the pelvis and performance of formal TME (Fig. 19.4). If the uterus is present and obscuring the visualization of the anterior cul-de-sac, a 2-0 polypropylene suture on a Keith needle can be inserted through the abdominal wall at the level of the pubic symphysis, passed through the uterus, and back out through the abdominal wall where it is tightened and clamped to the drapes. The assistant grasps the rectosigmoid junction through the left-sided trocar and retracts it anteriorly and cephalad. The surgeon pushes the rectum anteriorly with an open bowel grasper, much like the way one would retract with a St. Mark's deep pelvic retractor. The complete mesorectum is then mobilized with electrocautery working in the avascular loose areolar plane first posteriorly, then laterally, and then anteriorly. The posterior mobilization is extended as low as Waldeyer's fascia, curving up slightly at the edges in a crescent shape conforming to the round, smooth (albeit bilobed) posterior surface of the mesorectum. Laterally the peritoneum is incised on each side, extending across the midline at the cul-de-sac, several millimeters anterior to the fold at the peritoneal reflection. The rectum is pushed medially and anteriorly by the surgeon's left-hand instrument to demonstrate the avascular plane at the lateral aspect of the mesorectum. Care is taken distally to protect the paired sacral autonomic nerves ("nervi erigentes"), which arise from S2–S4 and contribute fibers to the inferior hypogastric plexus on either side of the rectum before innervating the bladder, prostate, and genitals. Finally the anterior dissection is performed posterior to Denonvilliers' fascia in males, avoiding the prostate and seminal

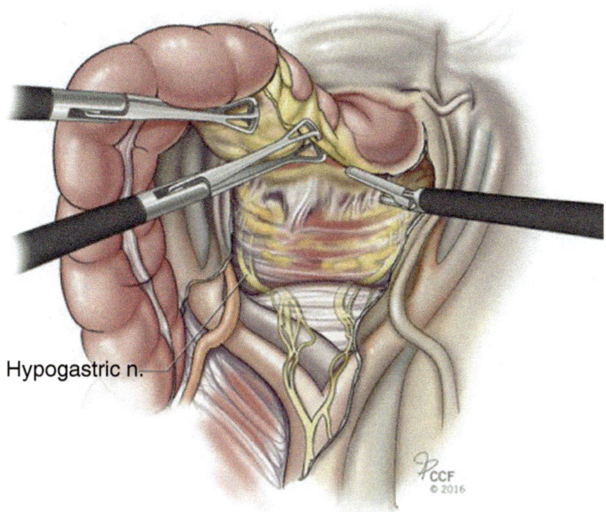

Fig. 19.4 Total mesorectal excision is completed using standard laparoscopic techniques

vesicles, or in the rectovaginal septum in females, and protecting the cavernous nerves which lie anterolaterally just beyond Denonvilliers' fascia. Again it is emphasized that when reaching the levator ani muscles at the distal extent of the dissection, further dissection toward the anorectal ring is avoided in order to preserve the cylindrical nature of the specimen and avoid "waisting" at the sphincters.

19.4.7 Perineal Dissection

Once the abdominal and pelvic portions of the operation are completed, it is the authors' preference to maintain insufflation, keep the trocars in place, and defer colostomy creation until after the perineal portion of the procedure has been completed and the perineal wound closed. For this reason, we do not employ prone positioning for the perineal dissection, unless the tumor extends posteriorly such that the coccygeal area cannot be reached in lithotomy. In these rare cases, the patient is turned prone. Normally, by desufflating the abdomen and placing the legs in a high lithotomy position (Fig. 19.5), an excellent view of the perineum can be obtained [16]. The area is normally re-prepped with betadine and re-draped. Liberal use of additional prep solution is applied as needed. Separate suction tubing and electrocautery are passed off for use on the perineum. An elliptical incision is marked on the perineum extending from the base of the transverse perineal body to the tip of the coccyx, extending just inside the ischial tuberosities bilaterally. We use six tethering O-polyglactin sutures in the form of a Lone Star retractor to maintain adequate exposure of the perineum. Sutures are placed through the skin and subcutaneous tissue just lateral to the planned incision and then through a second bite 8 or 10 cm radial to the first before being tied down to evert the anal margin. The perineal incision is made with electrocautery, and dissection is carried out through the

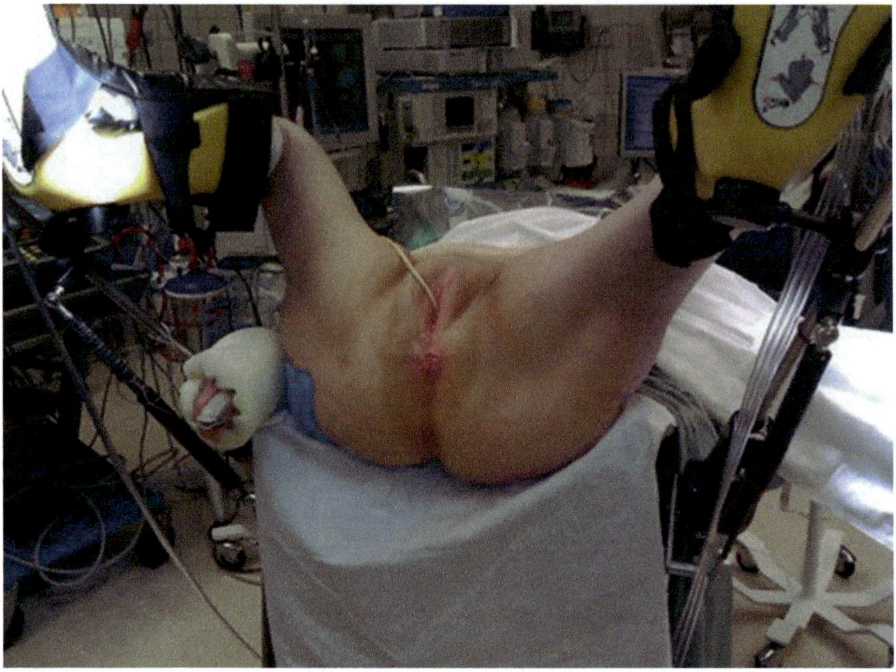

Fig. 19.5 Patient placed in high Trendelenberg position for perineal dissection

subcutaneous fat of the ischiorectal space, taking care to stay lateral to all fibers of the external sphincter. Once the skin has been incised circumferentially, two Allis clamps are placed on the anus for retraction. The specimen is retracted anteriorly, while dissection is directed toward the anterior surface of the tip of the coccyx. The pelvic floor may be seen bulging into the field from the abdominal insufflation at this location. The anococcygeal ligament is then divided, allowing entry to the pelvis as confirmed by a rush of air. The insufflation is then stopped until after the perineal wound has been closed. We do not remove the coccyx unless there is suspicion for a close margin (Fig. 19.6).

The lateral subcutaneous fat is divided through the ischioanal fossa toward the pelvic floor. Branches of the paired internal pudendal arteries may be encountered in this location but are easily controlled with cautery. The index finger of the non-dominant hand is inserted into the pelvis through the defect at the coccyx and hooks the levator ani muscles from above, serving as a guide for transection. The mesorectum should not be bluntly swept off by the levators from above, but rather the muscle should be divided at this location to ensure the specimen remains cylindrical. Once the levators have been divided bilaterally, only the anterior attachments remain. In female patients, the distal vagina is often angled well posterior of the introitus, and frequent digital vaginal exams are required to assure the appropriate plane is maintained. This dissection is greatly facilitated by having made every effort to separate the vagina from the anterior mesorectum laparoscopically. In men,

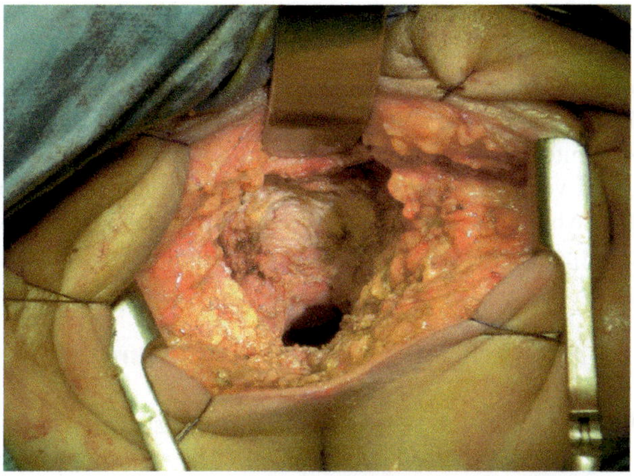

Fig. 19.6 Demonstration of excellent view permitted in this position

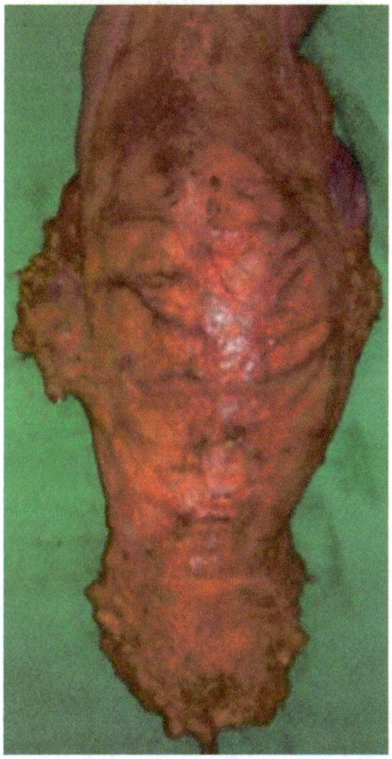

Fig. 19.7 Macroscopically complete excision of the mesorectum and anus

a finger can be swept above the specimen, between the rectum and prostate, to serve as a guide as dissection proceeds from both sides as well as directly anterior. Occasionally, this dissection is made easier by everting the specimen through the perineal wound leaving only the anterior attachments in place and allowing gravity to help delineate the plane. After completing the dissection, the specimen is delivered through the perineum and inspected for gross margins and completeness of the mesorectal envelope (Fig. 19.7).

The perineal wound is copiously irrigated, along with the pelvis. Any bleeding from the pelvic sidewalls is easily visualized and controlled through the perineal defect. The wound is closed in layers with absorbable suture. The levators cannot be closed as they have been excised. The deep fatty layers are reapproximated with large bites, using O-polyglactin sutures. The perineal skin is closed with 2-0 interrupted vertical mattress sutures, which are left in place until they dissolve. We do not use biologic mesh or other foreign material, and myocutaneous flaps are reserved for larger perineal defects caused by extended resection.

19.4.8 Colostomy Creation and Closure

With the perineum closed, the abdomen is reinsufflated. The pelvis is irrigated a final time and hemostasis is ensured. The right lower quadrant 12 mm trocar site is closed with a O-polyglactin suture using a laparoscopic suture passer. The proximal staple line is grasped with a bowel grasper through the right-sided 5 mm trocar. Insufflation is maintained, while the left-sided incision is enlarged to accommodate the colostomy. The subcutaneous fat and anterior fascia are divided in a vertical fashion with cautery, and the rectus fibers are bluntly separated with a Kelly clamp. After enlarging the aperture in the posterior rectus sheath, the insufflation is stopped, and the colon is grasped with a Babcock clamp and exteriorized to skin level. The umbilical U-stitch is tied down, and the skin of the remaining trocar sites is closed with absorbable subcuticular sutures. The wounds are covered with a sterile towel, and the colostomy is matured by excising the staple line, everting the mucosa, and suturing the bowel wall to the dermis with absorbable suture.

19.4.9 Postoperative Care

Patients are admitted to a general surgical floor postoperatively unless comorbidities warrant overnight observation in intensive care. Antibiotics are not redosed beyond the operating room; DVT prophylaxis is continued in the form of pneumatic antiembolism stockings and subcutaneous heparin injections. The patient is immediately offered clear liquids to drink and ordered an IV PCA, IV ketorolac, and oral acetaminophen for pain. The Foley catheter is left in place and removed on postoperative day 1. Also on postoperative day 1, the patient is transitioned to oral pain medication and is offered a regular diet as tolerated.

19.5 Special Circumstances

19.5.1 The Large Perineal Defect

Occasionally, a bulky distal rectal tumor or anal cancer requires a wide perineal resection that cannot be closed primarily without undue tension. In these circumstances, it is advisable to enlist the help of a plastic surgeon for closure of the defect.

A variety of flap options are available including gracilis and rectus abdominis myocutaneous flaps. The need for a flap does not universally exclude the possibility of performing the operation laparoscopically, but operative plans from both teams should be discussed prior to surgery. Rectus abdominis flaps do require open surgery.

19.5.2 T4 Tumors

Invasion of adjacent pelvic organs by T4 rectal cancers is best treated by en bloc resection of the rectum and the involved structures to obtain a negative oncologic margin. The most simple of these to manage is a distal rectal tumor with involvement of the posterior wall of the distal vagina. In this situation, the abdominal and pelvic portions of the operation are performed exactly as described above, except that the anterior dissection terminates above the level of tumor invasion. The perineal incision therefore extends from the perineal skin to encompass the posterior introitus and the posterior vaginal wall to just above the tumor. Depending on the age and lifestyle of the patient and the amount of the vagina resected, the defect may be closed primarily or with a tissue flap. Pelvic exenterations requiring APR with multivisceral resection of the bladder and/or prostate are typically done in an open fashion at our institution.

19.5.3 Reoperative Pelvis

Resection of a previous coloanal anastomosis due to anastomotic complications, poor function, or local recurrence is often best treated by APR. We have performed laparoscopic APR in many patients, but in some cases, it is performed after the index operation was done in an open fashion. The principles remain the same, especially with regard to reestablishing normal anatomy. Depending on the technique of the original surgeon, the IMA may or may not be present. If preserved, the vessel provides a path into the retrorectal TME plane and greatly facilitates safe dissection. If formal TME has previously been performed however, a more difficult pelvic dissection is often required. In the setting of recurrent cancer, a safe radial margin is paramount, and any uncertainty in differentiating cancer from scar should be addressed by conversion rather than risk cutting through tumor.

19.5.4 Intersphincteric Perineal Dissection

Occasionally, rectal cancer patients in whom anterior resection is technically feasible are best treated with a permanent colostomy due to lifestyle issues or impaired continence. In this situation, the authors favor laparoscopic APR over a low, stapled rectal stump or Hartmann procedure. It is important to remember in this setting, however, that any resection of the levators is unnecessary from an oncologic standpoint and that perineal wound complications can be minimized by performing an intersphincteric dissection and simply closing the external sphincters. This intersphincteric APR is more commonly used in benign disease.

References

1. Miles WE. A method of performing abdominoperineal excision for carcinoma of the rectum and of the terminal portion of the pelvic colon. Lancet. 1908;2:1812–3.
2. Lange MM, Rutten HJ, van de Velde CJ. One hundred years of curative surgery for rectal cancer: 1908-2008. Eur J Surg Oncol. 2009;35(5):456–63. doi:10.1016/j.ejso.2008.09.012.
3. Heald RJ, Smedh RK, Kald A, Sexton R, Moran BJ. Abdominoperineal excision of the rectum--an endangered operation. Norman Nigro Lectureship. Dis Colon Rectum. 1997;40(7):747–51.
4. Sackier JM, Berci G, Hiatt JR, Hartunian S. Laparoscopic abdominoperineal resection of the rectum. Br J Surg. 1992;79(11):1207–8.
5. Larach SW, Salomon MC, Williamson PR, Goldstein E. Laparoscopic assisted abdominoperineal resection. Surg Laparosc Endosc. 1993;3(2):115–8.
6. Veldkamp R, Kuhry E, Hop WC, Jeekel J, Kazemier G, Bonjer HJ, et al. Laparoscopic surgery versus open surgery for colon cancer: short-term outcomes of a randomised trial. Lancet Oncol. 2005;6(7):477–84. doi:10.1016/S1470-2045(05)70221-7.
7. Fleshman J, Sargent DJ, Green E, Anvari M, Stryker SJ, Beart RW, Jr., et al. Laparoscopic colectomy for cancer is not inferior to open surgery based on 5-year data from the COST Study Group trial. Ann Surg. 2007;246(4):655–62; discussion 62–4. doi:10.1097/SLA.0b013e318155a762.
8. Bonjer HJ, Deijen CL, Abis GA, Cuesta MA, van der Pas MH, de Lange-de Klerk ES, et al. A randomized trial of laparoscopic versus open surgery for rectal cancer. N Engl J Med. 2015;372(14):1324–32. doi:10.1056/NEJMoa1414882.
9. Kang SB, Park JW, Jeong SY, Nam BH, Choi HS, Kim DW, et al. Open versus laparoscopic surgery for mid or low rectal cancer after neoadjuvant chemoradiotherapy (COREAN trial): short-term outcomes of an open-label randomised controlled trial. Lancet Oncol. 2010;11(7):637–45. doi:10.1016/S1470-2045(10)70131-5.
10. van der Pas MH, Haglind E, Cuesta MA, Furst A, Lacy AM, Hop WC, et al. Laparoscopic versus open surgery for rectal cancer (COLOR II): short-term outcomes of a randomised, phase 3 trial. Lancet Oncol. 2013;14(3):210–8. doi:10.1016/S1470-2045(13)70016-0.
11. Schlussel AT, Lustik MB, Johnson EK, Maykel JA, Champagne BJ, Goldberg JE, et al. A population-based comparison of open versus minimally invasive abdominoperineal resection. Am J Surg. 2015;209(5):815–23. doi:10.1016/j.amjsurg.2014.12.021.
12. West NP, Finan PJ, Anderin C, Lindholm J, Holm T, Quirke P. Evidence of the oncologic superiority of cylindrical abdominoperineal excision for low rectal cancer. J Clin Oncol. 2008;26(21):3517–22. doi:10.1200/JCO.2007.14.5961.
13. Holm T, Ljung A, Haggmark T, Jurell G, Lagergren J. Extended abdominoperineal resection with gluteus maximus flap reconstruction of the pelvic floor for rectal cancer. Br J Surg. 2007;94(2):232–8. doi:10.1002/bjs.5489.
14. Keller DS, Stulberg JJ, Lawrence JK, Delaney CP. Process control to measure process improvement in colorectal surgery: modifications to an established enhanced recovery pathway. Dis Colon Rectum. 2014;57(2):194–200. doi:10.1097/DCR.0b013e3182a62c91.
15. Delaney CP, Brady K, Woconish D, Parmar SP, Champagne BJ. Towards optimizing perioperative colorectal care: outcomes for 1,000 consecutive laparoscopic colon procedures using enhanced recovery pathways. Am J Surg. 2012;203(3):353–355.; discussion 5-6. doi:10.1016/j.amjsurg.2011.09.017.
16. Keller DS, Lawrence JK, Delaney CP. Prone jackknife position is not necessary to achieve a cylindrical abdominoperineal resection: demonstration of the lithotomy position. Dis Colon Rectum. 2014;57(2):251. doi:10.1097/DCR.0000000000000047.

Reduced Port Laparoscopic Abdominoperineal Resection

20

Seong Hyeon Yun and Kyung Uk Jung

Abstract

In the past decade, single-incision laparoscopic surgery (SILS) has shown acceptable results in a number of surgical interventions including colorectal procedures for benign and malignant diseases. However, the acceptance of SILS in the lower rectum has been hampered by its technical difficulties and concern over oncological outcome. More recently, increased experience, safety, and feasibility of SILS for rectal lesions in short-term outcomes have started to be reported. Many of them adopted an additional port for traction or transection of the rectum in the case of a very low rectal lesion, which is generally called "reduced port laparoscopic surgery." SILS or reduced port laparoscopic abdominoperineal resection (RPLAPR) is a relatively new technique in the minimally invasive surgery era, and there are only a few reports on this topic. In this chapter, we introduce the surgical technique of SILS or RPLAPR in our center and short-term outcomes with a literature review.

Keywords

Reduced port laparoscopic surgery • Single-port laparoscopic surgery • Rectal cancer • Reduced port laparoscopic APR • Single-port laparoscopic APR

S.H. Yun (✉)
Department of Surgery, Samsung Medical Center, Sungkyunkwan University School of Medicine, 81, Irwon-ro, Gangnam-gu, Seoul 135-710, Republic of Korea
e-mail: shyunmd@skku.edu

K.U. Jung
Department of Surgery, Kangbuk Samsung Hospital, Sungkyunkwan University School of Medicine, 29, Saemunan-ro, Seoul 110-746, Republic of Korea

G. Dapri, J.H. Marks (eds.), *Surgical Techniques in Rectal Cancer*,
https://doi.org/10.1007/978-4-431-55579-7_20

20.1 Introduction and History

Traditionally, the surgical incision represented the extent of the operation. A larger incision is generally more painful and cosmetically inferior and has more potential for causing complications related to the presence of the wound. Laparoscopic surgery, which is designed to reduce abdominal wall, surgical trauma, and morbidities related to a large incision, is shown to be safe and feasible in rectal surgery with several large prospective randomized trials [1–3]. Although the current guidelines of the National Comprehensive Cancer Network (version 3, 2015) recommend laparoscopic surgery for rectal malignancy only in a clinical trial setting [4], many institutes have adopted laparoscopy as a standard procedure for rectal cancer already.

Even after laparoscopic surgery was accepted as an alternative method to an open procedure, the efforts to reduce the incisions have continued. Since Esposito et al. reported laparoscopic appendectomy with only one trocar in 1998 [5], which was the first report of single-incision laparoscopic surgery (SILS), SILS has shown acceptable results in a number of surgical interventions including colorectal procedures for benign and malignant diseases [6–10].

However, the acceptance of SILS in the lower rectum has been hampered by its technical difficulties and concern over of oncological outcome related to the completeness of total mesorectal excision (TME) and circumferential resection margins. More recently, increased experience, short-term outcomes, safety, and feasibility of SILS for rectal cancer have started to be reported [11–24]. Many surgeons have adopted one additional port for traction or transection of the rectum in case of very low rectal lesions. This is generally called "reduced port laparoscopic surgery" [11, 13, 15, 16, 21, 22].

Although there are few reports on SILS or reduced port laparoscopic abdominoperineal resection (RPLAPR) [11, 16, 17, 19, 20], the APR is a more suitable candidate for the single-port technique than lower anterior resection. In performing an APR, contrary to the lower anterior resection which requires secure transection of the distal rectum and an anastomosis, there is no need to be concerned with difficult stapling or overlapping of staple lines due to the inadequate angle of the stapler. Furthermore, the perineal approach, which is an inevitable step of the APR, facilitates dissection of very low part of the rectum.

In this chapter, we introduce the surgical technique of SILS or RPLAPR and short-term outcomes in our center with a literature review.

20.2 Indications

APR was once the principal procedure for lower rectal or anal cancer; however, the number of APR has been quite reduced with the introduction of preoperative chemoradiation therapy and sphincter-saving procedures such as intersphincteric resection, TATA, or transanal endoscopic microsurgery for rectal malignancies.

Now the most common indications for APR in the current laparoscopic era include:

- Very low rectal cancer which invades the sphincteric complex
- Low rectal cancer with poor sphincter function which significantly decreases the patient's quality of life
- Anal cancer which does not resolved or recurred after chemoradiation therapy

20.3 Preoperative Assessment and Preparation

System assessment should be done to determine the preoperative stage of malignant lesions, including physical examination, colonoscopy, biopsy, measurement of carcinoembryonic antigen, and abdominopelvic computed tomography (CT) scan. Chest CT and positron-emission tomography scan also can be used to evaluate extraperitoneal metastasis. Transrectal ultrasonography and magnetic resonance imaging provide more precise information of sphincter invasion than a CT scan. Taking a detailed history of bowel habits and distal rectal exam may be helpful to determine the patient's sphincter function.

Bowel preparation is dependent on the surgeon's preference. We usually give a full mechanical bowel preparation with polyethylene glycol solution the day before surgery.

After acquiring informed consent for the surgery, the surgeon or a qualified enterostomal therapist marks the future colostomy site. It is placed in the right lower quadrant, within the rectus muscle borders, avoiding the skin fold, costal margin, bony prominences, belt or waist line, and previous scars or incisions. It should be marked before the patient goes to the operating room, with careful examination under sitting, standing, and lying position. The optimal placement of the stoma enhances the postoperative quality of life and reduces the skin and stoma complications. It must be emphasized that the proper performance of this step will greatly impact the patient's postoperative quality of life.

20.4 Operative Technique

20.4.1 Position

After induction of general anesthesia, the patient is positioned in the modified lithotomy position using adjustable Allen stirrups. Both arms should be alongside the body to achieve sufficient space for the surgeon and the camera operator. We place the main port in the left lower quadrant (LLQ), at the future colostomy site, and the surgeon and the assistant stand on the right side of the patient. The main monitor is located in the opposite side, near the patients' left leg (Fig. 20.1). The position of the surgeon and the camera operator can be changed during the

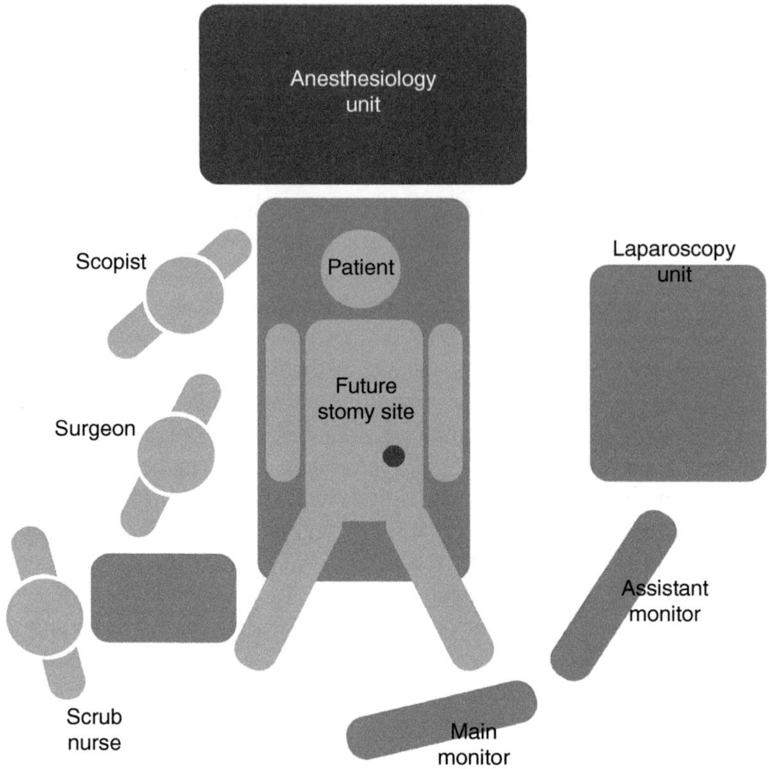

Fig. 20.1 Operating room setting at the initial step of the abdominal phase

abdominal phase depending on the procedure. The hip joint angle should be flat during the abdominal phase not to restrict the range of motion of laparoscopic device, especially during the dissection of the splenic flexure. The buttocks should be at the end of the bed, and palpation of the tip of the coccyx should be possible without putting a hand between the patients' body and the table. A pad under the sacrum makes the perineum project beyond the table and provides a better view during the perineal phase. We do not employ prone jackknife or left lateral position for the perineal phase and just proceed in the lithotomy position. Flexion of the hip joint and taking the legs upward with Allen stirrups provide enough space for the surgeon during the perineal phase.

Air hugger is applied on the chest of the patient to prevent hypothermia, and the bilateral sequential compression devices are placed on the calves to prevent thrombotic complication. A Foley catheter is inserted and passed over the thigh so as not to disturb the surgical field during the perineal phase.

After anesthesia, careful digital rectal exam is necessary to confirm the plan to sacrifice the sphincter complex. Then the abdomen and perineum are soaped and draped. The table position during the main portion of the procedure is steep Trendelenburg position with the left side up (Fig. 20.2).

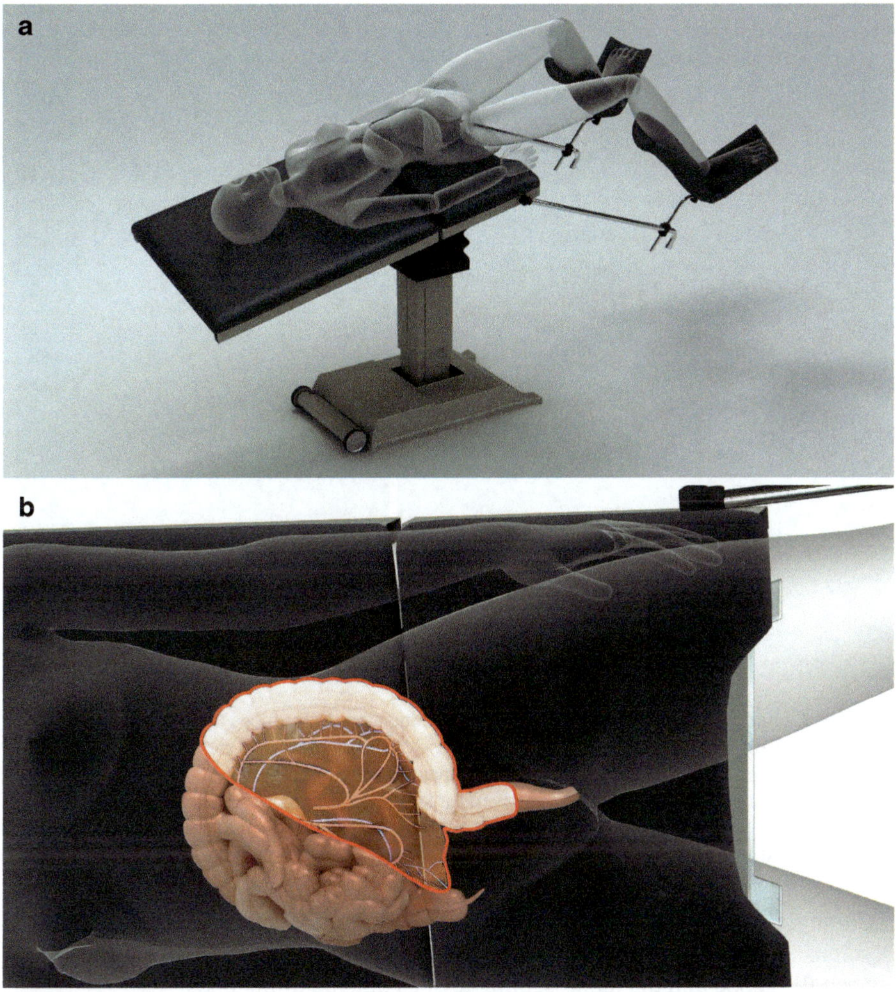

Fig. 20.2 Basic patient position: Steep Trendelenburg position with left side up is the basic operation setup during the abdominoperineal resection. (**a**) Patient position on the operative table. (**b**) Intraperitoneal organ and the surgical field (small-bowel loops were retracted caudal and downward)

20.4.2 Camera and Instruments

We normally use a 12 mm rigid laparoscope with a 30° optic. However, a flexible scope with 0° optic is also suitable. Any kind of scope which is familiar to the surgeon and the camera operator can be used. The experience of the camera operator is as important as the surgeons', and it is the key of the SILS or RPL procedure. A skillful camera operator not only can offer and maintain an optimal operative field but also can avoid unnecessary collisions with the instruments of the surgeon. Using

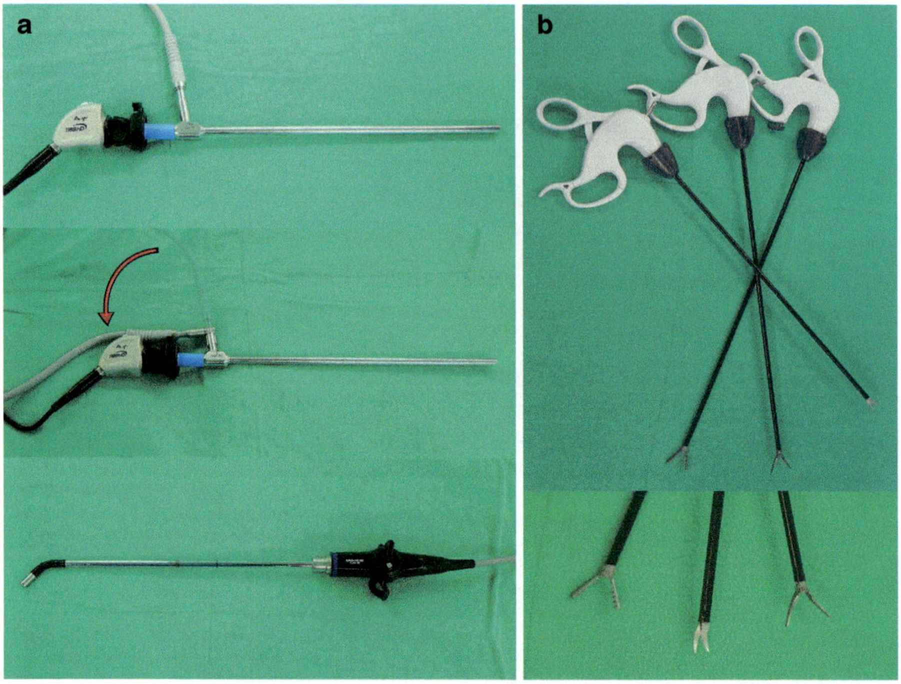

Fig. 20.3 Commonly used instruments for single-incision or reduced port laparoscopy. (**a**) Laparoscopic cameras. Top, 30° 10 mm rigid scope with conventional light source. Middle, 30° 10 mm rigid scope with right-angle converter connected to light cable: this is very useful during the single-port surgery for prevention of inadvertent touch to the surgeon's instruments when compared to the conventional light cable. Bottom, three-dimensional scope with flexible tip. (**b**) Commonly used straight laparoscopic instruments (grasper, dissector, and scissors)

a right-angle connector for the light cable or an all-in-one scope such as the Endoeye (Olympus Corporation, Tokyo, Japan) (Fig. 20.3a) can help to reduce clashing between the scope and the laparoscopic devices outside of the body.

Flexible instruments are not necessary. We use conventional straight instruments, as for conventional laparoscopy, in all cases (Fig. 20.3b). A multifunctional advanced energy-based device (EBD) is especially useful during single- or reduced port laparoscopic colorectal surgery, because it reduces the frequency of changing the instruments and reduces scope contamination by surgical smoke. LigaSure™ (Covidien, Mansfield, MA, USA) with the monopolar tip or Thunderbeat (Olympus) are representatives of this type of energy-based device and are useful not only for vessel or tissue sealing but also ordinary surgical maneuvers, such as grasping or dissection.

20.4.3 Port Preparation

There are various kinds of access ports for SILS on the market including SILS port (Covidien), OCTO port (Darim, Seoul, Korea), TriPort or QuadPort (Olympus), and GelPOINT (Applied Medical, Santa Margarita, CA, USA). We used a custom-made

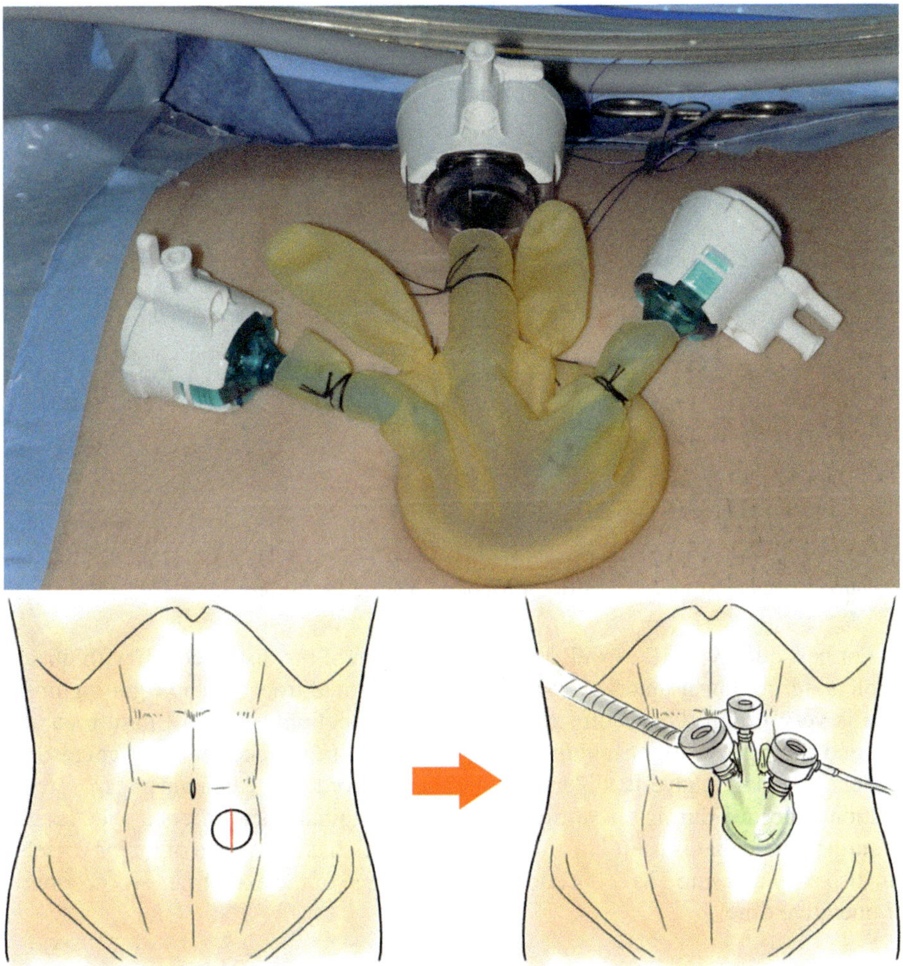

Fig. 20.4 Custom-made glove port consisting of powder-free left-hand surgical glove and three disposable trocars and installed feature in future colostomy site

glove port initially, tried some of the aforementioned commercial ports, and then returned to our original one. Our custom-made glove port consists of a powder-free left-hand medical use glove, Latex Biogel® Surgeons (Mölnlycke Health Care, Gothenburg, Sweden), and the three or four Separator® Access System (Applied Medical). Usually, two 12 mm diameter trocars and one 5 mm diameter trocar with short shafts are used. A 12 mm diameter trocar in the thumb is for the laparoscope, and the others are for the instruments (Fig. 20.4). The trocars of the custom-made glove port can be pushed into the hole of skin incision and serve as the guidance when inserting the instruments, to avoid hitting the fascia on insertion. Otherwise, they stay outside of the hole and don't occupy the space around the shaft of instrument. Consequently, the instruments move more freely and the collisions in the hole can be minimized (Fig. 20.5). For an additional port, a 12 mm trocar is usually used.

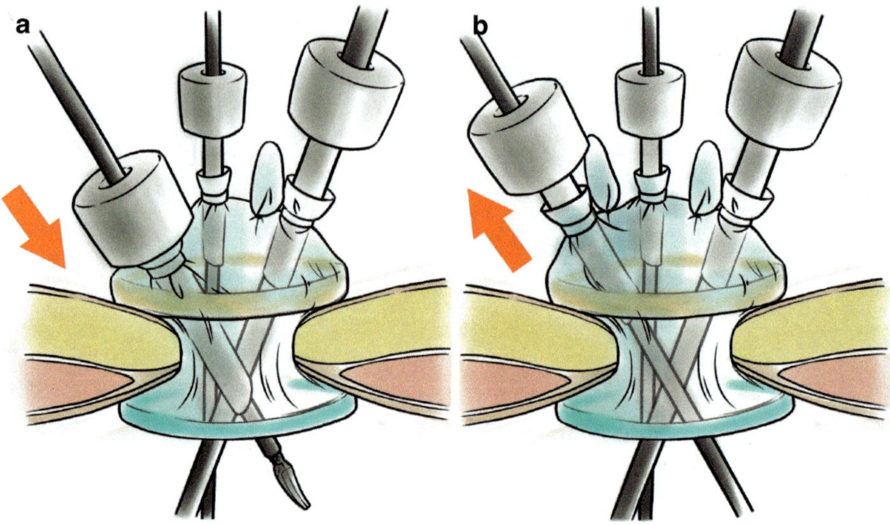

Fig. 20.5 Principle of reduced collision in custom-made glove port. (**a**) Trocar in the hole during the introduction of instruments. (**b**) Trocar out of the hole during the procedure

For best quality TME as well as optimal division of the distal rectum with linear staplers during lower anterior resection, one additional trocar in the right inguinal area is very useful. Under direct laparoscopic inspection, a 5 or 12 mm trocar is inserted through the right inguinal area, just lateral to the deep inferior epigastric vessels. To avoid inadvertent bleeding, hernia, and cord injury in male patient, great caution is needed during trocar placement. This inguinal trocar offers a wide range of surgical field that is useful in not only for dissection and division of major vessels but also easy and safe TME. An additional advantage of the extra trocar is reduction of operative time.

20.4.4 Procedure

20.4.4.1 The Abdominal Phase

The skin incision is made at the future colostomy site, which is marked preoperatively as mentioned above. A disc of skin, usually 2.5–3.5 cm in diameter reflecting the patients' body stature, is excised and the subcutaneous fat is dissected. A vertical incision is made in the rectus sheath using electrocautery, and the muscle is separated. Care should be taken not to injure the epigastric vessels. After the posterior rectus sheath and peritoneum are opened, an Alexis® Wound Retractor (Applied Medical) is inserted. In most cases, the appropriate size is S. A custom-made glove port is applied over the wound retractor, and then pneumoperitoneum is established.

The surgeon and the camera operator stand on the right side of the patient and start with the laparoscopic exploration of the peritoneal space from the liver to the pelvis. It is important not to skip over the exploration. Although preoperative

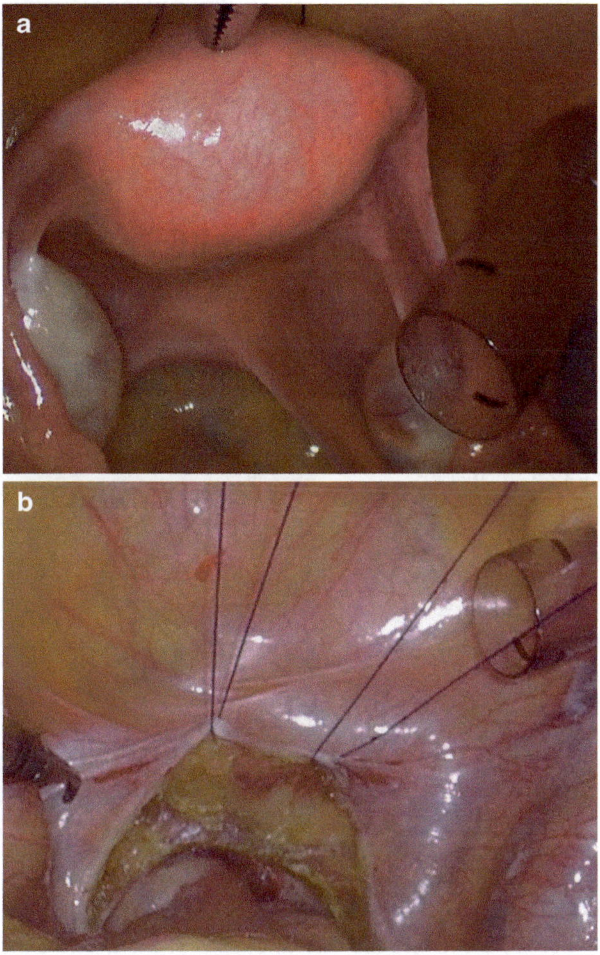

Fig. 20.6 Transabdominal traction with thread sling. (**a**) The uterus is lifted up in female patient. (**b**) Anterior portion of peritoneal reflection is lifted up in male patient

imaging techniques are highly developed, it is not uncommon to find an unexpected metastasis such as peritoneal seeding during the exploration.

The patient is placed in a steep Trendelenburg position with right side down (Fig. 20.2). The small bowel is moved toward the left upper abdomen and nudged with an X-ray detectable surgical gauze. Placing one or two gauzes over the ligament of Treitz and the proximal jejunum helps to retract the small bowel and to protect them from injury during the dissection and ligation of inferior mesenteric artery (IMA) and vein (IMV). Transabdominal suspension of the uterus (in women) or of the soft tissue around the anterior peritoneal reflection (in men) is applied using nonabsorbable suture with a straight needle (Fig. 20.6).

The sigmoid mesocolon is grasped with an instrument in the surgeon's nondominant hand and lifted up anteriorly to the left lateral side. The energy-based device is in the right hand of the surgeon, which is inserted through the right inguinal port. The IMA is identified, and the parietal peritoneum at the base of the sigmoid

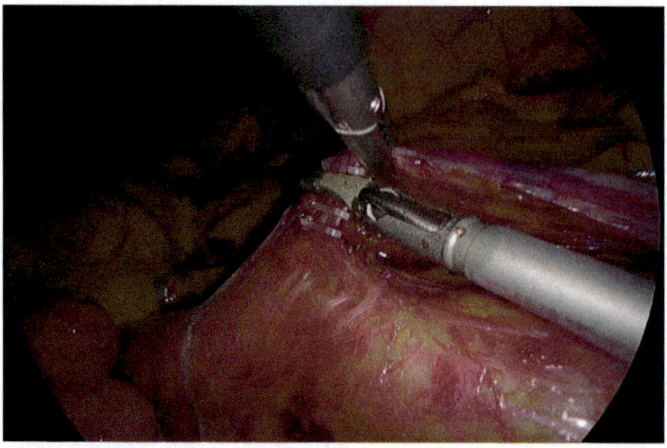

Fig. 20.7 Ligation of inferior mesenteric artery: The distal portion of the inferior mesenteric artery is lifted, and the vessel is divided with advanced energy-based device

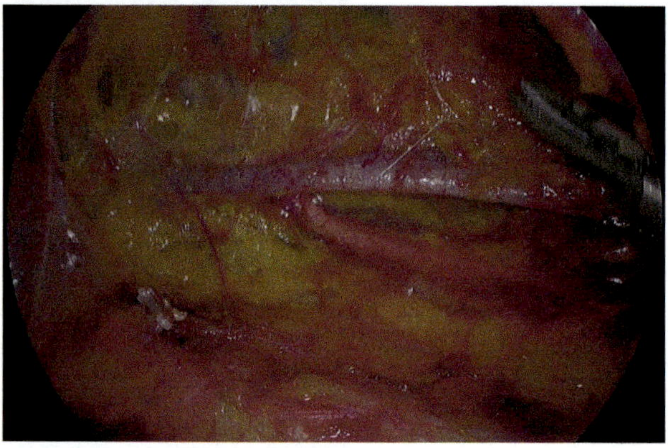

Fig. 20.8 Medial-to-lateral mobilization of sigmoid colon: Sigmoid mesocolon was lifted up and the underlying gonadal vessels are preserved along the avascular plane

mesocolon is incised at the level of the IMA origin and then extended downward to the pelvis, alongside the lateral border of the aorta. Unlike in conventional laparoscopic surgery, in which good traction-countertraction is maintained during the dissection at the level of aortic bifurcation, great caution is needed during reduced port surgery not to make an injury to the left iliac vein. The sigmoid mesocolon should be lifted up and pulled toward the surgeon with the nondominant hand in order to avoid this type of injury. The lymph node-bearing soft tissue around the IMA is dissected taking care not to damage the preaortic sympathetic nerve plexus. The IMA is ligated with surgical clips, 1 cm distal to its origin, then coagulated, and divided with the energy device (Fig. 20.7).

The sigmoid mesocolon is then taken off from the retroperitoneum in a medial-to-lateral fashion until one encounters the white line of Toldt. If the dissection plane is exactly right, there is no structure to bleed and electrocoagulation is not necessary. As the dissection progresses laterally, the left gonadal arteries and veins should be identified on the retroperitoneal side. The ureter, which crosses under the gonadal vein at the level of the inferior pole of the kidney, is usually found at the medial and posterior side of the gonadal vessels (Fig. 20.8).

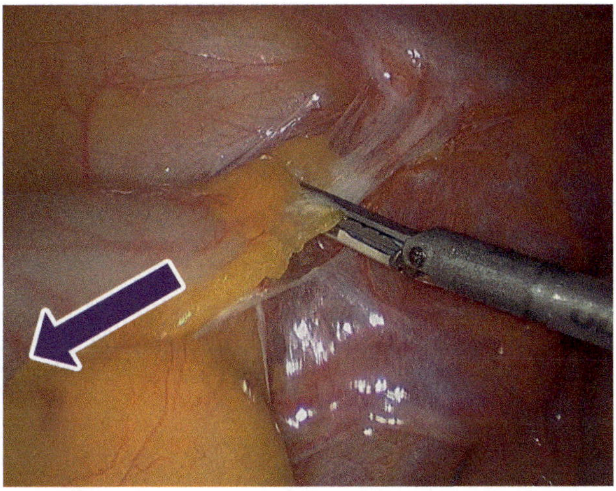

Fig. 20.9 Division of the lateral attachment of sigmoid colon: In this procedure, the mesocolon or epiploic appendage is pulled toward the surgeon with nondominant hand, and the attachment is divided with the energy-based device entered from the right inguinal additional port

The lateral attachment of the sigmoid colon is opened and connected to the dissection from the medial side (Fig. 20.9). In this procedure, pulling the mesocolon or epiploic appendages is very useful for better exposure and prevention of bowel injury or the bleeding from the mesocolon. The peritoneal incision is extended downward, and then it is continued to the cul-de-sac alongside the medial border of both ureters.

The mesorectal plane between the fascia propria of the rectum and the presacral fascia is entered at the level of the sacral promontory, with care to preserve hypogastric nerves. TME is established through the avascular plane using electrocautery and the energy device. Waldeyer's fascia is opened at the mid sacral level (Fig. 20.10). Going deep at this point on the sacral side can injure the presacral venous plexus and cause significant bleeding. If the bleeding is minor, compression with gauze is helpful to achieve hemostasis. During the left lateral dissection, the upper rectum is lifted up and pulled to the surgeon side with a grasper on the nondominant hand of the surgeon. It is helpful to lift up and push to the opposite side of the surgeon during the right lateral dissection. The posterior dissection is ended at the level of the coccyx.

The dissection is continued laterally, dividing the lateral ligament using energy devices (Fig. 20.11). Grasping the rectal wall and retracting to the opposite side are enough to achieve the plane in most cases. However, the additional port is used when it is difficult to proceed with the operation for any reason. It is generally located in right suprapubic area, on the lateral side of right epigastric vessels, as mentioned earlier in this chapter (Fig. 20.12).

The lateral peritoneal incisions are connected anteriorly at the rectouterine pouch (in women) or the rectovesical recess (in men). A curvilinear incision is made along the peritoneal reflection for the anterior aspect of total mesorectal excision with the energy-based device from the right suprapubic or inguinal port. At this point, the mesocolon of the upper rectum is pulled up for better exposure. The dissection is continued to the rectovaginal septum (in women) or the Denonvilliers' fascia (in

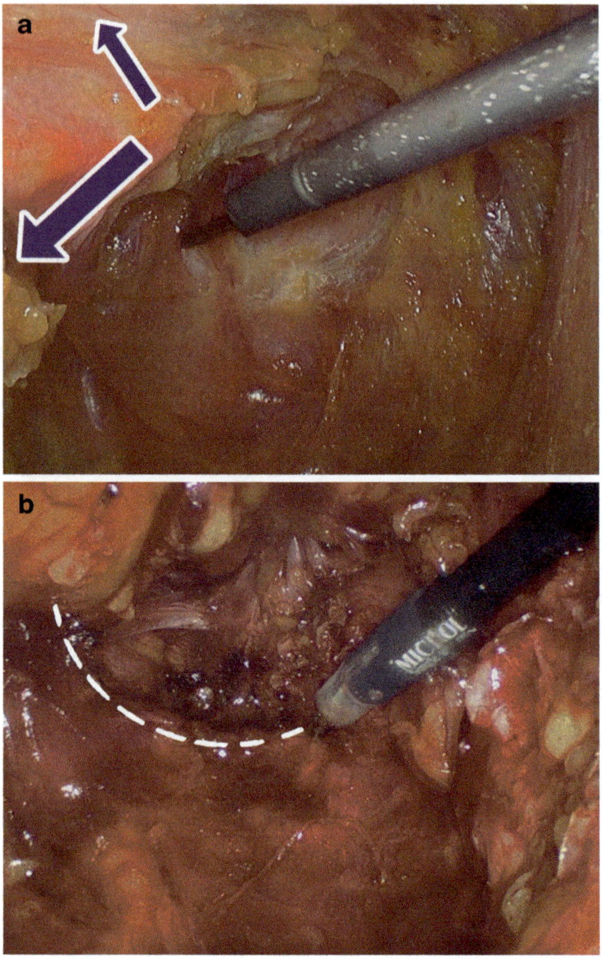

Fig. 20.10 Posterior dissection during total mesorectal excision and division of levator ani muscle. (**a**) Posterior mobilization along the total mesorectal excision plane. (**b**) Division of the levator ani muscle from the abdominal phase: levator ani muscle below the dotted arrow is remained

men). As the dissection progresses to the lower part of the rectum, a fan retractor may be helpful for better exposure. Injury of the pelvic splanchnic nerves at this point causes erectile dysfunction in men, so try not to expose the seminal vesicles unless the tumor is located in the anterior wall. When the pelvic floor is reached circumferentially around the rectum, pelvic dissection from the abdominal side is completed. In order to obtain a sufficient circumferential margin, it is helpful to divide the levator ani and pelvic floor muscles as much as possible if the good surgical field is maintained (Fig. 20.10b).

Then the descending colon and mesocolon are dissected cephalad until the length of the mobilized colon seems to be enough to make a colostomy without any tension. Proximal division can be performed with linear stapler inserted from the 12 mm right inguinal trocar (Fig. 20.13a). It is helpful to estimate the length of

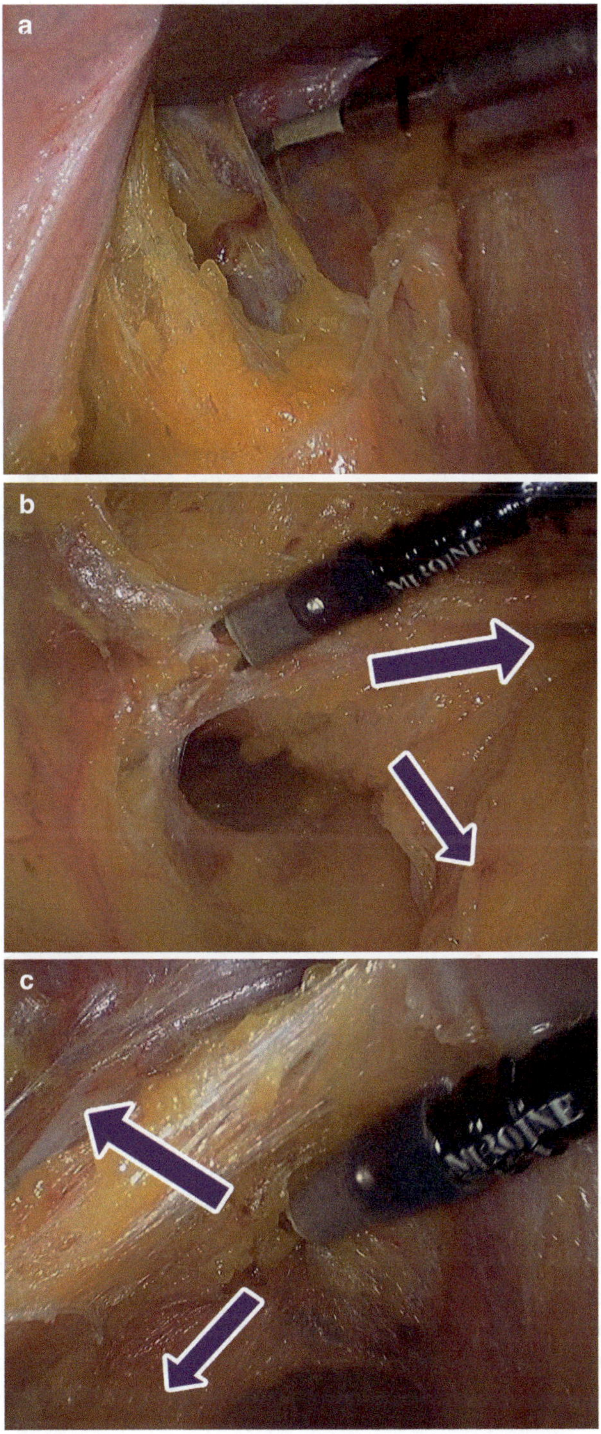

Fig. 20.11 Anterior and lateral dissection during the total mesorectal excision. (**a**) Anterior: fan retractor is useful for better exposure. (**b**) Right side: arrow indicates the direction of traction with the instrument of nondominant hand of surgeon thorough the single port at stoma site. (**c**) Posterior dissection during total mesorectal excision and division of the levator ani muscle

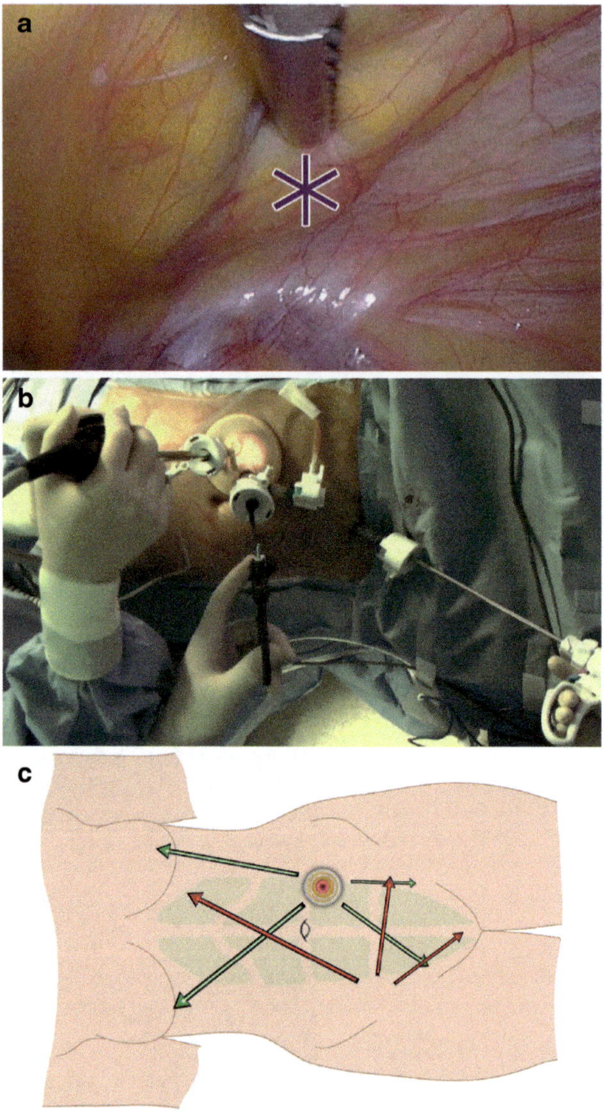

Fig. 20.12. Additional port in the right inguinal area. (**a**) Insertion of additional trocar under the direct vision: * indicates the insertion site of additional trocar. (**b**) External view of single port plus one trocar during the surgery. (**c**) Range of motion through the single port and the additional trocar

proximal colon for colostomy by checking the tension when the proximal colon is pulled through the single port, which is the future stoma site. If there is tension, further descending colon or some degree of splenic flexure mobilization is necessary to eliminate the tension to safely create the stoma (Fig. 20.13b). While full mobilization of the splenic flexure is not a routine procedure, it should be considered whenever the remnant colonic length seems to be short. Placing the patient in a steep reverse Trendelenburg position facilitates the splenic flexure dissection. In

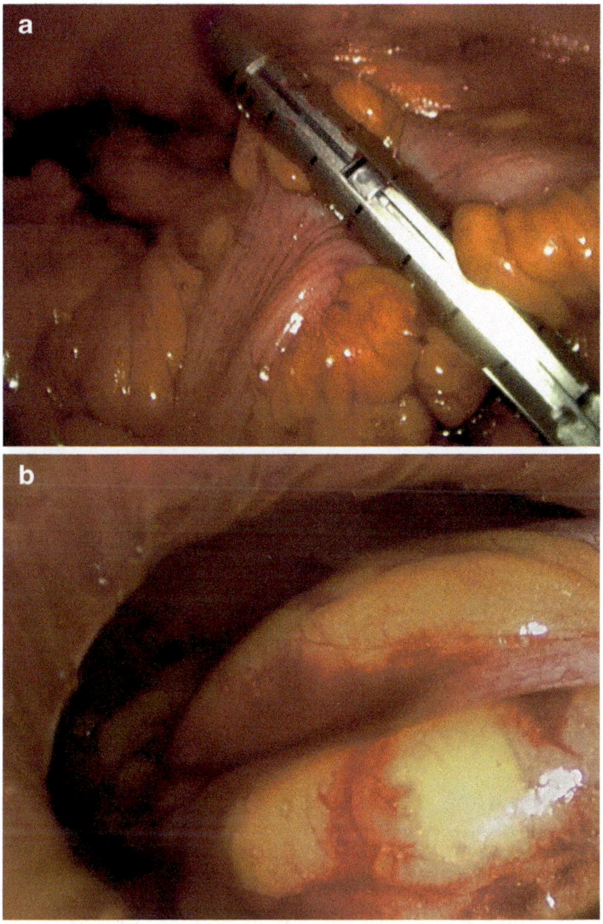

Fig. 20.13 Proximal division of the colon. (**a**) Division of colon with linear stapler. (**b**) Estimation of proximal colon length through the future stoma site (single port)

most cases, the mobilization of the splenic flexure can be achieved from the patients' left side. However, moving to the space between the legs of the patient is helpful in some difficult cases (Fig. 20.14).

After dividing the sigmoid colon at the proximal margin, the abdomen is deflated and the abdominal phase is ended.

20.4.4.2 The Perineal Phase

Perineal dissection is performed in the same lithotomy position without intraoperative repositioning, with flexion of the hip joint. The surgeon goes between the patients' legs, usually sitting on a stool. The anus is closed using a purse-string suture, and the perineum is prepped again if there has been any spillage during the operation.

A circular incision is made that extends from the midpoint of the perineal body to a point midway between the coccyx and the anus. The subcutaneous tissue is

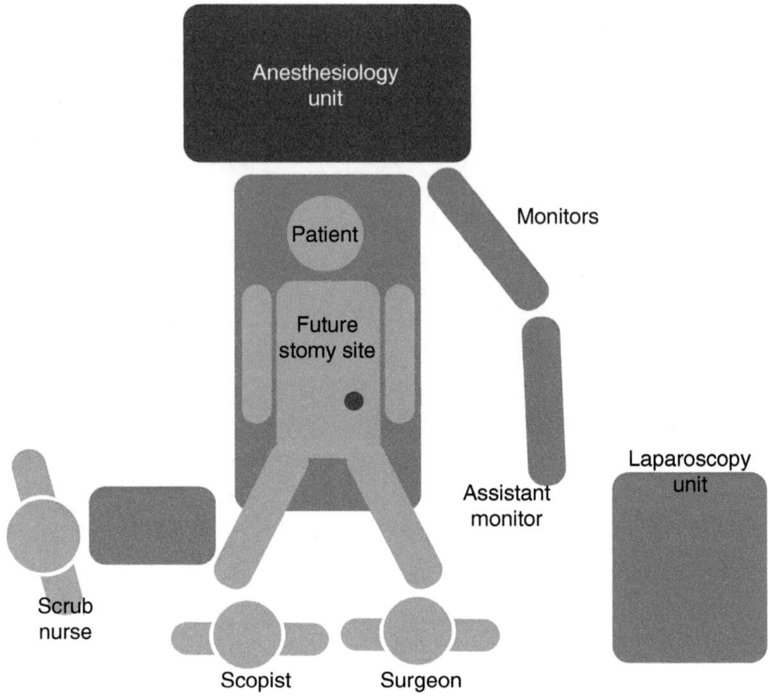

Fig. 20.14 Operating room setting during the mobilization of the splenic flexure

dissected using electrocautery, and the ischiorectal space is entered. The assistant from the abdominal side or beside the surgeon can aid the dissection with Richardson Retractor (Fig. 20.15). Perineal dissection is usually started posteriorly. With palpation of the coccyx as a guide, the posterior dissection is directed anterior to the coccyx, and the anococcygeal raphe is opened. After the pelvis is entered, the dissection is continued laterally. The levator muscle is divided at the most lateral side. After complete division of all attachments posteriorly and laterally, the specimen is extracted through the perineal wound. With traction of the specimen, the transverse perinei and rectourethralis muscles are divided anteriorly, caring not to injure the urogenital structures.

The specimen is removed and the pelvis is irrigated with warm saline. A closed suction drain can be inserted from the perineal side to the pelvic cavity, and the wound is closed. The right inguinal trocar site can be used for the site of closed suction drainage after completion of perineal closure (Fig. 20.16). We do not use a biologic mesh or in situ muscle flap routinely. If the remnant musculature is too short to oppose, the muscle is just pulled as close as it can get. Then the subcutaneous fat in the ischiorectal space is closed in multiple-layered fashions with absorbable suture. The skin is closed with surgical staplers.

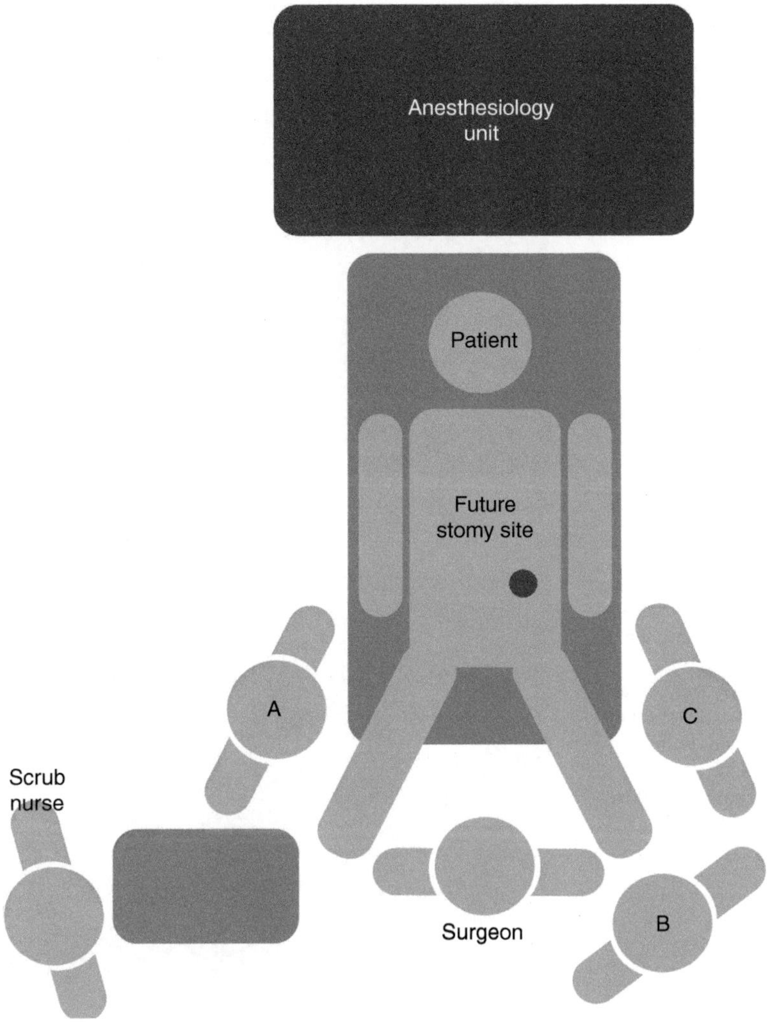

Fig. 20.15 Operating room setting during the perineal phase. A, B, and C are possible assistant's position

20.4.4.3 Stoma Formation and Wound Closure

At the end of the perineal phase, the perineal wound is completely closed, and the pneumoperitoneum can be achieved again. The surgeon moves to the patients' left side. Laparoscopic exploration is performed. All the bleeding is controlled and the peritoneal cavity is irrigated when necessary (Fig. 20.16). The additional port is removed and the fascia and skin are closed. The end of the sigmoid or descending colon is held with a grasper and the abdomen is deflated. The wound retractor is

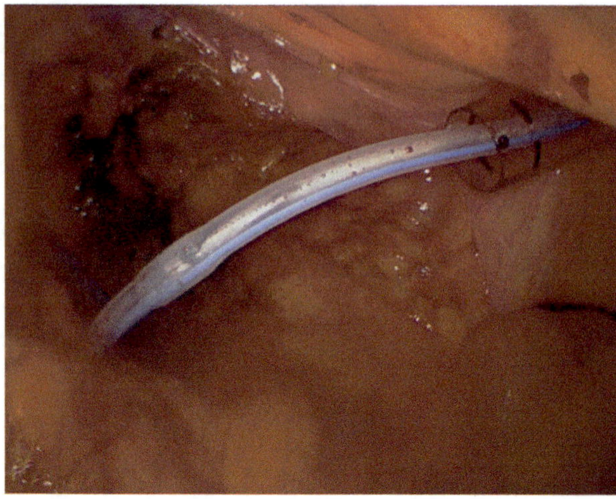

Fig. 20.16 Pelvic floor after completion of the perineal procedure and the drain insertion through the right inguinal port

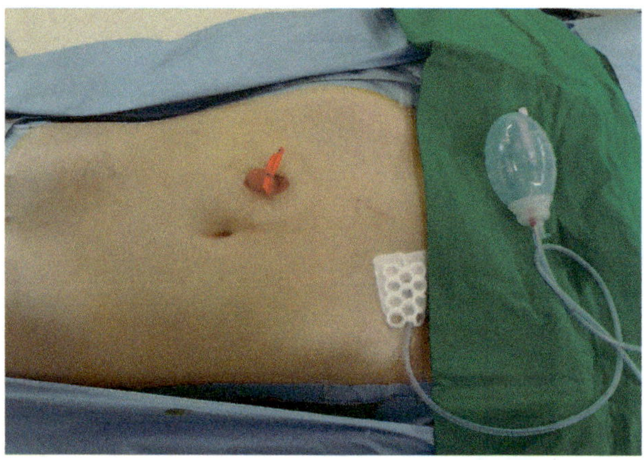

Fig. 20.17 Final abdominal state: stoma at the left lower quadrant and Jackson-Pratt drain through the right inguinal area. This photo was taken from the patient with loop ileostomy with total proctocolectomy and ileal pouch-anal anastomosis

removed, and the colon is drawn out through the wound to make the colostomy. If the wound is too big, the fascia is closed until it becomes a suitable size to prevent parastomal hernia. Generally, two finger breadths are enough. Care should be taken not to distort the direction of the mesocolon when withdrawing the bowel. We do not adopt an extraperitoneal tunneling procedure. The colon is fixed to the posterior and anterior rectal sheath, respectively. Then the stapled end of the colon is opened and the colostomy is matured.

After completion of the whole procedure, there remains only one or no scars in the abdomen. Only the permanent colostomy in LLQ is left (Fig. 20.17).

20.4.4.4 Technical Tips for Successful Single-Port or Reduced Port Colorectal Surgery

1. Set the target at the top:
   (a) Use the gravity as a hidden assistant.
   (b) Proper positioning of the target is essential for successful surgery.
2. Change the concept of traction and countertraction:
   (a) In single-port surgery, the instrument in the nondominant hand should take over the roles of both the assistant's instruments.
   (b) For better exposure, it is useful to lift up or push if the attached area and gravity are in same direction; on the contrary, it is helpful to pull the target if the attachment and gravity are in opposite direction.
3. Crossing the instruments is useful for better exposure.
4. The combination of a pulling, pushing, and rotating action with the nondominant hand can offer better exposure.
5. Transabdominal traction with thread or sling is useful during the pelvic dissection.

20.5 Outcomes

With a decade of experience, short-term data showed results from SILS or RPL in colonic malignancy comparable to results of conventional laparoscopy. Maggiori et al. and Makino et al. suggested that there may be potential benefits associated with SILS over conventional laparoscopy with decreased hospital day and reduced maximal pain score in their systematic review [6, 10]. However, due to the complexity of the procedure, there are few reports on SILS or RPL that include rectal lesions. There are several case series with low evidence level, and only one systematic review has focused on rectal SILS exclusively [14].

Current data of APR with SILS or RPL, one of the most complicated procedures in the colorectal arena, are sparser. After the first appearance in the case series of Bulut et al. in 2011 [25], SILS or RPLAPR was reported by Ali et al. [24] and Lauritsen et al. [20] as case reports, respectively. Until now, there is only one case series by Hua-Feng et al. [23], and no comparative study or systemic review which is focused on SILS or RPLAPR alone. However, we can infer its short-term outcome from the reports including other procedures.

Table 20.1 shows short-term results from existing series of SILS or RPLAPR. There was no mortality reported, and the results seem to be acceptable. There is no long-term follow-up data, so the oncologic integrity of this procedure is still not determined. However, new techniques always begin with low level of evidence and are proven to be safe and effective only after many years. SILS is a procedure at the cutting edge of minimally invasive technique and still developing. We should keep an eye on its progress and evolving long-term outcomes data.

Table 20.1 Short-term outcomes of existing case series of SILS or RPLAPR

	Hua-Feng et al. [23]	Vestweber et al. [17]	Bulut et al.[a] [16]	Sirikurnpiboon and Jivapaisarnpong [19]	Yun et al.[b]
Patient number	20	10	8 (out of 25 SILS rectal surgery)	10 (out of 10 SILS rectal surgery)	14
Age (year) mean ± SD (range)	67.45 ± 10.89 (45–81)	61.6 ± 16.3 (31–88)	69 (49–87)	69 ± 11.76 (52–86)	75 (33–75)
Body mass index (kg/m^2)	–	26.5 ± 4.5 (22–36)	24 (19–32)	21.77 ± 4.48 (15.00–30.00)	22.5 (16.8–27.3)
Diagnosis	Neoplasm	UC (1) Neoplasm (9)	Neoplasm	Neoplasm	Neoplasm
Operating time (min) mean ± SD (range)	138.55 ± 9.32 (125–155)	254.6 ± 83.7 (99–409)	280 (136–397)	269 ± 41.75 (200–300)	255 (157–595)
Conversion to open (n)	No	2	No	No	1
Length of hospital stay (days)	4.25 ± 0.97 (3–6)	16.0 ± 13.2 (7–28)	7 (4–39)	7 (5–10)	11 (8–46)
Complication	2	–	6 (out of all 25)	4 (out of all 10)	2
CRM (mm)	–	–	10 (1–25)	All negative	Positive in 1 patient

[a]The numbers are presented as median (range)
[b]Unpublished data, the numbers are presented as median (range)

References

1. Kang SB, Park JW, Jeong SY, Nam BH, Choi HS, Kim DW, et al. Open versus laparoscopic surgery for mid or low rectal cancer after neoadjuvant chemoradiotherapy (COREAN trial): short-term outcomes of an open-label randomised controlled trial. Lancet Oncol. 2010;11(7):637–45. doi:10.1016/s1470-2045(10)70131-5.
2. Green BL, Marshall HC, Collinson F, Quirke P, Guillou P, Jayne DG, et al. Long-term follow-up of the Medical Research Council CLASICC trial of conventional versus laparoscopically assisted resection in colorectal cancer. Br J Surg. 2013;100(1):75–82. doi:10.1002/bjs.8945.
3. van der Pas MH, Haglind E, Cuesta MA, Furst A, Lacy AM, Hop WC, et al. Laparoscopic versus open surgery for rectal cancer (COLOR II): short-term outcomes of a randomised, phase 3 trial. Lancet Oncol. 2013;14(3):210–8. doi:10.1016/s1470-2045(13)70016-0.
4. The National Comprehensive Cancer Network. http://www.nccn.org/professionals/physician_gls/pdf/rectal.pdf. Accessed 27 Jun 2015.
5. Esposito C. One-trocar appendectomy in pediatric surgery. Surg Endosc. 1998;12(2):177–8.
6. Maggiori L, Gaujoux S, Tribillon E, Bretagnol F, Panis Y. Single incision laparoscopy for colorectal resection: a systematic review and meta-analysis of more than a thousand procedures. Color Dis. 2012; doi:10.1111/j.1463-1318.2012.03105.x.

7. Poon JT, Cheung CW, Fan JK, Lo OS, Law WL. Single-incision versus conventional laparoscopic colectomy for colonic neoplasm: a randomized, controlled trial. Surg Endosc. 2012; doi:10.1007/s00464-012-2262-z.
8. Reibetanz J, Kerscher A, Kim M, Wierlemann A, Germer CT, Krajinovic K. Early-elective single-incision laparoscopic sigmoidectomy for perforated diverticulitis using a totally reusable single-port device. Surg Innov. 2012;19(1):45–9. doi:10.1177/1553350611413610.
9. Waters JA, Rapp BM, Guzman MJ, Jester AL, Selzer DJ, Robb BW, et al. Single-port laparoscopic right hemicolectomy: the first 100 resections. Dis Colon Rectum. 2012;55(2):134–9. doi:10.1097/DCR.0b013e31823c0ae4.
10. Makino T, Milsom JW, Lee SW. Feasibility and safety of single-incision laparoscopic colectomy: a systematic review. Ann Surg. 2012;255(4):667–76. doi:10.1097/SLA.0b013e31823fbae7.
11. Tokuoka M, Ide Y, Takeda M, Hashimoto Y, Matsuyama J, Yokoyama S, et al. Single-incision plus one-port laparoscopic abdominoperineal resection with bilateral pelvic lymph node dissection for advanced rectal cancer: a case report. Int Surg. 2015;100(1):15–20. doi:10.9738/intsurg-d-14-00232.1.
12. Perdawood SK, Lund T. Extralevator versus standard abdominoperineal excision for rectal cancer. Tech Coloproctol. 2015;19(3):145–52. doi:10.1007/s10151-014-1243-8.
13. Bae SU, Baek SJ, Min BS, Baik SH, Kim NK, Hur H. Reduced-port laparoscopic surgery for a tumor-specific mesorectal excision in patients with colorectal cancer: initial experience with 20 consecutive cases. Ann Coloproctol. 2015;31(1):16–22. doi:10.3393/ac.2015.31.1.16.
14. Lolle I, Rosenstock S, Bulut O. Single-port laparoscopic rectal surgery – a systematic review. Dan Med J. 2014;61(7):A4878.
15. Jung KU, Yun SH, Cho YB, Kim HC, Lee WY, Chun HK. Single incision and reduced port laparoscopic low anterior resection for rectal cancer: initial experience in 96 cases. ANZ J Surg. 2014; doi:10.1111/ans.12775.
16. Bulut O, Aslak KK, Rosenstock S. Technique and short-term outcomes of single-port surgery for rectal cancer: a feasibility study of 25 patients. Scand J Surg. 2014;103(1):26–33. doi:10.1177/1457496913495387.
17. Vestweber B, Galetin T, Lammerting K, Paul C, Giehl J, Straub E, et al. Single-incision laparoscopic surgery: outcomes from 224 colonic resections performed at a single center using SILS. Surg Endosc. 2013;27(2):434–42. doi:10.1007/s00464-012-2454-6.
18. Sourrouille I, Dumont F, Goere D, Honore C, Elias D. Resection of rectal cancer via an abdominal single-port access: short-term results and comparison with standard laparoscopy. Dis Colon Rectum. 2013;56(11):1203–10. doi:10.1007/dcr.12345678787890.
19. Sirikurnpiboon S, Jivapaisarnpong P. Single-access laparoscopic rectal surgery is technically feasible. Minim Invasive Surg. 2013;2013:687134. doi:10.1155/2013/687134.
20. Lauritsen ML, Bulut O. Single-port access laparoscopic abdominoperineal resection through the colostomy site: a case report. Tech Coloproctol. 2012;16(2):175–7. doi:10.1007/s10151-011-0694-4.
21. Hirano Y, Hattori M, Douden K, Shimizu S, Sato Y, Maeda K, et al. Single-incision plus one port laparoscopic anterior resection for rectal cancer as a reduced port surgery. Scand J Surg. 2012;101(4):283–6.
22. Hara M, Sato M, Takayama S, Imafuji H, Ogawa R, Takeyama H. Laparoscopic intersphincteric resection with a SILS port for very low rectal cancer: a case report. Surg Laparosc Endosc Percutan Tech. 2012;22(3):e138–41. doi:10.1097/SLE.0b013e318248b446.
23. Hua-Feng P, Zhi-Wei J, Gang W, Xin-Xin L, Feng-Tao L. A novel approach for the resection of low rectal cancer. Surg Laparosc Endosc Percutan Tech. 2012;22(6):537–41. doi:10.1097/SLE.0b013e31826d67e4.
24. Ali S, Moftah M, Ajmal N, Cahill RA. Single port-assisted fully laparoscopic abdominoperineal resection (APR) with immediate V-RAM flap reconstruction of the perineal defect. Updat Surg. 2012;64(3):217–21. doi:10.1007/s13304-012-0158-z.
25. Bulut O, Nielsen CB, Jespersen N. Single-port access laparoscopic surgery for rectal cancer: initial experience with 10 cases. Dis Colon Rectum. 2011;54(7):803–9. doi:10.1007/DCR.0b013e3182147b4d.

21 Single-Port Laparoscopic Abdominoperineal Resection

Giovanni Dapri

Abstract

Single-port laparoscopy (SPL) gained interest in the last decade, thanks to the attraction of performing minimally invasive surgery through natural orifices. In front of diseases where a tumor has to be removed, frequently the access site has to be enlarged at the end of SPL. Hence, the rationale of performing SPL in the suprapubic area and under the bikini line is for the resulting scar to be easily covered by the bikini and cosmetically acceptable. In this chapter, the SPL abdominoperineal resection, through a suprapubic access, is described.

Keywords

Single port • Laparoscopy • Abdominoperineal resection

21.1 Introduction

Single-port laparoscopy (SPL) gained interest in the last decade [1], thanks to the attraction of performing minimally invasive surgery through natural orifices [2]. The umbilicus, due to its embryological nature, has been considered as the main single-access site to perform SPL [3]. On the other hand, in diseases where a large tumor has to be removed, frequently the umbilical access site has to be enlarged at the end of SPL, and the final result can appear cosmetically inferior. Moreover, the risk of umbilical ventral hernia increases. SPL in the suprapubic area and under the bikini line results cosmetically acceptable [4] and it has been reported to be feasible and safe [4, 5]. In this chapter, the SPL abdominoperineal resection is described.

G. Dapri, M.D., Ph.D.
Department of Gastrointestinal Surgery, European School of Laparoscopic Surgery, Saint-Pierre University Hospital, 322, Rue Haute, 1000 Brussels, Belgium
e-mail: giovanni@dapri.net

G. Dapri, J.H. Marks (eds.), *Surgical Techniques in Rectal Cancer*,
https://doi.org/10.1007/978-4-431-55579-7_21

21.2 Preoperative Preparation and General Anesthesia

Patient is asked not to eat for at least 8 h prior to the procedure.

General anesthesia is induced intravenously (i.v.) with 0.2 mg/kg sufentanil, 2 mg/kg propofol, and 0.6 mg/kg rocuronium or 0.15 mg/kg cisatracurium. After tracheal intubation, anesthesia is maintained with 5–6% desflurane or 2% sevoflurane. In case of rapid sequence induction, 2 mg/kg etomidate or 2 mg/kg propofol and 1 mg/kg succinylcholine are used i.v., and a 0.2 mg/kg sufentanil and 0.1 mg/kg rocuronium are administered after the intubation.

Antibiotic and DVT prophylaxis are applied as well.

An arterial catheter, a central line, and a urinary catheter are placed.

21.3 Tools

21.3.1 Abdominal Table

- One scalpel, two tissue forceps, one monopolar electrode, two Farabeuf retractors, two Kocher-Ochsner curved forceps, one Mayo scissors, two Mayo-Hegar needle holders, two Pean-Rochester curved forceps, and one purse-string suture device (DAPRI purse-string suture device, Karl Storz—Endoskope, Tuttlingen, Germany), one monopolar electrode
- Sutures: one polydioxanon 1 (PDS 1, round tip, 1/2c, 36 mm), five polyglactin 1 (Vicryl 1, round tip, 1/2c, 27 mm), three polyamide 2/0 (Ethilon 2/0, straight needle, 60 mm), three polyglactin 2/0 (Vicryl 2/0, round tip, 1/2c, 36 mm), one polyglactin 3/0 (Vicryl 3/0, round tip, 1/2c, 26 mm), one poliglecaprone 4/0 (Monocryl 4/0, triangular tip, 3/8c, 16 mm), and four polyglactin rapide 3/0 (Vicryl Rapide 3/0, triangular tip, 1/2c, 22 mm)
- One reusable 11-mm rigid trocar
- One reusable 13-mm rigid trocar or one non-reusable 12-mm trocar
- Two reusable 6-mm flexible trocars and rigid mandrils (DAPRI flex trocars, Karl Storz—Endoskope)
- One straight 10-mm, 30°, and regular length scope (Karl Storz—Endoskope)
- One straight 5-mm, 30°, and long length scope (Karl Storz—Endoskope)
- One reusable bicurved grasping forceps (DAPRI grasping forceps I, Karl Storz—Endoskope) (Fig. 21.1a)
- One reusable monocurved grasping forceps (DAPRI grasping forceps IV, Karl Storz—Endoskope) (Fig. 21.1b)
- One reusable monocurved coagulating hook (DAPRI coagulating hook, Karl Storz—Endoskope) (Fig. 21.1c)
- One reusable monocurved dissecting forceps (DAPRI dissecting forceps, Karl Storz—Endoskope) (Fig. 21.1d)
- One reusable monocurved RoBi® bipolar grasping forceps (DAPRI bipolar grasping forceps, Karl Storz—Endoskope) (Fig. 21.1e)
- One reusable monocurved RoBi® bipolar scissors (DAPRI bipolar scissors, Karl Storz—Endoskope) (Fig. 21.1f)

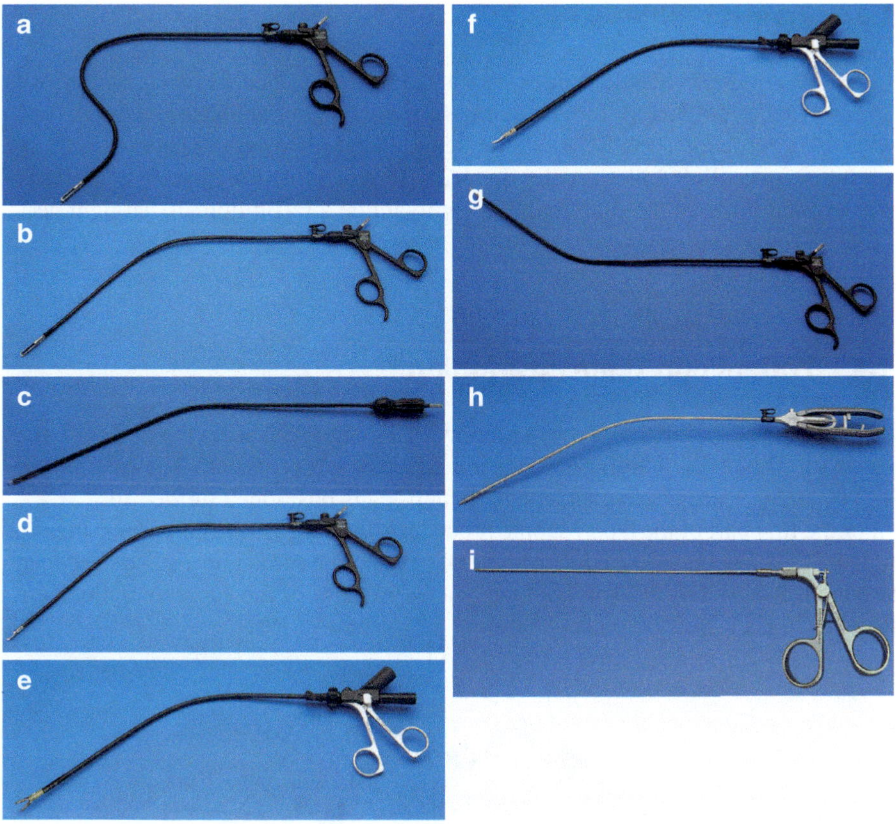

Fig. 21.1 (**a–i**) Reusable instruments according to DAPRI (Karl Storz—Endoskope, Tuttlingen, Germany): bicurved grasping forceps I (**a**), monocurved grasping forceps IV (**b**), monocurved coagulating hook (**c**), monocurved dissecting forceps (**d**), monocurved RoBi® bipolar grasping forceps (**e**), monocurved RoBi® bipolar scissors (**f**), monocurved scissors (**g**), monocurved needle holder I (**h**), straight 1.8-mm trocarless grasping forceps (**i**)

- One reusable straight 5-mm clip applier
- One reusable monocurved scissors (DAPRI scissors, Karl Storz—Endoskope) (Fig. 21.1g)
- One reusable monocurved needle holder (DAPRI needle holder I, Karl Storz—Endoskope) (Fig. 21.1h)
- One reusable monocurved suction and irrigation cannula (Karl Storz—Endoskope)
- One reusable straight grasping forceps
- One reusable Veress needle
- One reusable straight 1.8-mm trocarless grasping forceps (DAPRI trocarless grasping forceps, Karl Storz—Endoskope) (Fig. 21.1i)
- One non-reusable articulating–linear stapler
- Colostomy set

21.3.2 Perineal Table

- One Mayo-Hegar needle holder, two tissue forceps, one Mayo scissors, two Pean-Rochester curved forceps, one scalpel, one monopolar electrode, two Farabeuf retractors, one Beckman retractor, and two Doyen retractors
- Sutures: one silk 0 (silk 0, round tip, 1/2c, 26 mm), four polyglactin 2/0 (Vicryl 2/0, round tip, 1/2c, 36 mm), and three polyamide 2/0 (Ethilon 2/0, straight needle, 60 mm)
- Two suction drains

21.4 Patient and Team Positioning

The patient is placed in a supine position, with the arms alongside the body and the legs apart. The arms, ankles, and legs are secured and protected. These latter are well secured to the operative table, and the left leg is positioned further up.

For the first part of the laparoscopic procedure, the surgeon stands to the patient's right and the camera assistant to the surgeon's right. The scrub nurse stands between the patient's legs. The video monitor is placed in front of the surgeon and camera assistant (Fig. 21.2).

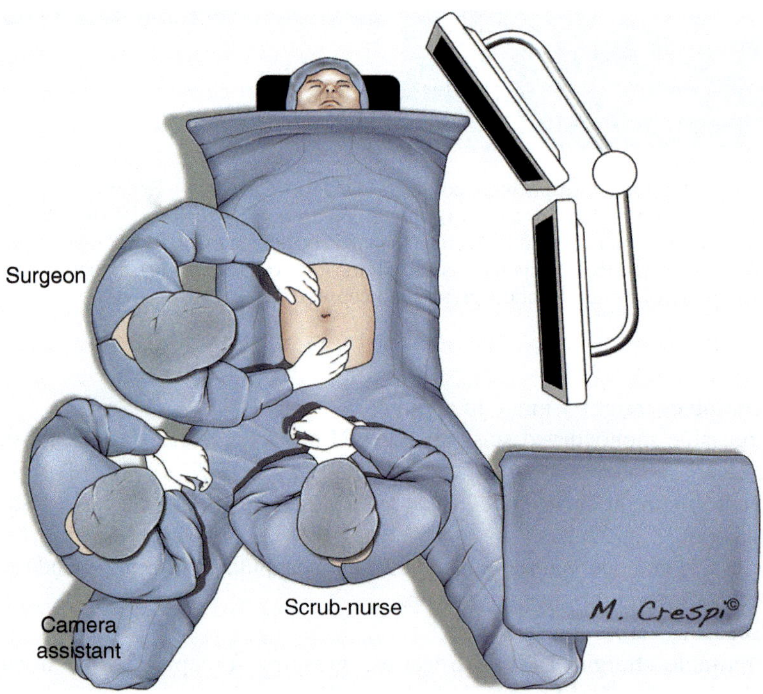

Fig. 21.2 Single-port laparoscopy: patient and team positioning. The copyright holder of this figure is the author.

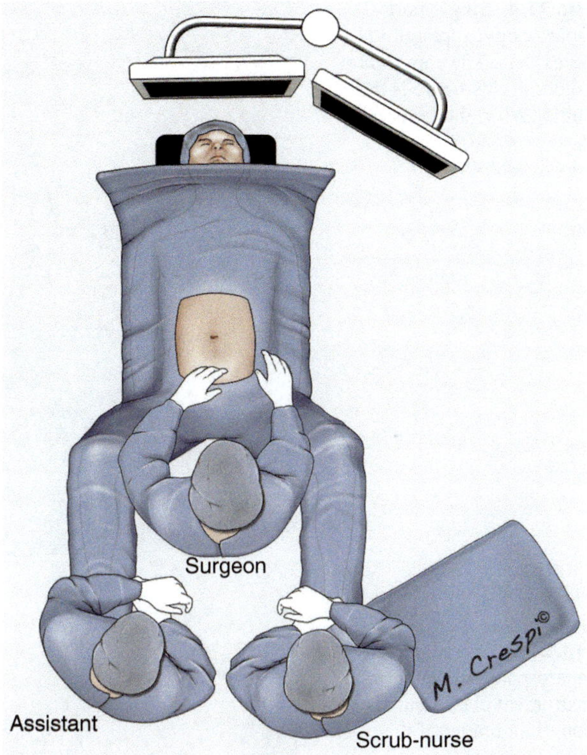

Fig. 21.3 Perineal approach: patient and team positioning. The copyright holder of this figure is the author.

Following the laparoscopic total mesorectal excision (TME), the camera assistant moves to the surgeon's left and the scrub nurse to the surgeon's right.

During the perineal resection, the surgeon stands between the patient's legs, the assistant to the surgeon's left, and the scrub nurse to the surgeon's right. The video monitor is placed in front of the surgeon and assistant (Fig. 21.3).

21.5 Technique

21.5.1 Single-Port Laparoscopy

A 3.5-cm transverse skin incision is made 1 cm above the pubic symphysis on the right side of the rectus abdominis muscle (Fig. 21.4). The underlying fascia is vertically divided in a pararectal fashion for 1.5 cm, which exposes the rectus abdominis muscle. The muscle is medially retracted, and a purse-string suture using PDS 1 is placed in the fascia, going inside and outside, respectively, at the 5, 7, 9, 11, 1, and 3 o'clock positions. The peritoneal sheet is entered through a 1-cm vertical incision, and a new purse-string suture using Vicryl 1 is placed, going inside and outside, respectively, at the 5, 7, 9, 11, 1, and 3 o'clock positions. Both sutures are kept externally with Pean-Rochester curved forceps.

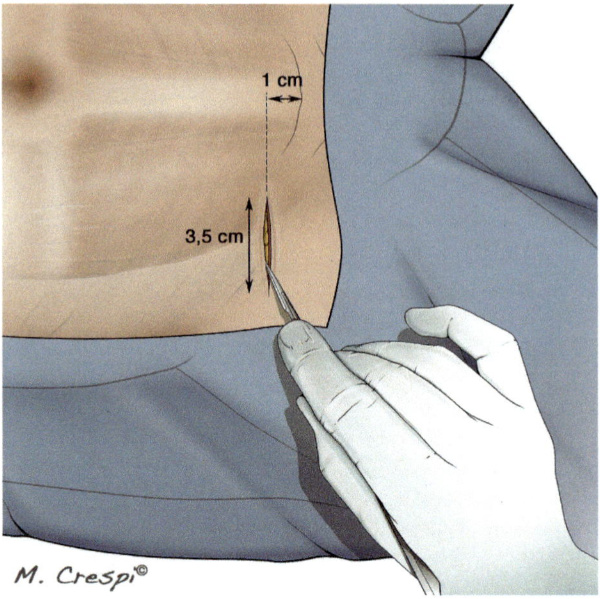

Fig. 21.4 Single-port laparoscopy: suprapubic access site. The copyright holder of this figure is the author. All rights reserved

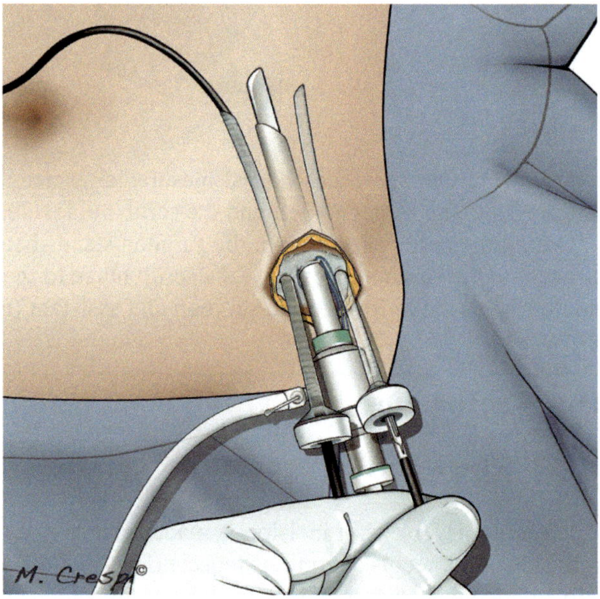

Fig. 21.5 Single-port laparoscopy: trocar and instrument placement. The copyright holder of this figure is the author. All rights reserved

An 11-mm rigid trocar (or a 12-mm non-reusable trocar) is inserted into both purse-string sutures in order to accommodate the 10-mm 30° scope, and the pneumoperitoneum is created.

A 6-mm flexible trocar is inserted at the 12 o'clock position with respect to the patient's head, outside the purse-string sutures and on the same vertical line as the previous trocar, for the insertion of the bicurved grasping forceps I (Fig. 21.5). The

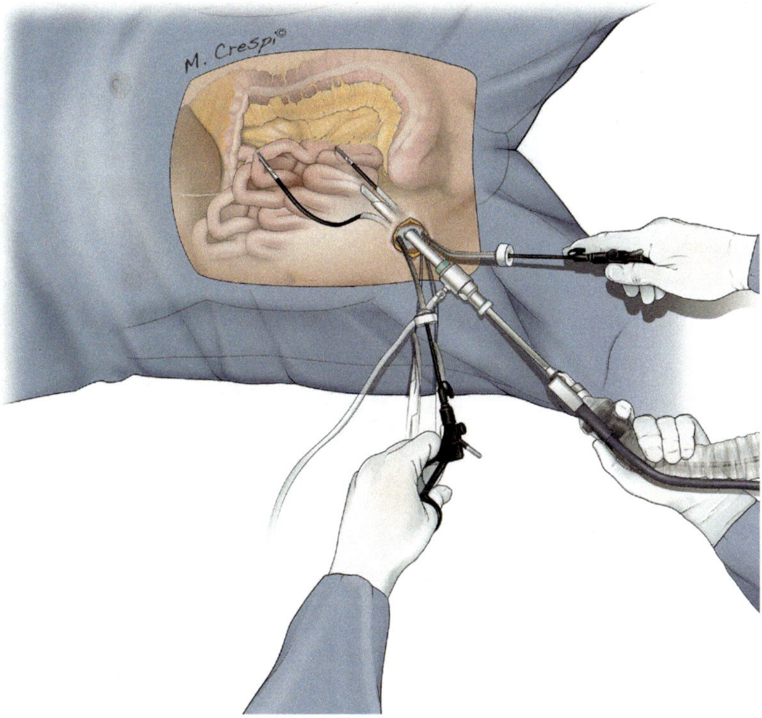

Fig. 21.6 Single-port laparoscopy: placement of the small bowel on the right liver. The copyright holder of this figure is the author. All rights reserved

grasping forceps is inserted following its curves at 45° with respect to the abdominal wall.

Another 6-mm flexible trocar is inserted at the 6 o'clock position with respect to the patient's head, outside the purse-string sutures and on the same vertical line as the previous trocars, for the insertion of other instruments (Fig. 21.5), such as the monocurved grasping forceps IV, the monocurved coagulating hook, the monocurved dissecting forceps, the monocurved bipolar forceps and scissors, the straight 5-mm clip applier, the monocurved scissors, the monocurved needle holder I, the monocurved suction and irrigation cannula, and the straight grasping forceps.

The abdominal cavity is explored and examined to rule out the presence of peritoneal metastases, superficial hepatic lesions, and free ascites.

The operating room table is placed in an accentuated Trendelenburg position with right-sided tilt.

The small bowel is moved into the right abdominal quadrants and above the right liver lobe, using the bicurved and the monocurved grasping forceps (Fig. 21.6).

The ligament of Treitz is identified in order to expose the root of the inferior mesenteric vein. The peritoneal sheet covering the root of this vein is incised by the monocurved coagulating hook until the Toldt's fascia is reached. The inferior

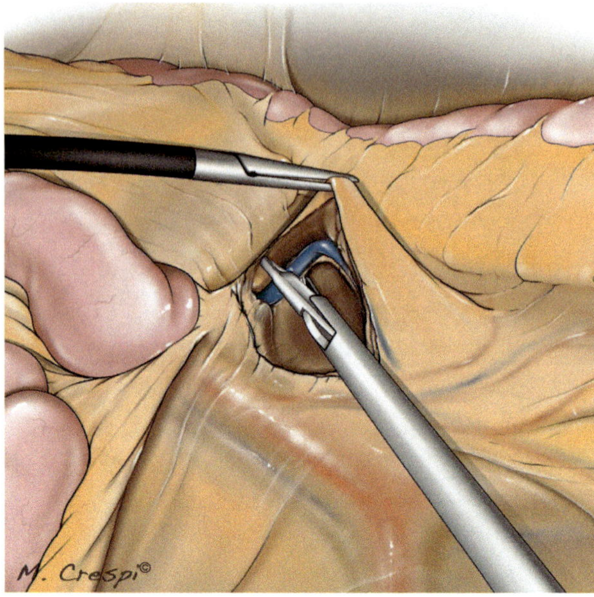

Fig. 21.7 Single-port laparoscopy: inferior mesenteric vein section. The copyright holder of this figure is the author.

mesenteric vein is isolated using the monocurved dissecting forceps and clipped by the 5-mm straight clip applier (Fig. 21.7).

The left mesocolon is separated from the Toldt's fascia in an avascular plane using the monocurved coagulating hook or the monocurved suction cannula.

The surgeon works with curved instruments without crossing hands and without interference with the camera assistant's hand (Fig. 21.8).

The peritoneal sheet is incised along the abdominal aorta by the monocurved coagulating hook, reaching the origin of the inferior mesenteric artery. The root of the artery is freed using the monocurved coagulating hook and the monocurved dissecting forceps, clipped by the 5-mm straight clip applier, and divided by the monocurved scissors (Fig. 21.9).

The left mesocolon is freed from the Toldt's fascia (Fig. 21.10), respecting the left Gerota's fascia and proceeding in the direction of the pancreatic tail.

The procedure is continued with mobilization of the left mesocolon reaching the promontory (Fig. 21.11). The upper mesorectum is incised and dissected from the presacral fascia in an avascular plane, using the monocurved coagulating hook and the monocurved bipolar grasping forceps and scissors (Fig. 21.12).

For the rest of the TME, the camera assistant moves to the surgeon's left and the scrub nurse to the surgeon's right. To improve the pelvic field's exposure, one temporary percutaneous suture using a straight Ethilon 2/0 needle is passed from the suprapubic area into the uterine fundus (female) (Fig. 21.13). Moreover, a straight 1.8-mm trocarless grasping forceps can be inserted percutaneously by a skin puncture (created by a Veress needle) in the left flank, or another straight Ethilon 2/0 needle can be passed in the pericolic fatty tissue, helping in the rectosigmoid colon retraction.

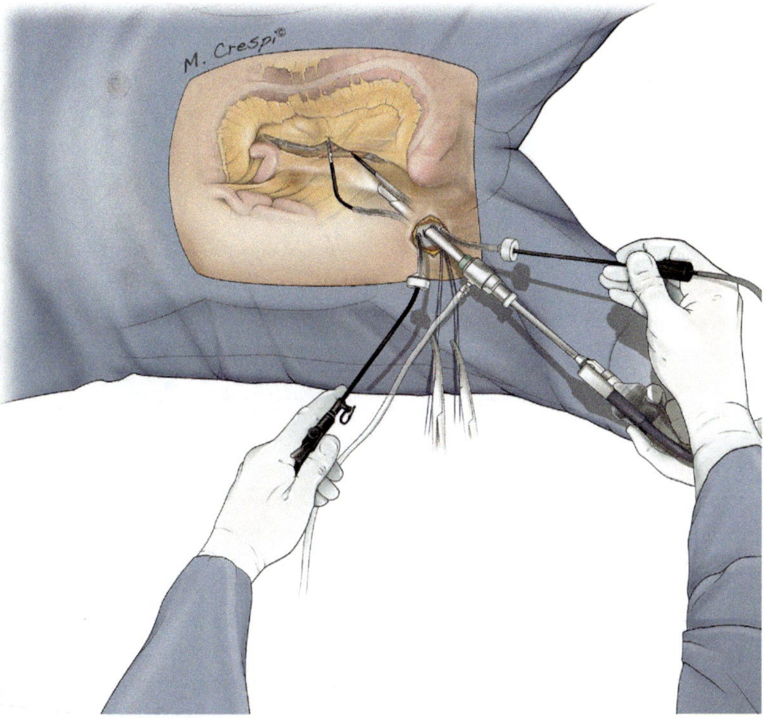

Fig. 21.8 Single-port laparoscopy: left mesocolic dissection and surgeon's ergonomy.

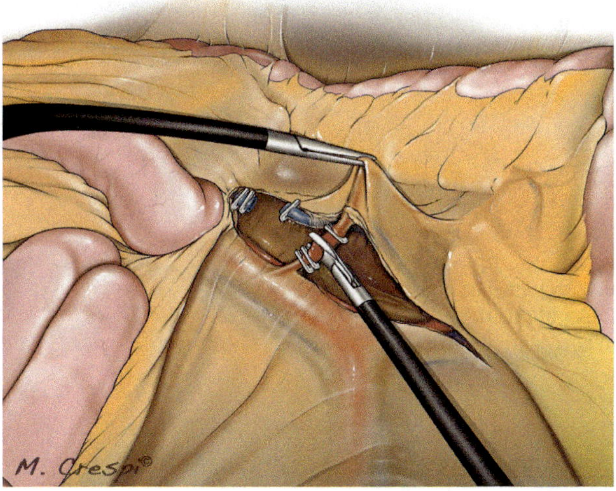

Fig. 21.9 Single-port laparoscopy: inferior mesenteric artery section

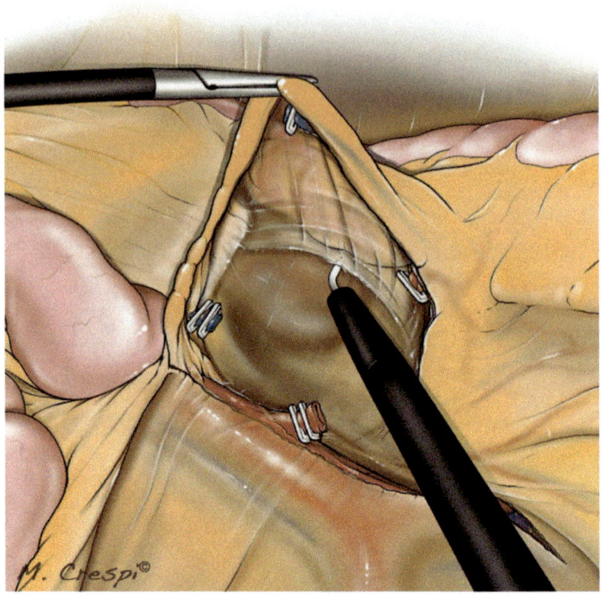

Fig. 21.10 Single-port laparoscopy: mesocolic dissection respecting the Toldt's fascia. The copyright holder of this figure is the author.

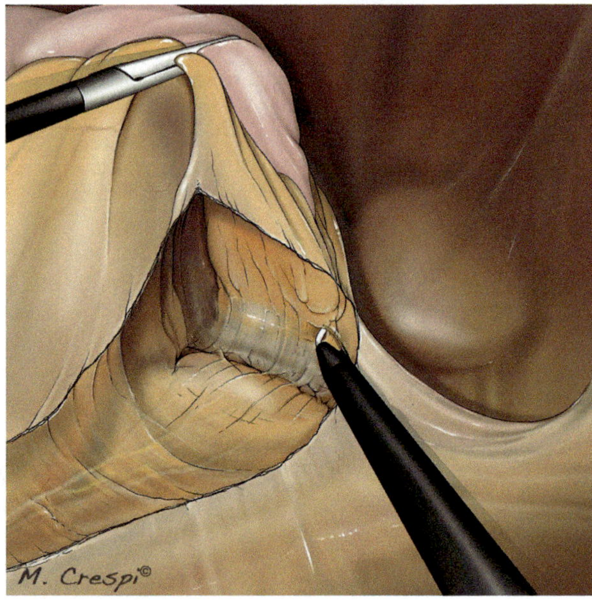

Fig. 21.11 Single-port laparoscopy: upper mesorectum. The copyright holder of this figure is the author.

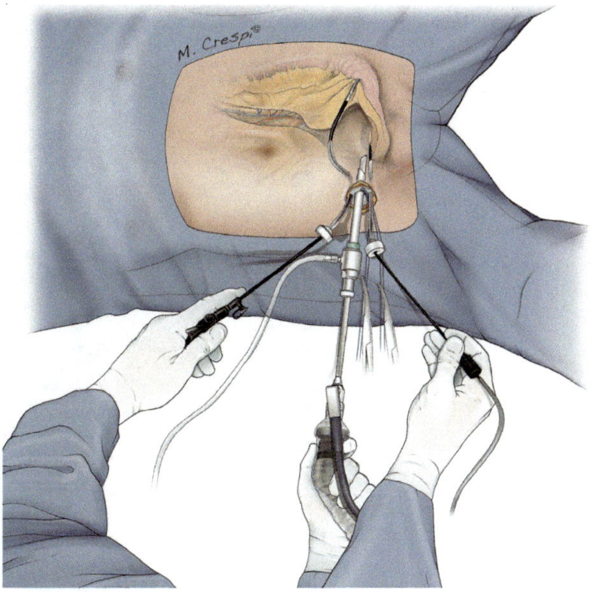

Fig. 21.12 Single-port laparoscopy: mobilization under surgeon's ergonomy.

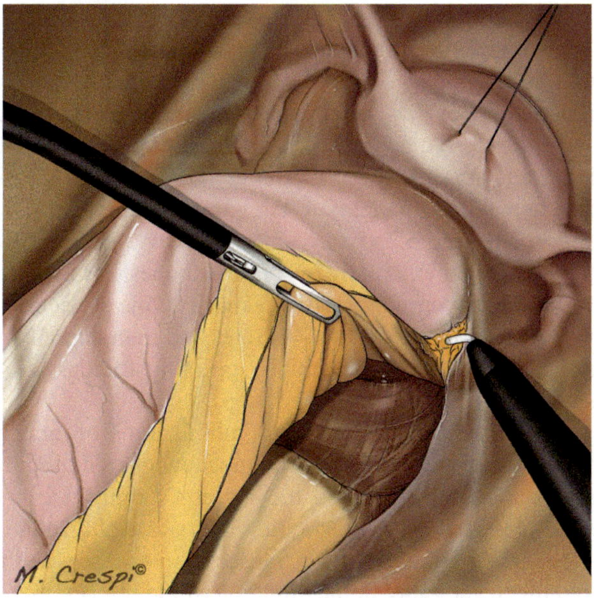

Fig. 21.13 Single-port laparoscopy: uterus retraction and right lateral mobilization of the rectum.

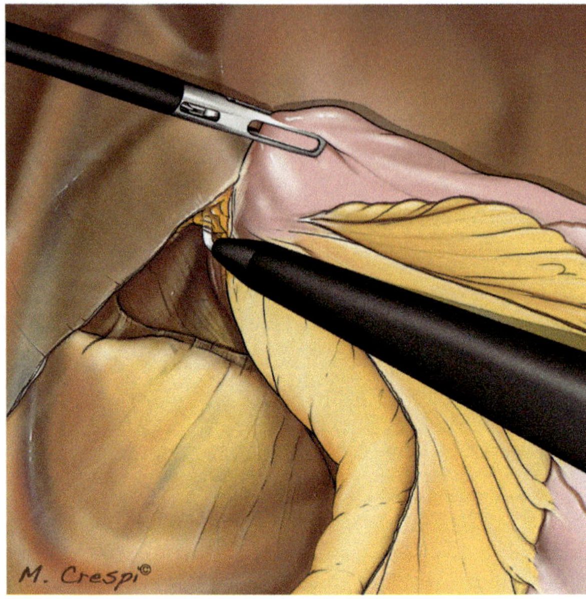

Fig. 21.14 Single-port laparoscopy: left lateral mobilization of the rectum.

The middle mesorectum is dissected posteriorly and then laterally, using both the coagulating hook and bipolar instruments (Figs. 21.13 and 21.14). The anterior peritoneal sheet is opened by the monocurved coagulating hook, and the plane anterior to the rectum and posterior to the seminal vesicles/rectoprostatic fascia (male) (Fig. 21.15) or uterine cervix (female) (Fig. 21.16) is dissected. At this step in both male and female patients, a temporary suprapubic percutaneous suture (straight Ethilon 2/0 needle) is passed into the pelvic peritoneal reflexion (Figs. 21.17 and 21.18) and kept externally by a Pean-Rochester curved forceps.

Once the lower mesorectum is reached, the dissection continues, first posteriorly to reach both the levator ani muscles and then laterally and anteriorly (Figs. 21.19 and 21.20). Monocurved bipolar grasping forceps and scissors are continuously used and exchanged during this step.

The procedure continues with mobilization of the sigmoid and left colon from the peritoneal attachments, using the monocurved coagulating hook or scissors. The camera assistant returns to the surgeon's right and the scrub nurse between the patient's legs. Usually it is not necessary to mobilize the splenic flexure.

The level of the left colon transection is chosen, and the mesocolon is dissected from this level going in the direction of the inferior mesenteric vein root, using the monocurved coagulating hook and bipolar tools.

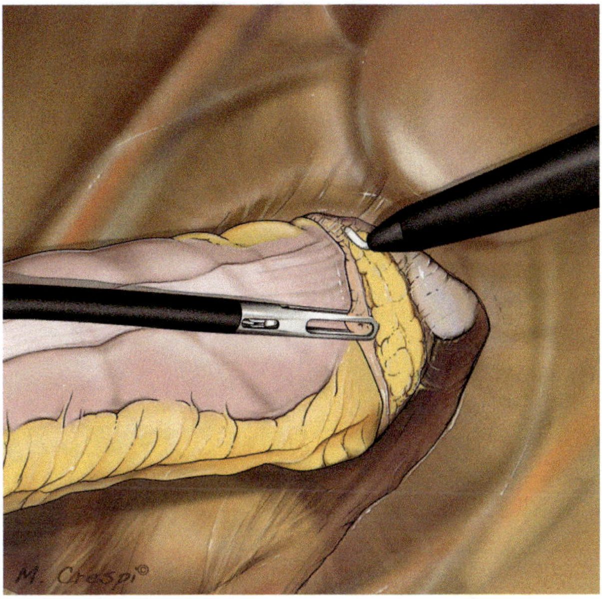

Fig. 21.15 Single-port laparoscopy: anterior mobilization of the middle rectum in male patient.

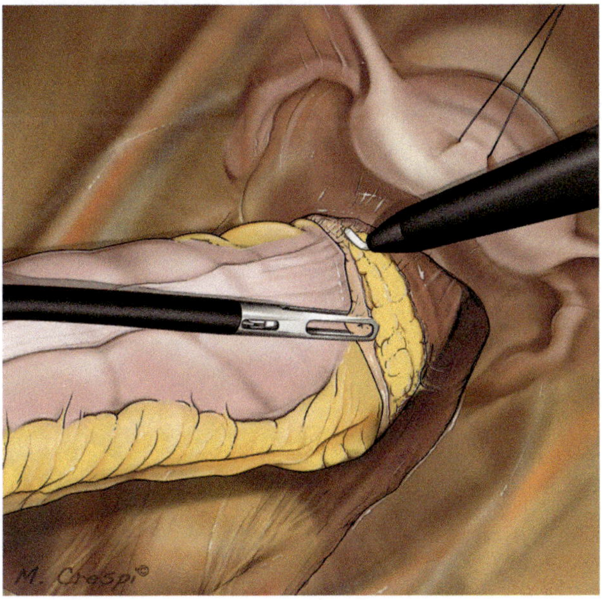

Fig. 21.16 Single-port laparoscopy: anterior mobilization of the middle rectum in female patient.

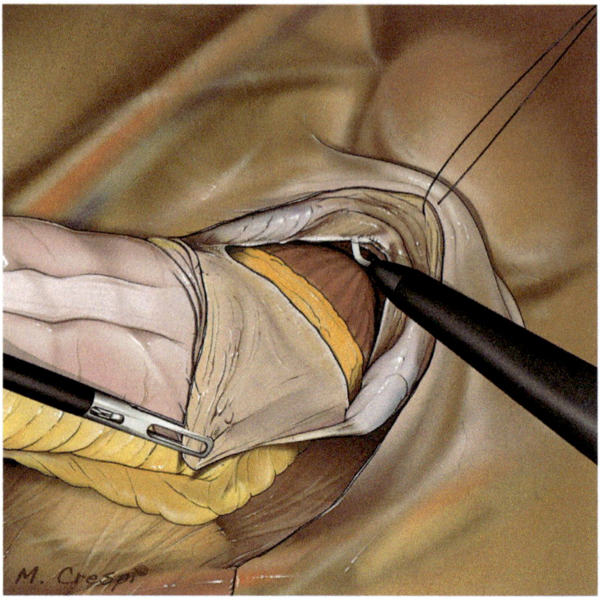

Fig. 21.17 Single-port laparoscopy: anterior mobilization of the low rectum in male patient. The copyright holder of this figure is the author. All rights reserved

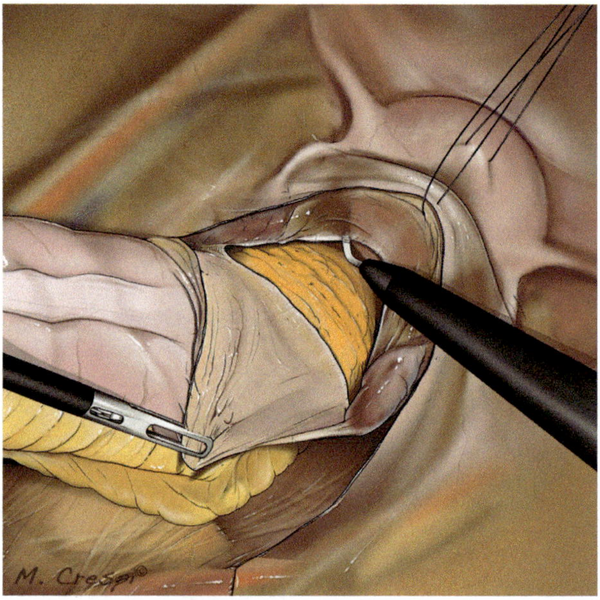

Fig. 21.18 Single-port laparoscopy: anterior mobilization of the low rectum in female patient. The copyright holder of this figure is the author. All rights reserved

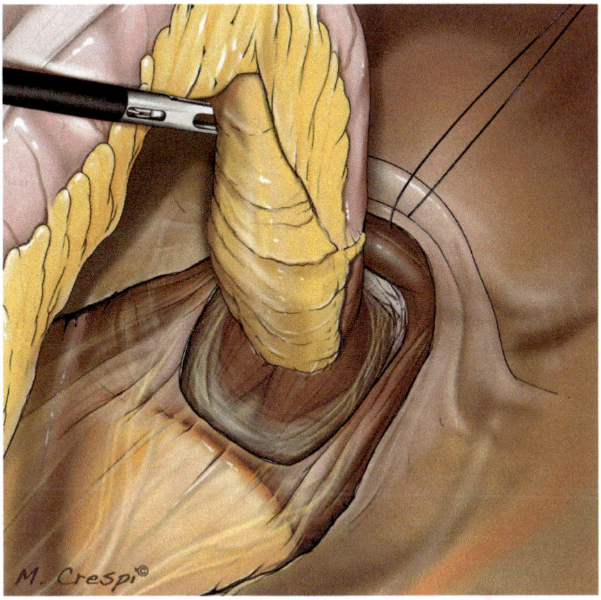

Fig. 21.19 Single-port laparoscopy: complete mobilization of the rectum in male patient. The copyright holder of this figure is the author. All rights reserved

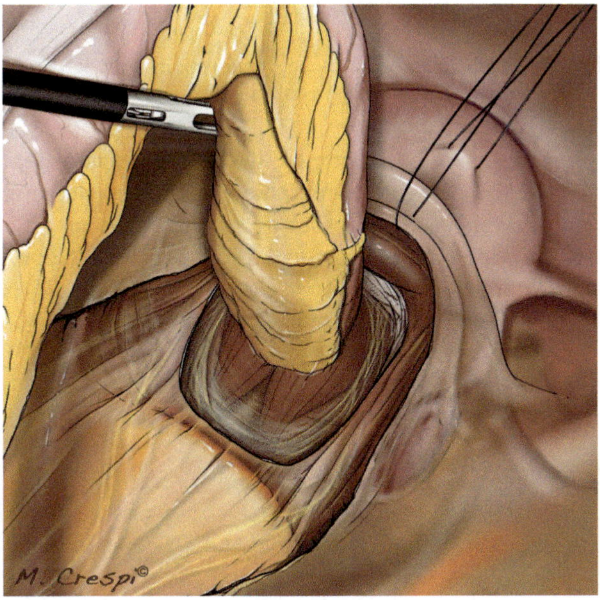

Fig. 21.20 Single-port laparoscopy: complete mobilization of the rectum in female patient. The copyright holder of this figure is the author. All rights reserved

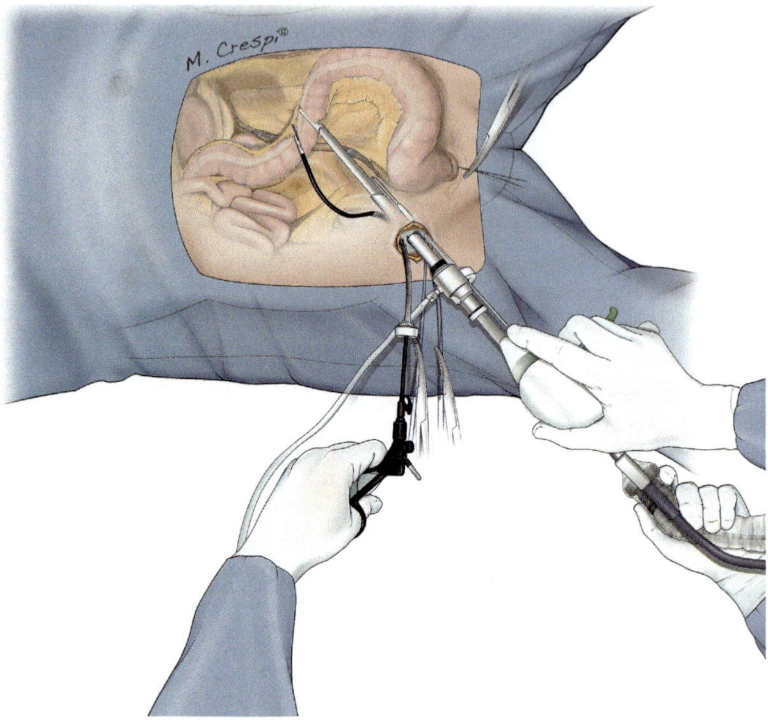

Fig. 21.21 Single-port laparoscopy: transection of the left colon using a linear stapler under a 5-mm scope view.

For the left colon sectioning, the 11-mm trocar is replaced by a reusable 13-mm trocar (if the 12-mm non-reusable trocar is inserted at the beginning, this replacement is not needed), in order to accommodate an articulating linear stapler. The 10-mm scope is switched for a 5-mm 30° long scope, which is inserted into the 6-mm flexible trocar at the 6 o'clock position (Fig. 21.21). The linear stapler encircles the left colon and is fired.

21.5.2 Perineal Approach

Both patient's legs are positioned up (gynecologic positioning). The cutaneous ani has already been closed by a purse-string suture using silk 0, after the patient was positioned on the operative table and anesthetized and before placing any sterile towels. In this way, the risk of any infection is avoided.

After having performed the laparoscopic abdominal step, the skin around the anus is incised in ellipse pattern. The fatty tissue is dissected until the muscular plane of the levator ani is reached (Fig. 21.22). The dissection is performed starting on the left side, then on the right side, and finally inferiorly and anteriorly. Once the levator ani plane is exposed, an incision anteriorly to the coccyx is made, going deeply in the previous plane dissected by laparoscopy.

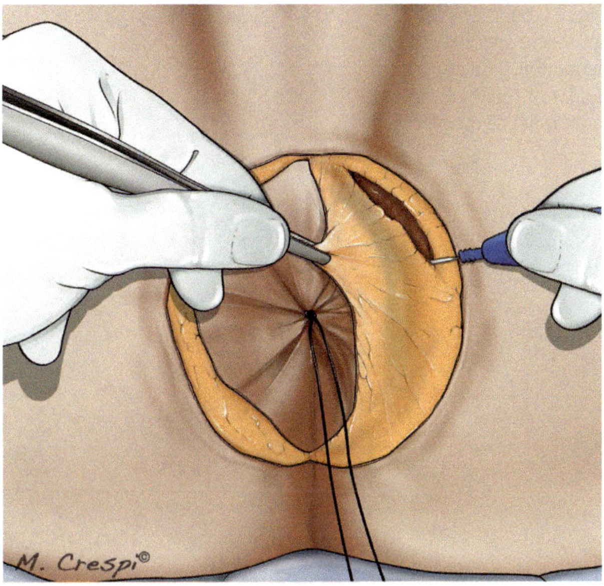

Fig. 21.22 Perineal approach: beginning of the dissection.

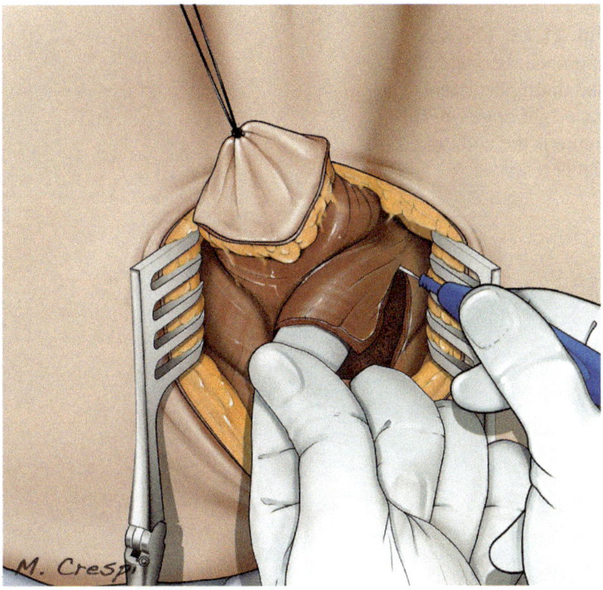

Fig. 21.23 Perineal approach: mobilization of the anorectal bloc.

A dissection in the levator ani muscles is performed on the left side of the patient (Fig. 21.23) and then on the right side, staying laterally to the anal sphincter. Finally, the anterior muscle plane is freed.

Once the anal portion is completely freed, the rectosigmoid colon is removed transanally (Fig. 21.24). Two perineal drains are positioned in the pelvic space (Fig. 21.25). The perineal fatty tissue is closed by Vicryl 2/0 sutures and the skin by Ethilon 2/0 sutures (Fig. 21.25).

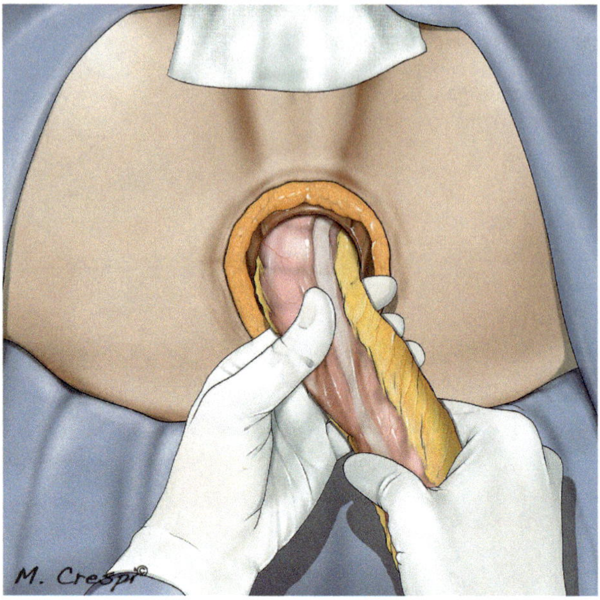

Fig. 21.24 Perineal approach: specimen's extraction. The copyright holder of this figure is the author. All rights reserved

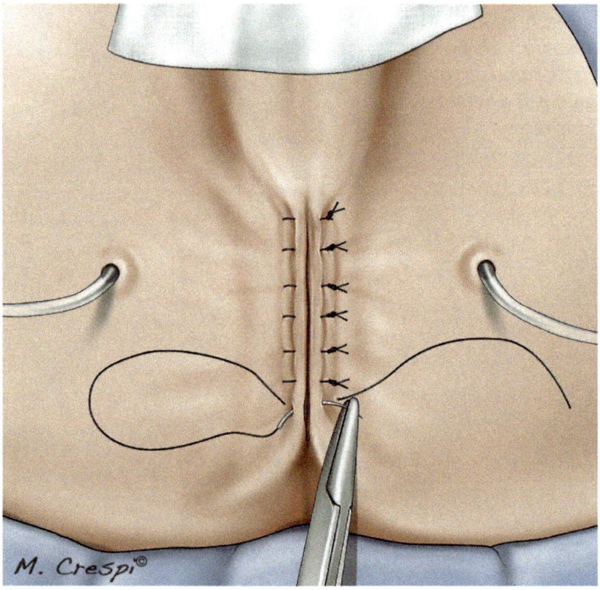

Fig. 21.25 Perineal approach: perineal closure and drain placement. The copyright holder of this figure is the author. All rights reserved

21.5.3 End of Procedure and Colostomy

The monocurved needle holder is introduced beside the bicurved grasping forceps (Fig. 21.26). The parietal pelvic peritoneum is closed by a running suture using Vicryl 2/0 (a preformed knot at its extremity is useful to gain operative time), after having removed the temporary percutaneous Ethilon 2/0 sutures (Fig. 21.27).

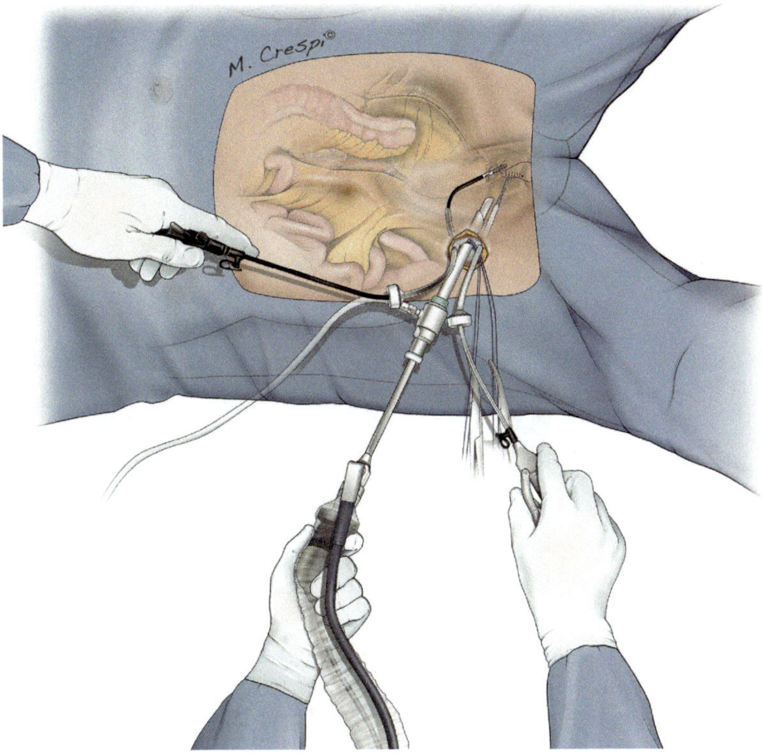

Fig. 21.26 Single-port laparoscopy: surgeon's ergonomy (Fig. 21.26). during pelvic peritoneum closure (Fig. 21.27).

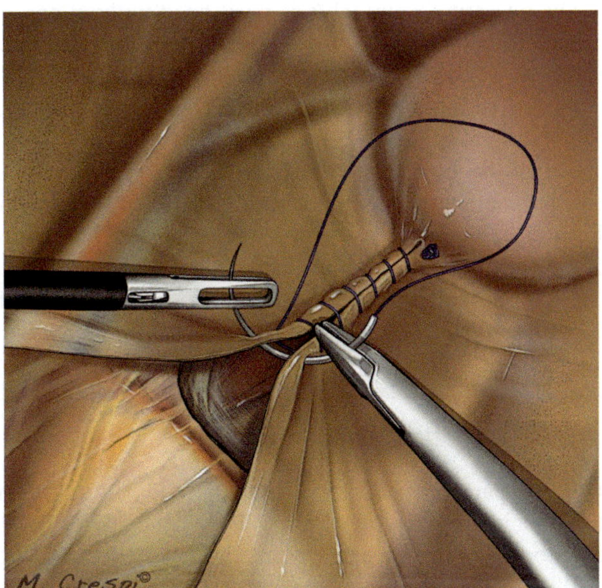

Fig. 21.27 Single-port laparoscopy: surgeon's ergonomy (Fig. 21.26). during pelvic peritoneum closure (Fig. 21.27).

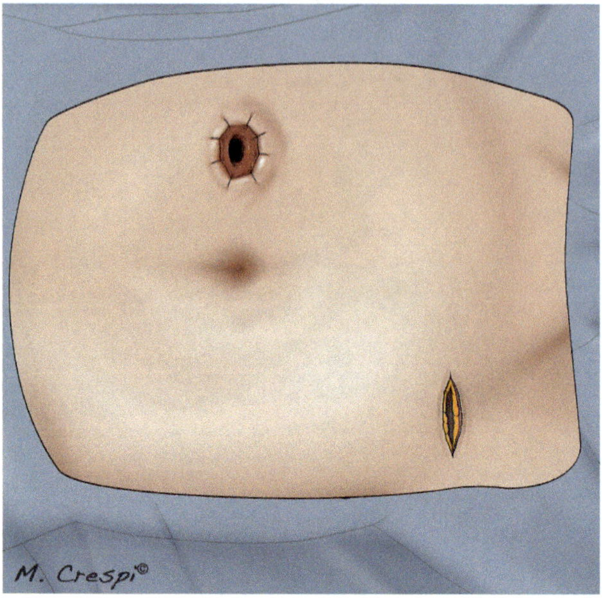

Fig. 21.28 Final view of the procedure: colostomy in the left flank and suprapubic access.

The distal left colon is taken up by the bicurved grasping forceps in the direction of the chosen colostomy site. The peritoneal sheet from the parietal wall until the chosen colostomy site is dissected and fixed by a Vicryl 2/0 running suture to the left colon, in order to cover this latter in part.

The skin, at the chosen colostomy site, is incised and both fascia and peritoneal sheet opened. The colic stump (maintained closed) is fixed to the posterior and anterior abdominis muscle fascia by Vicryl 3/0 sutures.

The operating room table is positioned without any Trendelenburg and tilt, and the small bowel is gently moved out of the right abdominal quadrants and over the left colon. No drain is left in the abdominal cavity.

The curved instruments are retrieved following the curves at 45° with respect to the abdominal wall.

Both purse-string sutures are retrieved together with the three trocars. The peritoneal sheet and the rectus abdominis muscle fascia are meticulously and separately closed by converging Vicryl 1 running sutures. The suprapubic cutaneous scar is joined by Monocryl 4/0 intradermic sutures.

The colic stump in the left flank is opened, fixing the mucosa to the skin by Vicryl Rapide 3/0 (Fig. 21.28). The colostomy pouch is placed.

21.6 Postoperative Care

One gram paracetamol is given i.v. at the end of the surgical procedure. Postoperative analgesia is given following the WHO visual analog pain scale (VAS). In the recovery room, the following scheme is followed: for VAS between 1 and 3, 1 g paracetamol i.v. is pushed; for VAS between 4 and 8, 100 mg tramadol i.v. is used; and for VAS greater than 8, 1 mg piritramide i.v. is incremented.

The arterial catheter is removed in the recovery room.

Once the patient leaves the recovery room, pain is assessed every 6 h, with 1 g paracetamol administered i.v. if VAS is between 1 and 3 and 100 mg tramadol administered i.v. if VAS is between 4 and 8.

Antibiotic prophylaxis is prescribed if necessary and DVT prophylaxis until discharge of the patient from the hospital. The urinary catheter is removed after 5 days. The patient is allowed to drink water after 24 h and to tolerate a light diet from the third postoperative day. The management of the colostomy is started after 48 h. If there are no complications, the two perineal drains are removed on the seventh postoperative day, and the patient can be discharged.

Upon discharge, 1 g paracetamol perorally or 50 mg tramadol perorally is prescribed only if needed.

Office visits are scheduled at 10 days and 1 and 3, 6, and 12 months after the procedure.

References

1. Dapri G. Single-incision laparoscopy: a review of the indications, techniques and results after more than 700 procedures. Asian J Endosc Surg. 2014;7(2):102–16.
2. Mathias JM. NOTES: a new way of performing surgery using natural body orifices. OR Manager. 2007;23(7):1,12–3.
3. Canes D, Desai MM, Aron M, Haber GP, Goel RK, Stein RJ, Kaouk JH, Gill IS. Transumbilical single-port surgery: evolution and current status. Eur Urol. 2008;54(5):1020–9.
4. Dapri G. Suprapubic single-incision laparoscopic left hemicolectomy: an alternative non-visible scar. Ann Surg Oncol. 2014;21(3):841–2.
5. Dapri G, Carandina S, Mathonet P, Himpens J, Cadière GB. Suprapubic single-incision laparoscopic right hemicolectomy with intracorporeal anastomosis. Sug Innov. 2013;20(5):484–92.

Robotic-Assisted Abdominoperineal Resection

22

Paolo Pietro Bianchi, Giampaolo Formisano, and Giuseppe Giuliani

Abstract

In 1908, Sir Ernest Miles reported his first attempt to develop a radical operation for rectal cancer, publishing his experience with abdominoperineal resection (APR).

The introduction of the embriologically based concept of total mesorectal excision (TME) and the increasing use of intersphincteric resection in combination with neoadjuvant chemoradiotherapy have further contributed to improve oncological outcomes and have significantly reduced the need of APR even for low rectal cancers.

Nevertheless, APR is still strictly indicated in patients with type IV low rectal cancer (<6 cm from the anal verge), defined as transanal tumors with external anal sphincter or levator ani muscle invasion.

Though randomized trials have shown that minimally invasive TME is oncologically as safe as open surgery, it is technically a demanding procedure and has a steep learning curve. Robotic surgery, thanks to its technological advantages, may potentially overcome these limitations especially in lower mesorectal dissection and, potentially, in transabdominal levator ani transection. This might help to reduce CRM positivity and, ultimately, local recurrence rates for ultralow rectal cancer-requiring APR.

Keywords

Robotic surgery • Robotic abdominoperineal resection • Rectal cancer • Robotic-assisted total mesorectal excision

P.P. Bianchi, M.D. (✉) • G. Formisano, M.D. • G. Giuliani, M.D.
Department of General and Minimally-Invasive Surgery, International School of Robotic Surgery, Misericordia Hospital, Via Senese 169, 58100 Grosseto, Italy
e-mail: paolopietro.bianchi@fastwebnet.it

G. Dapri, J.H. Marks (eds.), *Surgical Techniques in Rectal Cancer*,
https://doi.org/10.1007/978-4-431-55579-7_22

22.1 Introduction

The first attempt to develop a radical operation for rectal cancer dates back to 1908, when Sir Ernest Miles reported the first 12 cases of abdominoperineal resection (APR) [1].

With the intention to reduce the local recurrence rates in an era of perineal-only procedures, Miles focused his attention on the lymphatic drainage of the rectum by distinguishing three patterns, upward, lateral, and downward, thus supporting the theory that lymphatic drainage can occur in all directions ("cylindrical concept"). Miles sustained that recurrence could be decreased by removing the pelvic colon, its mesentery, the rectum, and as much of the lymphatic drainage as possible: these are the basis of the APR with a combined transabdominal and perineal approach [2].

The introduction of the embriologically based concept of total mesorectal excision (TME) by Heald [3, 4] and the increasing use of intersphincteric resection in combination with neoadjuvant chemoradiotherapy have further contributed to improve oncological outcomes and have significantly reduced the need of APR even for low rectal cancers [5, 6].

Nevertheless, APR rate is still high though consistently variable: it ranges from 5 to 55% in the United Kingdom and from 6 to 100% in the United States, depending on the local expertise of institutions or areas [7]. According to classification of low rectal cancer proposed by Rullier et al. [7], APR is strictly indicated in patients with type IV of low rectal cancer (<6 cm from the anal verge), defined as transanal tumors with external anal sphincter or levator ani muscle invasion.

As far as the abdominal phase is concerned, minimally invasive TME is gaining increasing worldwide acceptance since three randomized controlled trials have proven that it is oncologically as safe as open surgery [8–10]. However, minimally invasive TME is technically demanding and has a steep learning curve: robotic surgery may potentially overcome these limitations in lower dissection and difficult pelvis.

Moreover, though levator ani division has been traditionally carried out via a perineal approach, some reports of robotic transabdominal pelvic floor excision have been recently published [11–13], thus highlighting another interesting field of investigation for future studies.

Technical details of full-robotic APR will be discussed in this chapter.

22.2 Surgical Technique

All procedures were performed with the da Vinci Si Surgical Platform (Intuitive Surgical Inc., Sunnyvale, CA, USA) with a full-robotic single-docking technique.

22.2.1 Patient Positioning

The patient is placed in lithotomy position with arms alongside the body and is carefully secured with shoulder supports on both sides of the neck to prevent sliding.

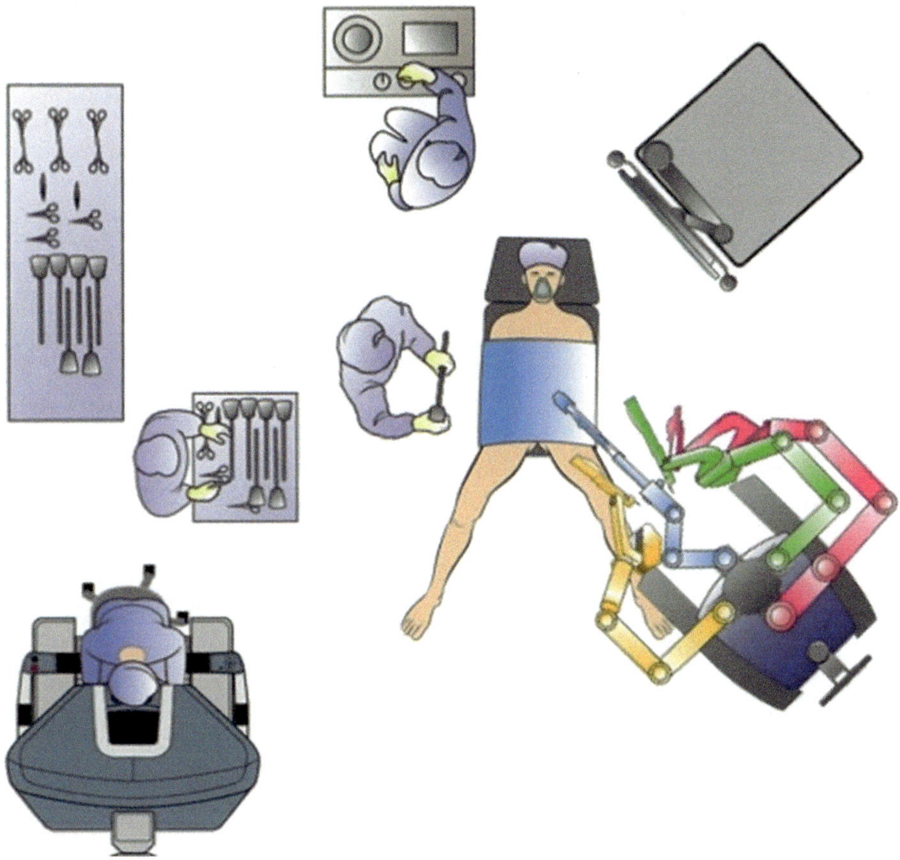

Fig. 22.1 OR setup for robotic abdominoperineal resection

The preparation is concluded by the insertion of a Foley catheter and a nasogastric tube. A body warmer and a compression device for deep venous thrombosis prophylaxis are used, and antibiotic prophylaxis is administered.

The first assistant stands on the patient's right side. The scrub nurse is at the lower right side of the table, and the assistant's monitor is located at the patient's left shoulder. The cart is placed at the patient's left side and is docked from the left lower quadrant over the left hip with an angle of approximately 45°. OR setup is shown in Fig. 22.1.

22.2.2 Port Placement

A Veress needle is inserted in the left hypochondrium (Palmer's point) for the induction of a 12-mmHg pneumoperitoneum. Anatomic landmarks are then identified and marked, together with the midpoint between pubic symphysis and the xyphoid process (real navel).

Fig. 22.2 Trocar layout

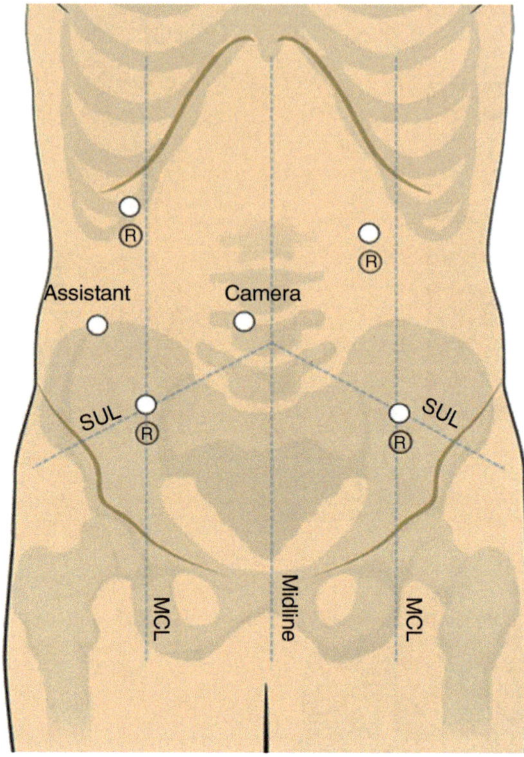

The trocars are placed as follows (Fig. 22.2):

- A 12-mm standard laparoscopic trocar for robotic camera (0–30°) is placed about 2 cm lateral and 2–3 cm above the real umbilicus.
- One 8-mm robotic trocar (R1) on the right lower quadrant, at the intersection between the spinoumbilical line (SUL) and the midclavicular line (MCL).
- One 8-mm robotic port in the right upper quadrant (R3 during vascular control), slightly lateral to the right MCL, and 2–3 cm below the costal margin.
- One 8-mm robotic port robotic arm (R3 during TME) in the left upper quadrant, 4–5 cm below the costal margin, and 4–5 cm lateral to the midline.
- One 8-mm robotic port (R2) in the left lower quadrant, 2 cm lateral to the MCL.
- A 12-mm standard laparoscopic trocar is placed in right flank, 2–3 cm lateral to the right MCL, as assistant port for graspers and/or suction–irrigator device.

22.2.3 Robot Positioning and Docking

A complete exploration of the abdominal cavity is performed to rule out peritoneal seeding. If present, adhesions are freed, and an intraoperative liver ultrasonography is carried out with a laparoscopic-dedicated probe to complete the intraoperative staging of the disease. The patient is then placed in a 20–25° Trendelenburg position with a 20–25° right tilt: the greater omentum and the

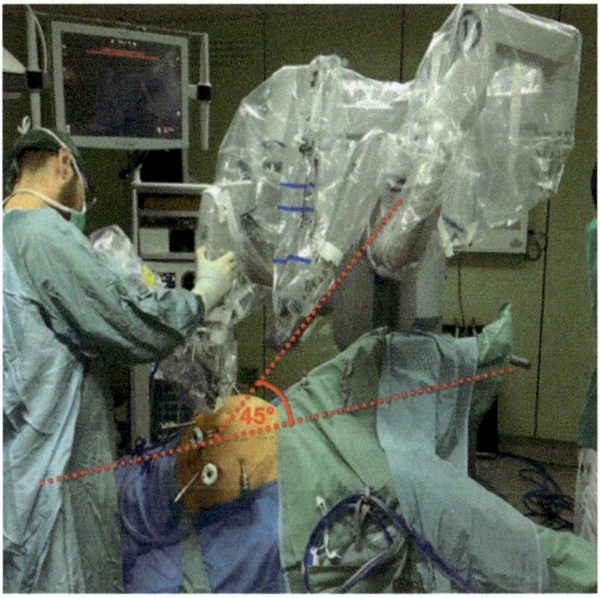

Fig. 22.3 Patient and cart position

small bowel loops are retracted out of the pelvic area into the right upper quadrant laparoscopically.

The robotic cart is then approximated and docked from the left hip of the patient. To adjust the positioning correctly, the following steps are carried out:

- Align the camera arm with the center column.
- Position the setup joint in the "sweet spot" by placing the blue arrow on the camera arm in the middle of the blue bar located on the camera arm setup joint.
- Move the cart to the patient so that a straight line passes through the center column, the camera arm, the left anterior superior iliac spine, and the camera trocar.
- When the camera arm joins the camera trocar, the robotic cart is in the correct position and does not require further adjustments.

Then robotic arms are then connected to the trocars, starting from the camera, and patient positioning will not be changed during all the steps of the procedure. Robotic instruments are then inserted under visual control (Fig. 22.3).

22.3 Step-by-Step Review of Critical Elements of the Procedure

Full-robotic single-docking APR is essentially based on four steps:

1. Vascular control
2. Sigmoid colon mobilization
3. Total mesorectal excision (TME)
4. Perineal phase and specimen extraction

22.3.1 Vascular Control

The procedure starts with the following arm setup (Fig. 22.4):

- R1: Cautery hook (right iliac fossa)
- R2: ProGrasp™ Forceps (left iliac fossa)
- R3: Bipolar forceps (right hypochondrium)

R1 and R3 are the operative arms, whereas R2 is used for stable retraction. The assistant trocar is used for suction/irrigator, clip applier, swab introduction, or additional retraction if needed.

The assistant grasper and the robotic ProGrasp™ Forceps in R2 lift anteriorly and laterally the sigmoid colon and upper rectum to expose the root of the sigmoid mesocolon and the upper mesorectum. The peritoneum is then incised at the level of the sacral promontory, to obtain the avascular presacral plane, with the cautery hook in arm 1: after the superior hemorrhoidal artery identification, the inferior mesenteric artery is obtained. The robotic monopolar hook on arm 1 and bipolar grasper on arm 3 work synergically for the dissection of the IMA, which is freed by the surrounding lymphatic tissue, providing a wide locoregional lymphadenectomy and preserving the main trunks of the hypogastric plexus.

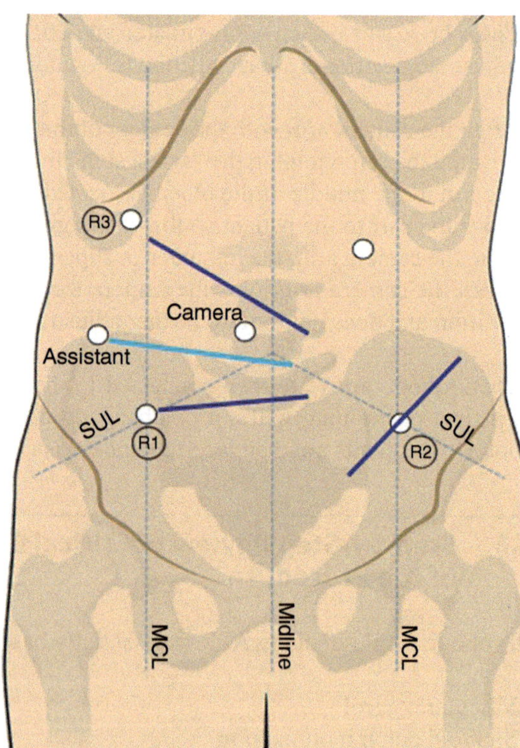

Fig. 22.4 Arm setup for vascular control and sigmoid mobilization. R1, cautery hook (right iliac fossa); R2, ProGrasp™ Forceps (left iliac fossa); R3, bipolar forceps (right hypochondrium). R1 and R3 are the operative arms, whereas R2 is used for retraction. The assistant trocar is used for suction/irrigator, clip applier, swab introduction, or additional retraction if needed

The IMA is then isolated and a high tie of IMA is performed by application of Hem-o-lok® (Teleflex, Weck, Morrisville, NC, USA) clips.

22.3.2 Sigmoid Mobilization

After the vascular control, a medial-to-lateral dissection is carried out preserving the left gonadal vessels and the left ureter. With the sigmoid colon retracted medially by the assistant, the dissection continues cephalad along the white line of Toldt up to the descending colon. The dissection is extended inferiorly up to the psoas muscle where the left ureter crosses the iliac vessels.

22.3.3 Total Mesorectal Excision

During this step, arm 3 is moved and connected to the left hypochondrium trocar to achieve optimal access to the mesorectum, whereas arm 1 and arm 2 remain in their original position (Fig. 22.5). R1 and R3 are the operative arms, whereas R2 is used

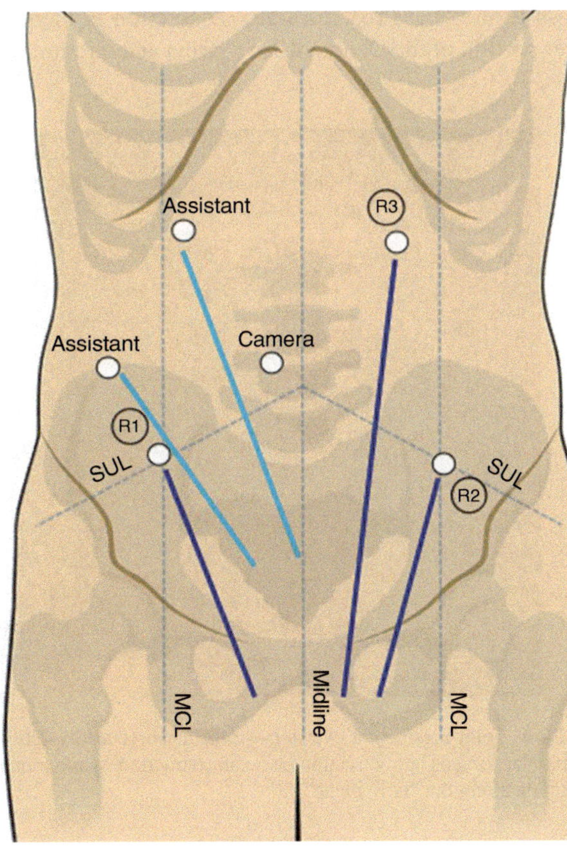

Fig. 22.5 Arm setup for total mesorectal excision (TME). Arm 3 is moved and connected to the left hypochondrium trocar to achieve optimal access to the mesorectum, whereas arm 1 and arm 2 remain in their original position. Two assistant trocars are now available for suction/irrigator and additional retraction on pelvic sidewalls if needed

to expose the pelvic area with lateral traction on pelvic sidewalls or anterior/upward traction on the Douglas peritoneal reflection, vaginal wall, or seminal vesicles/Denonvillier's fascia.

An additional assistant trocar is now available, i.e., robotic trocar in right hypochondrium, in order to maximize the assistance with cranial retraction on the sigmoid colon and simultaneous suction/irrigation or additional gentle pelvic sidewall retraction. Frequent repositioning of R2 to maintain adequate countertraction will allow the dissection plane to be continued up to the level of the pelvic floor. R3 should be used with the wrist joint in an L shape to allow for a larger surface area of retraction on the mesorectum and can be protected with a swab to avoid tears on the proper mesorectal fascia.

TME is carried out according to Heald's principles through the so-called holy plane. This step is fundamental to avoid the transection of the hypogastric nerve plexus (nervi erigentes of Eckardt) and sacral venous plexus located deep in the parietal layer within the presacral space. Dissection starts on the posterior aspect of the mesorectal envelope: the right lateral and the anterior plane are then subsequently dissected up to the seminal vesicles (Figs. 22.6 and 22.7) in a counterclockwise fashion. The left lateral pelvic fascia is then dissected up to its lower portion (Fig. 22.8) to allow for the identification of the pelvic nerve plexus and to gain access to the "bare rectum area." Dissection is then completed anteriorly on the lower portion of the Denonvillier's fascia and circumferentially below the reflection

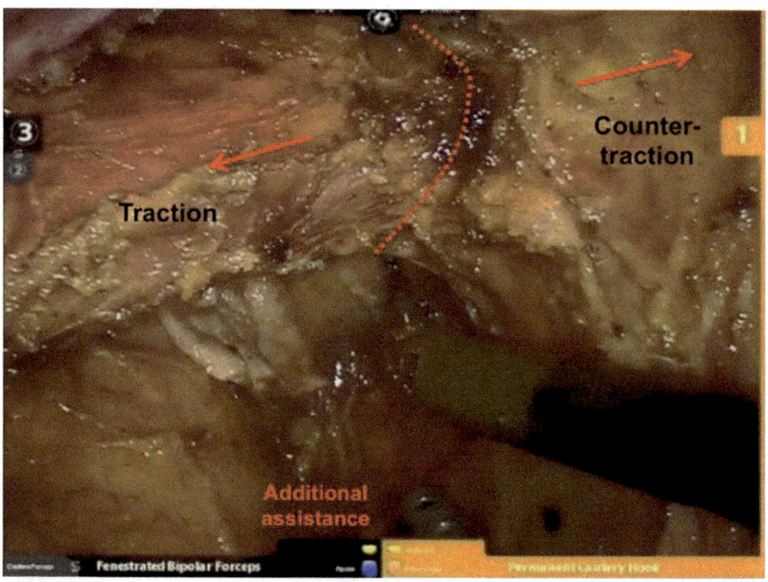

Fig. 22.6 Total mesorectal excision—right mesorectal dissection. R2 and R3 (Cadiere Forceps and bipolar forceps apply traction and countertraction, while monopolar hook on R1 continues the dissection along the "holy plane")

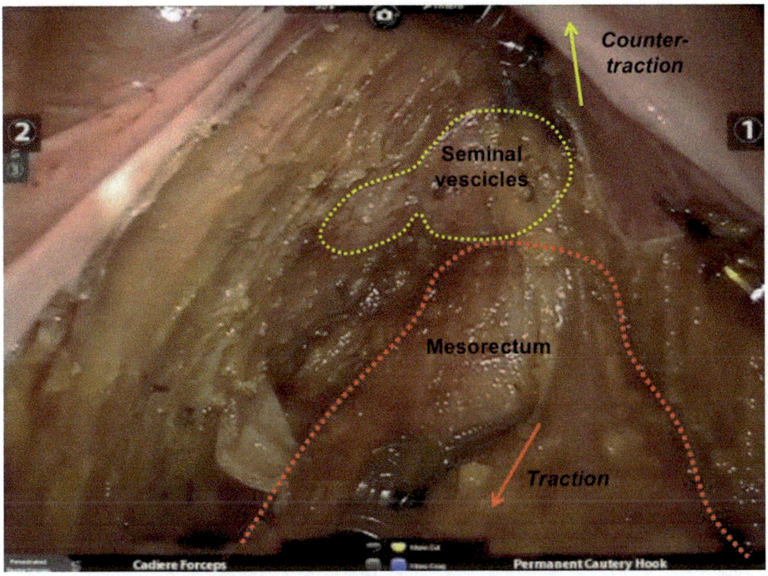

Fig. 22.7 Total mesorectal excision—anterior mesorectal dissection

Fig. 22.8 Total mesorectal excision—left mesorectal dissection

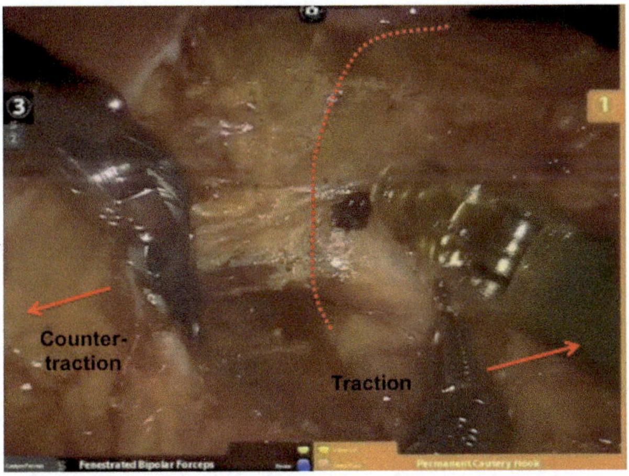

of the mesorectal fascia to gain access to the levator ani plane (Fig. 22.9). The pelvic floor is then incised with a transabdominal robotic approach in a cylindrical fashion, in order to avoid the "coning" effect.

During the dissection of the lower mesorectum, it may be helpful to shift to a 0° or 30° up camera in order to achieve better visualization. R1 and R3 instruments may be inverted as well for easier and more ergonomic access to the left lower transection.

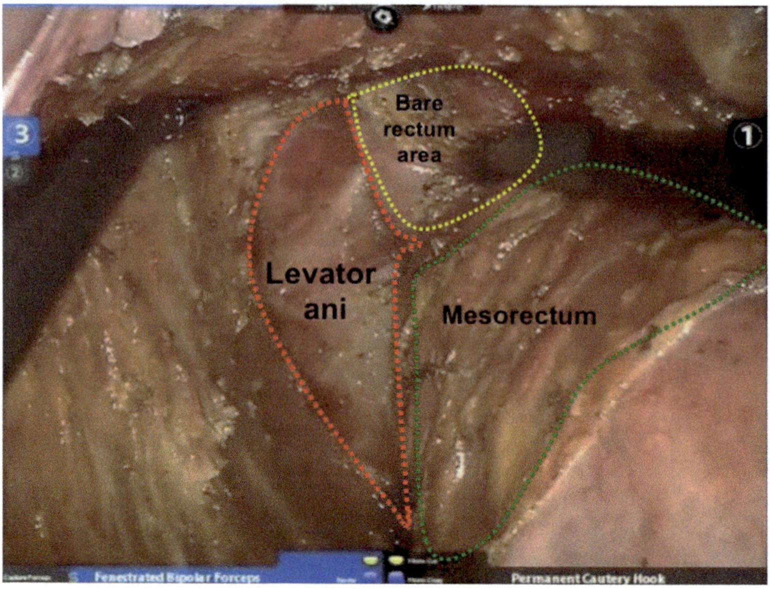

Fig. 22.9 Final view of the pelvic floor after TME

After the completion of perineal dissection, a sigmoid extraperitoneal colostomy is performed. The sigmoid mesentery is dissected through bipolar coagulation and staples if necessary, following the IMA stump. The correct site of colonic transection is confirmed by ICG fluorescence and performed with laparoscopic linear stapler by the assistant at the operating table.

22.3.4 Perineal Phase and Specimen Extraction

Anal closure with purse-string sutures is followed by an elliptical cutaneous incision 2–3 cm from the anal margin, and the subcutaneous fat is divided laterally. Adipose tissue in the ischiorectal fossa is removed, and the pelvic floor is identified just anteriorly to the coccyx, at the level of the incision performed transabdominally, working circumferentially from posterior to anterior and resulting in en bloc resection of the tumor and the adjacent pelvic floor without opening the interface between the tumor and the levator ani. Posterior vaginal resection or removal of the Denonvillier's fascia is performed en bloc with the specimen if any tumor infiltration is evident. Care should be taken not to damage the pelvic urethra. The specimen is then extracted transanally (Fig. 22.10), and the pelvic defect is closed in a standard fashion.

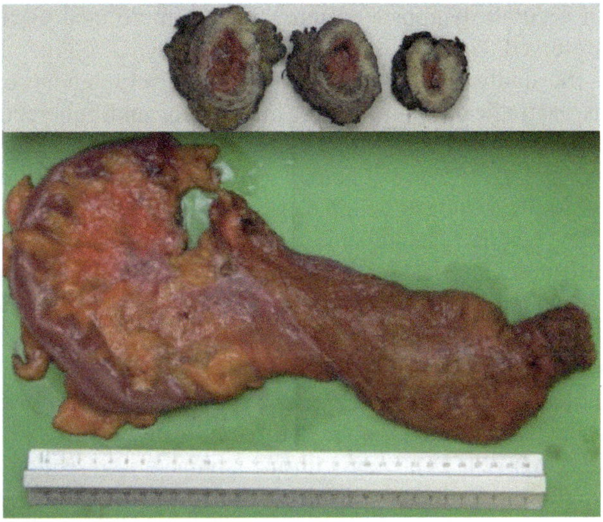

Fig. 22.10 Final view of the resected specimen. Abdominoperineal excision

22.4 Literature Review and Personal Remarks

Accurate tumor staging, neoadjuvant chemoradiation, and intersphincteric resections with manual coloanal anastomosis, even with the transabdominal and transanal approach or robotic transabdominal intersphincteric resection [14–19], have significantly contributed to increase the number of sphincter-saving procedures in low rectal tumors. However, direct sphincter infiltration and the inability to obtain a negative distal margin (a colocutaneous anastomosis results in poor quality of life) are absolute contraindications for sphincter preservation, and an APR remains the only surgical option for these patients [5, 7].

To date, three randomized controlled trials have demonstrated the oncological equivalence of laparoscopic approach if compared to its open counterpart [8–10]. Nevertheless, the technical limitations of conventional laparoscopic instruments make lower rectal dissection a technically demanding procedure to perform, and robotic surgery can potentially play a major role.

Three main issues need to be underlined when analyzing a minimally invasive abdominoperineal excision: IMA ligation with hypogastric nerve preservation, the quality of mesorectal dissection according to Quirke grading system in the lower rectum, and the circumferential resection margin at the level of levator ani plane.

First of all, IMA ligation with hypogastric nerve preservation can be facilitated by the robotic approach, thanks to the several technological features and better three-dimensional visualization. Moreover, though no evidence exists about long-term advantages of high vs. low tie of IMA for low and ultralow rectal cancer [20], an accurate lymphadenectomy can be performed even if the left colic artery is preserved.

Secondly, the lower rectum has a relatively thin mesorectal envelope, because of its anatomical coning toward the levator and puborectalis muscles. This feature, together with the poor visibility and challenging surgical exposure in deep and narrow pelvis, is a possible explanation for the high circumferential margin (CRM) positivity of tumors within 5 cm of the anal verge. Numerous reports confirm higher CRM positivity in abdominoperineal resections (APRs) when compared to anterior resections for rectal cancer that is a valid surrogate end point (together with mesorectal plane) for local recurrence and disease-free survival [21–23]. Robotic surgery may potentially overcome these pitfalls in lower mesorectal dissection, thanks to a stable three-dimensional camera platform, EndoWrist™ technology, tremor filtering, and motion scaling. Several retrospective case series and comparative studies have demonstrated the feasibility and safety of robotic low and ultralow anterior resection [24, 25], even with intersphincteric resection and coloanal anastomosis. Moreover, preliminary results of the randomized controlled ROLARR (robotic versus laparoscopic resection for rectal cancer) trial are encouraging: a potential reduction of the conversion rates in low anterior resection, obese and male patients (though not statistically significant) and the high oncological safety and quality of robotic mesorectal excision (with a very low percentage of CRM involvement—5.1% in the robotic group and 6.3% in the laparoscopic group—among a group of surgeons with low experience in robotic TME and a mean number of only 25 procedures performed per surgeon prior to enrollment vs. 91.5 performed with the laparoscopic approach) are the main consistent findings. Three-year local recurrence rates and disease-free and overall survival are awaited to draw more definitive conclusions.

Finally, several studies have concluded that APRs have worse oncological outcomes when compared to sphincter-saving operations. The high reported CRM positivity at the level of the levator ani and puborectalis muscles has pushed the scientific community to the development of the so-called extralevator abdominoperineal excision (ELAPE) [26, 27], with the aim of reducing R1 resections and, ultimately, local recurrence rates. It is still a matter of debate whether this procedure represents a new concept or it is a simple reintroduction of the original principles developed by Sir Ernest Miles nearly 100 years ago, with the procedure performed in a prone or jackknife position. Nevertheless, robotic surgery could potentially provide a more comfortable and technically superior operative environment for transabdominal levator ani transection.

Though many published series of robotic-assisted TME for rectal cancer include patients submitted to APR, only few papers, to date, have selectively analyzed the results of robotic APR. The available literature about robotic APR is summarized in Table 22.1 [11–13, 28, 29].

To date, our personal experience includes 25 robotic-assisted APR (17 male/8 female; mean age, 63 years) performed from July 2009 to June 2015. Mean operative time was 360 ± 63.7 min (range, 256–555). Neither conversion to open surgery nor intraoperative complications was observed.

Table 22.1 Results of robotic-assisted abdominoperineal resections

Authors	*n*	OT	POC	HS	CRM+	30 D-M	LN	APR/ELAPE	TALAT	CR
Marecik SJ [11]	5	343	0	5.8	0	0	12.4	ELAPE	Yes	0
Kang [12]	6	335	3	5	0	Na	Na	ELAPE	Yes	0
Alimoglu [28]	7	Na	2	8.1	0	0	Na	APR	No	0
Eriksen [29]	10	318	1	8	Na	0	Na	Na	Na	0
Kim [13, 18]	21	197 ± 29	4	7.6 ± 1.6	0	0	20 ± 8	ELAPE (67%), APR (33%)	Yes	0
Bianchi (2015) unpublished data	25	360 ± 63.7	4[a]	6.6 ± 1.4	2	0	17 ± 6.7	APE	Yes	0

OT operative time, *POC* postoperative complications, *HS* hospital stay, *CRM+* positive circumferential resection margins, *30-day M* 30-day mortality, *LN* number of retrieved lymph nodes, *APR/ELAPE* standard abdominoperineal resection/extralevator abdominoperineal excision, *TALAT* transabdominal levator ani transection, *CR* conversion rate, *Na* not available data

[a]Clavien–Dindo grade I–II: perineal wound infection

Twenty-two out of 25 patients (88%) underwent neoadjuvant chemoradiotherapy. Two specimens (8%) showed a CRM involvement (defined as CRM $\leq$ 1 mm): in one case, CRM involvement was due to a metastatic lymph node adherent to the proper mesorectal fascia. Mean lymph node yield was 17 ± 6.7 (range, 4–34).

All patients were submitted to a perioperative fast-track program. Recovery of bowel function and length of stay were 2.2 ± 0.8 days (range, 1–4) and 6.6 ± 1.4 days (range, 4–9), respectively. According to the Clavien–Dindo classification system, the overall complication rate for grade I–II and III–IV was 16% and 0%, respectively. Perineal wound infection was the only complication recorded in grade I–II group, and no reinterventions were observed.

Median follow-up was 36.5 months. Three-year local recurrence rate, disease-free survival, and overall survival were 3.8%, 62%, and 100%, respectively. One death was recorded at 5 years in a patient who underwent lung metastasectomy 24 months after primary surgery and died due to disease progression (unpublished data).

In conclusion, robotic-assisted APR can be safely performed for the treatment of malignant ultralow rectal disease, thanks to improved maneuverability and its excellent three-dimensional visual platform, especially in lower mesorectal dissection and transabdominal levator ani transection. This may potentially help to reduce CRM positivity and, ultimately, local recurrence rates for ultralow rectal cancer requiring APR.

References

1. Miles WE. A method of performing abdomino-perineal excision for carcinoma of the rectum and of the terminal portion of the pelvic colon (1908). CA Cancer J Clin. 1971;21(6):361–4.
2. Campos FG, Habr-Gama A, Nahas SC, Perez RO. Abdominoperineal excision: evolution of a centenary operation. Dis Colon Rectum. 2012;55(8):844–53. doi:10.1097/DCR.0b013e31825ab0f7.
3. Heald RJ, Husband EM, Ryall RD. The mesorectum in rectal cancer surgery—the clue to pelvic recurrence? Br J Surg. 1982;69(10):613–6.
4. Heald RJ, Ryall RD. Recurrence and survival after total mesorectal excision for rectal cancer. Lancet (London). 1986;1(8496):1479–82.
5. Holm T. Ultra low resection versus abdomino-perineal excision in low rectal cancer. Rec Results Cancer Res. 2014;203:57–67. doi:10.1007/978-3-319-08060-4_7.
6. Holm T. Controversies in abdominoperineal excision. Surg Oncol Clin N Am. 2014;23(1):93–111. doi:10.1016/j.soc.2013.09.005.
7. Rullier E, Denost Q, Vendrely V, Rullier A, Laurent C. Low rectal cancer: classification and standardization of surgery. Dis Colon Rectum. 2013;56(5):560–7. doi:10.1097/DCR.0b013e31827c4a8c.
8. Jayne DG, Thorpe HC, Copeland J, Quirke P, Brown JM, Guillou PJ. Five-year follow-up of the Medical Research Council CLASICC trial of laparoscopically assisted versus open surgery for colorectal cancer. Br J Surg. 2010;97(11):1638–45. doi:10.1002/bjs.7160.
9. Bonjer HJ, Deijen CL, Abis GA, Cuesta MA, van der Pas MH, de Lange-de Klerk ES, et al. A randomized trial of laparoscopic versus open surgery for rectal cancer. N Engl J Med. 2015;372(14):1324–32. doi:10.1056/NEJMoa1414882.

10. Jeong SY, Park JW, Nam BH, Kim S, Kang SB, Lim SB, et al. Open versus laparoscopic surgery for mid-rectal or low-rectal cancer after neoadjuvant chemoradiotherapy (COREAN trial): survival outcomes of an open-label, non-inferiority, randomised controlled trial. Lancet Oncol. 2014;15(7):767–74. doi:10.1016/s1470-2045(14)70205-0.
11. Marecik SJ, Zawadzki M, Desouza AL, Park JJ, Abcarian H, Prasad LM. Robotic cylindrical abdominoperineal resection with transabdominal levator transection. Dis Colon Rectum. 2011;54(10):1320–5. doi:10.1097/DCR.0b013e31822720a2.
12. Kang CY, Carmichael JC, Friesen J, Stamos MJ, Mills S, Pigazzi A. Robotic-assisted extralevator abdominoperineal resection in the lithotomy position: technique and early outcomes. Am Surg. 2012;78(10):1033–7.
13. Kim JC, Kwak JY, Yoon YS, Park IJ, Kim CW. A comparison of the technical and oncologic validity between robot-assisted and conventional open abdominoperineal resection. Int J Color Dis. 2014;29(8):961–9. doi:10.1007/s00384-014-1916-9.
14. Marks J, Mizrahi B, Dalane S, Nweze I, Marks G. Laparoscopic transanal abdominal transanal resection with sphincter preservation for rectal cancer in the distal 3 cm of the rectum after neoadjuvant therapy. Surg Endosc. 2010;24(11):2700–7. doi:10.1007/s00464-010-1028-8.
15. Marks J, Nassif G, Schoonyoung H, DeNittis A, Zeger E, Mohiuddin M, et al. Sphincter-sparing surgery for adenocarcinoma of the distal 3 cm of the true rectum: results after neoadjuvant therapy and minimally invasive radical surgery or local excision. Surg Endosc. 2013;27(12):4469–77. doi:10.1007/s00464-013-3092-3.
16. Marks JH, Frenkel JL, D'Andrea AP, Greenleaf CE. Maximizing rectal cancer results: TEM and TATA techniques to expand sphincter preservation. Surg Oncol Clin N Am. 2011;20(3):501–520., viii–ix. doi:10.1016/j.soc.2011.01.008.
17. Park SY, Choi GS, Park JS, Kim HJ, Choi WH, Ryuk JP. Robotic-assisted transabdominal intersphincteric resection: a technique involving a completely abdominal approach and coloanal anastomosis. Surg Laparosc Endosc Percutan Tech. 2013;23(1):e5–10. doi:10.1097/SLE.0b013e318275b27a.
18. Kim JC, Lim SB, Yoon YS, Park IJ, Kim CW, Kim CN. Completely abdominal intersphincteric resection for lower rectal cancer: feasibility and comparison of robot-assisted and open surgery. Surg Endosc. 2014;28(9):2734–44. doi:10.1007/s00464-014-3509-7.
19. Yoo BE, Cho JS, Shin JW, Lee DW, Kwak JM, Kim J, et al. Robotic versus laparoscopic intersphincteric resection for low rectal cancer: comparison of the operative, oncological, and functional outcomes. Ann Surg Oncol. 2015;22(4):1219–25. doi:10.1245/s10434-014-4177-5.
20. Cirocchi R, Trastulli S, Farinella E, Desiderio J, Vettoretto N, Parisi A, et al. High tie versus low tie of the inferior mesenteric artery in colorectal cancer: a RCT is needed. Surg Oncol. 2012;21(3):e111–23. doi:10.1016/j.suronc.2012.04.004.
21. Quirke P, Durdey P, Dixon MF, Williams NS. Local recurrence of rectal adenocarcinoma due to inadequate surgical resection. Histopathological study of lateral tumour spread and surgical excision. Lancet (London). 1986;2(8514):996–9.
22. Quirke P, Steele R, Monson J, Grieve R, Khanna S, Couture J, et al. Effect of the plane of surgery achieved on local recurrence in patients with operable rectal cancer: a prospective study using data from the MRC CR07 and NCIC-CTG CO16 randomised clinical trial. Lancet (London). 2009;373(9666):821–8. doi:10.1016/s0140-6736(09)60485-2.
23. Nagtegaal ID, Quirke P. What is the role for the circumferential margin in the modern treatment of rectal cancer? J Clin Oncol. 2008;26(2):303–12. doi:10.1200/jco.2007.12.7027.
24. Bianchi PP, Ceriani C, Locatelli A, Spinoglio G, Zampino MG, Sonzogni A, et al. Robotic versus laparoscopic total mesorectal excision for rectal cancer: a comparative analysis of oncological safety and short-term outcomes. Surg Endosc. 2010;24(11):2888–94. doi:10.1007/s00464-010-1134-7.
25. Formisano G, Marano A, Bianchi PP, Spinoglio G. Challenges with robotic low anterior resection. Minerva Chir. 2015.

26. Nagtegaal ID, van de Velde CJ, Marijnen CA, van Krieken JH, Quirke P. Low rectal cancer: a call for a change of approach in abdominoperineal resection. J Clin Oncol. 2005;23(36):9257–64. doi:10.1200/jco.2005.02.9231.
27. Holm T, Ljung A, Haggmark T, Jurell G, Lagergren J. Extended abdominoperineal resection with gluteus maximus flap reconstruction of the pelvic floor for rectal cancer. Br J Surg. 2007;94(2):232–8. doi:10.1002/bjs.5489.
28. Alimoglu O, Atak I, Kilic A, Caliskan M. Robot-assisted laparoscopic abdominoperineal resection for low rectal cancer. Int J Med Robot. 2012;8(3):371–4. doi:10.1002/rcs.1432.
29. Eriksen JR, Helvind NM, Jakobsen HL, Olsen J, Bundgaard M, Harvald T, et al. Early results after robot-assisted colorectal surgery. Dan Med J. 2013;60(12):A4736.

Part III

Transanal Laparoscopy and Robot-Assisted

Transanal Endoscopic Microsurgery (TEM) and Transanal Minimally Invasive Surgery (TAMIS)

23

Amanda Feigel and Patricia Sylla

Abstract

Transanal endoscopic surgery (TES) is an innovative minimally invasive approach with an ever increasing range of applications ranging from local excision of rectal neoplasms to repair of complex rectovisceral fistulas, completion proctectomy, and even transanal total mesorectal excision. Patients experience the benefits of a minimally invasive approach including shorter length of hospital stay, reduced postoperative pain and morbidity, and faster recovery relative to radical rectal resection. Well-documented advantages of this approach over traditional transanal excision include improved visualization and reach for lesions in the proximal rectum and improved capacity to complete full-thickness excision with reduced specimen fragmentation and margin positivity. TES is currently indicated for a variety of benign rectal pathologies, carefully selected early rectal cancer with low histopathological risk for lymph node metastasis, and palliation of locally advanced rectal tumors. The transanal endoscopic microsurgery (TEM) and transanal endoscopic operation (TEO) system are metal platforms with a fixed camera allowing for stability of operative and optical field that can provide transanal access to lesions up to 20 cm from the anal verge, but that afford limited range of motion due to their rigid design. Transanal minimally invasive surgery (TAMIS) platforms are shorter, more pliable, and disposable, which are compatible with standard laparoscopic equipment, but require a second operator to control the camera. Far more published data exists regarding the procedural efficacy and long-term oncologic safety of rigid TES platforms for carefully selected rectal lesions. In the absence of randomized trials directly comparing the various TES approaches, the preliminary TAMIS data published to date suggests equivalent outcomes to TEM and TEO in selected patients.

A. Feigel, M.D. • P. Sylla, M.D., F.A.C.S., F.A.S.C.R.S. (✉)
Division of Colon and Rectal Surgery, Department of Surgery, Icahn School of Medicine at Mount Sinai, One Gustave L. Levy Place, New York, NY 10029, USA
e-mail: patricia.sylla@mountsinai.org

G. Dapri, J.H. Marks (eds.), *Surgical Techniques in Rectal Cancer*,
https://doi.org/10.1007/978-4-431-55579-7_23

Keywords
Transanal excision (TAE) • Transanal endoscopic surgery (TES) • Transanal endoscopic microsurgery (TEM) • Transanal endoscopic operation (TEO) • Transanal minimally invasive surgery (TAMIS) • Rectal cancer

23.1 Introduction: From Radical Rectal Resection to Local Excision

The gold standard in the oncologic resection of rectal cancer has been firmly established as requiring radical en bloc sharp dissection of the rectum and mesorectum along the mesorectal fascia, a technique termed total mesorectal excision (TME) as first described by Dr. Heald and colleagues in 1982 [1]. In combination with the selective use of neoadjuvant chemoradiation (CRT) for locally advanced tumors, widespread adoption of TME technique, has resulted in substantial decrease in local recurrence rates following curative resection of rectal cancer [2, 3]. TME is performed in conjunction with sphincter-preserving low anterior resection (LAR) or abdominoperineal resection (APR), for tumors with threatened circumferential margins (CRM) and/or involving the anal sphincter muscles. While curative resection with APR comes at the price of a permanent end colostomy, both APR and LAR result in operative mortality ranging from 2% to 5% and significant perioperative morbidity ranging 18–55% [4–7], including infectious and wound-related complications in addition to substantial urinary and sexual dysfunction. Sphincter-preserving LAR for low and mid-rectal cancers that have been treated with CRT usually require coloanal anastomoses and a diverting loop ileostomy with the added morbidity from anastomotic and parastomal complications, and short- and long-term functional disturbances in defecatory function [8, 9]. It is important to note that recent advances in minimally invasive approaches to perform pelvic surgery, including multiport laparoscopy and robotic surgery, while impactful in reducing pain, length of hospital stay (LOS) and overall recovery, have not had a substantial impact on perioperative or functional morbidity relative to open TME [4–7, 10]. It is in this background of high morbidity rates related to TME that interest in local excisional approaches for rectal tumors has evolved and blossomed. This is particularly true for patients with benign rectal lesions not amenable to endoscopic removal by colonoscopy, in whom, in the absence of local excision strategies, TME would be offered as last resort.

Until the more recent introduction of transanal endoscopic platforms, local excision techniques for rectal tumors have included transanal local excision (TAE or Park's operation), transcoccygeal, and transsphincteric excision. TAE predates endoscopy and radical excision. Still TAE remains as a strategy to perform full-thickness excision of lesions in the distal rectum that could not be removed endoscopically during colonoscopy, thereby eliminating the need for radical resection and stoma creation. Procedures are performed using conventional anoscopes to expose the rectum and resect lesions as a disc or circumferentially and in a submucosal or full-thickness fashion, followed by suture closure of rectal defects. The mesorectum is entirely preserved, with no attempt of harvesting lymph nodes. The morbidity of

TAE has been shown to be substantially lower than that of radical resection, with complication rates ranging from 5% to 25% [11–13]. Furthermore the scope of morbidities is generally less significant than radical surgery, mostly consisting of bleeding, transient urinary retention and transient fecal incontinence. However, this type of local excision is limited to the distal 6–8 cm of the rectum at best, with limited exposure and visualization of the surgical field through standard anoscopes and increased risk of specimen fragmentation and positive resection margins [13].

Popularized by Kraske for resection of rectal cancer in the mid and distal rectum in the late nineteenth century [14], transsacral resection, which is more accurately described as a transcoccygeal resection, has been used for larger and more proximal rectal lesions that could not be accessed via TAE. This approach consists of resection of the coccyx and incision of the anococcygeal ligament to provide exposure to the posterior rectum. The adjacent mesorectum can be removed en bloc with tumors of the posterior rectum, but this remains a limited sleeve rectal resection. The rectal defect is closed with sutures. This approach can be complicated by the development of a fecal fistula from the rectum to the posterior midline incision, with a reported incidence ranging from 5% to 20% [15, 16]. Transsphincteric excision was first described by York Mason in 1970 as an alternative to extend a local excision approach for tumors in the mid and distal rectum. This technique involves complete division of the posterior anal sphincter complex and posterior rectal wall followed by reapproximation of the divided muscles following resection [17]. This procedure has been associated with higher risk of fecal incontinence due to sphincter dysfunction relative to the transcoccygeal approach [17].

As local excision techniques gained popularity in the management of benign rectal lesions as well as early rectal cancer [18], long-term oncologic outcomes of TAE for T1 and T2 rectal cancers raised major concerns regarding the oncologic adequacy of local excision, particularly due to reports of higher local recurrence rates. In a series of 260 patients with T1 or T2 rectal cancer treated with either TAE or radical resection, Mellgren et al. reported an 18% vs. no local recurrence rate following local excision vs. radical resection of T1 tumors, although 5-year survival was similar in both groups [19]. In another retrospective series of 74 T1 rectal cancers treated with TAE, Paty et al. reported a similarly high local recurrence rate of 17%, with a 74% 10-year survival [20]. It is important to note that none of these earlier retrospective series on local excision for T1 and T2 rectal cancers incorporated strict selection criteria based on tumor size or histological features which are now known to represent strong prognostic factors for lymph node involvement. Another source of heterogeneity in those earlier series includes the lack of standardization of surgical techniques with TAE and TEM procedures often grouped together.

23.2 Transanal Endoscopic Surgery

Transanal endoscopic microsurgery (TEM, Richard Wolf Company, Tubingen, Germany) was developed by Buess in 1983 to perform endoscopic resection of rectal polyps deemed too proximal for access by TAE, too large or distal for access by standard colonoscopy, and otherwise managed with proctectomy [21]. Remarkably this device predated the laparoscopic revolution that would emerge later in that decade. The original beveled rigid TEM metal multiport platform represents a substantial technological advance over TAE and flexible endoscopy by providing stable rectal distention with CO_2, magnified 3D stereoscopic visualization of rectal lesions, and adapted angled instruments for dissection and suture closure of rectal defects within the narrow confines of a 4 cm-wide platform. Other ergonomic advantages include an anchoring arm that locks the platform onto the operating table, stabilizing the operating platform and permitting a single operator to perform either submucosal or full-thickness rectal dissection by triangulating two or three instruments through the platform. The technology has remained largely unaltered over the last 30 years except for modifications in the stereoscopic system for better adaptability with standard videolaparoscopic towers. The transanal endoscopic operation platform (TEO, Karl Storz GmbH, Tuttlingen, Germany) was subsequently introduced in the era of laparoscopic surgery, as an alternative metal platform with an adapted 3 mm 2D scope compatible with a conventional laparoscopic camera and video tower. It should be noted that because of the similarity between TEM and TEO rigid metal platforms, many series do not necessarily distinguish between the two rigid platforms and may use the terms TEM and TEO interchangeably, or refer to them as TEM or TES rigid platforms.

Over time, with the growing experience with the platforms and ample data supporting the safety profile and significantly lower postoperative pain, morbidity, and faster recovery relative to low anterior resection [22–24], indications for local excision using TEM and TEO have expanded from large rectal adenomas not amenable to complete endoscopic resection, incompletely resected adenomas with dysplasia or intramucosal adenocarcinoma, small low-risk carcinoids, and other benign rectal pathologies (Table 23.1). However until recently, universal adoption of TES was limited by the perceived long learning curve required to master TEM/TEO technique and the relatively high cost of the capital investment required for the specialized instrumentation [25, 26]. With a growing interest in single-incision laparoscopy and the introduction of disposable multichannel platforms (SILS Port, Medtronic, Elizabeth, NJ, Gelpoint Path, Applied Medical, Rancho Santa Margarita, CA), the

Table 23.1 Applications for TEM and TAMIS

Applications
Rectal adenoma
Early rectal cancer
Palliation of advanced rectal tumors
Carcinoid tumor
Retrorectal tumors
Rectourethral, rectovaginal and rectovesicular fistula repair
Anastomotic leak
Drainage of pelvic abscess
Anastomotic stricture
Rectal foreign body removal
Completion proctectomy
Transanal NOTES

concept of performing transanal minimally invasive surgery (TAMIS) was introduced in 2009, as an alternative setup to the more rigid platforms [27]. This approach utilizes standard laparoscopic equipment, and although two operators rather than one are required, one holding the laparoscopic camera and the other performing the procedure, benefits include wider access and lower costs of disposable platforms that do not depend on the use of specialized instrumentation. TAMIS platforms are also shorter and more pliable than the longer rigid ones, thereby increasing the freedom of motion externally and limiting instrument collision internally. Limitations however include the shorter length of the platforms which limits the proximal reach of, particularly beyond the second or third Haustral valves [28]. While a number of case series have been published demonstrating the preliminary feasibility and safety of TAMIS, these studies are relatively small and the data short term, with no long-term oncologic results [28–32].

23.3 TES Compared to TAE and TME

Several studies have demonstrated equivalent or superior outcomes of TEM for rectal cancer as compared with other methods of local excision [11, 12, 21, 33, 34]. A recent meta-analysis by Clancy et al. reviewed six studies that compared outcomes from TAE and TEM [13]. Cohorts were highly heterogeneous and included a mix of adenomas and adenocarcinomas as well as tumors of various stages. There were no differences in overall complication rates, but TEM was associated with higher negative margin rates (OR 5.28), reduced specimen fragmentation (OR 0.10), and lower rates of local recurrence (OR 0.25) when compared with conventional transanal excision [13]. However, studies included in this meta-analysis were retrospective, with varying definitions of specimen fragmentation and local recurrence. Although randomized studies comparing local excision techniques are lacking, superior oncologic outcomes with TEM are presumably secondary to the better visualization and more precise dissection that can be accomplished with this approach as compared to TAE. Despite this evidence, TAE is still more commonly used than TEM or TAMIS in many centers because of lack of specific training in TES, low volume of cases, and higher costs related to these procedures [11].

Although originally developed to treat benign disease, indications for TEM have expanded over the last 30 years to include the curative treatment of rectal adenocarcinoma via full-thickness endoscopic excision in select cases. Selection of appropriate tumors for local excision rather than radical resection remains a topic of controversy. Unacceptably high local recurrence rates in heterogeneous cohorts treated with TEM alone are still quoted, despite their inherent biases. These earlier retrospective case series reported mixed data from TAE and TEM cohorts and did not use current staging modalities including pelvic MRI. Further, T1 tumors were not sub-analyzed based on histopathologic features that are now known to be of prognostic significance for lymph node metastasis and local recurrence [18–20, 35]. More contemporary TEM series have demonstrated comparable oncologic outcomes in select cohorts with low-risk T1 tumors relative to radical resection with

TME [36]. Authors have adopted standard preoperative staging and detailed pathologic review in order to identify patients with very low risk of occult nodal disease who would in effect likely be overtreated by radical surgery, thus incurring unnecessary morbidity [22, 37, 38]. These carefully selected T1 rectal tumors can usually be safely offered TEM alone as curative therapy. Moreover, there is mounting evidence to support the use of TEM in combination with adjuvant or neoadjuvant chemotherapy for more advanced lesions [39, 40]. Marks et al. reported on True Natural Orifice Transluminal Endoscopic Surgery (NOTES) TME resection with splenic flexure release, high ligation of IMA, and side-to-end handsewn coloanal anastomosis in four patients [41].

23.4 Indications for TES

23.4.1 Rectal Adenoma

TEM was originally designed to perform rectal mucosectomy or full-thickness resection of large adenomas of the mid and proximal rectum deemed endoscopically unresectable by standard polypectomy and out of reach by TAE. This is particularly relevant in centers that do not offer endoscopic submucosal dissection (ESD) or endoscopic mucosal resection (EMR). For adenomas not found or suspected to harbor an invasive component, en bloc ESD can be performed for large flat carpeting villous lesions using TEM and creation of large full-thickness defects can be avoided. Relative to conventional polypectomy and EMR, TEM facilitates more complete resection of larger adenomatous lesions. A retrospective review of 292 patients undergoing excision of adenomas larger than 2 cm via either TEM or EMR demonstrated that early recurrences were substantially higher in the EMR group (31.0% vs. 10.2%, $p < 0.001$) [42]. This was accounted for by a higher incidence of incomplete adenoma resection via EMR after a single intervention; however, if permitted additional endoscopic attempts within six months, the long-term efficacy of resection appears equal. A systematic review of the literature describing EMR or TEM resection for large rectal adenoma further supported an increased early recurrence rate for EMR (11.2% vs. 5.4%, $p = 0.04$) [43].

Full-thickness resection of incompletely resected adenomas with dysplasia or intramucosal carcinoma is another well-suited application of TES that not only provides a definitive diagnosis but that can also be curative, thereby avoiding overtreatment by radical surgery and the unnecessary morbidity associated with proctectomy.

Compared to standard transanal excision, TES has also been associated with superior results with respect to local control of adenomas. As demonstrated in their systematic review of 927 local resections performed by either TEM or TAE for rectal neoplasia (both benign and malignant indications), Clancy et al. found that TEM was associated with higher negative margin rates (OR, 5.281; 95% CI, 3.201–8.712; $p < 0.001$), lower rate of specimen fragmentation (OR, 0.096; 95% CI, 0.044–0.209; $p < 0.001$), and lower recurrence rate (OR, 0.248; 95% CI,

0.154–0.401; $p < 0.001$) relative to TAE [13]. A major limitation of the meta-analysis was the fact the studies were retrospective, with no consensus on the definition of specimen fragmentation defined and significant variations in the follow-up period for assessment of local recurrence. Although randomized studies comparing local excision techniques are lacking, the superior rates of local control achieved with TEM is presumably secondary to the better visualization and more precise dissection that can be accomplished with this endoscopic approach relative to TAE.

With respect to strictly benign indications, in a subgroup 78 rectal adenomas from a larger retrospective series of rectal tumors excised using either TEM or TAE, Moore et al. demonstrated that despite lesions being of similar size (14 ± 21.5 cm^2 in TEM vs. 15 ± 22.7 cm^2, $p = 0.95$), local excision by TEM was associated with a higher rate of negative resection margins (83% vs. 61%, $p = 0.03$), lower rate of specimen fragmentation and lower recurrence rate (3 vs. 32%, $p = 0.003$) [11]. The largest retrospective series on TEM/TEO excision rectal adenomas using either mucosectomy or full-thickness excision ($N = 91$–353 patients), for adenomas of median diameter 3 cm or less, local recurrence rates at a median of 2 or more years typically range from 4% to 10%, confirming excellent local control using this minimally invasive approach. Most importantly, the reported mortality rate of TES is uniformly under 1% with morbidity ranging from 3% to 8% [44–47]. Several large series demonstrated that resection margin positivity was the strongest predictor for local recurrence [46, 47]. Several TEM series have also investigated the efficacy of TEM for rectal lesions larger than 3 cm. While giant rectal lesions, namely, near-circumferential or completely circumferential tumors, are often described to require conversion to laparotomy due incomplete resection and/or closure of rectal defects, in the hands of experienced operators, TEM was found to result in good local control rates and low morbidity for rectal tumors even larger than 5 cm. In a retrospective review of 233 rectal adenomas with median diameter of 5 cm (1–12 cm) resected full-thickness using TEM, Allaix et al. reported a 11.1% positive margin rate and a 5.6% overall local recurrence rate at a median follow-up of 110 months [47]. However, the rate of positive margins was 8.9% vs. 20.9% for lesions less than 5 cm in diameter vs. 5 cm or more, respectively ($p = 0.047$). While both tumor diameter and margin positivity correlated with local recurrence on univariate regression analysis, only margin positivity remained an independent risk factor for local recurrence [47]. Similarly, in series from Levic ($N = 30$) and Schafer ($N = 33$) on outcomes of TEM for adenomas larger than of 4 × 4 cm and larger than 5 cm in diameter, respectively, the incidence of positive resection margins was 17.9% and 18%, respectively, with local recurrence rates as high as 26.3% and 12%, respectively, although in the series by Levic, 5/10 of the TEM local recurrences consisted in invasive carcinomas [48, 49]. Overall these findings support the use of TES to resect large rectal adenomas as an alternative minimally invasive strategy to avoid proctectomy, although the incidence of underlying invasive adenocarcinoma is increased with larger tumors [47, 48, 50], the rate of local recurrence increases proportionally to the size of the lesions and does the technical difficulty of closing full-thickness rectal wall defects [49].

Despite the evidence of superior local control achieved with TEM, TAE is still more commonly used than TEM in many centers due to lack of specific training, low volume of cases, and higher costs related to these procedures [11]. The introductions of more readily available TAMIS platforms have however helped diffuse this technique more widely and rendered this approach more mainstream. To date, the published TAMIS experience with rectal adenomas is more limited but growing quickly. Among the 323 cases reported across 14 TAMIS series published between 2010 and 2015, 158 consisted of adenomas [28, 30–32, 51–58]. The overall margin positivity rate across benign and malignant lesions removed with TAMIS ranged from 0% to 16%, but was below 10% among the largest TAMIS series [10, 28, 31]. Morbidity across series was also similar to historical TEM and TEO rates and ranged from 0% to 25% [28, 30–32, 51–58]. Noticeable among TAMIS series is the fact that there is limited to no data on resection of larger lesions (>3 cm) and limited data on resection of lesions in the upper rectum, which may relate to the fact that disposable transanal platforms are typically shorter than the rigid TEM and TEO platforms, making it more challenging to negotiate prominent rectal valves and expose lesions that may lie behind them with the laparoscope and rigid instruments.

23.4.2 Early Rectal Cancer

Common indications for TES include malignant rectal polyps, defined as containing a focus of neoplastic cells confined to the mucosa (considered pTis in AJCC staging), correctly defined as high-grade dysplasia (HGD), but still often referred to as intramucosal carcinoma. These lesions are associated with a $\leq 2\%$ risk of lymph node metastasis, and therefore local excision in the form of polypectomy and EMR is usually curative provided negative margins are achieved [59, 60]. Early rectal cancer (ERC) consists of invasive adenocarcinoma extending into but not beyond the submucosa, i.e., staged as T1, and are typically found within a pedunculated or sessile adenoma, or an a ulcerated lesion. The extent of invasion can be further characterized by the depth of penetration of the carcinoma into the polyp stalk or submucosa for pedunculated and sessile lesions, respectively [61]. A low-risk ERC contained in a pedunculated polyp is defined as Haggit level 1, 2, or 3, where the carcinoma invades through the muscularis mucosa into the submucosa but is confined to the head, neck, or stalk, respectively. Routine snare polypectomy is an acceptable curative strategy for these pedunculated ERC which are typically incidentally found on pathologic review following endoscopic removal [62]. For ERC contained in small flat rectal polyps and ulcerated lesions, the depth of T1 invasion into the submucosal layer needs to be further characterized based on the Kikuchi classification where Sm1 represents invasion into the upper third, Sm2 into the middle third, and Sm3 into the deepest third [63]. Deeper submucosal invasion correlates with increased risk of lymphovascular invasion (LVI), and polypectomy alone for Sm3 and high-risk Sm2 lesions is associated with higher risk of lymph node metastasis and local recurrence [63]. Kikuchi and Nascimbeni independently determined from large samples of T1 colorectal cancers undergoing radical resection that Sm1, Sm2 and Sm3 depth of tumor invasion was associated with a 0–3, 8–10 and

23–25% risk of lymph node metastasis respectively [63, 64]. Therefore, complete polypectomy or EMR of a low-risk ERC, i.e., <3 cm sessile or ulcerated Sm1 pT1 well or moderately well differentiated adenocarcinoma with no LVI, does not require further treatment [62]. For larger and more distal ERC, TAE and TES provide improved transanal access, exposure, and chance of achieving negative margins. In addition, when polypectomy or EMR results in positive or indeterminate resection margins for otherwise low-risk ERC, TAE and TES with full-thickness excision of the polypectomy site is particularly well suited to complete the excision, achieve a cure, or identify an unsuspected deeper invasive component.

Routine use of local excision including TES in the curative resection of T1 rectal cancers has been controversial however because of unacceptably high rates of local recurrence reported in early series on local excision using TAE and TEM relative to radical resection rates. The high risk of locoregional recurrence is directly correlated to the risk of lymph node metastasis, which is not addressed by any of the local excision techniques. While standard preoperative staging of patients with biopsy proven rectal cancer with CEA, stating CT scans and pelvic MRI with or without endorectal ultrasound (ERUS) can exclude patients with T2 and more advanced rectal tumors, the challenge resides in selecting T1 tumors that are associated with the lowest risk of lymph node metastasis and that will be cured with R0 local resection alone.

Across earlier series, local recurrence rates for T1 rectal cancer treated with local excision ranges widely, from 0% to 26%, reflecting the heterogeneity of cohorts treated with either TAE or TEM, with variations in preoperative tumor staging modality, extent of resection (mucosectomy or full thickness), adequacy of resection (R0 vs. R1 resection, en bloc vs. fragmentation, etc.), tumor size and detailed histopathologic analysis to stratify outcomes based on risk factors for occult nodal disease and hence, local recurrence [36, 37, 65–67]. This contrasts with local recurrence rates of 6% or less for T1 tumors treated with radical proctectomy with TME [62]. More contemporary published series, however, have demonstrated that with careful preoperative staging to rule out locally advanced tumors and distant disease, and when T1 rectal tumors are carefully sub-analyzed based on histopathologic features that are now known to be of prognostic significance for lymph node metastasis and local recurrence, a select subgroup of T1 lesions are amenable for local excision by TES with acceptable oncologic outcomes.

Histopathological risk factors for local recurrence following local excision of T1 tumors, by either ESD or full-thickness TES or TAE have been extensively studied. In addition to Kikuchi depth of submucosal involvement, other important histopathologic risk factors for locoregional failure include tumor size, positive resection margins (R1 resection), poor differentiation grade, LVI, and the presence of tumor budding [63, 68–71]. In a retrospective review of 353 patients who underwent radical resection for sessile T1 rectal lesions, Nascimbeni et al. reported a 13% overall incidence of lymph node metastasis [64]. Independent predictors of metastasis based on multivariate analysis included penetration into the deep submucosa or sm3 ($p = 0.001$), LVI ($p = 0.005$) and lesions in the lower third of the rectum ($p = 0.007$). Two additional studies reviewing large prospectively collected databases have also found LVI, poor differentiation, and depth of invasion (T2 lesions, or extension into the muscularis propria) to be significantly related to nodal involvement [63, 72, 73].

Along with LVI, the depth of submucosal invasion is one of the strongest predictors of lymph node metastasis and local recurrence. The depth of submucosal invasion according to the Kikuchi classification has been shown to be predictive of local recurrence following TEM, with depth greater than sm1 being highly predictive of local recurrence [74]. In a cohort of 48 patients who underwent TEM for T1 cancer, at a median follow-up of 54 months, 10.4% developed local recurrence. Of these, none of 26 patients with sm1 lesions developed recurrence, while 5 of 22 patients with sm2–3 lesions recurred, suggesting that T1 sm2–3 lesions carry the same risk for lymph node involvement as T2 tumors and are not suitable for treatment with local excision alone [69]. This finding corroborates the prior finding that the extent of submucosal invasion is highly associated with the likelihood of positive lymph nodes, with sm1 lesions having a 0–3% chance of lymph node positivity, whereas T1 sm2–3 and T2 lesions have 15–25% lymph node positivity [75].

Tumor budding refers to the presence of small discrete clusters of tumor cells (less than five cells) at the invasive tumor edge [76]. Tumor budding is a strong prognostic factor for locoregional and distant metastasis in colorectal cancer and is associated with worse overall and disease-free survival [77]. In a series of 251 submucosally invasive colorectal carcinomas that underwent radical resection, high tumor grade, LVI, and tumor budding were independently associated with lymph node metastasis [78]. Relative to patients without any of the above risk factors, patients with one, two, or three risk factors had significantly higher rates of nodal involvement (1% vs. 21% vs. 36%). These results suggest that local excision with polypectomy, EMR, ESD, or TEM with R0 resection margins would be oncologically adequate for T1 colorectal carcinoma with no evidence of LVI, tumor budding or poor differentiation [78, 79].

As previously demonstrated by the increased incidence of positive resection margins with TES for large rectal adenomas, TES excision for rectal tumors greater than 4 cm in diameter is usually considered a risk factor for local recurrence. In addition, in a series of 62 patients with T1 rectal tumors, Doornebosch et al. reported a 31% local recurrence rate at 3 years following TEM, with significantly higher local recurrence for tumors larger than 3 cm relative to tumors smaller than 3 cm (39% vs. 11%). Local recurrence was lowest in the subgroup of tumors less than 3 cm with no evidence of sm3 submucosal invasion (7%). In addition, the 3-year local recurrence for tumors less than 3 cm without budding was 10% compared with 38% in tumors greater than 3 cm and with budding [68].

With respect to current consensus and guidelines for the management of early rectal cancer, the 2012 NCCN guidelines currently recommend TES as an alternative approach for the management of selected T1 rectal tumors ([80] Table 23.2). According to these guidelines, candidates' lesions include those with no radiographic evidence of lymph node involvement based on preoperative ERUS and/or pelvic MRI, tumors less than 3 cm in diameter and less than 30% of the rectal circumference, well to moderately well differentiated, and within 8 cm of the anal verge. These guidelines are based on several recent series where T1 tumors were carefully selected based on the above histopathological features, with local

Table 23.2 NCCN guidelines for transanal excision of rectal cancer [80]

T1 lesion
Well to moderately differentiated adenocarcinoma
No lymphovascular invasion
No perineural invasion
Less than 3 cm in diameter
Occupying less than 1/3 circumference of the lumen
Mobile, non-fixed
Within 8 cm of the anal verge
Anticipated clear margin (>3 mm)

recurrence rates approaching those of radical surgery with TME. Heintz et al. conducted a retrospective study of all TEM cases performed between 1985 and 1996 and classified T1 tumors as low risk vs. high risk, where low-risk features included good to moderate differentiation and absence of LVI [22]. Using these strict criteria, they could demonstrate a 4.4% local recurrence rate with TEM relative to 2.9% following radical surgery. On the other hand, TEM for high-risk tumors was associated with a 33% risk of recurrence following TEM, relative to 18.2% following radical resection. Several similar studies have demonstrated local recurrence rates ranging from 0% to 10% when strict selection criteria for TEM excision of T1 tumors were used [36, 37, 66, 81]. In a prospective series of 66 T1 rectal cancer cases, Borschitz et al. reported similar differences in local recurrence rates when T1 tumors were stratified according to histopathological features following TEM [37]. Local recurrence rates were 6% vs. 39% in low- vs. high-risk tumors. Another prospective cohort of 110 patients with T1 rectal cancers selected for TEM on the basis of good to moderate differentiation, size less than 3 cm, and distance of 8 cm or less from the anal verge demonstrated no local recurrence at a median follow-up of up to 82 months (range 48–144) [36, 38, 82].

Over the last decade, ESD was developed as an alternative to EMR to facilitate performance of en bloc submucosal resection of large adenomas as well as superficial colorectal cancer (intramucosal adenocarcinoma or T1 sm1 cancers). ESD has been associated with low morbidity, good R0 resection rates and local recurrence rates as well as good short and long-term oncologic outcomes [83, 84]. Although there are no studies comparing TEM and ESD for adenomas, a recent retrospective comparison 30 ESD and 33 TEM cases for resection of non-polypoid rectal mucosal adenocarcinomas or submucosally invasive adenocarcinomas, demonstrated no significant differences in en bloc resection rates or R0 resection rates (96.7 vs. 97%), procedural or postoperative complications, or need for additional treatment such as radical resection or adjuvant treatment. ESD was associated with shorter operative time and length of hospital stay, and no local recurrence or distant metastases were noted over the study period [83]. Compared with conventional EMR, ESD is technically more difficult with an exceedingly long learning curve with has been a major obstacle for wider adoption. At this time, TES remains the preferred approach for en bloc excision of large rectal adenomas, malignant polyps, and carefully selected T1 rectal cancers.

23.4.3 High-Risk T1 and T2 Rectal Cancers

As previously demonstrated, TES excision of high-risk T1 rectal cancer has been associated with local recurrence rate as high as 33% when pT1 tumors were demonstrated to harbor high-risk histopathological factors [22, 37]. With respect to T2 rectal tumors, the majority of series reporting on long-term oncologic outcomes following local excision of rectal cancer did not differentiate between type of local excision and combined data from TAE and TEM approach. In their series of 261 patients treated with TAE or radical resection (RR) for T1 or T2 rectal cancer not treated with adjuvant therapy, Mellgren et al., the local recurrence rate in the cohort of unselected T1 rectal tumors was 18% vs. 0% for T1 tumors in the TAE vs. RR group, and 47% vs. 10% for T2 tumors in the TAE vs. RR group [19]. The estimated 5-year survival was similar for T1 tumors between the groups (72% vs. 80%), but it was significantly lower for T2 tumors (65% vs. 81%) in the TAE vs. RR group [19]. A more contemporary series by Elmessiry that included both TAE and TEM, reported outcomes of unselected T1 and T2 rectal adenocarcinomas treated with LE ($N = 74$) or radical resection with TME (RR = 79) without the use of adjuvant treatment. Although no statistically significant difference in local recurrence (18.4% vs. 5.1%) or 3-year DFS (84.2% vs. 94.9%) was noted between LE vs. RR groups for pT1 tumors, local recurrence was significantly higher with LE vs. RR (42.3% vs. 7.5%) with significantly worse 3-year DFS (61.5% vs. 87.5%) but no difference in overall survival between the groups [85].

The 5-year local recurrence rates following TEM excision for T2 lesions, including TEM, not treated with neoadjuvant or adjuvant therapy, ranges from 19.5% to as high as 36% [19, 86]. In a series of 17 vs. 83 pT2 rectal tumors resected with TEM vs. RR and where no patients received adjuvant therapy, local recurrence was 19.5% vs. 9.4% in the TEM vs. RR group ($p = 0.035$) but the 3-year DFS was similar between the two groups [86]. In their series of 40 T2 rectal tumors treated with TEM alone with no further surgery or adjuvant therapy, at a median follow-up of 59 months, the local and distant recurrence rate was 35% and 30%, respectively [37]. Among patients with high-risk histopathological features such as poorly differentiated or LVI, the local recurrence rate was as high as 50% [37]. Overall, although local recurrence rates in series where T2 tumors were strictly resected full-thickness dissection with TEM were substantially lower than those reported in mixed TAE and TEM series, such unacceptably high recurrence rates relative to historical outcomes with radical resection preclude the use of local excision for the curative resection of T2 rectal tumors without neoadjuvant or adjuvant treatment.

Based on the above findings, when histopathologic analysis of resected TES specimens demonstrates R1 resection margins or when tumors are staged as a pT1 with adverse pathologic features or upstaged to pT2, patients should undergo immediate salvage radical surgery [74]. Several retrospective series have reported on outcomes of patients who, rather than immediate resection, received adjuvant CRT, typically in patients who either declined immediate radical resection or who were considered medically unfit. These series include patients treated with neoadjuvant and/or adjuvant therapy with significant heterogeneity in selection criteria, regimens (CRT or radiation alone), with variability in local and distant recurrence rates, and on long-term oncologic outcomes, which was further impacted by whether or not patients ultimately underwent salvage radical surgery [67, 87]. In one study by Ramirez et al. where six high-risk pT1 and 24 pT2 rectal cancers resected using TEM were treated with 50.4 Gy of adjuvant radiation, local recurrence was noted in three (10%) at a mean follow-up of 71 with a 5-year cancer-specific survival of 93%, relative to 8% recurrence rate, and 98% CSS in 54 patients who underwent TEM for low-risk pT1 rectal tumors [81].

The role of neoadjuvant CRT has been increasingly explored both in combination with local excision of T2 and T3 tumors, and more recently, in the non-operative management of rectal cancer. Lezoche et al. reported their group's long-term outcomes from a randomized trial of 100 preoperatively staged T2 N0 rectal cancers treated with neoadjuvant CRT and subsequently randomized to TEM vs. laparoscopic TME [39]. At a median follow-up of 9.6 years, the local recurrence was 6% vs. 8% in the TEM vs. RR group [39]. Moreover, the surgical morbidity was lower in the TEM group. Other groups have since cautioned about the relative incidence of TEM wound-related complications in radiated patients, ranging 0–60.9% and which include dehiscence associated with severe and refractory pain [87–89]. The prospective multicenter ACOSOG Z6041 phase II trial recently reported the 3-year oncologic outcome from 72 patients with preoperative staged T2 N0 cancers located within the distal 8 cm of the rectum and treated with FOLFOX and 54 Gy of radiation followed by local excision using TAE or TES [40, 90]. Complete pathologic response was noted in 44% and 64% of tumors were downstaged (ypT0–1) with 39% incidence of CRT related toxicity [40]. The 3-year DFS for the intention-to-treat group was 88.2% and 86.9% for the per-protocol group. Overall organ sparing could be achieved in 66% of patients, and the authors concluded that neoadjuvant therapy followed by local excision should be reserved for those with cT2 N0 lesions that are not otherwise amenable to anterior resection [90]. The CARTS study recently investigated the pathologic response of 51 cT1–3 N0 rectal tumors treated with capecitabine and 50–54 Gy of radiation followed TEM resection [91]. Among the 47/51 tumors that demonstrated sufficient clinical downstaging to proceed with TEM (ycT0–2), 30 were staged ypT0–1 with negative resection margins and were observed. There was a 42% incidence of toxicity and 3.6% mortality rate related to CRT. At a median follow-up 17 months, four local recurrences were noted in one patient with ypT1, and three patients with ypT2 tumors who declined radical resection. Overall, organ sparing could be achieved in 55% of patients with CRT [91].

Most recently, advocates of organ-preserving strategies have investigated the outcomes of non-operative management for rectal tumors that have demonstrated complete clinical regression following neoadjuvant therapy. The "watch-and-wait" approach has been most extensively evaluated by Habr-Gama et al. in a cohort of 69 patients with cT2–T4, N0–N2 tumors treated with intensive CRT regimens, achieving a 68% rate of complete clinical response when assessed 10–12 weeks following completion of treatment based on imaging, endoscopy, and DRE confirming the absence of residual tumor or other mucosal irregularity [92]. These 47 patients were subsequently observed and a sustained complete clinical response was observed in

51% of the entire cohort at 3 years posttreatment. The remaining 49% with evidence of recurrent disease underwent immediate or salvage surgery with either TEM or radical surgery. Several European series have corroborated the findings from the Habr-Gama group [93, 94]. With more aggressive CRT regimens, the rates of complete clinical response have exceeded the historical 20–30% rate, although this occurs at the expense of increase toxicity and possibly overtreatment early rectal tumors that ultimately require salvage radical resection.

Ultimately, the oncologic adequacy of TES with or without neoadjuvant treatment is dependent on accurate tumor staging, careful patient selection, and intensive postoperative surveillance in order to promptly identify local recurrences and salvage patients with radical resection, particularly in patients receiving neoadjuvant treatment. There is no consensus on neoadjuvant treatment regimen or surveillance protocols following TES or following neoadjuvant CRT with complete clinical response. Another challenge is posed by the accuracy of postradiation imaging in detecting residual or recurrent disease, which is notoriously difficult to interpret due to radiation-induced fibrosis and inflammation.

While the evidence in support of the role of TEM as part of a multimodal organ-sparing strategy for T2 N0 rectal cancer, current NCCN guidelines recommend that treatment with neoadjuvant treatment with or without local excision be used only in the experimental setting [80].

23.4.4 Radical Resection and Salvage Surgery for Recurrence Following TES

In the event that more advanced pathology or positive resection margins are uncovered following local excision of a presumed low-risk rectal cancer, multiple studies have found no significant difference in oncologic outcomes when local excision is followed by completion radical resection TME compared to performing TME as initial therapy [67]. This scenario is common and results from inaccurate preoperative staging due to limitations of our current imaging modalities for low rectal tumors in particular, and insufficient tumor sampling which can limit assessment of prognostic histopathological features. In many cases of suspected early rectal cancers where the alternative would require APR and grossly overtreat early rectal tumors, local excision techniques including full-thickness TES have been increasingly used as excisional biopsy and guide further therapy. In a case-matched study by Levic et al., 25 patients who underwent TEM followed by interval radical resection 14–90 days later based on findings of unsuspected adverse pathological findings were compared to 25 patients who underwent TME as primary treatment [95]. The groups were well matched with respect to tumor staging, omission of neoadjuvant treatment, and subsequent use of adjuvant treatment. No differences in operative time or intraoperative complications were noted between the groups, suggesting that prior TEM did not greatly increase the technical difficulty of interval TME. However more patients in the primary TME group had a complete or near-complete mesorectal fascia although that difference did not reach statistical significance [95]. Overall, no differences in local and distant recurrence rates were noted between the groups [95]. A similar study comparing 17 patients undergoing TEM followed by laparoscopic TME (LTME) within 8 weeks of TEM due to adverse histological factors were compared to 34 patients who underwent primary LTME with no significant differences in tumor stage, tumor location, demographics, or preoperative treatment [96]. A significantly higher rate of APR was performed in the post-TEM LTME group, and prior TEM was the only independent predictor of APR. Although post-TEM LTME procedures required longer operative time that primary LTME procedures, the perioperative morbidity, and quality of mesorectal excision was similar between the groups.

The issue of the quality of TME achieved following full-thickness TEM excision has been a source of concern however. In a retrospective review of 36 TEM cases that underwent interval completion TME 0.5–8.7 weeks later for adverse pathological features without neoadjuvant therapy, 53% of radical resections were graded as "difficult" mostly due to bleeding and/or fibrosis at the TEM site, with a 17% incidence of major postoperative complications and 19.4% incidence of incomplete mesorectal excision [97]. The R0 resection rate was 94.5% and adjuvant CRT or radiation was given to 30.5% of patients following interval TME. At a median follow-up of 49.2 months, only one local recurrence but five distant recurrences occurred with an 85% 5-year OS but only 74% disease-specific survival. The authors found that full-thickness TME for distal rectal tumors, and a > 7 weeks interval to completion TME, correlated with an inferior mesorectal specimen [97]. In conclusion, although there is some evidence that interval TME following full-thickness TES may be technically more challenging, more morbid, and may decrease the likelihood of achieving sphincter preservation relative to primary therapy with TME, oncologic outcomes appear similar, particularly in the setting of adjuvant therapy.

On the other hand, when radical resection is undertaken later as salvage therapy for local recurrence following local excision, outcomes are generally poor. Baron et al. evaluated 21 patients who underwent immediate LAR or APR following TEM because of adverse histopathological features and compared their outcome to another group of 21 patients who underwent salvage LAR or APR for local recurrence [98]. Although the T stage of primary tumors was similar between the groups, the DFS of the immediate reoperation group was 94.1% vs. only 55.5% for the salvage group [98]. Similarly, a retrospective study of 50 patients who underwent salvage surgery to treat a local recurrence following local excision for T1 and T2 rectal tumors reported that 55% of 49 resectable patients required an extended pelvic dissection with en bloc resection [99]. Overall, 44% of patients received adjuvant CRT following local excision, and another subset received adjuvant treatment either before or after salvage surgery. Although a 96% R0 resection rate could be achieved with aggressive salvage surgery, 29 patients recurred or died of disease, and the 5-year OS was 53% [99].

In the setting of the increasing use of organ-preserving strategies in the management of locally advanced low rectal tumors that would otherwise require APR, oncologic outcomes of patients with complete clinical response following CRT confirmed on local excision and subsequently observed have been under evaluation, including the outcomes of salvage resection in cases of local recurrence. In a prospective series by Pucciarelli et al., 63 patients with cT2/3 and N0/1 rectal tumors treated with CRT and restaged. If there was evidence of clinical response, local excision was performed followed by observation for ypT0–1 with tumor regression grade (TRG) ≤2 and negative margins. In cases of more advanced pathology, immediate TME was performed [100]. Overall, there were two local recurrences and two distant recurrences, and both local recurrences were treated with salvage TME with good oncologic outcomes. Overall, the organ salvage rate was 90.5%, and the estimated cumulative 3-year OS, DFS, and local disease-free survival was 91.5, 91, and 96.5%, respectively [100]. Finally, in the Habr-Gama watch-an-wait study mentioned earlier, where among a cohort of 69 patients in whom cT2–T4 rectal tumors were treated with CRT, 51% sustained complete clinical response at 3 years post-CRT [92]. Among the 33 patients who failed the watch-and-wait protocol, 22 with an incomplete response underwent immediate TME, while eight patients with initial clinical complete response developed local recurrence. Seven recurrences were amenable to salvage surgery, but three developed either local or systemic recurrence of systemic recurrences only with a 3-year OS and DFS of 90% and 72%, respectively. An additional four patients developed late recurrence, 100% of which could be salvaged with R0 resection with no evidence of disease at a median follow-up of 25.5 months [92].

Overall, cumulatively, these studies demonstrate that in the setting of the watch- and wait approach which incorporate aggressive surveillance protocol to ensure early detection of locoregional recurrence, salvage resection for early and late recurrences is associated with acceptable oncologic outcomes.

23.4.5 Palliation of Rectal Cancer

In medically unfit patients, locally advanced and symptomatic rectal cancer often requires palliation through fecal diversion, stenting, surgical debulking, cryosurgery, embolization and radiotherapy. Multimodal approach combining TEM and neoadjuvant treatment, or TEM without CRT, can be used in the palliative treatment of advanced rectal tumors and in patients who refuse radical surgery that would otherwise require a permanent colostomy.

Turler et al. described TES as an alternative method for rectal cancer palliation for bleeding and intestinal obstruction in a case series of 29 patients [101]. Rectal bleeding was controlled by coagulation or suture placement and obstruction was relieved by complete or near-complete excision of the mass. Preoperative symptoms of bleeding and intestinal obstruction were relieved in all cases. One patient experienced an intra-abdominal perforation, and the overall morbidity rate was reported to be 14%. Thirteen patients died from their rectal cancer within 3–58 months and eight patients remained without recurrence during postoperative surveillance [101]. Therefore, TES is a viable option for rectal cancer palliation in the appropriate setting and aligned with patient-specific goals of care.

23.4.6 Carcinoid Tumors

Carcinoid tumors of the gastrointestinal tract are a slow-growing neuroendocrine tumors (NET) for which the rectum is a common site of occurrence. A review of the SEER database from 1973 to 2008 revealed the incidence of all gastrointestinal NETs has increased over the past four decades with the highest rates in the small bowel and rectum [102]. Of the 19,699 patients with GI NETS, 6796 had lesions in the rectum, making this the second most common site of observed occurrence. Rectal carcinoids were most likely to be detected in the age group of 40–59 which is likely attributable to improved detection during and increased utilization of screening endoscopy. Despite being indolent, carcinoid tumors are malignant tumors whose risk of lymph node metastasis is directly related to tumor size and evidence of LVI. Staging of rectal carcinoids includes ERUS in addition to staging CT scans and surgical options for resection includes endoscopic resection with EMR or ESD, TAE, TES, and radical proctectomy. A multicenter study retrospectively reviewing nine prospective databases compiled a cumulative experience of 202 patients with rectal carcinoids treated by endoscopic surgery (n = 86), radical resection (n = 101), or transanal excision (n = 16); six patients (6%) were treated by TEM [103]. Multivariate analysis found size >1 cm and LVI to be independent predictors of nodal involvement ($p = 0.006$ and $p < 0.001$, respectively) leading to the conclusion that lesions with such characteristics should be managed via TME. Other meta-analyses have demonstrated that tumor size greater than 10 mm, T stage, and LVI were independently associated with an increased risk of metastatic disease [104, 105]. Although endoscopic treatment of small and superficial rectal carcinoids is associated with good local control and survival, worse outcomes are associated with increasing tumor size, advanced T stage, and presence of metastases [106]. Although there are no strict guidelines on the optimal surgical treatment for carcinoids, the consensus is that local excision, including endoscopic resection, is safe for carcinoid tumors less than 10 mm, with no invasion of the muscularis propria and no ulceration [107]. TES is particularly well suited for treating rectal carcinoids, either for primary full-thickness excision of small rectal carcinoids with no high-risk features on preoperative imaging or for completion resection of lesions incompletely removed endoscopically (with indeterminate of positive resection margins).

The two largest retrospective series of TEM as a modality for treatment of rectal carcinoids either used for initial resection or following incomplete endoscopic excision included 27 and 24 patients in the Japanese and US publication, respectively [108, 109]. The average primary tumor size was 7.5–10.1 mm, and the residual tumor was 0.7–7.9 mm, and the distance from the anal verge was 8.5–9 cm. In the Japanese series, all tumors were localized with the submucosal layer, and R0 resection was achieved in all cases [108]. In the US series, one patient with a 15 mm rectal carcinoid underwent interval LAR [109]. At a mean follow-up of 30–70.6 months, all patients were alive and disease-free [108, 109].

23.4.7 Retrorectal Tumors

Retrorectal tumors are rare lesions, usually diagnosed and treated in children but that can remain asymptomatic until adulthood when they are typically diagnosed incidentally. Retrorectal tumors are classified as congenital, neurogenic, osseous, or miscellaneous and can be benign or malignant. In several small case series and reports, TES has been described as a minimally invasive transanal approach to remove these lesions. Although preliminary, this approach would represent a minimally alternative to the traditional transabdominal or transcoccygeal approach which typically requires coccygectomy. Advantages include excellent visualization and exposure of the presacral space through the transanal platforms to allow for precise dissection of these lesions off the coccyx [110]. Zoller et al. first reported using TEM to resect tail gut cysts in two adult patients in 2007 [111]. An additional case of a perineal inclusion cyst treated successfully with TEM resection was subsequently described [112]. The largest series included six patients with tailgut and duplication cysts resected transanally with TEM with no evidence of recurrence at 24 months postoperatively [113]. One patient in this series was found to have squamous cell carcinoma within the tailgut cyst that was treated with chemotherapy following the Nigro protocol without recurrence at 20 months. Serra-Aracil et al. described three cases of retrorectal tumors excised as part of a larger of a larger series describing atypical indications for TEM [114]. Retrorectal tumors included two peritoneal inclusion cysts and one epidermal cyst, with no recurrence noted during a follow-up ranging from 16 to 38 months. Overall, TES may serve as an alternative surgical approach for resection of small and benign retrorectal tumors based on proper patient selection and preoperative imaging. Benefits of this approach may include minimal surgical morbidity, improved cosmesis and faster recovering.

23.4.8 Rectovisceral Fistulae

TES has been described for repair of multiple rectovisceral fistulae including complex fistulas to the urethra, vagina, and bladder, particularly in cases of repeatedly failed local repair using a transrectal or transvaginal approach, and in order to avoid a major abdominal procedure. Repair of a rectourethral fistula utilizing a combined TEM and transurethral approach was initially described in two patients who developed complications from radical prostatectomy [115]. The fistula tract was excised endoscopically through the transanal platform and a full-thickness rectal advancement flap was used to close the defect. Transurethral repair through cystoscopy consisted in cauterization of the tract and closure of the defect with fibrin glue. Additional case reports have subsequently described transanal rectourethral fistula closure using TEM in eight patients with recurrence in two patients that ultimately required definitive closure with a gracilis muscle interposition flap [114, 116–119]. Atallah et al. reported the first successful case of TAMIS closure for a rectourethral fistula in a patient who developed the fistula following cryoablation of prostate cancer and who diverted with a loop ileostomy. Layered closure of the fistula tract with absorbable sutures was performed through the TAMIS platform, and the patient subsequently underwent stoma reversal with no recurrence 23 months post-closure [120].

There is a single published case series describing repair of rectovesicular fistula following radical prostatectomy using TEM in ten patients [121]. All patients had already undergone fecal diversion with placement of urinary drainage catheters and had undergone failed attempt at fistula closure using transanal suture repair. Patients were placed in prone position, and TEM procedures consisted in resection of the rectal mucosa and fistula tract into the bladder followed by closure of the bladder and rectal wall in multiple layers. Successful closure was achieved in five patients, while three patients developed recurrence within 8 weeks, all with a history of severe fibrosis at the fistula site from two to three prior fistula repairs. One patient was successfully treated with a gracilis interposition flap whereas the other two refused further intervention [121].

Rectovaginal fistulas that have failed conventional transrectal and/or transvaginal repair are also amenable to TEM repair, particularly when the fistulas are located higher up in the rectum and difficult to access through standard transanal approach. D'Ambrosio et al. conducted a retrospective review of 13 patients with rectovaginal fistula repaired by TEM over an 8 year period with a median follow-up of 25 months [122]. Fistulas occurred as a complication of transvaginal hysterectomy ($n = 7$), low anterior resection ($n = 5$), and following pelvic radiation ($n = 1$). All patients presented with prior fecal diversion. Nine patients experienced a failed attempt at transperineal fistula closure, of which four had multiple failed repairs with either transabdominal, transperineal or a combined approach. The procedure was performed in prone position for optimal visualization of the rectovaginal septum which is dissected through the TEM platform and further dissected bluntly after removing the proctoscope. Repair of the vaginal wall and rectal defect are then performed through the TEM platform. Only one patient developed recurrence and underwent repeat TEM repair which ultimately failed, and the patient declined to undergo further intervention [122]. The success of TEM in this series, particularly in the setting of multiple prior failed local repairs, highlights the potential for TES-based repair, particularly due to the enhanced exposure provided by these multiport platforms.

23.4.9 Colorectal Anastomotic Leak

Anastomotic leaks frequently complicate colorectal procedures, with rates ranging 3–25% with mortality as high as 22%, particularly following low colorectal and coloanal anastomoses [123, 124]. In the acute setting, in the absence of sepsis, colorectal anastomotic leaks can often be successfully managed conservatively with bowel rest, antibiotics, and percutaneous drainage. Provided patients remain stable and that urgent abdominal drainage and fecal diversion is not needed, transanal suture repair of small anastomotic defects has been described with success in selected patients [125]. TES platforms may provide a well-suited platform for improved access to colorectal anastomoses, drainage of presacral abscesses with or without primary repair of small anastomotic defects. Beunis et al. described an anastomotic leak case following laparoscopic rectosigmoid resection with an end-to-end stapled anastomosis for recurrent diverticulitis that was successfully repaired using TEM [126]. The anastomotic defect measured 1.5 cm and was closed primarily with interrupted sutures. Neither re-intervention nor fecal diversion was necessary. In the subacute setting, persistent anastomotic leaks can also be difficult to treat, particularly following rectal cancer resection in patients who have undergone CRT. Anastomotic defects and associated presacral abscesses often fail to heal despite repeated drainage, local debridement, direct suture repair, anorectal advancement flap repair, even with concurrent fecal diversion [127]. Options for definitive repair include takedown of the anastomosis and more distal coloanal anastomosis or permanent colostomy, which are associated with substantial morbidity and poor functional outcomes. TES may represent an alternative approach for local repair and was described by Sneider et al. in a patient with a persistent colorectal anastomotic leak 15 months post low anterior resection of a previously radiated rectal cancer. Through a TAMIS platform, a small defect was visualized along the linear staple line, which was opened and allowed endoscopic debridement of a chronic presacral abscess cavity followed by suture closure of the defect, with good long-term outcome [128]. While TEM serves as an excellent local adjunct to attempt to repair these problems transanally, the underlying issues of tissue fibrosis, limited mobility, and chronic infection remain. These factors together often make a transanal approach, even with the TES equipment, a nonviable option.

23.4.10 Pelvic Abscess

Transrectal drainage of pelvic abscesses complicating colorectal surgery represents an important therapeutic alternative in cases where the size and location of the pelvic abscess may pose a technical challenge and preclude safe transabdominal, transgluteal, or transperineal percutaneous drainage. When suitable, percutaneous drainage is always preferable to operative drainage given the added morbidity associated with reoperative procedures. TES has been described as an approach to transrectally drain abscesses in locations not amenable to percutaneous drainage. This technique was first reported in 2012 to describe the case of a patient with sepsis due to a pelvic abscess following a Hartmann procedure for perforated rectal cancer [129]. The abscess was approached using TEM by opening the rectal stump staple line to drain the purulent fluid. Local exploration was performed confirming no evidence of an enteric fistula or perforation and the cavity was irrigated. The stump was left open and a drainage catheter was placed. No further intervention was necessary. Serra-Aracil et al. reported the cases of TES drainage of pelvic abscesses from perforated diverticulitis, complicating a Hartmann procedure for ischemic colitis, and from an unknown etiology [114]. Two abscesses were approached using TEM and one with the TEO platform. The abscess was drained through a defect in the rectal wall and a drain was placed with subsequent resolution of the abscess.

23.4.11 Benign Strictures

Benign rectal strictures most commonly complicate stapled and handsewn colorectal anastomoses although other inflammatory etiologies include IBD, radiation, trauma, and iatrogenic causes. While endoscopic balloon dilatation or transanal dilatation are usually sufficient, a subset of strictures require additional intervention including strictureplasty, colorectal resection with coloanal anastomosis, or even proctectomy in severe cases. Transanal strictureplasty can be challenging when strictures are located in the upper rectum. TES can facilitate endoscopic access and permit strictureplasty under excellent visualization and exposure. Baatrup et al. described successful treatment of benign strictures using TEM for a series of six patients involving partial excision of the stricture [130]. Strictures were excised using a bipolar device with full-thickness posterior incision of the rectal wall for approximately one third of stricture circumference followed by transverse closure of the rectal defect. Satisfactory functional results were reported in five of the six patients. One additional case report described a hybrid approach using TEM for longitudinal stricture incision followed by endoscopic balloon dilation without evidence of luminal compromise at one-year follow-up [131].

23.4.12 Foreign Body Removal

The use of traditional bedside transanal extraction of foreign bodies is only successful for approximately 75% of patients, and the remainder must be removed operatively either via an exam under anesthesia or by laparoscopy or laparotomy [132]. There have been two case reports of successful foreign body extraction utilizing the TAMIS platform [133, 134]. This application of TES is appealing to avoid the morbidity associated with more aggressive abdominal exploration. TES also permits excellent endoscopic visualization and facilitates accurate assessment of the rectal mucosa to rule out full-thickness injury that would prompt additional treatment.

23.4.13 Transanal NOSE and NOTES

Transvaginal and transanal specimen extraction during left-sided colorectal resection, also termed NOSE (Natural Orifice Specimen Extraction), has been proposed as a strategy to help reduce the number of abdominal incision and incision-related complications including incisional pain, wound infection, and incisional hernia rate [135]. TES platforms have been used as a transanal portal not only for transanal specimen extraction but also to deliver the anvil intraperitoneally in preparation for stapled colorectal anastomosis [136, 137]. In a trial of 70 patients undergoing laparoscopic left colectomy for cancer and randomized to either conventional transabdominal or transanal specimen extraction and anvil insertion through the TEO platform, Leung et al. reports significantly lower pain scores and wound infection rate in the transanal group [136]. Other authors have also described performing rectal transection through TES platforms, in addition to specimen extraction and anvil insertion [138]. Limitation to widespread adoption of NOSE has been the steep learning curve.

One of the most exciting advances in transanal surgery has been the evolution of transanal Natural Orifice Transluminal Endoscopic Surgery (NOTES) techniques and platforms. First through the use of rigid TEM and TEO platform and soon thereafter through newly commercialized TAMIS platforms, transanal endoscopic proctectomy with TME, with and without laparoscopic abdominal assistance, was demonstrated to be feasible in experimental models, human cadavers, and quickly transitioned to clinical application in 2009 [139–142]. Through improved exposure via transanal platforms, CO_2 insufflation, and videoscopic setup, TES can further the extent of intersphincteric, rectal, and mesorectal dissection that was previously be performed through conventional transanal approach in combination with transabdominal TME [143, 144]. Since the first case report of laparoscopic-assisted transanal TME for rectal cancer [142], nearly 500 case reports and series of pure and hybrid transanal TME with LAR or APR for benign and malignant indications have been published to date, with acceptable morbidity and short-term oncologic safety profile [145–150]. Although no prospective comparative study or randomized controlled trial has yet been published, based on the reports published to date, proposed benefits of taTME include:

1. The ability to establish a tumor-free distal margin by initiating the dissection transanally
2. Improved exposure, visualization, and maneuverability around TME planes in a narrow pelvis relative to the abdominal approach
3. Elimination of an abdominal extraction site by extracting the specimen transanally when feasible
4. Potential reduction in OR time with simultaneous abdominal and transanal dissection

Further investigation of long-term functional and oncologic outcomes of taTME is necessary, particularly as it relates to laparoscopic and robotic TME.

One particularly attractive application of transanal NOTES using TES is completion proctectomy in patients with retained rectal stumps and severe diversion or Crohn's proctitis, rectovaginal or perineal fistulas, or with dysplasia. Pure transanal proctectomy without any abdominal incisions can be performed using TES platforms. Both Bremers and Liyanage described pure transanal proctectomy using TEM in a series of 9 and 16 patients, respectively, with retained stumps following surgery for IBD, collagenous colitis, lynch syndrome, dysplasia, anastomotic leaks, and radiation proctitis [151, 152] In both cases, intersphincteric dissection was initiated perianally followed by rectal mobilization with preservation of the mesorectum. Four patients required abdominal assistance, one patient developed a postoperative abscess, and four had delayed perineal wound healing. This approach demonstrates the feasibility and safety of pure transanal completion proctectomy in selected patients and can avoid the morbidity of abdominal incisions.

23.5 Patient Selection, Preoperative Planning, Assessment, and Preparation

23.5.1 Patient Selection

Historically, rectal tumor location higher than 8–10 cm was considered a relative contraindication to TES, particularly if anterior, due to the high chance of full-thickness excision resulting in peritoneal entry [153]. That is because inadvertent peritoneal entry during full-thickness TEM excision was previously considered to be a complication requiring immediate conversion to laparotomy with low anterior resection or fecal diversion in order to mitigate the risk of leak and infection [154, 155]. However, extensive recent data from experienced centers have demonstrated the feasibility and safety of performing transanal suture closure of upper rectal full-thickness defects without increased morbidity or adverse oncologic outcomes. Overall, only lesions within the reach of the 12–20 cm rigid proctoscope, and otherwise amenable to local excision, should be considered for full-thickness TES resection.

At the other extreme end of the rectum, TAMIS platforms do not permit access to rectal polyps located within 4 cm of the anal verge [32]. For lesions partially or entirely located within the distal 4 cm of the anorectal canal, the TEM and TEO platforms can often be pulled back maximally to permit exposure without losing excessive pneumorectum. This is in contrast to TAMIS where resection must be combined with a standard TAE approach for the distal part of the dissection.

With respect to rectal tumor size, nearly obstructing, near-circumferential, and circumferential tumors constitute a contraindication for TES. This is due to the anticipated difficulty in achieving R0 resection and safely closing giant rectal defects using a purely transanal approach, without resulting in rectal stenosis or incomplete closure [156].

23.5.2 Preoperative Planning

TES can be safely performed in the large majority of patients, including high-risk surgical patients, provided they are acceptable candidates for intervention under anesthesia. TES can also be safely performed in patients with morbid obesity (BMI ranging from 35 to 66) as reported in a recent case series without an increase in adverse events [157].

Potential candidates for TES must undergo a comprehensive evaluation to localize and stage rectal lesions. Preoperative workup must include a colonoscopy with biopsy and careful pathology review to locally stage malignant lesions and identify histopathological risk factors that might contraindicate local excision. In addition to comprehensive clinical evaluation, DRE is essential to assess baseline sphincter tone, and for low palpable rectal tumors, DRE is useful to assess fixity, location in relation to the anorectal ring as well as exact location along the rectal wall. Presence of a tight rectal stricture precluding safe insertion of a rigid or disposable TES platform would exclude patients from consideration for TES. A low baseline anal sphincter tone on DRE indicative of impaired sphincter function may preclude further sphincter dilatation with TES, and the potential risk for at least transient worsened fecal incontinence should be discussed with patients preoperatively.

Rigid or flexible proctoscopy is also needed preoperatively to determine the exact distance from the anal verge, tumor size and extent of rectal wall involvement, and orientation along the rectal wall. This assessment is essential to determine the extent and feasibility of the planned resection, anticipate potential operative challenges and mitigate complications, and optimize patient positioning and available instrumentation to complete TES procedures safely.

23.5.3 Preoperative Staging

Early rectal cancers that are under evaluation for TES should also be staged as per standard of care which include carcinoembryonic antigen (CEA), CT scans of the chest, abdomen, and pelvis to rule out distant spread and a pelvic MRI and/or endorectal ultrasound (ERUS). While the T-stage accuracy of ERUS is largely operator dependent with reported accuracy ranging from 63% to 95% across studies, accuracy rates in assessing nodal status only range 65–81% [158]. Overall, ERUS is relatively less accurate at differentiating between T1 and T2 lesions, with one multi-institutional study reporting a 57% accuracy, relative to rates as high as 88% accuracy in identifying T1 lesions in individual center studies [159, 160]. Despite the accuracy obtained by highly skilled practitioners, a recent study showed that the results of ERUS rarely changed the management plan for patients undergoing TES when used in conjunction with CT scan and pelvic MRI [161].

Pelvic MRI has supplanted ERUS as the preferred modality for rectal cancer staging. Unfortunately all of these methods have significant difficulty in differentiating a T1 from an early T2 cancer. Although standard MRI imaging has comparably low sensitivity and specificity as ERUS for lymph node assessment, it provides critical assessment of CRM, tumor location in relation to anal sphincters, prostate, vagina, and even the peritoneal reflection, all essential for accurate local staging [162]. Newer radiographic technologies, such as 3 T MRI, may improve nodal staging in rectal cancer by providing morphologic details beyond nodal size, which is not a reliable predictor of lymph node involvement [163].

23.5.4 Preoperative Preparation and Operative Setup

Patients typically undergo full mechanical bowel preparation and/or administration of enemas prior to surgery in order to clear the rectum, allow adequate visualization, and prevent fecal peritoneal contamination in the event of full-thickness resection with peritoneal entry. Enemas and/or full mechanical bowel preparation are also used selectively based on anticipation of the possibility of full-thickness excision with peritoneal entry. Standard perioperative parenteral antibiotic prophylaxis as well as thromboembolic prophylaxis is also administered. A Foley catheter is usually inserted if procedures are anticipated to require longer than 2 h, although in combination with low intraoperative fluid strategy, insertion may not be mandatory. General anesthesia with complete muscle paralysis is usually recommended for TES in order to avoid abdominal wall contractions during procedures, thereby minimizing CO_2 leakage and maintaining a working pneumorectum. A recent case series reported the feasibility and safety of TAMIS under spinal anesthesia in 25 patients with rectal lesions located in the mid and upper rectum [32]. However, the insufflation of the bowel with CO2 can lead to loss of diaphragmatic excursion and respiratory problems with this approach.

Depending on the tumor location along the rectum and TES platform used, patients are either placed in the supine, prone, or lateral decubitus position (Fig. 23.1). Patients are either placed in lithotomy position using stirrups or prone using split leg operating tables. By design, TEM and TEO platforms are beveled at their tip, with the 30° angled camera fixed at the superior aspect of the platform. By convention, rectal lesions should be in a dependent position, directly opposite the operating camera for optimal visualization and instrument triangulation. Therefore, anterior rectal lesions are managed with patients in prone position, whereas posterior lesions are managed in lithotomy and lateral lesions with patients in lateral

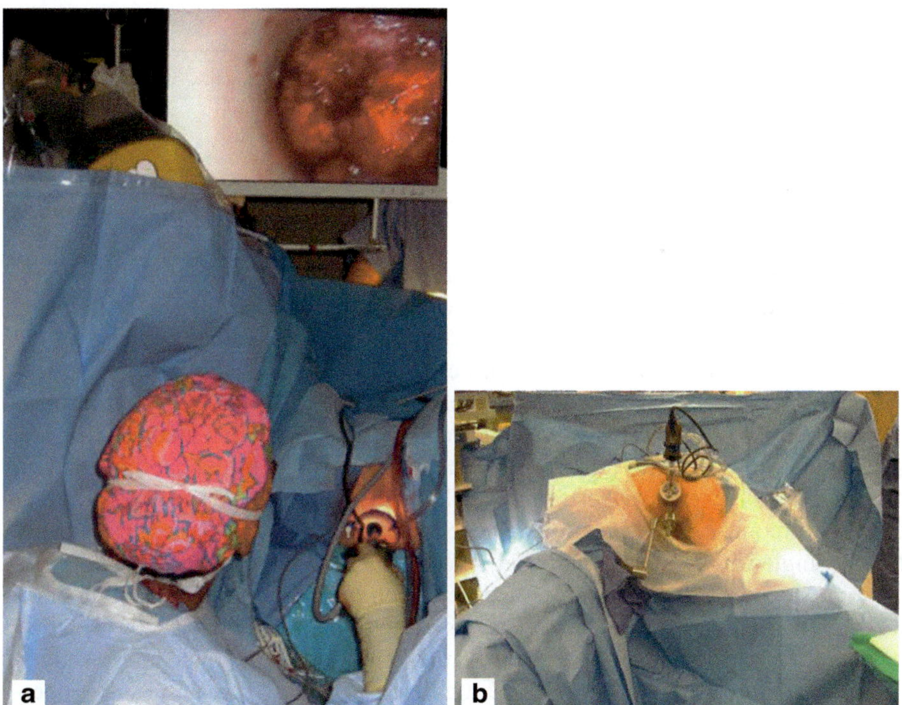

Fig. 23.1 TES setup. Patients are positioned in lithotomy (**a**) or prone position (**b**). The monitor is placed in an ergonomically favorable position, typically between the patient's legs

decubitus positioning. Most experienced TEM and TEO operators however will perform the majority of these procedures with patients in lithotomy regardless of the location of the lesion [164]. TAMIS is usually performed with patients in lithotomy position, and the use of a deflectable-tip scope and articulating instruments greatly facilitates exposure and visualization during these procedures [30].

One relative indication for placing patients in prone position includes anticipation of peritoneal entry during full-thickness excision of high-risk rectal lesions [96]. High-risk lesions for peritoneal entry include anterior and lateral lesions located in the upper rectum or rectosigmoid, as well as circumferential or near-circumferential lesions [165–168]. Peritoneal entry through large rectal wall defects can result in the rapid accumulation of CO_2 into the abdominal cavity and collapse of loss of the pneumorectum. In such cases, closure of the rectal wall defect can be very difficult due to poor exposure. Preemptively positioning of patients in prone position can mitigate the extent of CO_2 leakage into the abdominal cavity and help maintain a stable pneumorectum to facilitate closure of the full-thickness rectal wall defect [169].

Prior to insertion of the TES platform, anal blockade with a local anesthetic is performed followed by gentle dilatation of the anus to prevent rectal trauma. The typical CO_2 pressure needed to maintain an adequate pneumorectum ranges 9–18 mmHg, although high pressures might be needed to compensate for CO_2 leakage.

23.6 TES Procedures

23.6.1 Instrumentation

The original TEM platform (Richard Wolf, Tubingen, Germany) consists in a 4 cm-wide rigid beveled proctoscope that comes in two lengths (12 and 20 cm) to allow for ease of operation in different parts of the rectum (Table 23.3). The proctoscope has a detachable faceplate that provides an airtight seal to maintain insufflation of the rectum and that is equipped with a binocular stereoscope with 3D visualization with up to sixfold magnification. Alternatively, in the most recent version of the TEM platform, a 10 mm HD laparoscope can be used rather than the stereoscope. The proctoscope can accommodate three 5 mm channels for dissecting instruments. The rigidity of the metal proctoscope limits hand movement and instrument separation, resulting in collisions and crossing of instruments that can be overcome by rotational movements and the use of specialized instruments that are angled at their tip. In addition, novel articulating laparoscopic instruments can help negotiate difficult angles and help with reach. The TEM setup includes its own combined pump and insufflation system to maintain consistent distention of the rectum, even during smoke evacuation and fluid suctioning. The system is secured to the operating table with an articulated arm, which creates a stable operating platform. The 20 cm TEM proctoscope is the longest transanal platform commercially available, providing access to the upper rectum and even the rectosigmoid colon.

Table 23.3 Commercially available TES platforms (in the USA)

Transanal technique	Platform name (manufacturer)	Type	Platform radius (mm)	Platform length (cm)	Proximal reach (cm)	Working channels	Specialized equipment required
Transanal endoscopic microsurgery	TEM (Richard Wolf)	Rigid	40	12–13.7 and 20	15–20	3	Yes
Transanal endoscopic operation	TEO (KARL STORZ)	Rigid	40	7.5, 15 (20 unavailable in US)	7.5–15	3	Yes
Transanal minimally invasive surgery	TAMIS-SILS (Medtronic)	Flexible	20	4	8–10	2	No
Transanal minimally invasive surgery	TAMIS-GelPOINT Path (Applied Medical)	Flexible	40	4.5	8–10	2–3	No
Transanal minimally invasive surgery	TAMIS-TriPort (Olympus)	Flexible	48	12.5	8–10	3	No

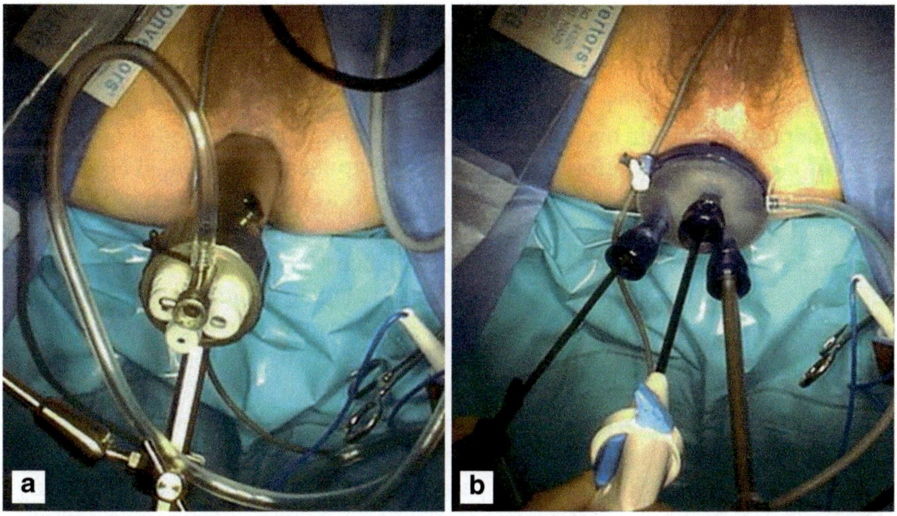

Fig. 23.2 TES set up. (**a**) TEO platform with a single operator, (**b**) TAMIS platform in position with two operators

The transanal endoscopic operation (TEO) platform (Karl Storz GmbH, Tuttlingen, Germany) is another 4 cm-wide rigid transanal endoscopic surgical platform that incorporates a 5 mm angled fiber-optic laparoscope and adapted angled tip laparoscopic dissecting instruments (Fig. 23.2a). This system comes in two lengths

(7.5 and 15 cm), with a faceplate with three ports in addition to the dedicated camera port (12, 5, and 5 mm), that accommodate conventional laparoscopic instruments. The system also includes an articulated arm holder to secure the system to the operating table. Insufflation is provided with a standard CO_2 insufflator and tubing, and the laparoscope is compatible with standard laparoscopic HD camera and video towers. The TEO system does not have a built-in system for smoke evacuation, which is achieved by standard laparoscopic suctioning or venting through small valves on the platform itself. This system is lower in cost than the TEM system and seeks to decrease the operating room setup time and lessen the learning curve for TEM with the use of more familiar laparoscopic equipment.

Three commercial devices, the Gelpoint Path (Applied Medical, Rancho Santa Margarita, CA, Fig. 23.2b) and SILS Port (Medtronic), and the Triport (Olympus, Center Valley, PA), have been most commonly used for TAMIS in the USA (Table 23.3). Other single-incision laparoscopic platforms have been used for TAMIS, including several platforms that are not currently commercially available in the USA. One group described using a simpler and cost-effective transanal access device consisting of a surgical glove assembled onto a wound retractor inserted transanally, in combination with laparoscopic trocars and instruments [170]. By virtue of being disposable, less costly and more widely available, as well as faster to setup in the operating room, TAMIS has been more rapidly incorporated in colorectal surgical practices than TEM or TEO. TAMIS platforms have three channels that can accommodate standard laparoscopic instruments ranging from 5 to 15 mm, including both rigid and flexible-tipped scopes [28]. TAMIS requires a second operator to hold the laparoscope, while another operator performs the procedure. The use of extra-long straight laparoscopes, deflectable-tip laparoscopes, and conventional endoscopes can help overcome some of the limitations of maneuvering a rigid scope through TAMIS platforms and reduce instrument collision [171]. High-definition and 3D imaging can also be incorporated to improve image quality and depth of perception. In addition, articulating laparoscopic instruments that were designed for use in single-incision laparoscopy can be incorporated in TEM, TEO, and TAMIS procedures in an effort to facilitate reaching difficult angles. TAMIS platforms are not anchored to the operating room table and often get dislodged from the anus during procedures, resulting in CO_2 leakage. The port can be sutured to perianal skin to avoid dislodgement and minimize leakage [27].

Recently, high-flow CO_2 insufflation units (Olympus) have been used in conjunction with TES platforms for active smoke evacuation. These insufflators provide automatic smoke evacuation and high-speed CO_2 insufflation that responds quickly to CO_2 leaks resulting from suctioning, maintaining a stable pneumorectum and stable field of view. The AirSeal insufflation system (SurgiQuestInc, Milford, CT, USA) uses a cannula though which a continuous flow circuit occurs, evacuating CO_2 and smoke, and recirculating filtered and high-pressure CO_2, maintaining a stable pneumorectum. The 5–12 mm cannula can only be used through TAMIS platforms and has been described as a useful tool to maintain a stable pneumorectum [172].

Robotic TAMIS has been described with the first clinical case of robotic transanal endoscopic resection reported in 2012 [173]. Several small case series have since reported preliminary outcomes of robotic transanal endoscopic resection of rectal lesions [174, 175]. Despite a cumbersome robotic setup and increased costs associated with robotic procedures, the preliminary data demonstrates feasibility of this approach with proposed advantages including more of ergonomic dissection and suturing.

23.6.2 Procedural Steps

Following insertion of the transanal platform with staple pneumorectum achieved with CO_2, the lesion is visualized and the rectal mucosal around the lesion is scored with electrocautery circumferentially in order to map out a 5–10 mm resection margin depending on whether this is a benign vs. malignant lesion (Fig. 23.3a). The scoring of a 5–10 mm circumferential margin is usually sufficient to achieve

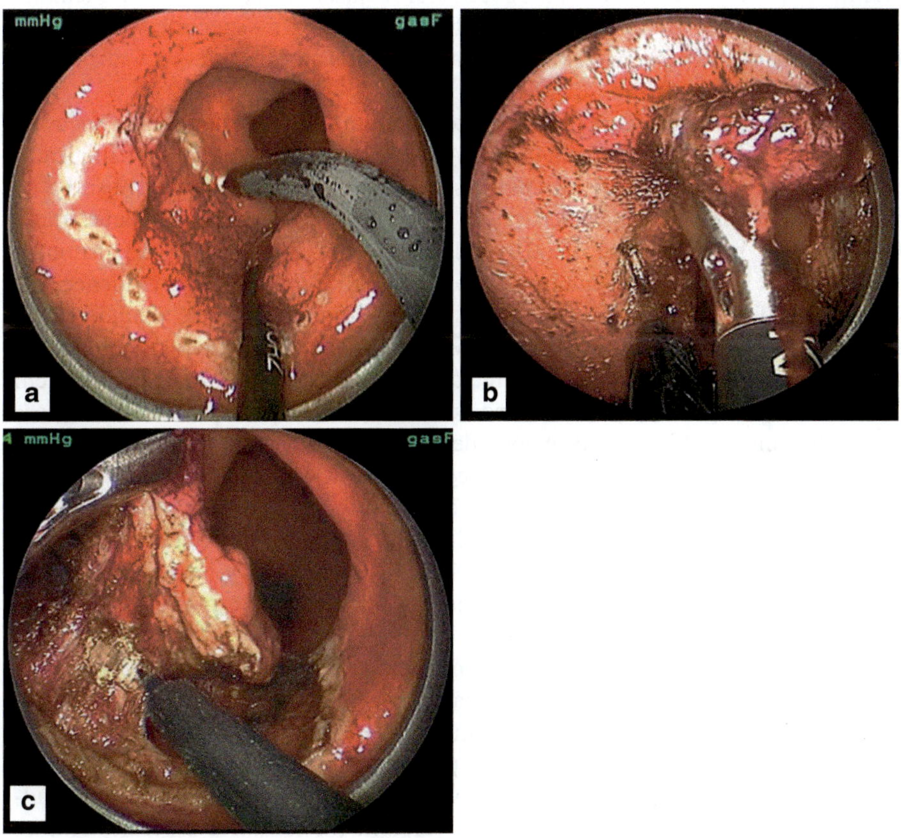

Fig. 23.3 TES procedural steps. (**a**) The lesion is scored circumferentially with monopolar cautery to mark the circumferential margins. Submucosal (**b**) or full-thickness (**c**) dissection is carried out endoscopically

R0 resection [176]. Monopolar cautery and bipolar and ultrasonic energy devices are then used to perform either submucosal or full-thickness resection depending on the anticipated pathology (Fig. 23.3b, c). Submucosal dissection can be facilitated by submucosal injection during EMR and ESD, and care must be taken to avoid injury to the underlying muscularis propria. Full-thickness TES dissection is carried out until the perirectal or mesorectal fat if visualized for anterior and lateral lesions or posterior rectal lesions, respectively. Others have performed sleeve resections for near-circumferential and circumferential rectal tumors. However, more extensive rectal dissection may be associated with higher morbidity, including bleeding, suture line dehiscence and leak, complex perirectal infections, and inadvertent injuries to surrounding organs, as well as postoperative urinary retention [45, 177]. In addition, wider rectal dissection, including partial mesorectal dissection, may complicate or compromise the quality of interval TME, if subsequent warranted. Several authors have described detrimental residual inflammation and fibrosis along the mesorectal plane up during interval TME up to 3 months after prior TES [97]. Placement of stay sutures along the rectal wall adjacent to the lesion can facilitate retraction and exposure during the dissection and assist with specimen orientation. In the event of intraoperative bleeding, hemostasis can be achieved with laparoscopic clips or sutures.

The specimen is subsequently extracted transanally and oriented for accurate pathologic assessment (Fig. 23.4a, b). Although most operators systematically close all full-thickness rectal wall defects using running or interrupted absorbable monofilament sutures, in selected cases, particularly for submucosal defects and full-thickness posterior and distal rectal defects not associated with peritoneal entry, the rectal wall defect can be left open (Fig. 23.5a, b). There is evidence that leaving rectal wall defects open does not increase the incidence of wound-related complications [31, 178]. In a recent TAMIS series of 75 patients who underwent partial or full-thickness resection for rectal lesions located an average 6.4 ± 2.3 cm from the anal verge, the authors found no differences in postoperative complications between the 40 patients whose defects were left open relative to the 35 patients whose defects were suture closed [31]. However, it should be noted that only 6% of the 35 open rectal wall defects were located anteriorly compared to 28% of 38 closed rectal wall defects. Clearly, for larger, full-thickness lesions, and in particular for high-risk lesions where peritoneal entry has occurred or is suspected, closure of rectal defects should be performed to minimize the risk of leak and infectious complications.

Prior to closure, particularly in the event of an incomplete bowel preparation and ongoing fecal contamination of the rectal wound, the area can be irrigated with dilute iodopovidone. A variety of suture materials are described including glycolide and trimethylene carbonate (Maxon), polydioxanone (PDS), and polyglactin (Vicryl) [164]. Intracorporeal suturing devices and techniques can be used, including extracorporeal knot tiers. In order to overcome the technical difficulty of knot

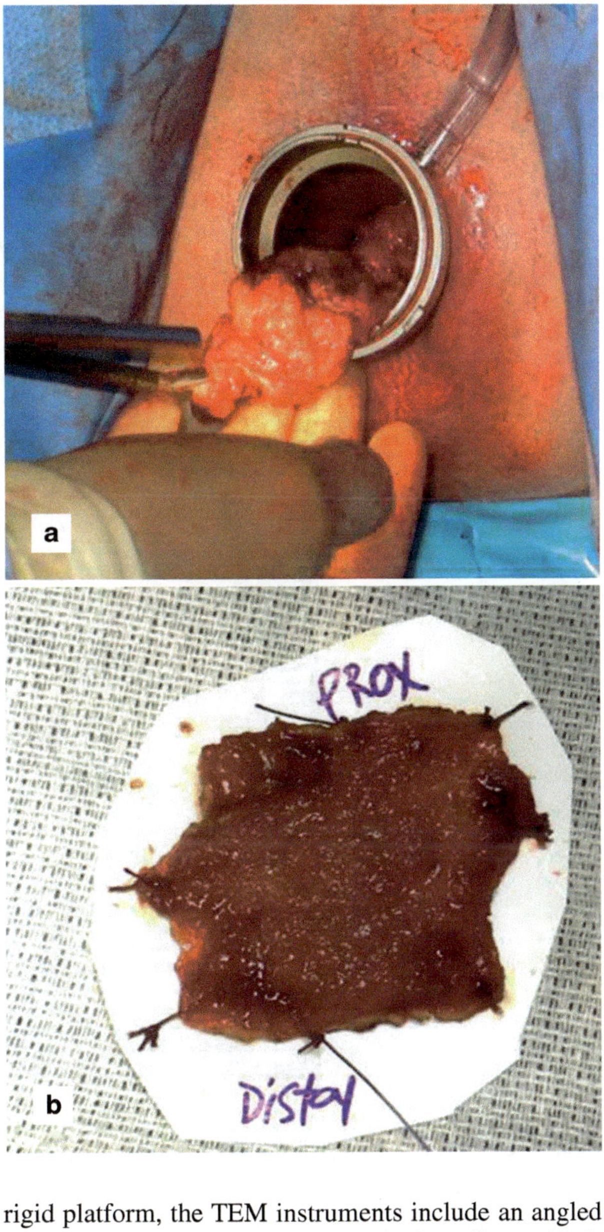

Fig. 23.4 (**a**) Transanal specimen extraction. (**b**) The specimen is oriented with sutures in preparation for pathological assessment

tying thorough a transanal rigid platform, the TEM instruments include an angled needle holder, and sutures can be secured with specialized anchoring clips and bullets. Alternatively, a V-Loc barbed absorbable suture (Medtronic) can be used to avoid knot tying [179, 180]. Finally, disposable automated suturing devices can facilitate knot tying including the Endo Stitch device (Medtronic) and the Cor-Knot

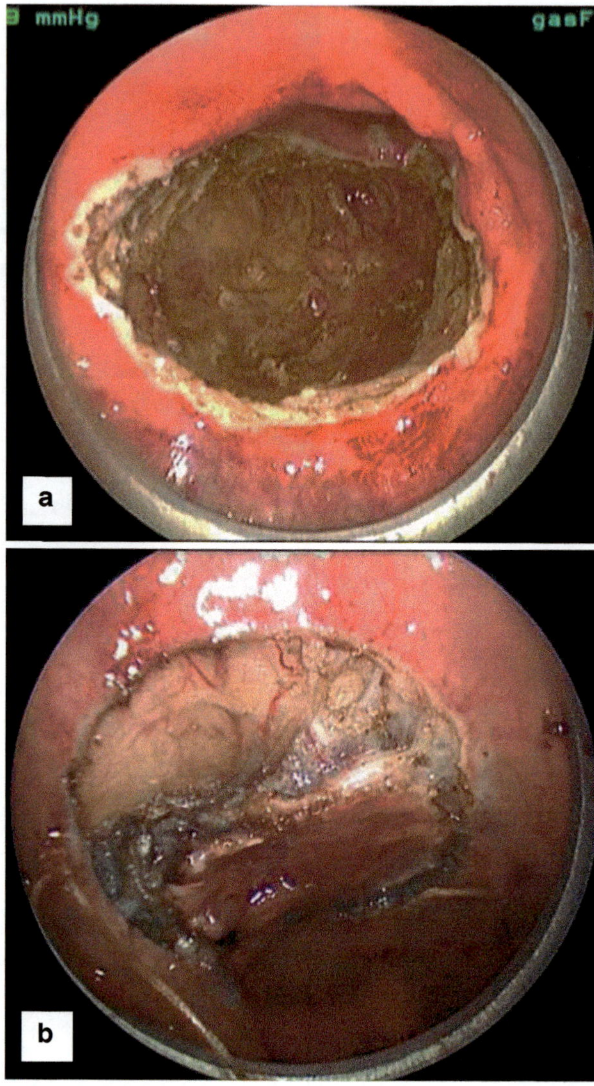

Fig. 23.5 Rectal wall defect following full-thickness transanal endoscopic resection of a posterior (**a**) and anterior (**b**) rectal lesion

device (LSI Solutions, Victor, NY (Fig. 23.6)). If peritoneal entry occurs, care must be taken to complete full-thickness rectal wall closure with sutures to reduce the risk of anastomotic dehiscence and peritonitis (Fig. 23.7). Some authors advocate closing the defect in two layers [164]. In cases where there is intraoperative concern that the closure is not airtight, diagnostic laparoscopy should be performed. Postoperatively, further investigation with a Gastrografin enema would be recommended in order to rule out a leak.

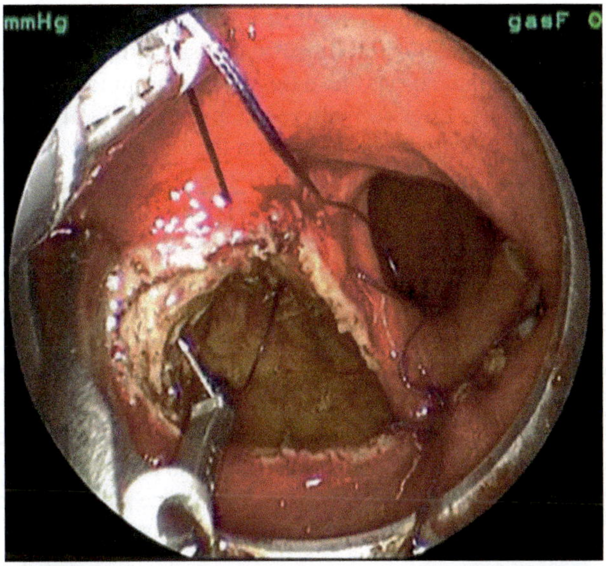

Fig. 23.6 Suture closure of full-thickness posterior rectal wall defect using absorbable sutures

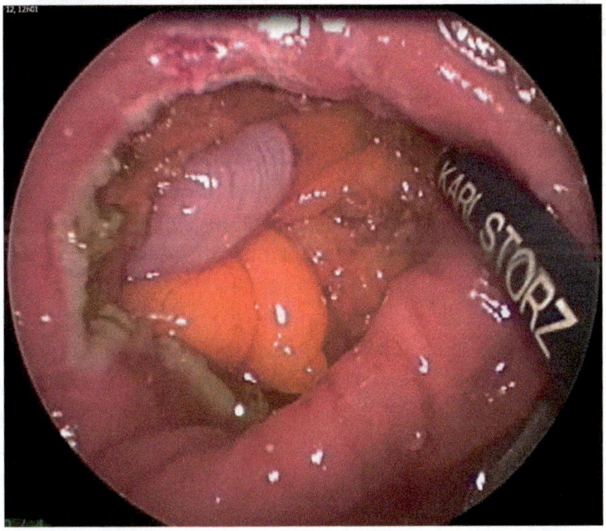

Fig. 23.7 Full-thickness transanal endoscopic dissection of a large upper rectal lesion complicated by peritoneal entry. The sigmoid colon can be seen through the full-thickness rectal defect which was closed transanally with sutures

23.7 Postoperative Care and Surveillance

Although practice among individual surgeons varies, overnight admission for observation is commonly recommended for patients who have undergone TES with full-thickness rectal resection, particularly when peritoneal entry was either noted and repaired, or when it was suspected, such as with occurrence of pneumoperitoneum or crepitus. Postoperative antibiotics are not routinely recommended for small or submucosal excisions, nor is routine imaging, in the absence of clinical indications. In cases where submucosal dissection was performed or full-thickness resection of a rectal lesion was well below the peritoneal reflection, patients can usually discharged on the same day [181].

There are no strict guidelines for postoperative surveillance specific to patients who have undergone TES for carcinoid tumors, adenomas, or rectal adenocarcinoma. Current practice follows standard NCCN guidelines for rectal cancer surveillance, including clinical evaluation, CEA, and endoscopic surveillance by flexible sigmoidoscopy every 3–4 months for the first 3 years, and then every 6 months until year 5 [80, 182]. Other standard surveillance imaging includes yearly CT scans until year 5, surveillance colonoscopy at 1 year followed by 3 years post-resection. There is no NCCN guideline for surveillance pelvic MRI. However, following TES excision of T1 tumors with high-risk histopathological features and more advanced rectal tumors that are not subsequently undergoing interval TME and are either observed or treated with adjuvant therapy followed by observation, surveillance pelvic MRI either yearly or twice yearly is advocated for five years in order to rule out locoregional recurrence.

23.8 Intraoperative Complications

Although rare, TES can result in visceral organ injury, including injury to structures anterior to the rectum including the vagina, prostate, bladder, and urethra. In addition, peritoneal entry can result in inadvertent injury to the colon and small bowel during attempted suture closure of the rectal defect. In their series of 402 TEM cases, Guerrieri et al. have reported two cases of urethral injury during TEM resection of anterior-based rectal lesions [82]. Injuries can result in delayed rectovisceral fistulas and pelvic and perirectal abscesses.

The most common intraoperative complications are related to technical difficulties establishing or maintaining adequate pneumorectum during the case. CO_2 leakage during TES results in suboptimal rectal distention and exposure and must be corrected. Typical causes of CO_2 leakage include dislocation or malpositioning of the transanal platform, leakage around the platform due to a patulous anus, which necessitates either suture fixation to the perianal skin (TAMIS) or partial suture closure of the anal orifice around the platform (TEM/TEO). It is also important to verify that the platform has been correctly assembled, and that inner and outer rubber TEM/TEO ports have not been damaged or displaced. Finally, the patient should remain completely paralyzed until completion of the case. In the case of sudden loss of pneumorectum well into the case, it is important to ensure that there hadn't been leakage of CO_2 from an unrecognized rectal defect into the peritoneal cavity which would require closure.

23.8.1 Peritoneal Entry

Despite an increasing number of published reports on this intraoperative occurrence, peritoneal entry (PE) during TES, either unplanned or anticipated based on location and/or extent of the rectal lesion, remains an area of controversy regarding further management as well as infectious and oncologic implications of PE. Earlier TEM reports considered PE to be a major complication requiring conversion to abdominal procedure with abdominal lavage, radical resection with or without fecal diversion due to concern of peritonitis from bacterial contamination [154, 155]. From an oncologic standpoint, PE during TEM excision of a rectal cancer was also thought to increase the risk of tumor cell spillage and thus the risk of peritoneal tumor implants [165]. Recent TEM/TEO series have reported an incidence of PE ranging 0–32.5%, but across large TEM series by the most experienced centers with more than 300 included patients, that rate of PE ranges 5–10.7% [25, 183]. The studies have demonstrated that PE occurred more commonly during full-thickness resection of lesions located in the upper rectum, anteriorly or laterally along the rectal wall, and during resection of circumferential or near-circumferential rectal lesions [166–168]. With regard to the morbidity associated with PE, several studies have reported no increased morbidity or increased risk of infectious complications relative to TEM cases without PE [46, 167, 169]. Finally, several studies have demonstrated no adverse short or long-term oncologic outcomes in patients in whom peritoneal entry occurred during TEM excision of rectal tumors [165, 169]. Morino et al. followed 13 patients with rectal adenocarcinoma in whom peritoneal perforation occurred during TEM [169]. At a median follow-up of 48 months (range 12–150), no cases of liver or peritoneal metastasis occurred. Two patients with T2 and T3 tumors developed local recurrence and subsequently died of lung metastases.

Based on these studies, tumor location 10 cm or more from the anal verge is no longer considered a contraindication to TEM surgery, as long as full-thickness suture closure of rectal defects can be achieved transanally by experienced operators [165–167, 169, 184].

Entry into the peritoneal cavity, with subsequent difficulty maintaining adequate pneumorectum and visualization, presents a considerable technical challenge to the surgeon (Fig. 23.7). Therefore, for lesions where a high risk of PE is anticipated, patients are preemptively placed in prone position to help mitigate the loss of pneumorectum resulting from leakage of CO_2 into the peritoneal cavity [169]. This maneuver permits the surgeon to maintain a stable pneumorectum and facilitate adequate closure of the rectal wall defect. Other strategies to compensate for loss of pneumorectum into the peritoneal cavity include decompressing the pneumoperitoneum with a Veress needle or trocar. Over time, and in experienced centers as demonstrated in the largest TEM and TEO series, conversion rates following peritoneal entry have steadily decreased, with conversion rates ranging from 0% to 40% but averaging 10% or less [169].

Much less has been published regarding the experience of peritoneal entry during TAMIS. The systematic TAMIS review of 390 procedures reported inadvertent PE in only four cases (1.025%), and the average distance of rectal lesions from the anal verge was 7.6 cm [138]. All four cases of PE occurred during dissection of upper rectal lesions and two (50%) could be closed transanally, while the others required abdominal conversion. Only three TAMIS series that include 32–75 patients, have reported an incidence of PE ranging from 2% to 9.4% [28, 30, 31].

Among the seven cases of PE during TAMIS across all three studies, six (86%) required conversion to laparoscopy or laparotomy from inability to effectively close the rectal wall defect. This may reflect the long learning curve required for managing these complex rectal lesions and the currently small experience with TAMIS to date. But it may also reflect technical limitations of shorter TAMIS platforms, which do not always permit adequate retraction and exposure of the proximal rectum [184]. Molina et al. reviewed their experience with incidence of PE among various TES modalities including 51 TEO, 21 TEM, and 6 TAMIS cases. A 28.2% incidence of PE was reported during resection of high-risk anterior/lateral lesions located an average of 13.1 cm from the anal verge. PE occurred in 4/6 TAMIS cases and 18/72 TEM/TEO cases. Although transanal suture closure of rectal wall defects associated with PE could be performed in 90.9% of all cases, this could be accomplished with TEM and TEO platforms, but not with TAMIS platforms. All four TAMIS cases with PE were converted to TEO for suture closure, due to the inability to maintain adequate exposure through the shorter TAMIS platforms. Conversion to laparoscopy LAR and Hartmann's procedure was required in 2/18 (11.1%) TEM/TEO cases with PE, which is consistent with previously reported TEM conversion rates [185, 186].

23.8.2 Conversion

Conversion to standard transanal excision (TAE) or LAR may be required in cases where more advanced pathology is encountered, adequate exposure of rectal lesions cannot be achieved or maintained, full-thickness rectal wall defect closure cannot be completed, or in cases of major intraoperative complication such as major bleeding or organ injury. Conversion is more likely to occur with proximal and circumferential rectal lesions and is also strongly related to the operator's experience with advanced TES techniques. In larger series of experienced TES surgeons, conversion rates range 0–5.3% [46, 185, 186]. In the largest multicenter TES series published to date, among 693 combined TEM and TEO cases, conversion to conventional TAE or abdominal procedures was required in 4.3%, and the 30-day morbidity was 11.1%, with hemorrhage and suture dehiscence being the most common surgical complications, and urinary tract infection being the most common nonsurgical complication [25].

23.8.3 Positive Resection Margins

Positive resection margins are an important predictor of local recurrence for both benign and malignant rectal lesions and, along with specimen fragmentation, constitute an important metric of the quality and efficacy of local excision including TAE and TEM. As previously reviewed, positive resection margins strongly correlate with local recurrence of rectal adenomas. In a series of 80 rectal adenomas resected with TEM, Speake et al. reported a 10% recurrence rate in patients with positive margins vs. no recurrence in patients with negative resection margins [187]. With respect to rectal cancers resected using TEM, positive margin rates range across TEM and TEO series from less than 2% to as high as 8.8% [65, 67, 81, 183, 186]. Across TAMIS series, rates of positive margins also vary but have generally been 6% or less for larger series that typically include both benign and malignant pathologies [28, 30, 31].

23.9 Postoperative Complications

TES has experienced a renewed interest over the past decade with the development of newer and more accessible transanal platforms, extended applications for both benign and malignant indications, and the recent development of transanal NOTES. TES has built on over three decades of published data that has firmly established the safety of this approach, primarily derived from large TEM and TEO series. A major advantage of TES is the exceedingly low morbidity and mortality rates relative to TME. Mortality across TEM, TEO, and TAMIS series has remained under 1%, and 30-day morbidity rates range 6–23% in the largest TEM/TEO series with cohort size ranging from 262 to 693 patients relative to historical TME 30-day mortality and morbidity rates ranging 2–5 and 18–55%, respectively (Table 23.4, [4–7, 185]). In additional, the majority of TES-related complications are relatively minor and transient and major complications are noted in 10% or less of cases [23, 25, 183, 185, 186, 188].

The most common surgical complication following TES is hemorrhage, which is reported in 1–13% of patients, and is usually managed non-operatively. The most common nonsurgical complication is urinary retention which is transient and occurs in 5–10% of patients [24, 183, 185, 186]. Other surgical complications include suture line dehiscence, which can occur following excision of large rectal lesions, although the incidence is rare. Suture dehiscence can range from minor defects usually managed expectantly with antibiotics and bowel rest, to major defects with leakage and sepsis, requiring return to the operating room for washout and fecal

Table 23.4 Transanal endoscopic surgery complications

Intra- and postoperative bleeding
Complex peritoneal entry
CO_2 leakage
Organ injury
Rectovisceral fistula (rectovaginal and rectourethral)
Urinary retention
Conversion (transanal or abdominal)
Suture line dehiscence/anastomotic leak
Perirectal or pelvic abscess
R0 resection
Anorectal dysfunction (fecal incontinence)
Rectal stricture

diversion. In their prospective multicenter study of 588 patients who underwent TEM resection, Guerrieri et al. reported a 5.9% incidence of partial disruption or leak of the suture line that were all successfully managed non-operatively with antibiotics [189]. The incidence of rectal stenosis following TEM is also rare (3.6% or less) and found to be most commonly associated with initial presentation of a circumferential lesion or recurrence of disease [190]. Additional major TES complications include perirectal and presacral abscess and fistulas.

In the TAMIS literature, the published rate of perioperative complications range 0–25%, with bleeding and urinary retention being the most common complications [28, 29, 31, 52]. In a review of published TAMIS outcomes between 2010 and 2013, a total of 29 complications were reported among 367 patients (7.9%) treated for rectal neoplasms [29]. The incidence of bleeding and suture dehiscence was 2.7% and 0.5%, respectively, and conversion to either TAE, TEM, or laparoscopic abdominal approach was required in 2.3% of cases. There were no deaths reported following TAMIS, and the average length of hospital stay was only 1.9 days. In the absence of comparative studies evaluating rigid metal vs. TAMIS platforms, there is no data on differences in morbidity, mortality, or length of stay between approaches.

23.10 Postoperative Functional Outcomes

Several studies have demonstrated that patients without pre-existing anal sphincter dysfunction can experience a transient decrease in resting anal and contractile pressures following TES, with no impact on long-term anorectal function. Multiple small TEM studies have documented a transient decrease in sphincter resting pressures on anal manometry that was proportional to the duration of the procedure, with resting pressures returning to baseline 12 months postoperatively [24, 191, 192]. Alterations in resting anal sphincter pressures did not translate into any detrimental effects on continence. In a study of 41 TEM patients, Cataldo et al. found no significant changes in the Fecal Incontinence Severity Index (FISI) or Fecal Incontinence Quality of Life (FIQL) scores 6 weeks postoperatively relative to preoperative scores [193]. A recent study that longitudinally assessed anorectal function and quality of life score in 102 TEM patients preoperatively and at 6, 12, 26, and 52 weeks postoperatively, found that the general quality of life scores (EQ-5D) were significantly lower at 6 and 12 weeks, but returned toward baseline at 26 weeks. Similar to prior studies, anorectal function as assessed by colorectal functional outcome (COREFO) was worse at 6 weeks postoperatively, but returned to baseline at 12 weeks postoperatively [194]. However, two TEM series reported persistent sphincter dysfunction following TEM in on long-term assessment using either St. Mark's fecal incontinence score or Wexner and Kamm incontinence scores [195, 196]. Dafnis et al. reported a 37% rate of various degrees of fecal incontinence in 48 patients at a median follow-up of 22 months following TEM and found a correlation with OR time [196]. Restivo et al. also reported a 28%

incidence of variable degrees of fecal incontinence at a median follow-up of 40 months among a cohort of 89 patients who underwent TEM. Preoperative radiotherapy and perioperative complications were found to be independent risk factor for functional disturbances [195].

Overall, all patients under evaluation for TES should have resting anal sphincter tone and squeeze assessed on DRE with selective use of anal manometry in patients with clinical evidence of dysfunction. Patients with anal sphincter dysfunction at baseline, in particular patients treated with neoadjuvant therapy, may develop further deterioration in fecal continence following TES, and the risks vs. benefits of TES in that setting should be carefully reviewed with patients during preoperative discussions.

By virtue of the prolonged stretching of the anal sphincter by 4 cm-wide rigid platforms, it has been hypothesized that softer and more pliable disposable transanal platforms may have a less detrimental impact on anorectal function. On the other hand, there is also concern that functional outcomes might be worse as compared to traditional rigid platform TES because of more extreme movements and stretch allowed by the flexible platform. Thus far, although published data is limited, short-term functional results following TAMIS have been comparable to historical TEM reports. One small prospective study conducted by Schiphorst et al. assessed functional outcomes in 37 patients following TAMIS using FISI score collected preoperatively and at 3, 6, 9, and 12 months postoperatively [55]. Among 17 patients with decreased preoperative fecal continence at baseline, improved FISI scores were noted in 88%, while among 18 patients with normal continence at baseline, no change in FISI scores were found in 83%, suggesting preserved long-term anorectal function following TAMIS procedures.

Conclusions

TES was developed as a minimally invasive alternative to proctectomy in the curative treatment of benign rectal neoplasms with acceptable oncologic results and substantially improved safety profile in carefully selected T1 rectal cancer. The recent introduction of TAMIS platforms has facilitated widespread adoption of TES and helped expand its application to more complex anorectal conditions. TES has most recently served as a portal to the most recent paradigm shift in rectal cancer resection, namely transanal NOTES TME. Further, although the use of TES for locally advanced rectal cancer is limited to the experimental and palliative settings, there is increasing evidence that in combination with neoadjuvant and/or adjuvant chemoradiation, TES may facilitate organ preservation and serve as an acceptable alternative to radical surgery for T2 or even T3 tumors demonstrating complete clinical response. Finally, a transanal endoscopic approach offers the possibility of entirely "incisionless" transanal colorectal resection, whereby rectal and/or colon dissection followed by specimen extraction is performed primarily through the anus. Future advances in surgical optics, multiport transanal platforms, and endoscopic instrumentation will help further expand the scope of transanal procedures.

References

1. Heald RJ, Husband EM, Ryall RD. The mesorectum in rectal cancer surgery—the clue to pelvic recurrence? Br J Surg. 1982;69:613–6.
2. MacFarlane JK, Ryall RD, Heald RJ. Mesorectal excision for rectal cancer. Lancet. 1993;341:457–60.
3. Marijnen CAM, Kapiteijn E, van de Velde CJH, Martijn H, Steup WH, Wiggers T, et al. Acute side effects and complications after short-term preoperative radiotherapy combined with total mesorectal excision in primary rectal cancer: report of a multicenter randomized trial. J Clin Oncol. 2002;20:817–25.
4. Guillou PJ, Quirke P, Thorpe H, Walker J, Jayne DG, Smith AMH, et al. Short-term endpoints of conventional versus laparoscopic-assisted surgery in patients with colorectal cancer (MRC CLASICC trial): multicentre, randomised controlled trial. Lancet (London). 2005;365:1718–26.
5. van der Pas MH, Haglind E, Cuesta MA, Fürst A, Lacy AM, Hop WC, et al. Laparoscopic versus open surgery for rectal cancer (COLOR II): short-term outcomes of a randomised, phase 3 trial. Lancet Oncol. 2013;14:210–8.
6. Fleshman J, Branda M, Sargent DJ, Boller AM, George V, Abbas M, et al. Effect of laparoscopic-assisted resection vs open resection of stage II or III rectal cancer on pathologic outcomes: the ACOSOG Z6051 randomized clinical trial. JAMA. 2015;314:1346–55.
7. Stevenson ARL, Solomon MJ, Lumley JW, Hewett P, Clouston AD, Gebski VJ, et al. Effect of laparoscopic-assisted resection vs open resection on pathological outcomes in rectal cancer: the ALaCaRT randomized clinical trial. JAMA. 2015;314:1356–63.
8. Snijders HS, Wouters MWJM, van Leersum NJ, Kolfschoten NE, Henneman D, de Vries AC, et al. Meta-analysis of the risk for anastomotic leakage, the postoperative mortality caused by leakage in relation to the overall postoperative mortality. Eur J Surg Oncol. 2012;38:1013–9.
9. Hendren SK, O'Connor BI, Liu M, Asano T, Cohen Z, Swallow CJ, et al. Prevalence of male and female sexual dysfunction is high following surgery for rectal cancer. Ann Surg. 2005;242:212–23.
10. Mirnezami AH, Mirnezami R, Venkatasubramaniam AK, Chandrakumaran K, Cecil TD, Moran BJ. Robotic colorectal surgery: hype or new hope? A systematic review of robotics in colorectal surgery. Color Dis. 2010;12:1084–93.
11. Moore JS, Cataldo PA, Osler T, Hyman NH. Transanal endoscopic microsurgery is more effective than traditional transanal excision for resection of rectal masses. Dis Colon Rectum. 2008;51:1026–30.
12. de Graaf EJR, Burger JWA, van Ijsseldijk ALA, Tetteroo GWM, Dawson I, Hop WCJ. Transanal endoscopic microsurgery is superior to transanal excision of rectal adenomas. Color Dis. 2011;13:762–7.
13. Clancy C, Burke JP, Albert MR, O'Connell PR, Winter DC. Transanal endoscopic microsurgery versus standard transanal excision for the removal of rectal neoplasms: a systematic review and meta-analysis. Dis Colon Rectum. 2015;58:254–61.
14. Classic articles in colonic and rectal surgery. Paul Kraske 1851–1930. Extirpation of high carcinomas of the large bowel. Dis Colon Rectum. 1984;27:499–503.
15. Bleeday R. Local excision of rectal cancer. World J Surg. 1997;21:706–14.
16. Killingback M. Local excision of carcinoma of the rectum: indications. World J Surg. 1992;16:437–46.
17. Mason AY. Surgical access to the rectum—a transsphincteric exposure. Proc R Soc Med. 1970;63(Suppl):91–4.
18. You YN, Baxter NN, Stewart A, Nelson H. Is the increasing rate of local excision for stage I rectal cancer in the United States justified? A nationwide cohort study from the National Cancer Database. Ann Surg. 2007;245:726–33.
19. Mellgren A, Sirivongs P, Rothenberger DA, Madoff RD, García-Aguilar J. Is local excision adequate therapy for early rectal cancer? Dis Colon Rectum. 2000;43:1064–71.

20. Paty PB, Nash GM, Baron P, Zakowski M, Minsky BD, Blumberg D, et al. Long-term results of local excision for rectal cancer. Ann Surg. 2002;236:522–9.
21. Buess G, Theiss R, Hutterer F, Pichlmaier H, Pelz C, Holfeld T, et al. Transanal endoscopic surgery of the rectum - testing a new method in animal experiments. Leber Magen Darm. 1983;13:73–7.
22. Heintz A, Mörschel M, Junginger T. Comparison of results after transanal endoscopic microsurgery and radical resection for T1 carcinoma of the rectum. Surg Endosc. 1998;12:1145–8.
23. de Graaf EJR, Doornebosch PG, Tollenaar RAEM, Meershoek-Klein Kranenbarg E, de Boer AC, Bekkering FC, et al. Transanal endoscopic microsurgery versus total mesorectal excision of T1 rectal adenocarcinomas with curative intention. Eur J Surg Oncol. 2009;35:1280–5.
24. Allaix ME, Rebecchi F, Giaccone C, Mistrangelo M, Morino M. Long-term functional results and quality of life after transanal endoscopic microsurgery. Br J Surg. 2011;98:1635–43.
25. Barendse RM, Dijkgraaf MG, Rolf UR, Bijnen AB, Consten ECJ, Hoff C, et al. Colorectal surgeons' learning curve of transanal endoscopic microsurgery. Surg Endosc. 2013;27:3591–602.
26. Maslekar S, Pillinger SH, Sharma A, Taylor A, Monson JRT. Cost analysis of transanal endoscopic microsurgery for rectal tumours. Color Dis. 2007;9:229–34.
27. Atallah S, Albert M, Larach S. Transanal minimally invasive surgery: a giant leap forward. Surg Endosc. 2010;24:2200–5.
28. McLemore EC, Weston LA, Coker AM, Jacobsen GR, Talamini MA, Horgan S, et al. Transanal minimally invasive surgery for benign and malignant rectal neoplasia. Am J Surg. 2014;208:372–81.
29. Martin-Perez B, Andrade-Ribeiro GD, Hunter L, Atallah S. A systematic review of transanal minimally invasive surgery (TAMIS) from 2010 to 2013. Tech Coloproctol. 2014;18:775–88.
30. Albert MR, Atallah SB, de Beche-Adams TC, Izfar S, Larach SW. Transanal minimally invasive surgery (TAMIS) for local excision of benign neoplasms and early-stage rectal cancer: efficacy and outcomes in the first 50 patients. Dis Colon Rectum. 2013;56:301–7.
31. Hahnloser D, Cantero R, Salgado G, Dindo D, Rega D, Delrio P. Transanal minimal invasive surgery for rectal lesions: should the defect be closed? Color Dis. 2015;17:397–402.
32. Lee T-G, Lee S-J. Transanal single-port microsurgery for rectal tumors: minimal invasive surgery under spinal anesthesia. Surg Endosc. 2014;28:271–80.
33. Buess G, Theiss R, Günther M, Hutterer F, Pichlmaier H. Endoscopic surgery in the rectum. Endoscopy. 1985;17:31–5.
34. Christoforidis D, Cho H-M, Dixon MR, Mellgren AF, Madoff RD, Finne CO. Transanal endoscopic microsurgery versus conventional transanal excision for patients with early rectal cancer. Ann Surg. 2009;249:776–82.
35. Whitehouse PA, Armitage JN, Tilney HS, Simson JNL. Transanal endoscopic microsurgery: local recurrence rate following resection of rectal cancer. Color Dis. 2008;10:187–93.
36. Guerrieri M, Gesuita R, Ghiselli R, Lezoche G, Budassi A, Baldarelli M. Treatment of rectal cancer by transanal endoscopic microsurgery: experience with 425 patients. World J Gastroenterol. 2014;20:9556–63.
37. Borschitz T, Heintz A, Junginger T. The influence of histopathologic criteria on the long-term prognosis of locally excised pT1 rectal carcinomas: results of local excision (transanal endoscopic microsurgery) and immediate reoperation. Dis Colon Rectum. 2006;49:1492–506. discussion 1500–5
38. Lezoche G, Guerrieri M, Baldarelli M, Paganini AM, D'Ambrosio G, Campagnacci R, et al. Transanal endoscopic microsurgery for 135 patients with small nonadvanced low rectal cancer (iT1–iT2, iN0): short- and long-term results. Surg Endosc. 2011;25:1222–9.
39. Lezoche E, Baldarelli M, Lezoche G, Paganini AM, Gesuita R, Guerrieri M. Randomized clinical trial of endoluminal locoregional resection versus laparoscopic total mesorectal excision for T2 rectal cancer after neoadjuvant therapy. Br J Surg. 2012;99:1211–8.
40. Garcia-Aguilar J, Shi Q, Thomas CR, Chan E, Cataldo P, Marcet J, et al. A phase II trial of neoadjuvant chemoradiation and local excision for T2N0 rectal cancer: preliminary results of the ACOSOG Z6041 trial. Ann Surg Oncol. 2012;19:384–91.

41. Marks JH, Lopez-Acevedo N, Krishnan B, Johnson MN, Montenegro GA, Marks GJ. True NOTES TME resection with splenic flexure release, high ligation of IMA, and side-to-end hand-sewn colonanal anastomosis. Surg Endosc. 2016;30:4626–31. doi:10.1007/s00464-015-4731-7.
42. Barendse RM, van den Broek FJ, van Schooten J, Bemelman WA, Fockens P, de Graaf EJ, Dekker E, TREND Study Group. Endoscopic mucosal resection vs transanal endoscopic microsurgery for the treatment of large rectal adenomas. Color Dis. 2012;14:e191–6.
43. Barendse RM, van den Broek FJC, Dekker E, Bemelman WA, de Graaf EJR, Fockens P, et al. Systematic review of endoscopic mucosal resection versus transanal endoscopic microsurgery for large rectal adenomas. Endoscopy. 2011;43:941–9.
44. Léonard D, Colin JF, Remue C, Jamart J, Kartheuser A. Transanal endoscopic microsurgery: long-term experience, indication expansion, and technical improvements. Surg Endosc. 2012;26:312–22.
45. Guerrieri M, Baldarelli M, Organetti L, Grillo Ruggeri F, Mantello G, Bartolacci S, et al. Transanal endoscopic microsurgery for the treatment of selected patients with distal rectal cancer: 15 years experience. Surg Endosc. 2008;22:2030–5.
46. de Graaf EJR, Doornebosch PG, Tetteroo GWM, Geldof H, Hop WCJ. Transanal endoscopic microsurgery is feasible for adenomas throughout the entire rectum: a prospective study. Dis Colon Rectum. 2009;52:1107–13.
47. Allaix ME, Arezzo A, Cassoni P, Famiglietti F, Morino M. Recurrence after transanal endoscopic microsurgery for large rectal adenomas. Surg Endosc. 2012;26:2594–600.
48. Levic K, Bulut O, Hesselfeldt P. Transanal endoscopic microsurgery for giant polyps of the rectum. Tech Coloproctol. 2014;18:521–7.
49. Schäfer H, Baldus SE, Hölscher AH. Giant adenomas of the rectum: complete resection by transanal endoscopic microsurgery (TEM). Int J Color Dis. 2006;21:533–7.
50. Serra-Aracil X, Caro-Tarrago A, Mora-López L, Casalots A, Rebasa P, Navarro-Soto S. Transanal endoscopic surgery with total wall excision is required with rectal adenomas due to the high frequency of adenocarcinoma. Dis Colon Rectum. 2014;57:823–9.
51. van den Boezem PB, Kruyt PM, Stommel MWJ, Tobon Morales R, Cuesta MA, Sietses C. Transanal single-port surgery for the resection of large polyps. Dig Surg. 2011;28:412–6.
52. Bridoux V, Schwarz L, Suaud L, Dazza M, Michot F, Tuech J-J. Transanal minimal invasive surgery with the Endorec(TM) trocar: a low cost but effective technique. Int J Color Dis. 2014;29:177–81.
53. Ragupathi M, Vande Maele D, Nieto J, Pickron TB, Haas EM. Transanal endoscopic video-assisted (TEVA) excision. Surg Endosc. 2012;26:3528–35.
54. Barendse RM, Doornebosch PG, Bemelman WA, Fockens P, Dekker E, de Graaf EJR. Transanal employment of single access ports is feasible for rectal surgery. Ann Surg. 2012;256:1030–3.
55. Schiphorst AHW, Langenhoff BS, Maring J, Pronk A, Zimmerman DDE. Transanal minimally invasive surgery: initial experience and short-term functional results. Dis Colon Rectum. 2014;57:927–32.
56. Lim S-B, Seo S-I, Lee JL, Kwak JY, Jang TY, Kim CW, et al. Feasibility of transanal minimally invasive surgery for mid-rectal lesions. Surg Endosc. 2012;26:3127–32.
57. Sevá-Pereira G, Trombeta VL, Capochim Romagnolo LG. Transanal minimally invasive surgery (TAMIS) using a new disposable device: our initial experience. Tech Coloproctol. 2014;18:393–7.
58. Gorgun IE, Gorgun IE, Aytac E, Costedio MM, Erem HH, Valente MA, et al. Transanal endoscopic surgery using a single access port: a practical tool in the surgeon's toybox. Surg Endosc. 2014;28:1034–8.
59. Gunderson LL, Jessup JM, Sargent DJ, Greene FL, Stewart AK. Revised TN categorization for colon cancer based on national survival outcomes data. J Clin Oncol. 2010;28:264–71.
60. Kim MN, Kang JM, Yang JI, Kim BK, Im JP, Kim SG, Jung HC, Song IS, Kim JS. Clinical features and prognosis of early colorectal cancer treated by endoscopic mucosal resection. J Gastroenterol Hepatol. 2011;26:1619–25.

61. Haggitt RC, Glotzbach RE, Soffer EE, Wruble LD. Prognostic factors in colorectal carcinomas arising in adenomas: implications for lesions removed by endoscopic polypectomy. Gastroenterology. 1985;89:328–36.
62. Tytherleigh MG, Warren BF, Mortensen NJM. Management of early rectal cancer. Br J Surg. 2008;95:409–23.
63. Kikuchi R, Takano M, Takagi K, Fujimoto N, Nozaki R, Fujiyoshi T, et al. Management of early invasive colorectal cancer. Risk of recurrence and clinical guidelines. Dis Colon Rectum. 1995;38:1286–95.
64. Nascimbeni R, Burgart LJ, Nivatvongs S, Larson DR. Risk of lymph node metastasis in T1 carcinoma of the colon and rectum. Dis Colon Rectum. 2002;45:200–6.
65. Doornebosch PG, Ferenschild FTJ, de Wilt JHW, Dawson I, Tetteroo GWM, de Graaf EJR. Treatment of recurrence after transanal endoscopic microsurgery (TEM) for T1 rectal cancer. Dis Colon Rectum. 2010;53:1234–9.
66. Mentges B, Buess G, Effinger G, Manncke K, Becker HD. Indications and results of local treatment of rectal cancer. Br J Surg. 1997;84:348–51.
67. Stipa F, Giaccaglia V, Burza A. Management and outcome of local recurrence following transanal endoscopic microsurgery for rectal cancer. Dis Colon Rectum. 2012;55:262–9.
68. Doornebosch PG, Zeestraten E, de Graaf EJR, Hermsen P, Dawson I, Tollenaar RAEM, et al. Transanal endoscopic microsurgery for T1 rectal cancer: size matters! Surg Endosc. 2012;26:551–7.
69. Morino M, Allaix ME, Caldart M, Scozzari G, Arezzo A. Risk factors for recurrence after transanal endoscopic microsurgery for rectal malignant neoplasm. Surg Endosc. 2011;25:3683–90.
70. Suzuki A, Togashi K, Nokubi M, Koinuma K, Miyakura Y, Horie H, et al. Evaluation of venous invasion by Elastica van Gieson stain and tumor budding predicts local and distant metastases in patients with T1 stage colorectal cancer. Am J Surg Pathol. 2009;33:1601–7.
71. Heafner TA, Glasgow SC. A critical review of the role of local excision in the treatment of early (T1 and T2) rectal tumors. J Gastrointest Oncol. 2014;5:345–52.
72. Chang HC, Huang SC, Chen JS, Tang R, Changchien CR, Chiang JM, et al. Risk factors for lymph node metastasis in pT1 and pT2 rectal cancer: a single-institute experience in 943 patients and literature review. Ann Surg Oncol. 2012;19:2477–84.
73. Saraste D, Gunnarsson U, Janson M. Predicting lymph node metastases in early rectal cancer. Eur J Cancer. 2013;49:1104–8.
74. Bach SP, Hill J, Monson JRT, Simson JNL, Lane L, Merrie A, et al. A predictive model for local recurrence after transanal endoscopic microsurgery for rectal cancer. Br J Surg. 2009;96:280–90.
75. Sengupta S, Tjandra JJ. Local excision of rectal cancer: what is the evidence? Dis Colon Rectum. 2001;44:1345–61.
76. Shinto E, Jass JR, Tsuda H, Sato T, Ueno H, Hase K, et al. Differential prognostic significance of morphologic invasive markers in colorectal cancer: tumor budding and cytoplasmic podia. Dis Colon Rectum. 2006;49:1422–30.
77. Syk E, Lenander C, Nilsson PJ, Rubio CA, Glimelius B. Tumour budding correlates with local recurrence of rectal cancer. Color Dis. 2011;13:255–62.
78. Ueno H, Mochizuki H, Hashiguchi Y, Shimazaki H, Aida S, Hase K, et al. Risk factors for an adverse outcome in early invasive colorectal carcinoma. Gastroenterology. 2004;127:385–94.
79. Mitrovic B, Schaeffer DF, Riddell RH, Kirsch R. Tumor budding in colorectal carcinoma: time to take notice. Mod Pathol. 2012;25:1315–25.
80. Benson AB, Bekaii-Saab T, Chan E, Chen Y-J, Choti MA, Cooper HS, et al. Rectal cancer. J Natl Compr Cancer Netw. 2012;10:1528–64.
81. Ramirez JM, Aguilella V, Valencia J, Ortego J, Gracia JA, Escudero P, et al. Transanal endoscopic microsurgery for rectal cancer. Long-term oncologic results. Int J Color Dis. 2011;26:437–43.
82. Guerrieri M, Baldarelli M, de Sanctis A, Campagnacci R, Rimini M, Lezoche E. Treatment of rectal adenomas by transanal endoscopic microsurgery: 15 years' experience. Surg Endosc. 2010;24:445–9.

83. Park SU, Min YW, Shin JU, Choi JH, Kim Y-H, Kim JJ, et al. Endoscopic submucosal dissection or transanal endoscopic microsurgery for nonpolypoid rectal high grade dysplasia and submucosa-invading rectal cancer. Endoscopy. 2012;44:1031–6.
84. Kawaguti FS, Nahas CSR, Marques CFS, Martins BC, Retes FA, RSS M, et al. Endoscopic submucosal dissection versus transanal endoscopic microsurgery for the treatment of early rectal cancer. Surg. Endoscopy. 2014;28:1173–9.
85. Elmessiry MM, Van Koughnett JA, Maya A, DaSilva G, Wexner SD, Bejarano P, et al. Local excision of T1 and T2 rectal cancer: proceed with caution. Color Dis. 2014;16:703–9.
86. Lee W, Lee D, Choi S, Chun H. Transanal endoscopic microsurgery and radical surgery for T1 and T2 rectal cancer. Surg Endosc. 2003;17:1283–7.
87. Allaix ME, Arezzo A, Giraudo G, Morino M. Transanal endoscopic microsurgery vs. laparoscopic total mesorectal excision for T2N0 rectal cancer. J Gastrointest Surg. 2012;16:2280–7.
88. Perez RO, Habr-Gama A, São Julião GP, Proscurshim I, Scanavini Neto A, Gama-Rodrigues J. Transanal endoscopic microsurgery for residual rectal cancer after neoadjuvant chemoradiation therapy is associated with significant immediate pain and hospital readmission rates. Dis Colon Rectum. 2011;54:545–51.
89. Marks JH, Valsdottir EB, DeNittis A, Yarandi SS, Newman DA, Nweze I, et al. Transanal endoscopic microsurgery for the treatment of rectal cancer: comparison of wound complication rates with and without neoadjuvant radiation therapy. Surg Endosc. 2009;23:1081–7.
90. Garcia-Aguilar J, Renfro LA, Chow OS, Shi Q, Carrero XW, Lynn PB, et al. Organ preservation for clinical T2N0 distal rectal cancer using neoadjuvant chemoradiotherapy and local excision (ACOSOG Z6041): results of an open-label, single-arm, multi-institutional, phase 2 trial. Lancet Oncol. 2015;16:1537–46.
91. Verseveld M, de Graaf EJ, Verhoef C, van Meerten E, Punt CJ, de Hingh IH, et al. CARTS Study Group. Chemoradiation therapy for rectal cancer in the distal rectum followed by organ-sparing transanal endoscopic microsurgery (CARTS study). Br J Surg. 2015;102:853–60.
92. Habr-Gama A, Sabbaga J, Gama-Rodrigues J, São Julião GP, Proscurshim I, Bailão Aguilar P, et al. Watch and wait approach following extended neoadjuvant chemoradiation for distal rectal cancer: are we getting closer to anal cancer management? Dis Colon Rectum. 2013;56:1109–17.
93. Maas M, Beets-Tan RGH, Lambregts DMJ, Lammering G, Nelemans PJ, Engelen SME, et al. Wait-and-see policy for clinical complete responders after chemoradiation for rectal cancer. J Clin Oncol. 2011;29:4633–40.
94. Dalton RSJ, Velineni R, Osborne ME, Thomas R, Harries S, Gee AS, et al. A single-centre experience of chemoradiotherapy for rectal cancer: is there potential for nonoperative management? Color Dis. 2012;14:567–71.
95. Levic K, Bulut O, Hesselfeldt P, Bülow S. The outcome of rectal cancer after early salvage TME following TEM compared with primary TME: a case-matched study. Tech Coloproctol. 2013;17:397–403.
96. Morino M, Allaix ME, Arolfo S, Arezzo A. Previous transanal endoscopic microsurgery for rectal cancer represents a risk factor for an increased abdominoperineal resection rate. Surg Endosc. 2013;27:3315–21.
97. Hompes R, McDonald R, Buskens C, Lindsey I, Armitage N, Hill J, Scott A, et al. Association of Coloproctology of Great Britain and Ireland Transanal Endoscopic Microsurgery Collaboration. Completion surgery following transanal endoscopic microsurgery: assessment of quality and short- and long-term outcome. Color Dis. 2013;15:e576–81.
98. Baron PL, Enker WE, Zakowski MF, Urmacher C. Immediate vs. salvage resection after local treatment for early rectal cancer. Dis Colon Rectum. 1995;38:177–81.
99. Weiser MR, Landmann RG, Wong WD, Shia J, Guillem JG, Temple LK, et al. Surgical salvage of recurrent rectal cancer after transanal excision. Dis Colon Rectum. 2005;48:1169–75.
100. Pucciarelli S, De Paoli A, Guerrieri M, La Torre G, Maretto I, De Marchi F, et al. Local excision after preoperative chemoradiotherapy for rectal cancer: results of a multicenter phase II clinical trial. Dis Colon Rectum. 2013;56:1349–56.

101. Türler A, Schäfer H, Pichlmaier H. Role of transanal endoscopic microsurgery in the palliative treatment of rectal cancer. Scand J Gastroenterol. 1997;32:58–61.
102. Tsikitis VL, Wertheim BC, Guerrero MA. Trends of incidence and survival of gastrointestinal neuroendocrine tumors in the United States: a seer analysis. J Cancer. 2012;3:292–302.
103. Shields CJ, Tiret E, Winter DC, International Rectal Carcinoid Study Group. Carcinoid tumors of the rectum: a multi-institutional international collaboration. Ann Surg. 2010;252:750–5.
104. Kasuga A, Chino A, Uragami N, Kishihara T, Igarashi M, et al. Treatment strategy for rectal carcinoids: a clinicopathological analysis of 229 cases at a single cancer institution. J Gastroenterol Hepatol. 2012;27:1801–7.
105. Kim MS, Hur H, Min BS, Baik SH, Lee KY, Kim NK. Clinical outcomes for rectal carcinoid tumors according to a new (AJCC 7th edition) TNM staging system: a single institutional analysis of 122 patients. J Surg Oncol. 2013;107:835–41.
106. Wang M, Peng J, Yang W, Chen W, Mo S, Cai S. Prognostic analysis for carcinoid tumours of the rectum: a single institutional analysis of 106 patients. Color Dis. 2011;13:150–3.
107. McDermott FD, Heeney A, Courtney D, Mohan H, Winter D. Rectal carcinoids: a systematic review. Surg Endosc. 2014;28:2020–6.
108. Kinoshita T, Kanehira E, Omura K, Tomori T, Yamada H. Transanal endoscopic microsurgery in the treatment of rectal carcinoid tumor. Surg Endosc. 2007;21:970–4.
109. Kumar AS, Sidani SM, Kolli K, Stahl TJ, Ayscue JM, Fitzgerald JF, et al. Transanal endoscopic microsurgery for rectal carcinoids: the largest reported United States experience. Color Dis. 2012;14:562–6.
110. Aranda-Narváez JM, González-Sánchez AJ, Montiel-Casado C, Sánchez-Pérez B, Jiménez-Mazure C, Valle-Carbajo M, et al. Posterior approach (Kraske procedure) for surgical treatment of presacral tumors. World J Gastrointest Surg. 2012;27(4):126–30.
111. Zoller S, Joos A, Dinter D, Back W, Horisberger K, et al. Retrorectal tumors: excision by transanal endoscopic microsurgery. Rev Esp Enferm Dig. 2007;99:547–50.
112. Serra-Aracil X, Gómez-Díaz C, Bombardó-Junca J, Mora-López L, Alcántara-Moral M, et al. Surgical excision of retrorectal tumour using transanal endoscopic microsurgery. Color Dis. 2010;12:594–5.
113. Duek SD, Gilshtein H, Khoury W. Transanal endoscopic microsurgery: also for the treatment of retrorectal tumors. Minim Invasive Ther Allied Technol. 2014;23:28–31.
114. Serra-Aracil X, Mora Lopez L, Alcantara-Moral M, Corredera-Cantarin C, Gomez-Diaz C, Navarro-Soto S. Atypical indications for transanal endoscopic microsurgery to avoid major surgery. Tech Coloproctol. 2014;18:157–64.
115. Wilbert DM, Buess G, Bichler KH. Combined endoscopic closure of rectourethral fistula. J Urol. 1996;155(1):256–8.
116. Quinlan M, Cahill R, Keane F, Grainger R, Butler M. Transanal endoscopic microsurgical repair of iatrogenic recto-urethral fistula. Surgeon. 2005;3:416–7.
117. Bochove-Overgaauw DM, Beerlage HP, Bosscha K, Gelderman WA. Transanal endoscopic microsurgery for correction of rectourethral fistulae. J Endourol. 2006;20:1087–90.
118. Andrews EJ, Royce P, Farmer KC. Transanal endoscopic microsurgery repair of rectourethral fistula after high-intensity focused ultrasound ablation of prostate cancer. Color Dis. 2011;13:342–3.
119. Pigalarga R, Patel NM, Rezac C. Transanal endoscopic microsurgery-assisted rectal advancement flap is a viable option for iatrogenic rectourethral fistula repair: a case report. Tech Coloproctol. 2011;15:209–11.
120. Atallah SB, de Beche-Adams TC, Larach S. Transanal minimally invasive surgery for repair of rectourethral fistula. Dis Colon Rectum. 2014;57:899.
121. Kanehira E, Tanida T, Kamei A, Nakagi M, Iwasaki M, Shimizu H. Transanal endoscopic microsurgery for surgical repair of rectovesical fistula following radical prostatectomy. Surg Endosc. 2015;29:851–5.
122. D'Ambrosio G, Paganini AM, Guerrieri M, Barchetti L, Lezoche G, Fabiani B, Lezoche E. Minimally invasive treatment of rectovaginal fistula. Surg Endosc. 2012;26:546–50.

123. Rickert A, Willeke F, Kienle P, Post S. Management and outcome of anastomotic leakage after colonic surgery. Color Dis. 2010;12:e216–23.
124. Phillips BR, Harris LJ, Maxwell PJ, Isenberg GA, Goldstein SD. Anastomotic leak rate after low anterior resection for rectal cancer after chemoradiation therapy. Am Surg. 2010;76:869–71.
125. Dauser B, Herbst F. Diagnosis, management and outcome of early anastomotic leakage following colorectal anastomosis using a compression device: is it different? Color Dis. 2014;16:435–9.
126. Beunis A, Pauli S, Van Cleemput M. Anastomotic leakage of a colorectal anastomosis treated by transanal endoscopic microsurgery. Acta Chir Belg. 2008;108:474–6.
127. Blumetti J, Chaudhry V, Prasad L, Abcarian H. Delayed transanal repair of persistent coloanal anastomotic leak in diverted patients after resection for rectal cancer. Color Dis. 2012;14:1238–41.
128. Sneider E, Maykel J. Management of anastomotic leak after low anterior resection with transanal endoscopic microsurgical (TEM) debridement and repair. J Surg Case Rep. 2012;2012:1.
129. Martins BC, Marques CF, Nahas CS, Hondo FY, Pollara W, Nahas SC, et al. A novel approach for the treatment of pelvic abscess: transrectal endoscopic drainage facilitated by transanal endoscopic microsurgery access. Surg Endosc. 2012;26:2667–70.
130. Baatrup G, Svensen R, Ellensen VS. Benign rectal strictures managed with transanal resection—a novel application for transanal endoscopic microsurgery. Color Dis. 2010;12:144–6.
131. Wolthuis AM, Rutgeerts P, Penninckx F, D'Hoore A. A novel hybrid technique using transanal endoscopic microsurgery and balloon dilation in the treatment of a benign complete colorectal anastomotic stricture. Endoscopy. 2011;43(Suppl 2 UCTN):E176–7.
132. Lake JP, Essani R, Petrone P, Kaiser AM, Asensio J, Beart RW Jr. Management of retained colorectal foreign bodies: predictors of operative intervention. Dis Colon Rectum. 2004;47:1694–8.
133. Atallah S, Albert M, Debeche-Adams T, Larach S. Transanal minimally invasive surgery (TAMIS): applications beyond local excision. Tech Coloproctol. 2013;17:239–43.
134. Cawich SO, Mohammed F, Spence R, Albert M, Naraynsingh V. Colonic foreign body retrieval using a modified TAMIS technique with standard instruments and trocars. Case Rep Emerg Med. 2015;2015:815616.
135. Franklin ME Jr, Liang S, Russek K. Integration of transanal specimen extraction into laparoscopic anterior resection with total mesorectal excision for rectal cancer: a consecutive series of 179 patients. Surg Endosc. 2013;27:127–32.
136. Leung AL, Cheung HY, Fok BK, Chung CC, Li MK, Tang CN. Prospective randomized trial of hybrid NOTES colectomy versus conventional laparoscopic colectomy for left-sided colonic tumors. World J Surg. 2013;37:2678–82.
137. Leroy J, Costantino F, Cahill RA, D'Agostino J, Morales A, Mutter D, et al. Laparoscopic resection with transanal specimen extraction for sigmoid diverticulitis. Br J Surg. 2011;98:1327–34.
138. Fuchs KH, Breithaupt W, Varga G, Schulz T, Reinisch A, Josipovic N. Transanal hybrid colon resection: from laparoscopy to NOTES. Surg Endosc. 2013;27:746–52.
139. Whiteford MH, Denk PM, Swanström LL. Feasibility of radical sigmoid colectomy performed as natural orifice translumenal endoscopic surgery (NOTES) using transanal endoscopic microsurgery. Surg Endosc. 2007;21:1870–4.
140. Sylla P, Willingham FF, Sohn DK, Gee D, Brugge WR, Rattner DW. NOTES rectosigmoid resection using transanal endoscopic microsurgery (TEM) with transgastric endoscopic assistance: a pilot study in swine. J Gastrointest Surg. 2008;12:1717–23.
141. Telem DA, Han KS, Kim MC, Ajari I, Sohn DK, Woods K, et al. Transanal rectosigmoid resection via natural orifice translumenal endoscopic surgery (NOTES) with total mesorectal excision in a large human cadaver series. Surg Endosc. 2013;27:74–80.
142. Sylla P, Rattner DW, Delgado S, Lacy AM. NOTES transanal rectal cancer resection using transanal endoscopic microsurgery and laparoscopic assistance. Surg Endosc. 2010;24:1205–10.

143. Marks J, Nassif G, Schoonyoung H, DeNittis A, Zeger E, Mohiuddin M, et al. Sphincter-sparing surgery for adenocarcinoma of the distal 3 cm of the true rectum: results after neoadjuvant therapy and minimally invasive radical surgery or local excision. Surg Endosc. 2013;27:4469–77.
144. Rullier E, Zerbib F, Laurent C, Bonnel C, Caudry M, Saric J, et al. Intersphincteric resection with excision of internal anal sphincter for conservative treatment of very low rectal cancer. Dis Colon Rectum. 1999;42:1168–75.
145. Lacy AM, Tasende MM, Delgado S, Fernandez-Hevia M, Jimenez M, De Lacy B, et al. Transanal total mesorectal excision for rectal cancer: outcomes after 140 patients. J Am Coll Surg. 2015;221:415–23.
146. Rouanet P, Mourregot A, Azar CC, Carrere S, Gutowski M, Quenet F, et al. Transanal endoscopic proctectomy: an innovative procedure for difficult resection of rectal tumors in men with narrow pelvis. Dis Colon Rectum. 2013;56:408–15.
147. Tuech JJ, Karoui M, Lelong B, De Chaisemartin C, Bridoux V, Manceau G, et al. A step toward NOTES total mesorectal excision for rectal cancer: endoscopic transanal proctectomy. Ann Surg. 2015;261:228–33.
148. Veltcamp Helbach M, Deijen CL, Velthuis S, Bonjer HJ, Tuynman JB, et al. Transanal total mesorectal excision for rectal carcinoma: short-term outcomes and experience after 80 cases. Surg Endosc. 2015;30(2):464–70.
149. Serra-Aracil X, Mora-López L, Casalots A, Pericay C, Guerrero R, Navarro-Soto S. Hybrid NOTES: TEO for transanal total mesorectal excision: intracorporeal resection and anastomosis. Surg Endosc. 2016;30:346–54.
150. Burke JP, Martin-Perez B, Khan A, Nassif G, de Beche-Adams T, Larach SW, et al. Transanal total mesorectal excision for rectal cancer: early outcomes in 50 consecutive patients. Color Dis. 2016;18(6):570–7.
151. Bremers AJ, van Laarhoven KJ, van der Kolk BM, de Wilt JH, van Goor H. Transanal endoscopic microsurgery approach for rectal stump resection as an alternative to transperitoneal stump resection. Br J Surg. 2013;100:568–71.
152. Liyanage C, Ramwell A, Harris GJ, Levy BF, Simson JN. Transanal endoscopic microsurgery: a new technique for completion proctectomy. Color Dis. 2013;15:e542–7.
153. Ganai S, Garb JL, Kanumuri P, Rao RS, Alexander AI, Wait RB. Mapping the rectum: spatial analysis of transanal endoscopic microsurgical outcomes using GIS technology. J Gastrointest Surg. 2006;10:22–31.
154. Lev-Chelouche D, Margel D, Goldman G, Rabau MJ. Transanal endoscopic microsurgery: experience with 75 rectal neoplasms. Dis Colon Rectum. 2000;43:662–7. discussion 667–8
155. Demartines N, von Flüe MO, Harder FH. Transanal endoscopic microsurgical excision of rectal tumors: indications and results. World J Surg. 2001;25:870–5.
156. Serra-Aracil X, Mora-Lopez L, Alcantara-Moral M, Caro-Tarrago A, Gomez-Diaz CJ, Navarro-Soto S. Transanal endoscopic surgery in rectal cancer. World J Gastroenterol. 2014;20:11538–45.
157. Kumar AS, Chhitwal N, Coralic J, Stahl TJ, Ayscue JM, FitzGerald JF, et al. Transanal endoscopic microsurgery: safe for midrectal lesions in morbidly obese patients. Am J Surg. 2012;204:402–5.
158. Baatrup G, Endreseth BH, Isaksen V, Kjellmo A, Tveit KM, Nesbakken A. Preoperative staging and treatment options in T1 rectal adenocarcinoma. Acta Oncol. 2009;48:328–42.
159. Ashraf S, Hompes R, Slater A, Lindsey I, Bach S, Mortensen NJ, et al. A critical appraisal of endorectal ultrasound and transanal endoscopic microsurgery and decision-making in early rectal cancer. Color Dis. 2012;14:821–6.
160. Starck M, Bohe M, Simanaitis M, Valentin L. Rectal endosonography can distinguish benign rectal lesions from invasive early rectal cancers. Color Dis. 2003;5:246–50.
161. Mondal D, Betts M, Cunningham C, Mortensen NJ, Lindsey I, Slater A. How useful is endorectal ultrasound in the management of early rectal carcinoma? Int J Color Dis. 2014;29:1101–4.

162. Bipat S, Glas AS, Slors FJM, Zwinderman AH, Bossuyt PMM, Stoker J. Rectal cancer: local staging and assessment of lymph node involvement with endoluminal US, CT, and MR imaging—a meta-analysis. Radiology. 2004;232:773–83.
163. Kim CK, Kim SH, Chun HK, Lee W-Y, Yun S-H, Song S-Y, et al. Preoperative staging of rectal cancer: accuracy of 3-Tesla magnetic resonance imaging. Eur Radiol. 2006;16:972–80.
164. Kunitake H, Abbas MA. Transanal endoscopic microsurgery for rectal tumors: a review. Perm J. 2012;16:45–50.
165. Baatrup G, Borschitz T, Cunningham C, Qvist N. Perforation into the peritoneal cavity during transanal endoscopic microsurgery for rectal cancer is not associated with major complications or oncological compromise. Surg Endosc. 2009;23:2680–3.
166. Gavagan JA, Whiteford MH, Swanstrom LL. Full-thickness intraperitoneal excision by transanal endoscopic microsurgery does not increase short-term complications. Am J Surg. 2004;187:630–4.
167. Marks JH, Frenkel JL, Greenleaf CE, D'Andrea AP. Transanal endoscopic microsurgery with entrance into the peritoneal cavity: is it safe? Dis Colon Rectum. 2014;57:1176–82.
168. Ramwell A, Evans J, Bignell M, Mathias J, Simson J. The creation of a peritoneal defect in transanal endoscopic microsurgery does not increase complications. Color Dis. 2009;11:964–6.
169. Morino M, Allaix ME, Famiglietti F, Caldart M, Arezzo A. Does peritoneal perforation affect short- and long-term outcomes after transanal endoscopic microsurgery? Surg Endosc. 2013;27:181–8.
170. Hompes R, Ris F, Cunningham C, Mortensen NJ, Cahill RA. Transanal glove port is a safe and cost-effective alternative for transanal endoscopic microsurgery. Br J Surg. 2012;99:1429–35.
171. McLemore EC, Coker A, Jacobsen G, Talamini MA, Horgan S. eTAMIS: endoscopic visualization for transanal minimally invasive surgery. Surg Endosc. 2013;27:1842–5.
172. Bislenghi G, Wolthuis AM, de Buck van Overstraeten A, D'Hoore A. AirSeal system insufflator to maintain a stable pneumorectum during TAMIS. Tech Coloproctol. 2015;19:43–5.
173. Atallah S, Parra-Davila E, deBeche-Adams T, Albert M, Larach S. Excision of a rectal neoplasm using robotic transanal surgery (RTS): a description of the technique. Tech Coloproctol. 2012;16:389–92.
174. Buchs NC, Pugin F, Volonte F, Hagen ME, Morel P, Ris F. Robotic transanal endoscopic microsurgery: technical details for the lateral approach. Dis Colon Rectum. 2013;56:1194–8.
175. Hompes R, Rauh SM, Ris F, Tuynman JB, Mortensen NJ. Robotic transanal minimally invasive surgery for local excision of rectal neoplasms. Br J Surg. 2014;101:578–81.
176. Allaix ME, Arezzo A, Arolfo S, Caldart M, Rebecchi F, Morino M. Transanal endoscopic microsurgery for rectal neoplasms. How I do it. J. Gastrointest Surg. 2013;17:586–92.
177. Paganini AM, Balla A, Quaresima S, D'Ambrosio G, Bruzzone P, Lezoche E. Tricks to decrease the suture line dehiscence rate during endoluminal loco-regional resection (ELRR) by transanal endoscopic microsurgery (TEM). Surg Endosc. 2015;29:1045–50.
178. Ramirez JM, Aguilella V, Arribas D, Martinez M. Transanal full-thickness excision of rectal tumours: should the defect be sutured? A randomized controlled trial. Color Dis. 2002;4:51–5.
179. Wilhelm P, Storz P, Axt S, Falch C, Kirschniak A, Muller S. Use of self-retaining barbed suture for rectal wall closure in transanal endoscopic microsurgery. Tech Coloproctol. 2014;18:813–6.
180. Arezzo A. To clip or not to clip? Invited comment on Wilhelm et al.: use of self-retaining barbed suture for rectal wall closure in transanal endoscopic microsurgery. Tech Coloproctol. 2014;18:841.
181. Ford SJ, Wheeler JMD, Borley NR. Factors influencing selection for a day-case or 23-h stay procedure in transanal endoscopic microsurgery. Br J Surg. 2010;97:410–4.
182. Nielsen LBJ, Wille-Jørgensen P. National and international guidelines for rectal cancer. Color Dis. 2014;16:854–65.
183. Allaix ME, Arezzo A, Caldart M, Festa F, Morino M. Transanal endoscopic microsurgery for rectal neoplasms: experience of 300 consecutive cases. Dis Colon Rectum. 2009;52:1831–6.

184. Molina G, Bordeianou L, Shellito P, Sylla P. Transanal endoscopic resection with peritoneal entry: a word of caution. Surg Endosc. 2016;30(5):1816–25.
185. Kumar AS, Coralic J, Kelleher DC, Sidani S, Kolli K, Smith LE. Complications of transanal endoscopic microsurgery are rare and minor: a single institution's analysis and comparison to existing data. Dis Colon Rectum. 2013;56:295–300.
186. Tsai BM, Finne CO, Nordenstam JF, Christoforidis D, Madoff RD, Mellgren A. Transanal endoscopic microsurgery resection of rectal tumors: outcomes and recommendations. Dis Colon Rectum. 2010;53:16–23.
187. Speake D, Lees N, McMahon RFT, Hill J. Who should be followed up after transanal endoscopic resection of rectal tumours? Color Dis. 2008;10:330–5.
188. Bignell MB, Ramwell A, Evans JR, Dastur N, Simson JNL. Complications of transanal endoscopic microsurgery (TEMS): a prospective audit. Color Dis. 2010;12:e99–103.
189. Guerrieri M, Baldarelli M, Morino M, Trompetto M, Da Rold A, Selmi I, et al. Transanal endoscopic microsurgery in rectal adenomas: experience of six Italian centres. Dig Liver Dis. 2006;38:202–7.
190. Barker JA, Hill J. Incidence, treatment and outcome of rectal stenosis following transanal endoscopic microsurgery. Tech Coloproctol. 2011;15:281–4.
191. Mora López M, Serra Aracil X, Hermoso Bosch J, Rebasa P, Navarro SS. Study of anorectal function after transanal endoscopic surgery. Int J Surg. 2015;13:142–7.
192. Kennedy ML, Lubowski DZ, King DW. Transanal endoscopic microsurgery excision: is anorectal function compromised? Dis Colon Rectum. 2002;45:601–4.
193. Cataldo PA, O'Brien S, Osler T. Transanal endoscopic microsurgery: a prospective evaluation of functional results. Dis Colon Rectum. 2005;48:1366–71.
194. Hompes R, Ashraf SQ, Gosselink MP, van Dongen KW, Mortensen NJ, Lindsey I, et al. Evaluation of quality of life and function at 1 year after transanal endoscopic microsurgery. Color Dis. 2015;17:54–61.
195. Restivo A, Zorcolo L, Dalia G, Cocco F, Cossu A, Scintu F, et al. Risk of complications and long-term functional alterations after local excision of rectal tumors with transanal endoscopic microsurgery (TEM). Int J Color Dis. 2015;31(2):257–66.
196. Dafnis G, Påhlman L, Raab Y, Gustafsson UM, Graf W. Transanal endoscopic microsurgery: clinical and functional results. Color Dis. 2004;6:336–42.

Transanal Laparoscopic TME with Multiport Abdominal Laparoscopy

24

María Fernández-Hevia and Antonio M. Lacy

Abstract

Transanal total mesorectal excision (TME) is a new approach in the treatment of rectal cancer. It has gained popularity in the last years, not only because of the novelty of the surgical technique but because it tries to resolve old problems in rectal surgery. The main advantage of the approach is that the decision of where the rectum is sectioned is made as the first manoeuvre.

Its indications are singularly low-mid-rectal cancer and unfavourable patients but can be expanded to high rectal cancer and other pathologies. One of the differences with laparoscopy or open surgery is that, during these approaches, the surgeon is working in a reduced space in the pelvis, and in addition to this, the same area is occupied by the rectum, so it is a really small space. In transanal TME, the surgeon is performing the dissection "down-to-up", winning space to work, so the view is better, the dissection of the anterior side is better than from above and especially, in difficult cases, you have the perception of a false wider pelvis, just because the rectum is retracted cranially. Transanal TME represents a new approach to perform an old technique.

M. Fernández-Hevia, M.D.
Department of Gastrointestinal Surgery, Institute of Digestive and Metabolic Diseases (ICMDM), Hospital Clínic, IDIBAPS, Centro de Investigación Biomédica en Red de Enfermedades Hepáticas y Digestivas (CIBERehd), Centro Esther Koplowitz, BIMA, University of Barcelona, Villarroel 170, 08036 Barcelona, Spain

A.M. Lacy, M.D. (✉)
Department of Gastrointestinal Surgery, Institute of Digestive and Metabolic Diseases (ICMDM), Hospital Clínic, IDIBAPS, Centro de Investigación Biomédica en Red de Enfermedades Hepáticas y Digestivas (CIBERehd), Centro Esther Koplowitz, BIMA, University of Barcelona, Villarroel 170, 08036 Barcelona, Spain

Founder AIS Channel, Departament of Surgery, Hospital Clínic, University of Barcelona, Barcelona, Spain
e-mail: alacy@clinic.ub.es

G. Dapri, J.H. Marks (eds.), *Surgical Techniques in Rectal Cancer*,
https://doi.org/10.1007/978-4-431-55579-7_24

Keywords
Rectal cancer • Transanal • TME • taTME • Down-to-up

24.1 Introduction

Rectal surgery has changed during the last century. The evolution of the technique and the introduction of new technology have allowed us to know rectal surgery as we understand it today. Since the abdominoperineal resection was introduced at the beginning of the twentieth century until minimally invasive surgery, there has been a long list of innovations [1, 2].

It is not the objective of the chapter remarks to recount them, but at least two must be highlighted. The sphincter-sparing surgery, which was described in 1931 by Abel, has decreased the number of definitive stomas in low rectal cancer [2], and, of course, total mesorectal excision (TME), described by Heald in 1979, has led to a marked improvement in the survival and recurrence in these patients [3].

Minimally invasive surgery in rectal cancer has had many detractors, and if it is compared with colon cancer, the introduction of it has been slower and some controversial points remain [4]. There are some randomized trials that have demonstrated that laparoscopic surgery is feasible and safe and with comparable oncological outcomes as open surgery. There is no doubt that laparoscopic surgery has many advantages demonstrated also in rectal surgery including less postoperative pain, shorter hospital stay and recovery time. In short-term outcomes of COLOR II trial, it has been reported that there are no statistically significant differences between laparoscopic and open surgery with respect to TME in high and middle rectal tumours, but a laparoscopic approach was superior in low rectal tumours probably due to the fact that laparoscopy gets a better view in this subset of patients [5, 6].

A challenge in rectal surgery, still present nowadays, is to work into the deep pelvis, especially difficult in narrow, obese patients or bulky tumours. Transanal approaches try to facilitate an alternative in these patients.

There are some techniques that have contributed to the development of transanal surgery. Of course, transanal endoscopic microsurgery (TEM) is one of the most important steps towards transanal TME [7]. The full-thickness resection of the rectal wall, indicated at the beginning just for benign lesions, has extended its purpose. The scope magnifies the view of the lesion, improving the quality of the surgery. The difficulty of the technique is working in a reduced space and the triangulation with the instruments, working most of the time in parallel. The experience in TEM facilitates performing transanal TME.

Natural orifice transluminal endoscopic surgery (NOTES) and natural orifice specimen extraction (NOSE) have contributed in the conception of transanal TME. Also they have contributed in improving the instruments and demystifying these approaches, helping us to accept the rectum and colon as a feasible access in colorectal surgery [8, 9]. NOTES using the rectum as access in colorectal surgery is intuitively better suited than other access routes since it does not require incisions in viscera not directly implicated in the process. It is also a universal way, which is not limited by patients' gender, and it may represent the natural evolution of minimally invasive colorectal surgery [9–12].

There are some groups from the mid-1990s that perform a combined surgery transanal and transabdominal (TATA) approach in low rectal cancer, combining the perineal dissection with laparoscopic TME. It has been compared with laparoscopic TME, and the outcomes towards the TATA approach have been favourable, because it decreases positive circumferential and distal margins [13, 14].

The first transanal TME resection assisted by laparoscopy was published in 2010 [15]. Since then, the number of publications of transanal TME has grown up exponentially in the last 2 years. There are only short-term outcomes published in the literature, and they demonstrate a safe technique with comparable short-term outcomes to laparoscopy or open surgery [16–22]. Transanal TME represents a new approach to perform an old technique.

24.2 Indications

Rectal cancer is an indication to transanal TME; there will not be any discussion about low and mid-rectal cancer. It is specially indicated in low rectal cancer, where a perineal dissection can be started with a retractor and continued with the TME. In mid-rectal cancer, it is a valid option overall in unfavourable patients. Obese patients with bulky mesorectum, large tumours or narrow pelvis present a challenge in rectal surgery; furthermore, we cannot forget patients with previous pelvic surgery (prostatectomy, gynaecological surgery, previous rectal surgery) where the planes can be distorted.

If we talk about high rectal cancer, then doubts can appear. In those patients, a subtotal mesorectal excision can be performed, and doing TME transanally can be more difficult compared with other approaches. But we are in the same dilemma: what happens with these difficult patients? Besides, is subtotal mesorectal excision always performed with other approaches? If we analyse the short-term outcomes of the COLOR II trial, we can see how the rate of subtotal or partial mesorectal excision is lower compared with the number of high rectal tumours, so we are overtreating these patients or performing surgery that is not so easy with the conventional surgery [6]. Transanal subtotal mesorectal excision is possible, and you decide exactly where you are going to section the rectum and a perpendicular section of the mesorectum can be done. Likely performing a subtotal mesorectal excision can be more difficult than a TME, and for that we consider the abdominal assistance essential.

Other options to use this approach are benign diseases such as inflammatory bowel disease (ulcerative colitis) and patients who undergo a "redo" anastomosis, with previous complications after rectal surgery (fistulae, chronic sinus, stenosis, anastomotic leakage) or Hartmann reversal with a short or very short rectal stump.

24.3 Technique

In this approach, there are two parts clearly differentiated, abdominal and transanal part. There are three different ways to propose the surgery:

(a) *One team.* If the transanal part were performed as the first step, the risk to perform with a pneumoretroperitoneum that can obstruct the dissection during the abdominal part would be higher. So, in this case, our recommendation is starting with the abdominal part, stopping the dissection in the highest part of the pelvis without opening the peritoneal reflection and continuing with the transanal part.

(b) *Two teams*. If there are two teams working at the same time, both parts can be done simultaneously. For this it is necessary to have two monitors, two laparoscopes and two independent fields. As warning, the pressure during the surgery should be higher in the transanal field than in the abdominal one, and when both fields are connected, the pressures must be equalized. Of course performing the surgery with two teams together decreases the operative time, but the main indication for this approach is making the surgery safer for the patient.

(c) *Pure NOTES*. There are some cases reported in the literature describing transanal TME, the division on the inferior mesenteric vessels, sigmoid colon mobilization and, also, splenic flexure mobilization performed all transanally without abdominal assistance. The number of patients reported is still low, but it demonstrates a trend in surgery. Advances in technology will allow the development in that field; at this moment, it is only indicated in selected patients by experienced surgeons [23, 24].

24.3.1 Setting Up

Patients receive mechanical bowel cleansing, and the stoma site is marked the day before. Antibiotic prophylaxis with 2 g of cefoxitin or 400 mg of ciprofloxacin and 500 mg of metronidazole in patients with allergy to penicillin is administrated intravenously before starting the surgery. Preventive measures for deep vein thrombosis are made (prophylactic heparin the day before, pneumatic stockings during surgery).

Patients are fixed and placed in lithotomy position with legs in padded and adjustable stirrups. The thorax is fixed to avoid displacements during surgery due to the extreme Trendelenburg position (Fig. 24.1).

The rectum is irrigated with diluted iodine solution and prepared in the usual way. Two fields are prepared for both abdominal and perineal access. A urinary catheter is inserted under sterile conditions.

The position of the surgeons and nurse during the surgery and the position of the main monitors are shown in Fig. 24.2. It is important, if two teams are working at the same time, for the team position during the surgery to interfere as little as possible.

Necessary materials to perform the surgery are the same as in conventional laparoscopic colorectal surgery, just adding the equipment for the transanal approach (transanal devices, retractor, dilators).

About transanal devices there are different options; there are some groups that have used classical devices (TEM (Richard Wolf GmbH, Knittlingen, Germany), TEO (Karl Storz GmbH, Tuttlingen, Germany)) and its instruments; the advantage of it is that there is only one surgeon in the transanal field. On the other hand, single-port devices have gained popularity with this technique, not only because they are easier to place but also because of its comfort during the surgery, allowing a good

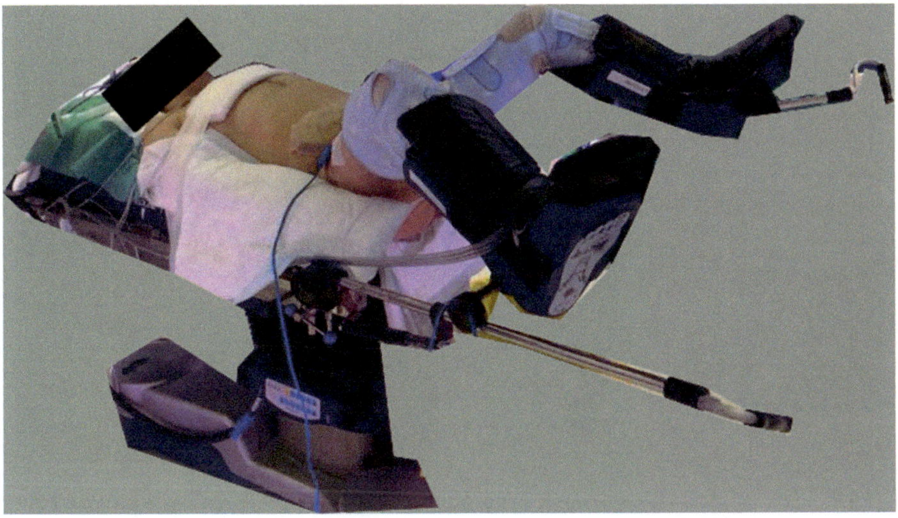

Fig. 24.1 Patient is fixed and placed in lithotomy position with legs in padded and adjustable stirrups. The thorax is fixed too

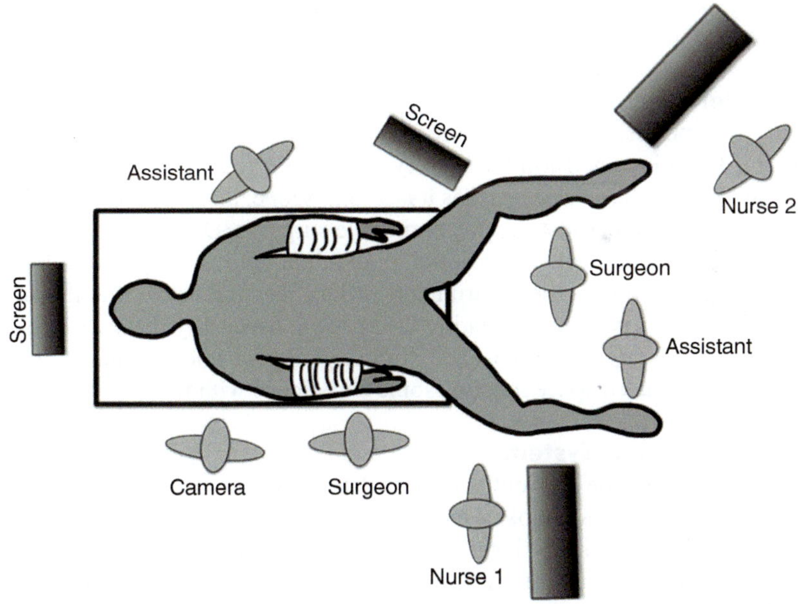

Fig. 24.2 Position into the surgery room: two teams are performing the procedure simultaneously. Abdominal team: the surgeon and camera are at the patient's right side, and the assistant is at the left side, and the nurse of the abdominal team is placed next to the patient's right leg and the screen is over the left leg. Transanal team: the surgeon and the assistant are between the patient's legs, and the nurse is next to the left leg and the screen is over the patient's head

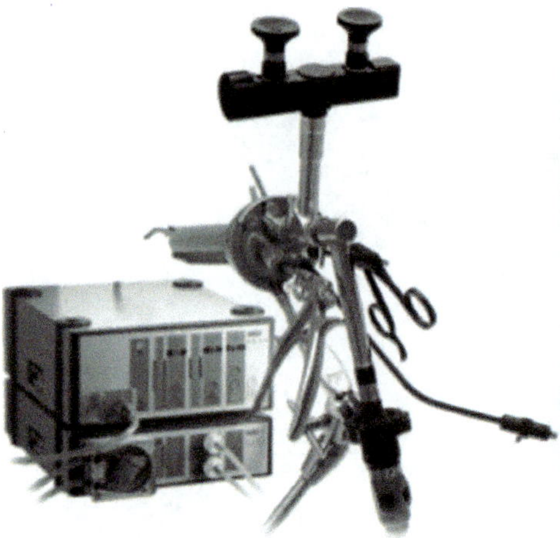

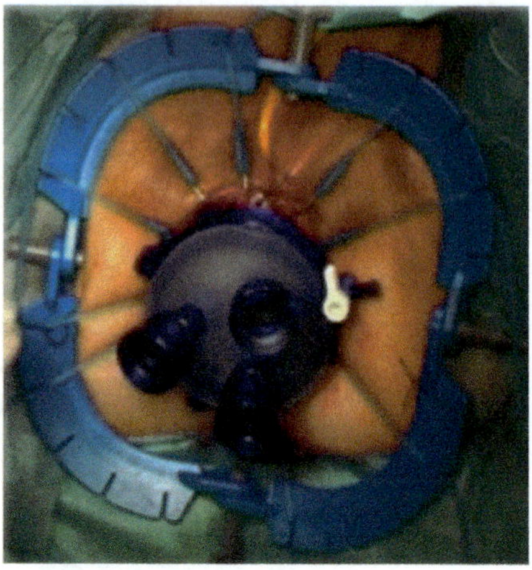

Fig. 24.3 In the left side, TEM system (Richard Wolf GmbH, Knittlingen, Germany) and, in the right side, a transanal GelPOINT platform (Applied Medical, Inc., Rancho Santa Margarita, CA, USA)

triangulation and the use of conventional laparoscopic instruments. With single-port devices, it is necessary to have an assistant for the camera (Fig. 24.3).

There are two important points to emphasize! One is the image and another is the insufflation system.

24.3.1.1 Image

There are two options, 3D or 2D. There is no doubt that 2D is more standard than 3D, and it is feasible to perform the surgery with it. It is mandatory to use an angulated scope (30° will be correct), and as it is a rigid scope, there will be no problems of crashing with the other instruments during the surgery. 3D systems, on the other hand, have the advantage of the perception of depth of field, so the camera does not need to be so close to the other instruments. It has been published that the advantages of 3D imaging include facilitating the surgery, especially difficult ones, and reducing surgeons' fatigue [25, 26]. The difficulty of this camera is the flexible tip, as the work in a reduced space requires some experience with these devices.

24.3.1.2 Insufflator System

We have two options, the conventional insufflators (with a discontinuous flow) or the devices with continuous smoke evacuation and carbon dioxide recirculation during surgery (AirSeal system insufflator, SurgiQuest Inc., Milford, CT, USA; Endoflator 40, Karl Storz GmbH, Tuttlingen, Germany). The conventional insufflators need to adapt to the pressure during the surgery, so the assistant can open the valve/catheter during the surgery to extract the smoke. The problem with these systems is that the flow variations do create a stable pressure in the pelvic cavity, and consequently there appear more movements of the rectum that can hinder the

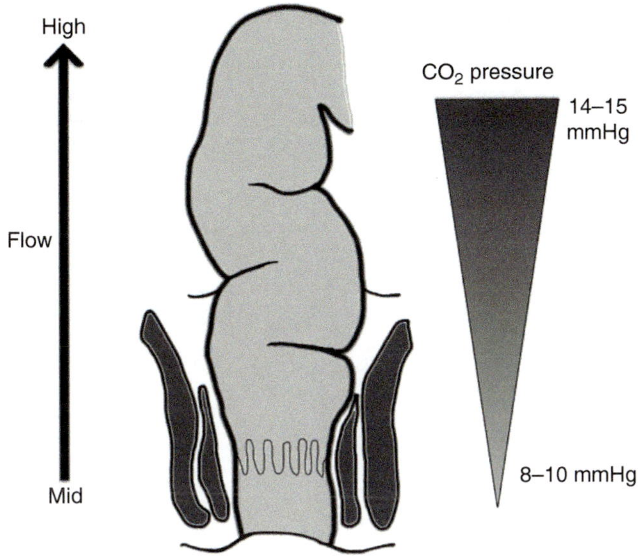

Fig. 24.4 The evolution of the pressure in function according to the height of the lesion. To start with pressure of 10 and mid-flow, but if the tumour is in the high rectum, a higher pressure and a higher flow will be needed, so as adapting it when the dissection is performed and the space is getting bigger

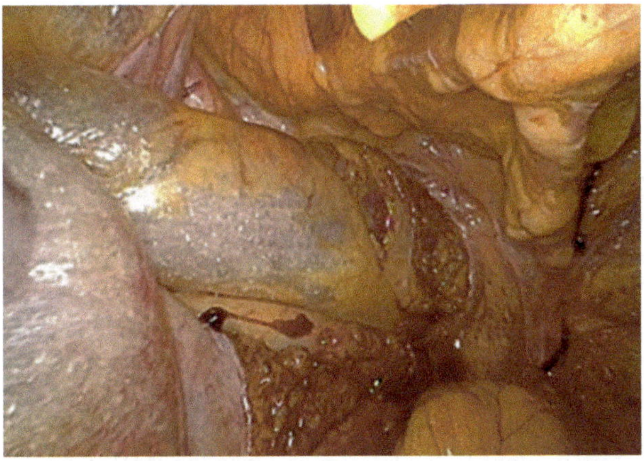

Fig. 24.5 Image during the abdominal part of transanal TME, the important pneumoretroperitoneum can be noticed . The solution is to wait until it is resorbed

surgery. Figure 24.4 tries to summarize the pressure with these devices and how it needs to be adapted when we are winning space.

The devices with continuous flow and smoke evacuation allow us to have a maintained pressure during the surgery. It is not necessary for it to adapt during the process and for the rectal movements to decrease significantly.

The main complication that the insufflators can produce is the pneumoretroperitoneum, which has been explained before; it is the reason to start with the abdominal part if only one team is performing the approach (Fig. 24.5).

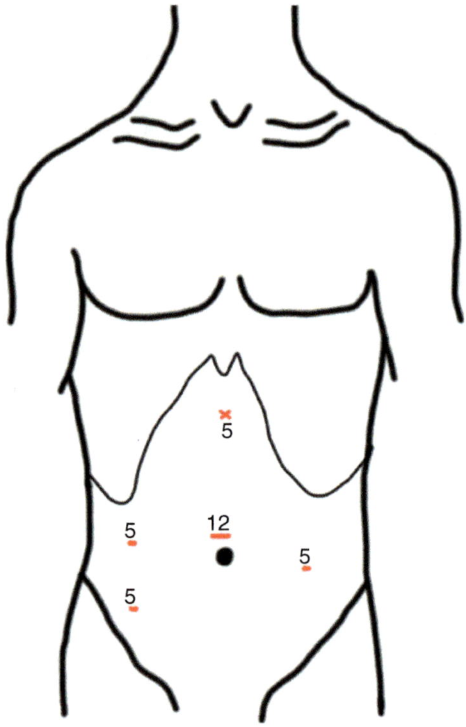

Fig. 24.6 Trocars' position. A 12 mm port at the umbilicus for the laparoscope, 5 mm port at low right quadrant for the surgeon's right hand, 5 mm port at right flank for the surgeon's left hand and 5 mm port at low left quadrant for the assistant. Another optional 5 mm at subxiphoid will be useful for splenic flexure mobilization

24.3.2 Abdominal Part

In the abdominal part, there are some essential steps. The position of the trocars are 12 mm at the umbilicus, 5 mm at low right quadrant, 5 mm at right flank and 5 mm port at low left quadrant (Fig. 24.6). The patient is positioned in the right side and in Trendelenburg position.

The first step is the division of the inferior mesenteric vessels (IMV) and opening the mesocolon distal to this. If the retroperitoneal plane is not opened, it is not mandatory to identify the left ureter. Once the IMV is dissected, the inferior mesenteric artery is sectioned using clips or a coagulation device. In the case of a low rectal cancer, and if it is possible, we try to respect the left colic artery to have a better vascularity, especially in elderly patients. The inferior mesenteric vein is dissected close to the Treitz ligament. The sigmoid and left colons are mobilized medial to lateral, and below the Toldt's fascia is opened.

Regarding splenic flexure mobilization, in our group, the decision to do it is made when we are going to perform the anastomosis; we mobilize it only if we need it to have a tension-free anastomosis. There are many groups that the mobilization of the splenic flexure is performed as the first manoeuvre routinely. We do not consider this essential in all cases, and we perform it at the end, because there are two groups working at the same time, and to do the splenic flexure, it is necessary to change the patient's position to anti-Trendelenburg. An additional trocar is used at subxiphoid (5 mm port). The gastrocolic ligament is opened to enter in the lesser sac, and it is sectioned until the splenic flexure. As usually the mobilization of the left colon has already been performed, we continue connecting the dissection of the mesocolon, always identifying the tail of the pancreas to avoid injuries at this level. After connecting the retroperitoneal plane with the lesser sac, we complete the mobilization lateral to medial by sectioning the adhesions with the spleen.

During the abdominal part, the highest part of rectum into the pelvis can be mobilized. It is recommended to not open the peritoneal reflection, trying to maintain the pressure into the transanal field. The traction from above to complete the TME at the high rectum facilitates in completing the surgery.

24.3.3 Transanal TME

We can divide this part into three different sections:

- Tumours in the low rectum where there is not enough space to insert the device (*2–3 cm over the dentate line*) and it is necessary to start by perineal dissection
- Tumours in low and mid-rectum where the device can be placed
- Tumours in the high rectum

24.3.3.1 Perineal Dissection

Sphincter-sparing surgery has changed the approach in the low rectum. We consider the classification published by Rullier in 2013 of low rectal cancer to be very interesting [27]. They propose a classical coloanal anastomosis, which was described by Marks in the TATA, in tumours 1 cm over the anal ring. A partial intersphincteric resection if the tumour is 1 cm below the anal ring or a total intersphincteric resection if the tumour is involving the internal sphincter is suggested. Abdominoperineal resection is limited to tumours invading the external sphincter [28].

After positioning a Lone Star retractor (CooperSurgical, Trumbull, CT, USA), exposing the anal canal and exploring the rectum, we can decide where we are going to section the rectum. So, rectal mucosa is sectioned with the electrocautery (it is usually protected to avoid burns to the distal rectal mucosa where the anastomosis will be performed), and if it is necessary, an intersphincteric resection is performed (Fig. 24.7).

The mucosa is closed with a running suture or a purse string using a monofilament 0 (PDS, prolene) with a 26 mm needle. Always remember cleaning with a solution of iodine after closing the lumen, to minimize the contamination and potential cell spillage.

As we know, how much is to be dissected to insert the device? If you have dissected enough space to put a gauze of 40x40, you will be able to place the device.

Introduce the transanal single-port device. It usually has three ports to work placed as an inverted triangle (Figs. 24.3 and 24.7). The camera is placed at 6

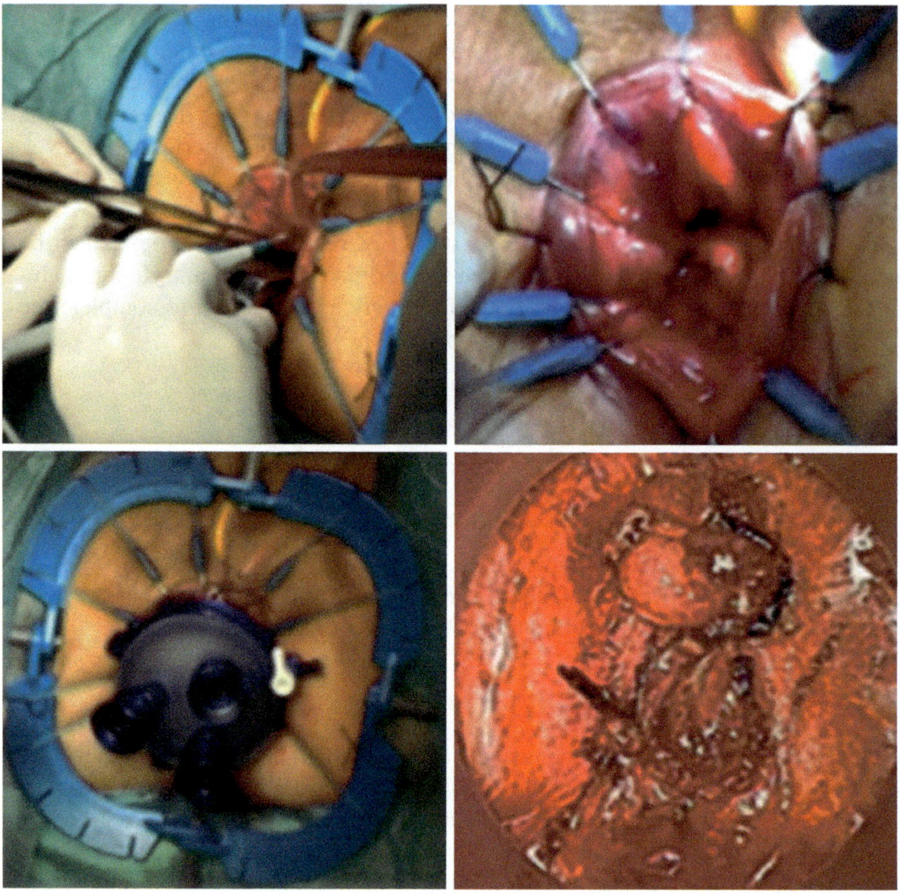

Fig. 24.7 Some images of the perineal dissection. Lone Star retractor facilitates the exposure of the anal canal. Once we have enough space, the device can be placed as you can see in the inferior left image, and the view inside the device with the rectum closed is the inferior right image

o'clock, and the surgeon works with the other ports. During the surgery, it may be necessary to change the position of the scope to the port at 10 o'clock to have a better visualization of the posterior side. If the device is angulated slightly, it may also help to improve the visualization.

24.3.3.2 Low-Mid-Rectal Tumours

In these cases, the transanal single-port device can be positioned before closing the rectal lumen. The ability to identify the lesion and decide which one is going to close the rectum is the main advantage of this technique; the first manoeuvre is to define where the rectum is going to be transected. If you do not have experience with performing stitches by laparoscopy, a possibility is performing the purse string by hand after removing the top of the device. A monofilament 0 is used to perform the purse string. It is very important to check if the suture is well closed, and if you are not sure, the best option is doing another stitch to ensure it. If the purse string is

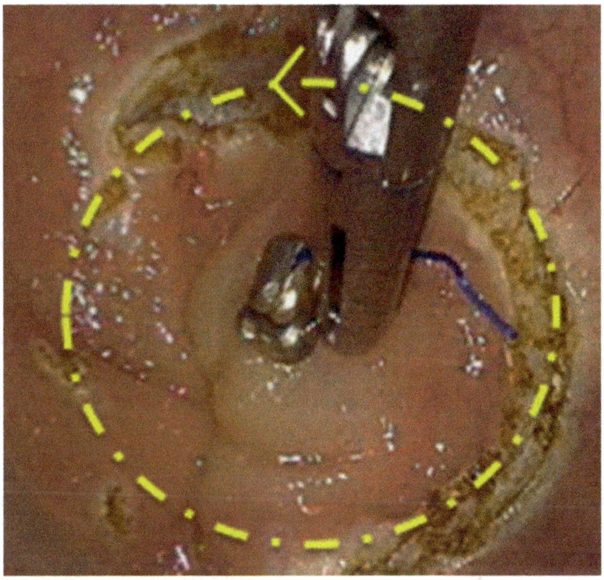

Fig. 24.8 Rectum closed and tattooed where it is going to be sectioned. Always perform the dissection circumferentially

open during the surgery, the risk of local contamination is higher as is the risk of malignant cell spillage.

While we are closing the rectum, it is important to not work with high flow and pressure, because it will cause distension of the colon. A trick will be occluding the colon in the abdomen, and if it has not been successful, then you can introduce a catheter to empty the colon before closing the suture.

After the mucosa is marked circumferentially, more or less 1 cm from the knot, all the points have to be connected with the hook, and the rectal wall is sectioned layer by layer until the mesorectal plane is entered (Fig. 24.8).

24.3.3.3 Mesorectal Dissection

The dissection after starting with the perineal approach must be carefully performed. The Waldeyer's fascia has to be sectioned as one of the first steps, and in patients with low rectal tumours or previous chemoradiotherapy, it can be difficult to find the correct plane. Besides, the mistakes at that point are going laterally to the endopelvic fascia, allowing the pneumorectum dissection more lateral and anterior than is needed, dissecting all the structures into the pelvis as well as increasing the risk of damage in the nerves. One of the differences with laparoscopy or open surgery is that during those approaches the surgeon is working in a reduced space; in addition, it is occupied by the same rectum, so it is a very small space. In transanal TME, accordingly, you are performing the dissection, you are winning space to work so the view is better and, especially, in difficult cases, you have the perception of a false wider pelvis, just because the rectum is retracted cranially.

Where do you start the dissection? The principal recommendation is to try to perform the surgery circumferentially and progressively, because if you focus on just one side, the rectum will be retracted to the opposite side; in that way you try to maintain the rectum at the centre, facilitating the process (Fig. 24.9). The anterior and the posterior sides have clear anatomical landmarks, but they are not so obvious in both lateral sidewalls.

Anterior Side

It is easier compared with the abdominal approach, and the anatomical landmarks are clear. In men, we will find the urethra, the Denonvilliers' fascia, the prostate and the seminal vesicles and, in women, the vagina and cervix. As it has been explained before, if during the dissection the lateral plane is not correct and you go too lateral to the endopelvic fascia, the pneumorectum can dissect the previous structures laterally and hinder the correct anterior plane. There are complications related with injuries in the urethra in that technique [17]. The dissection is continued cephalad until the peritoneal reflection. It is important to open the peritoneal reflection from below to maintain better the pelvic pressure and avoid variations of it (Fig. 24.10).

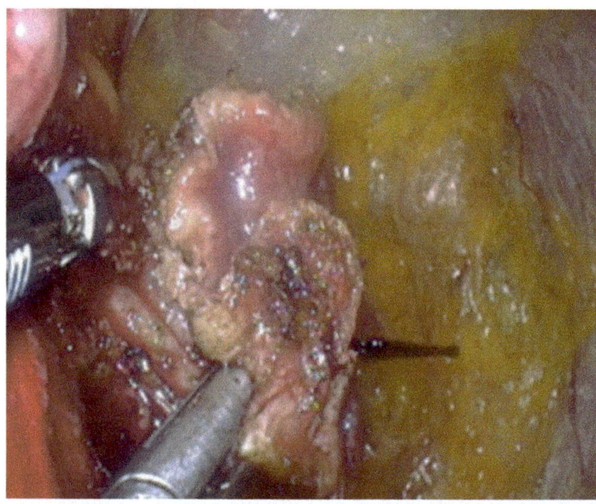

Fig. 24.9 Transanal view. The dissection of 270° has been performed (anterior, left lateral and posterior), and the rectum is retracted to the right side. It obstructs the dissection of that side

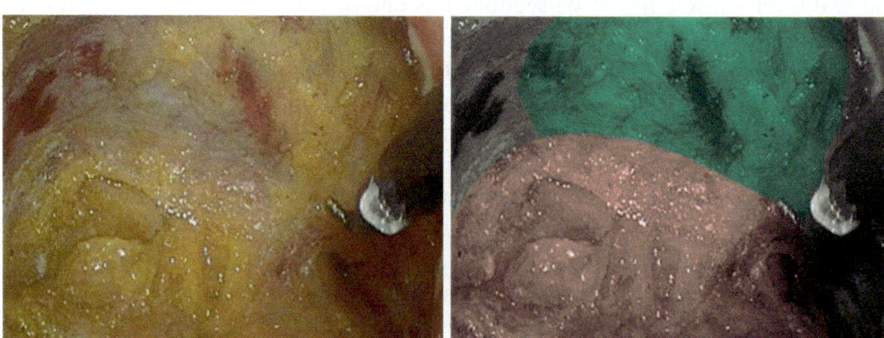

Fig. 24.10 Anterior side dissection. Left image is a real photo and, in the right image, there are the enhanced prostate-Denonvilliers' fascia (*blue*) and the mesorectum (*pink*)

Posterior Side

The anatomical references are the sacrum, the presacral vessels and its fascia. Injuries at that level can cause important haemorrhage. The angulation in the pelvis can vary in each person, and it is a point to consider. It is really easy to go deeper than necessary. During the dissection of that side, the position of the camera can be changed to the superior port or *the device angulated* to have a better view (Fig. 24.11).

Laterals

The anatomical references at these sides are not so clear. The limit of the mesorectum in both lateral sides is the endopelvic fascia, but it can be difficult to identify in many patients, especially in the radiated patients. The point of warning is the nerves and the potential problems if you are in the incorrect plane (Fig. 24.12). A trick is to have a good control of the anterior and the posterior parts, and the laterals will be drawn. It is really easy to perform a wide lateral dissection of the pelvis transanally with the potential vascular and ureteral injuries involved with it.

So after reviewing each option, which would be the best to start? Some groups recommend to start between 3 and 6 o'clock; our recommendation is to adapt the surgery to each patient and to perform the dissection circumferentially, and if you have a problem or a difficulty to find the correct plane in a side/point, change to the

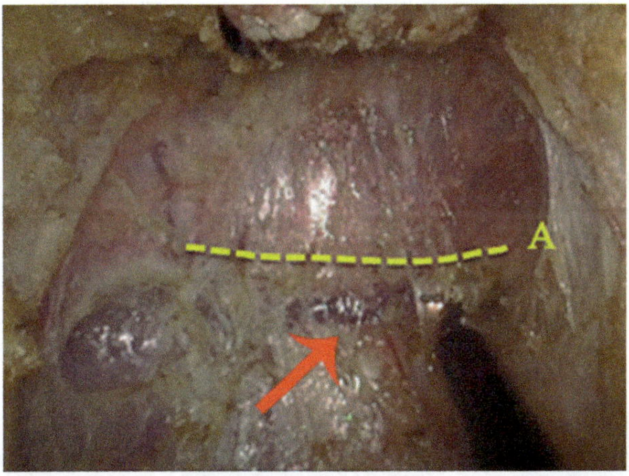

Fig. 24.11 Posterior side dissection. Real image during the dissection of the posterior side, at approximately 10 cm from the anal verge. At the level of the hook, a presacral vessel (*red arrow*) can be identified, and the correct plane is higher to this one (*yellow line*)

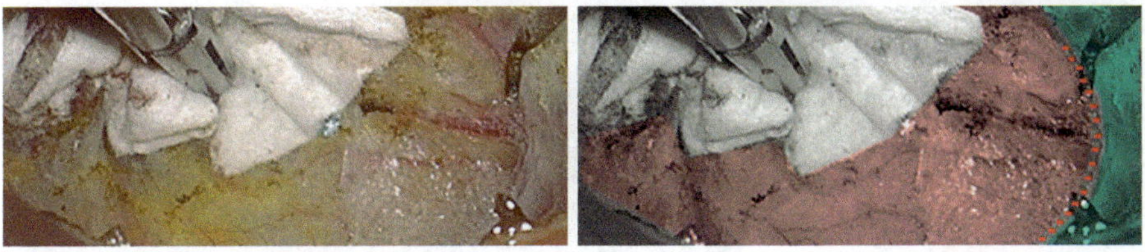

Fig. 24.12 Image during the transanal dissection at the left side, where the endopelvic fascia is visible. The left image is the real one, and in the right image, the *red line* corresponds to the endopelvic fascia, *pink* to the mesorectum and *green* to the incorrect plane

opposite and continue since then and you will find it. At the highest part of the pelvis, it is very important to gain the retraction from the abdomen, and it is a reason to work two teams at the same time to complete the dissection in the safest way.

24.3.3.4 High Rectal Tumours

In the case of high rectal cancer, the indication would be to perform a partial or subtotal mesorectal excision, respecting a distal margin of 5 cm. It is more difficult to perform a subtotal mesorectal excision than a TME, so in that case it is recommended to have previous experience in transanal TME. The device is inserted as in mid-rectal cancer and the rectum closed as well. The mesorectum must be transected perpendicular to the rectal lumen to avoid leaving tissue at the posterior part, and for that kind of dissection, it is better to use a coagulation device than the hook. Remember that the CO_2 pressure and flow that you need in these cases would be higher compared with low and mid-rectal cancer, when the dissection is starting.

24.3.3.5 Anastomoses

Handsewn Coloanal Anastomoses

It is performed as a classical anastomosis using absorbable suture (3/0), and the election anastomosis is a side to end, better than a mini-J pouch, or end to end, looking for the best functional outcomes later (Fig. 24.13).

Stapled Anastomosis

In our group, EEA 33 stapler 4.8 (Autosuture, Covidien, Medtronic, New Haven, CT, USA) is used to perform the anastomosis, because it has a longer spike which allows us to close the distal purse string over it and the size of the donuts are bigger compared with the conventional staplers. An option is to use conventional staplers and a catheter to elongate the spike and close the purse string over it. Furthermore, the anastomosis in transanal TME is different than the laparoscopic TME, where the distal rectum is not dissected and the corners after the section with the endostaplers in laparoscopy surgery are avoided.

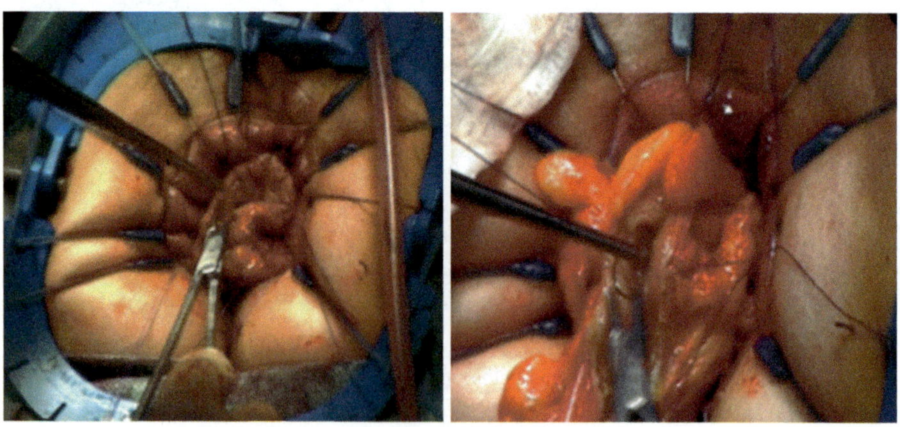

Fig. 24.13 There are some images of handsewn coloanal anastomosis

The distal purse string is performed using monofilament 0, and mid-/low rectal cancer is done by hand after removing the top of the device. The same device maintains the rectal lumen open, and the exposition is better. In high rectal cancer, it is better to perform the purse string before connecting both fields, because in that way the pressure into the pelvis is maintained and, if both fields are connected, it could be difficult to have a good distension of the distal rectal stump.

The anastomosis is checked to examine for bleeding. If bleeding is present and it is necessary, the device can be used, and some stitches can be placed (Figs. 24.14, 24.15, 24.16, and 24.17).

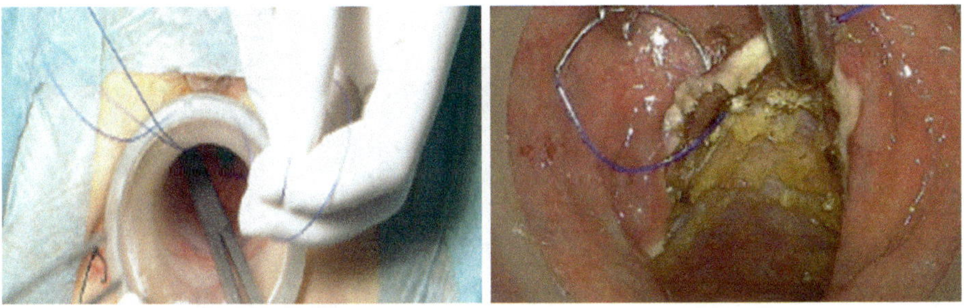

Fig. 24.14 Stapled anastomoses. Distal purse-string suture in the left image performed after removing the top of the device in mid-rectal lesions and in the right side performed transanally by endoscopy in high rectal lesions

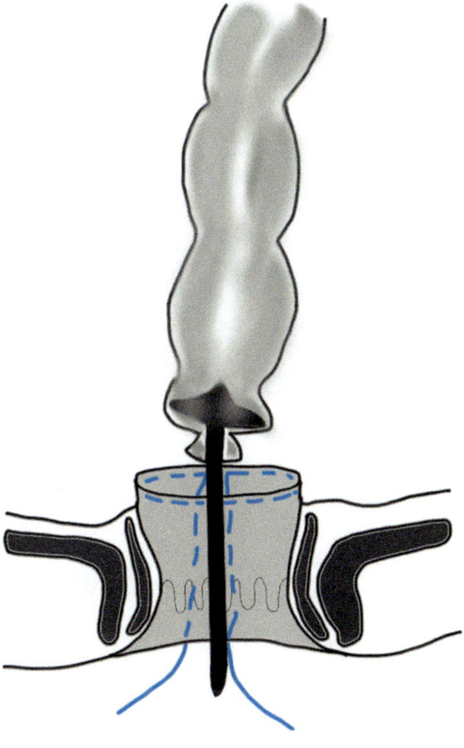

Fig. 24.15 Step 1. Stapled anastomosis. The anvil is inside the colon, and the distal purse string is performed in the distal rectal stump

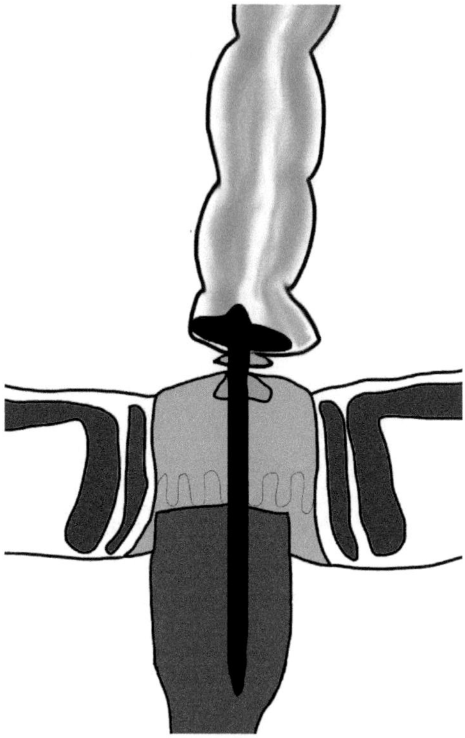

Fig. 24.16 Step 2. Stapled anastomosis. The distal purse string has been closed over the spike of the anvil in the colon, and the stapler has been joined up to it

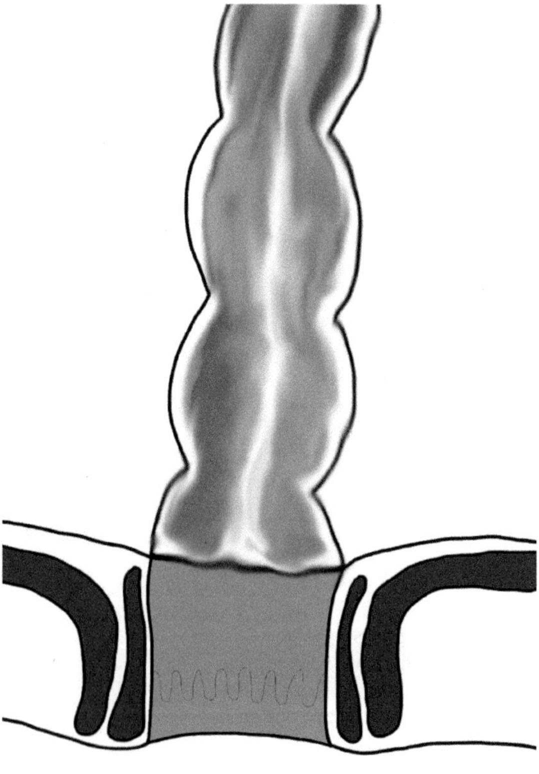

Fig. 24.17 Step 3. Scheme of this kind of stapled anastomosis

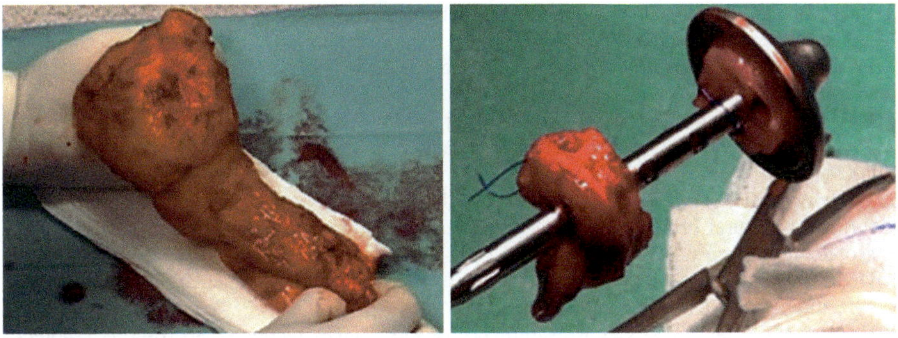

Fig. 24.18 Image of the specimen and the donuts

24.3.3.6 Specimen Extraction

Transanally

The specimen is extracted transanally always when it is feasible, and to facilitate it, the mesocolon is sectioned proximally to the vessels. The purse string is performed before this because, during the extraction, it may be necessary to completely remove the device and the mucosa can retract.

Transabdominal

In the case of a large tumour, a bulky mesentery or a size mismatch between the rectum and the specimen, an assistance incision is the elective choice to avoid injuries in the rectal stump and the anus.

24.3.3.7 Other Considerations

The decision to perform a diverting stoma must be made intraoperatively and in function of each patient. Generally a drainage tube into the pelvis is used and also another drainage tube, such as a Penrose or urinary catheter, through the rectum to decrease sphincter pressure. They will be removed into the first 24–48 h (Fig. 24.18).

References

1. Miles WE. A method of performing abdomino-perineal excision for carcinoma of the rectum and of the terminal portion of the pelvic colon (1908). CA Cancer J Clin. 1971;21:361–4.
2. Emhoff IA, Lee GC, Sylla P. Transanal colorectal resection using natural orifice translumenal endoscopic surgery (NOTES). Dig Endosc. 2014;26(Suppl 1):29–42.
3. Heald RJ. A new approach to rectal cancer. Br J Hosp Med. 1979;22:277–81.
4. Guillou PJ, Quirke P, Thorpe H, Walker J, Jayne DG, Smith AM, et al. Short-term endpoints of conventional versus laparoscopic-assisted surgery in patients with colorectal cancer (MRC CLASICC trial): multicentre, randomised controlled trial. Lancet. 2005;365(9472):1718–26.
5. Kang SB, Park JW, Jeong SY, et al. Open versus laparoscopic surgery for mid or low rectal cancer after neoadjuvant chemoradiotherapy (COREAN trial): short-term outcomes of an open-label randomized controlled trial. Lancet Oncol. 2010;11:637–45.
6. van der Pas MH, Haglind E, Cuesta MA, et al. Laparoscopic versus open surgery for rectal cancer (COLOR II): short-term outcomes of a randomised, phase 3 trial. Lancet Oncol. 2013;14:210–8.

7. Buess G, Theiss R, Gunther M, Hutterer F, Pichlmaier H. Transanal endoscopic microsurgery. Leber Magen Darm. 1985;15(6):271–9.
8. Franklin ME Jr, Ramos R, Rosenthal D, Schuessler W. Laparoscopic colonic procedures. World J Surg. 1993;17:51–6.
9. Knol J, D'Hondt M, Dozois EJ, Vanden Boer J, Malisse Received P. Laparoscopic-assisted Sigmoidectomy with transanal specimen extraction: a bridge to NOTES? Tech Coloproctol. 2009;13:65–8.
10. Whiteford MH, Denk PM, Swamstrom LL. Feasibility of radical sigmoid colectomy performed as natural orifice translumenal endoscopic surgery (NOTES) using transanal endoscopic microsurgery. Surg Endosc. 2007;21:1870–4.
11. Diana M, Wall J, Costantino F, et al. Transanal extraction of the specimen during laparoscopic colectomy. Color Dis. 2011;13(Suppl 7):23–7.
12. Franklin ME, Liang S, Russek K. Natural orifice specimen extraction in laparoscopic colorectal surgery: transanal and transvaginal approaches. Tech Coloproctol. 2013;17:S63–7.
13. Marks J, Mizrahi B, Dalane S, Nweze I, Marks G. Laparoscopic transanal abdominal transanal resection with sphincter preservation for rectal cancer in the distal 3 cm of the rectum after neoadjuvant therapy. Surg Endosc. 2010;24:2700–7. doi:10.1007/s00464-010-1028-8.
14. Denost Q, Adam JP, Rullier A, Buscail E, Laurent C, Rullier E. Perineal transanal approach: a new standard for laparoscopic sphincter-saving resection in low rectal cancer, a randomized trial. Ann Surg. 2014;260(6):993–9. doi:10.1097/SLA.0000000000000766.
15. Sylla P, Rattner DW, Delgado S, Lacy AM. NOTES transanal rectal cancer resection using transanal endoscopic microsurgery and laparoscopic assistance. Surg Endosc. 2010;24:1205–10.
16. Lacy AM, Rattner DW, Adelsdorfer C, Tasende MM, Fernández M, Delgado S, Sylla P, Martínez-Palli G. Transanal natural orifice transluminal endoscopic surgery (NOTES) rectal resection: "down-to-up" total mesorectal excision (TME)-short-term outcomes in the first 20 cases. Surg Endosc. 2013;27:3165–72.
17. Rouanet P, Mourregot A, Azar CC, Carrere S, Gutowski M, Quenet F, Saint-Aubert B, Colombo PE. Transanal endoscopic proctectomy: an innovative procedure for difficult resection of rectal tumors in men with narrow pelvis. Dis Colon Rectum. 2013;56:408–15.
18. Atallah S, Martin-Perez B, Albert M, deBeche-Adams T, Nassif G, Hunter L, Larach S. Transanal minimally invasive surgery for total mesorectal excision (TAMIS-TME): results and experience with the first 20 patients undergoing curative-intent rectal cancer surgery at a single institution. Tech Coloproctol. 2014;18(5):473–80. doi:10.1007/s10151-013-1095-7.
19. Velthuis S, Nieuwenhuis DH, Ruijter TE, Cuesta MA, Bonjer HJ, Sietses C. Transanal versus traditional laparoscopic total mesorectal excision for rectal carcinoma. Surg Endosc. 2014;28(12):3494–9. doi:10.1007/s00464-014-3636.
20. Fernández-Hevia M, Delgado S, Castells A, Tasende M, Momblan D, Díaz del Gobbo G, DeLacy B, Balust J, Lacy AM. Transanal total mesorectal excision in rectal cancer: short-term outcomes in comparison with laparoscopic surgery. Ann Surg. 2015;261(2):221–7. doi:10.1097/SLA.0000000000000865.
21. Muratore A, Mellano A, Marsanic P, De Simone M. Transanal total mesorectal excision (taTME) for cáncer located in the lower rectum: short- and mid-term results. EJSO. 2015;41:478–83.
22. Tuech JJ, Karoui M, Lelong B, De Chaisemartin C, Bridoux V, Manceau G, Delpero JR, Hanoun L, Michot F. A step toward NOTES total mesorectal excision for rectal cancer: endoscopic transanal proctectomy. Ann Surg. 2015;261(2):228–33. doi:10.1097/SLA.0000000000000994.
23. Leroy J, Barry BD, Melani A, et al. No-scar transanal total mesorectal excision: the last step to pure NOTES for colorectal surgery. JAMA Surg. 2013;148:226–30.
24. Chouillard E, Chahine E, Khoury G, Vinson-Bonnet B, Gumbs A, Azoulay D, Abdalla E. NOTES total mesorectal excision (TME) for patients with rectal neoplasia: a preliminary experience. Surg Endosc. 2014;28(11):3150–7. doi:10.1007/s00464-014-3573-z.
25. Wagner OJ, Hagen M, Kurmann A, Horgan S, Candinas D, Vorburger SA. Three-dimensional vision enhances task performance independently of the surgical method. Surg Endosc. 2012;26(10):2961–8.

26. Storz P, Buess GF, Kunert W, Kirschniak A. 3D HD versus 2D HD: surgical task efficiency in standardised phantom tasks. Surg Endosc. 2012;26(5):1454–60. doi:10.1007/s00464-011-2055-9.
27. Rullier E, Denost Q, Vendrely V, Rullier A, Laurent C. Low rectal cancer: classification and standardization of surgery. Dis Colon Rectum. 2013;56(5):560–7. doi:10.1097/DCR.0b013e31827c4a8c.
28. Marks JH, Lopez-Acevedo N, Krishnan B, Johnson MN, Montenegro GA, Marks GJ. True NOTES TME resection with splenic flexure release, high ligation of IMA, and side-to-end hand-sewn colonanal anastomosis. Surg Endosc. 2016;30:4626–31. doi:10.1007/s00464-015-4731-7.

Transanal Laparoscopic TME with Reduced Port Abdominal Laparoscopy

25

Ricardo Zorron

Abstract

Applications for natural orifice translumenal endoscopic surgery (NOTES) to access the abdominal cavity have increased in recent years. The modern rectal surgery evolves to a prioritization of the transanal access to allow natural orifice surgery. Despite potential advantages of transanal NOTES for colorectal diseases, it has not been widely applied in the clinical setting. This chapter discusses our experience with an evolving transanal technique for total mesorectal excision (TME), the so-called down-to-up total mesorectal excision for rectal cancer using reduced transabdominal laparoscopic assistance. Clinical experience and future trends in transrectal surgery are also discussed.

Keywords

Rectal cancer • Total mesorectal excision (TME) • Down-to-up transanal rectal resection • Natural orifice surgery NOTES

R. Zorron, M.D., Ph.D.
Center for Innovative Surgery- ZIC, Department of Surgery, Campus Charité Mitte / Campus Virchow-Klinikum, Charité – Universitätsmedizin Berlin, Campus Virchow Klinikum, Augustenburger Platz 1, 13353 Berlin, Germany
e-mail: Ricardo.Zorron@charite.de

G. Dapri, J.H. Marks (eds.), *Surgical Techniques in Rectal Cancer*,
https://doi.org/10.1007/978-4-431-55579-7_25

25.1 Introduction

Natural orifice translumenal endoscopic surgery (NOTES) has emerged in recent years as a promising new alternative to open and laparoscopic access for abdominal surgery. Potential benefits in avoiding the complications of surgical incisions encouraged the first successful series of clinical applications for transvaginal and transgastric NOTES [1, 2]. Access via the anal canal in the form of transrectal or transcolonic NOTES appears to be an attractive option for treating both colorectal and other abdominal diseases [3–5]. In fact, full-thickness rectal wall excision extending into the peritoneal cavity with hand-sewn closure by transanal endoscopic microsurgery (TEM) is not a new concept. Marks et al. showed the feasibility of the TATA (transanal transabdominal) procedure and standardized it for distal rectal tumors [6]. Technical obstacles such as the risk of infection, safe entrance into the abdominal cavity, and reliable closure of the bowel wall have been inhibiting factors that have prevented the progress of transrectal and transcolonic applications in particular. Our study group has developed innovative techniques in rigid and flexible transanal and perirectal access in animal studies and subsequently clinical pilot series in human subjects since 2009 [7–9].

Total mesorectal excision (TME) with high lymphadenectomy is the standard of care for curative resection of rectal cancer [10, 11], and there is currently good evidence showing that minimally invasive surgery has equivalent oncological outcomes [12]. In the case of transanal access for rectal cancer, the technique should maintain the principles and the dissection in the oncologic plane proposed by Heald [10]. In laparoscopic resection of rectal cancer of the middle and lower rectum, the distal part of the dissection is usually difficult and time-demanding, especially in obese male patients with a narrow pelvis. The integrity of the mesorectal fascia and free circumferential margins are demonstrated as the quality of the specimen in TME, thus representing an important prognostic factor for risk of local recurrence and overall survival [13]. However, the quality or totality of TME is inconstantly achieved. A study using postoperative magnetic resonance imaging to evaluate the completeness of mesorectal resection showed residual mesorectum in 36% of the patients which should receive complete TME [14]. The intraoperative correct assessment of margin-free limits of the resection is also challenging in low rectal tumors. The term transanal down-to-up technique, coined by our group in 2009 [16, 17], represents possibly a more direct and safe access for the last centimeters of the mesorectal dissection, in the right oncologic plane, with direct visualization of the distal limit of the tumor. This chapter describes the technique and clinical results of transanal down-to-up TME with reduced-port transabdominal assistance for patients with rectal cancer.

25.2 Evolution of the Technique

The history and progress of transrectal NOTES is undoubtedly due to the pioneering efforts of Gerhard Buess, who in the early 1980s described TEM (transanally endoscopic microsurgery), and it is still the standard therapy for most low rectal benign lesions [15]. Experimental programs with survival and cadaver studies were performed in recent years to evaluate the transrectal NOTES access, aiming to overcome technical and anatomical issues to NOTES colorectal surgery. Working with cadavers, Whiteford et al. demonstrated the feasibility of rectosigmoid resection using a rigid platform (TEM) [3]. He was able to perform rectal resection with adequate lymphadenectomy, transanal retrieval, and anastomosis and recognized the acute angle of the promontory as a true anatomic obstacle to perform rigid transrectal resections and the limited reach of the standard instruments.

Using a non-survival model in pigs, Sylla et al. described a technique using rigid transanal resection and NOTES transgastric access as an assistance to allow colonic mobilization [4], and Leroy et al. performed a combined technique (Totally NOTES) with flexible and rigid transrectal and flexible transgastric NOTES operating sigmoidectomy in pigs [5]. The survival follow-up in five animals demonstrated no signs of infections and no postoperative complications. Our group performed survival studies in swine model, solving problems of spatial orientation, insufflation, and development of instruments, and start of human casuistic was approved by our institutional review board for transcolonic NOTES clinical trials [7]. In these early series, the animals were operated through an incision at the dentate line, and progression of TME was successfully achieved using a standard flexible colonoscope (Figs. 25.1 and 25.2). No animal developed complications, and follow-up and sacrifice at 15 days showed sterile pelvic swabs and no abscess.

The term down-to-up TME was coined in 2009 to describe the technique of cephalad progression of mesorectal dissection in transanal rectal resections for rectal cancer [16, 17]. Originally, our technique proceeded the dissection using a flexible colonoscope to enter the presacral plane and dissect the mesorectum. In these cases the transanal access was made by entering the retrorectal space by an incision in the planned anastomosis level and then carrying the dissection using a colonoscope with endoscopic instruments. In the animal set, the progression of TME is fast and intuitive (Figs. 25.1 and 25.2). For human subjects, the status of the anatomy and neoadjuvant radiochemotherapy make the flexible dissection slow and challenging (Figs. 25.3 and 25.4). In the current state of technology, it is

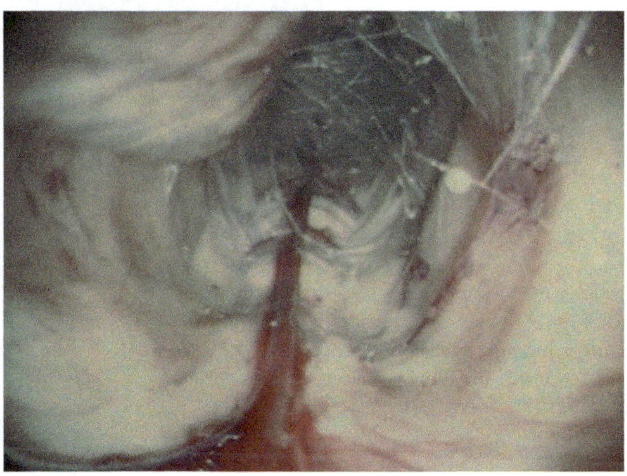

Fig. 25.1 Porcine survival study for perirectal flexible TME using a colonoscope. Endoscopic view of TME dissection with the colonoscope

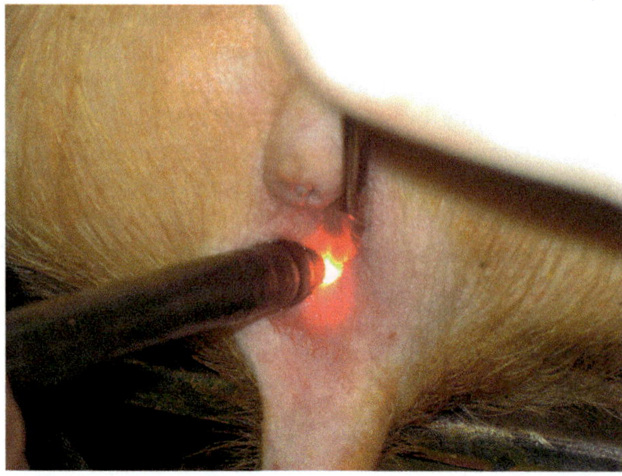

Fig. 25.2 Porcine survival study. Note the site of entrance just above the dentate line allowing a safe introduction for the retrorectal dissection

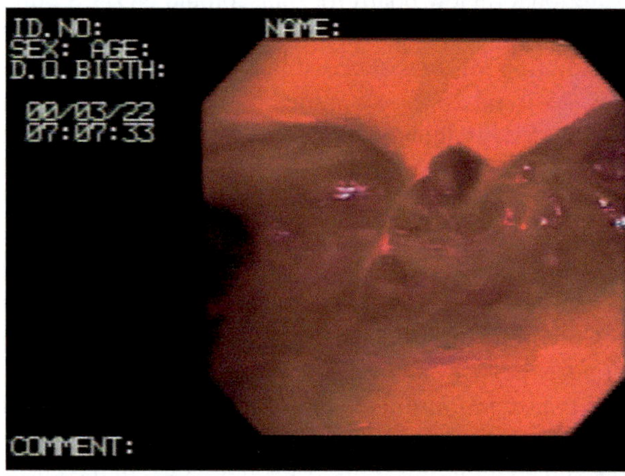

Fig. 25.3 Endoscopic view of flexible down-to-up TME for rectal cancer in a patient using a standard colonoscope. The endoscope is inserted directly in the presacral space, 3 cm above the dentate line, allowing flexible dissection in the anatomic oncologic plane from below

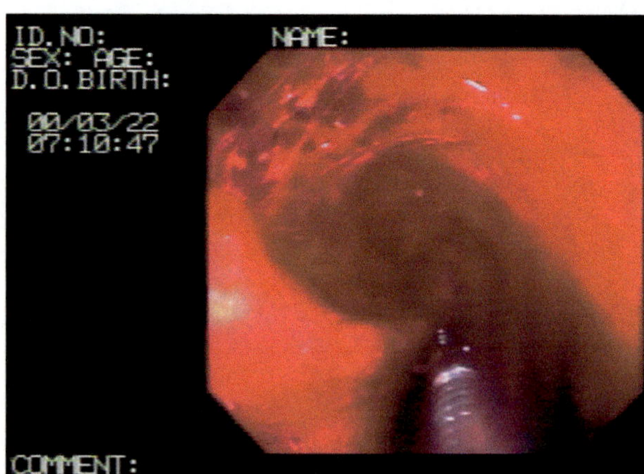

Fig. 25.4 Total mesorectal resection is progressively accomplished using endoscopic monopolar scissors inside the ideal oncologic plane of dissection

not possible to perform effective flexible TME dissection, but progress with flexible and robotic single site platforms can be a reasonable alternative to transanal single-port devices.

25.3 Clinical Indications

25.3.1 Indications

Transanal TME with reduced-port surgery can be indicated for most patients with middle and low rectal cancer (lower than 10 cm from linea dentata) with surgical indication for low anterior resection or intersphincteric resection. The usual status after neoadjuvant radiochemotherapy doesn't exclude the indication. Preoperative endorectal ultrasound and abdominal CT scan are mandatory to correctly evaluate TNM status.

25.3.2 Contraindications

- Presence of T4 disease before neoadjuvant therapy
- BMI higher than 35 kg/m^2
- Sphincteric invasion by the tumor or possibility to fail circumferential margins
- Clinical contraindications to capnoperitoneum

25.4 Surgical Technique

The technique used since 2009 was modified from flexible transanal surgery evolving to transanal single-port device with assistance of reduced-port abdominal laparoscopy. The technique can be performed using two simultaneous teams for the abdominal and for the transanal phases; most commonly it is performed as a sequence—first, transanal and then abdominal laparoscopy. The day before surgery, the patient receives mechanical bowel preparation by oral administration of fleet enema and a rectal cluster application the morning before surgery. The patient is placed in a Lloyd-Davies position, and sequential intermittent compression sleeves are applied to the legs. A single dose of antibiotic prophylaxis is given at the induction of anesthesia.

25.4.1 Transanal Phase

The surgeon and the camera assistant sit between the legs of the patient. The laparoscopic tower for the transanal phase is placed beside the left leg of the patient. The transanal port is insufflated to 10–12 mmHg of CO^2. The use of low-flow

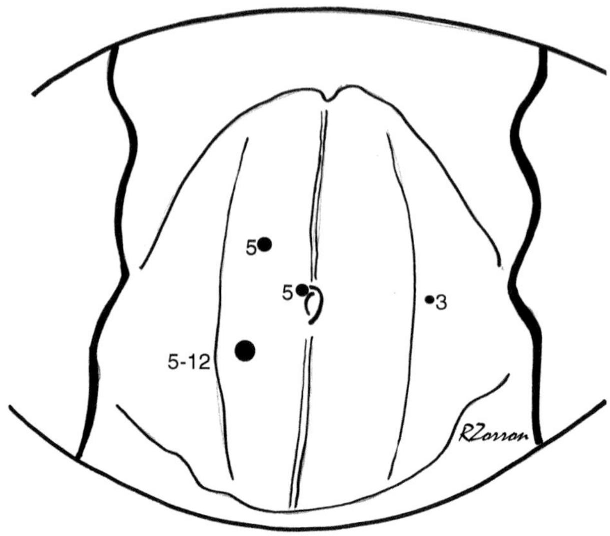

Fig. 25.5 Diagram illustrating disposition of the trocars for the abdominal phase of reduced-port down-to-up TME. If protective ileostomy is planned, alternatively a 12 mm trocar or an abdominal single-port device can be inserted instead of the 5 mm on the right abdominal area

insufflation of maximal 1 L/min is imperative to reduce the common "breathing" of the rectal wall by reducing the rhythmic contractions. A stable alternative is the addition of the AirSeal® System (Dach Medical, Salzburg, Austria), which allows for a stable and durable operative field, with the benefit of reducing the disturbance of smoke in the small space.

The strategy is different regarding the height of the tumor (Figs.25.5 and 25.6). For lower tumors, we start placing a Lone Star retractor and perform the incision cephalad to the dentate line (Figs. 25.7 and 25.8). An intersphincteric resection, if indicated, can also be performed. After the full-thickness section of the rectal wall circumferentially, a purse-string suture is placed below the tumor to avoid tumor cell spillage. The region is washed with iodopovidone solution as a cytocidal measure. The transanal single port (GelPOINT® Analpath, Applied Medical, Rancho Santa Margarita, California) is introduced and fixated to the skin with four unabsorbable sutures (Fig. 25.9). Pneumorectum is created using a pressure of 10–12 mmHg with reduced continuous flow (less than 1 L/min, or installing the AirSeal®) to avoid contractions of the bowel. In the case of more proximal tumors, the transanal device is first inserted, and a purse-string suture is placed from 3 to 4 cm above the dentate line to allow the complete resection of the mesorectum. Then a full-thickness incision is performed circumferentially through hook monopolar dissection below the suture to allow a further stapled anastomosis.

Standard dissection with the hook cautery is achieved by entering the correct avascular plane (Figs. 25.10 and 25.11). We recommend to start the dissection in the posterior mesorectal plane and then after completion to the anterior mesorectal plane and only with these two previously adequate managed to start the lateral dissections. This allows a reduced possibility of misunderstanding the anatomy

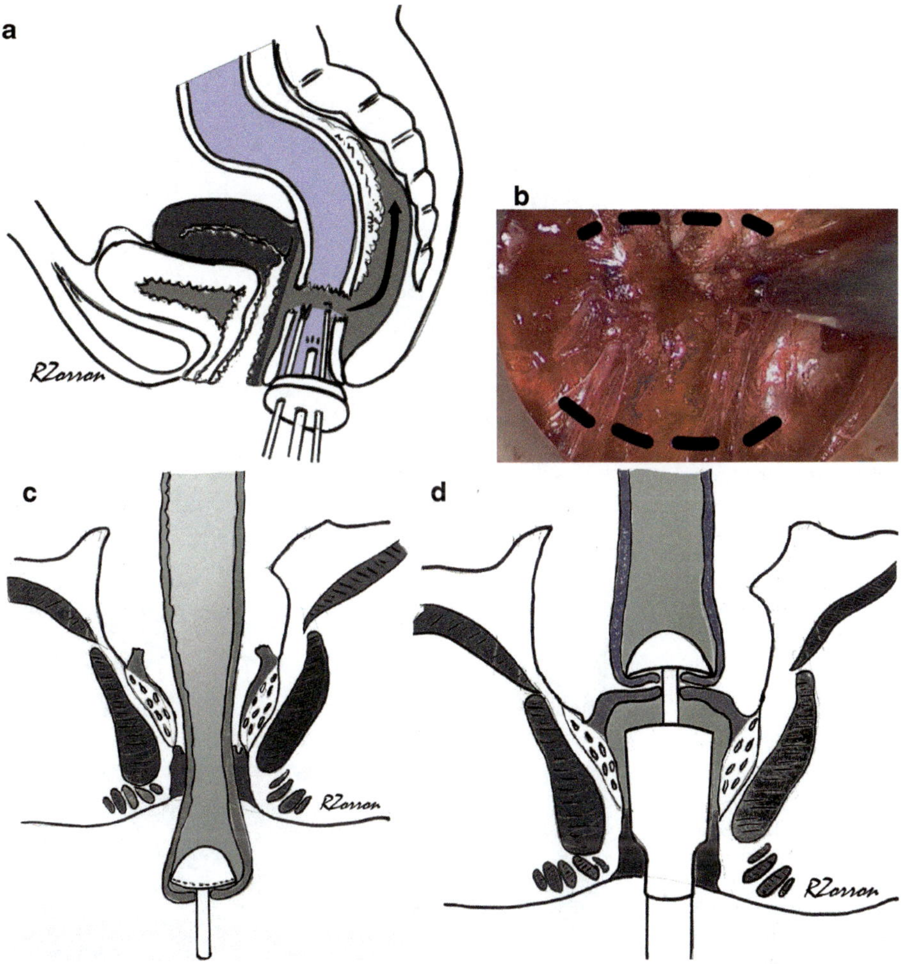

Fig. 25.6 (**a**) Transanally insertion of a disposable single-port access device. The port is inserted transanally, and circular intraluminal full-thickness incision allows entry into the presacral space and dissection in the anatomic oncologic plane from below. A laparoscopic camera, a 5 mm grasper, and a laparoscopic hook were inserted through the port to allow intraluminal dissection. (**b**) The inferior limits of the tumor were identified, and the lower limit of resection was chosen. Full-thickness circular incision reached the plane between presacral fascia and rectal fascia posteriorly, and the posterior wall of the vagina anteriorly. (**c**) Schematic view. After transanal extraction of the closed specimen, preparation of the proximal colon and anvil outside. If abdominal single port is used, this part can be performed by the transabdominal team. (**d**) Anastomosis can be performed by stapling using a long anvil or by coloanal hand-sewn technique

and accidentally entering the mesorectum or the rectum, especially in the previously irradiated pelvis. After full mobilization of the mesorectum, the peritoneum is entered, and the specimen is pushed inside, allowing the transection of remaining attachments.

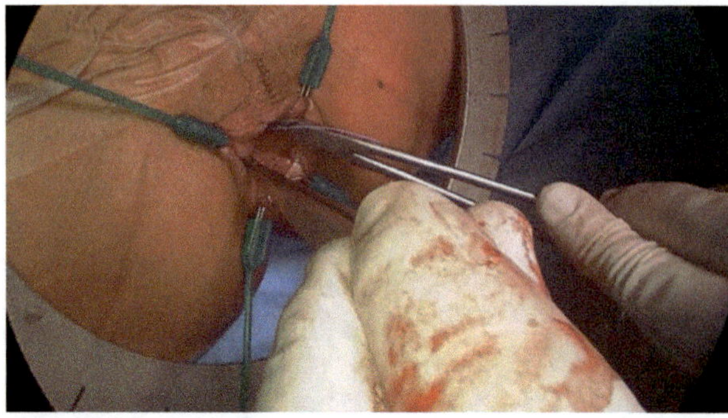

Fig. 25.7 Method 2 for starting down-to-up TME, performing the purse-string suture using the Lone Star retractor

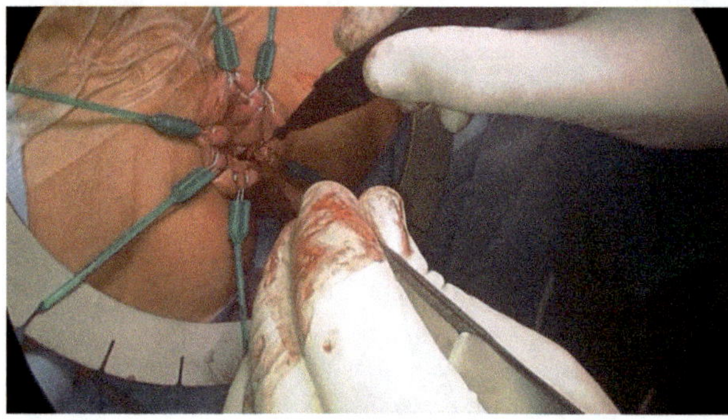

Fig. 25.8 For lower rectal tumors, it is appropriate to first perform the circular incision using the Lone Star type device for safe tumor resection margin. In some cases, direct incision at the dentate line and intersphincteric dissection can be indicated

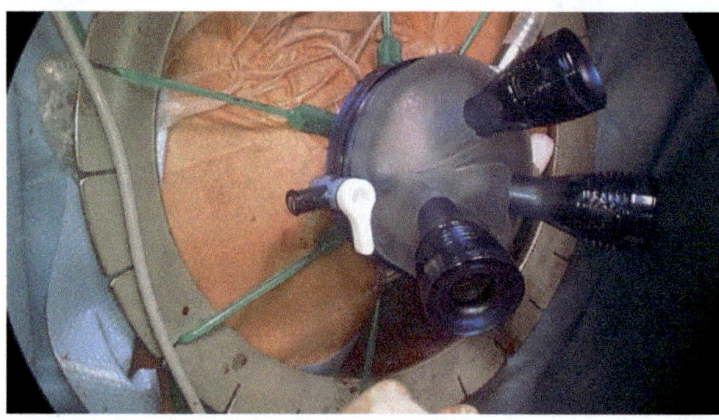

Fig. 25.9 Method 1 for starting down-to-up TME. For middle rectal tumors, the perianal single-port device is inserted, and the circular full-thickness incision is performed using transanal laparoscopic instruments

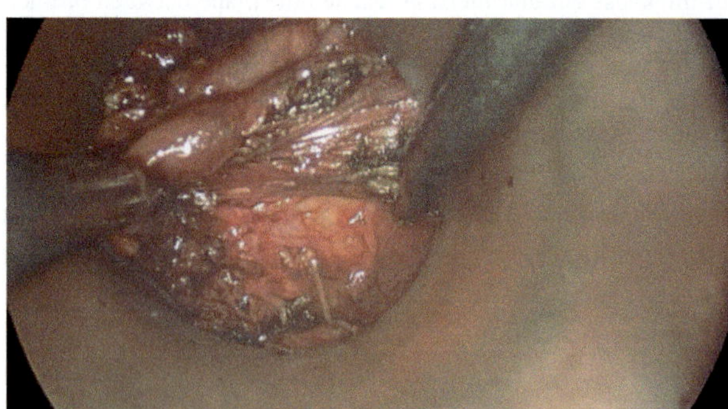

Fig. 25.10 Beginning of down-to-up TME from the posterior aspect, dissecting the presacral fascia from the mesorectal fascia

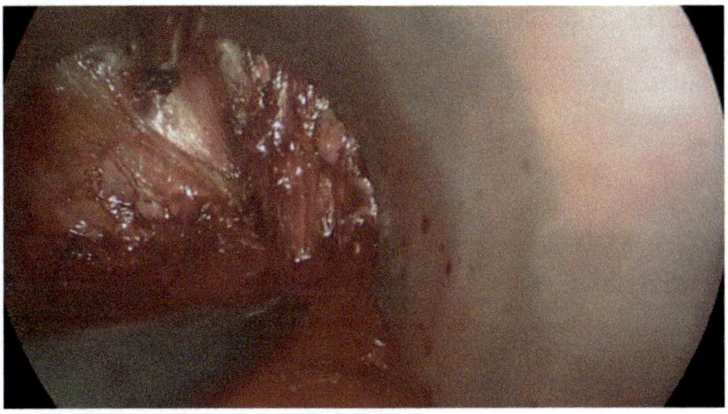

Fig. 25.11 Anterior progression of the dissection separating from vagina or prostate anteriorly

25.4.2 Reduced-Port Abdominal Phase

If a surgical team and equipment are available, the simultaneous work of the abdominal phase can be performed. A second independent laparoscopic tower is positioned at the left side of the patient. The surgeon stands on the right side of the patient and the first assistant cranial to him or at the left side, depending of the dissection site (pelvis versus colonic flexures). Limitations for the simultaneous operation by two teams are evident when there is the need for extreme head's up or down, for mobilizing the flexure and progress with the pelvic dissection. In some instances, it could be difficult or impossible for the other team to work depending on the positioning. Extensive retrorectal dissection should be avoided by the abdominal team to allow adequate "down-to-up" dissection by the transanal team. According to oncological principles, the ligation of the inferior mesenteric artery has to be high and including all troncular lymph nodes, but not necessarily timely before the transanal access. The concept of "previous" ligation of the artery has still weak evidence-based recommendation.

An umbilical 5 mm trocar is inserted by Hasson's open technique and pneumoperitoneum at 14 mmHg by a standard laparoflator is initiated. The AirSeal (AirSeal® iFS Intelligent Flow System, SurgiQuest, CT, USA) device is used preferentially via transanal to enable the stability of the insufflation during dissection, avoiding the typical "breathing" of the lumen. As the two cavities (perirectal and abdominal) communicate after the progression of the dissection both sides, the abdominal insufflation shall be interrupted to allow the unilateral transanal insufflation. A second 5 mm trocar is installed in the right lower abdomen in the previously demarcated area for the ileostomy and the third 5 mm trocar at the mamilar line in left abdomen (Fig. 25.5). As protective ileostomy is often indicated, a 12 mm trocar can be used instead of 5 mm, allowing the use of 10 mm instruments. A 3 mm trocar (KarlStorz, Tuttlingen, Germany) in the left abdomen can be added for mobilizing a difficult splenic flexure. Mostly in our cases, as it is not possible for the abdominal surgeon to stay between the legs for flexure mobilization (because of the transanal team), we usually use the camera at the left side trocar.

The sigmoid colon is retracted with the left hand trocar, and an incision is made in the peritoneum of the mesocolon using a 5 mm LigaSure™ device

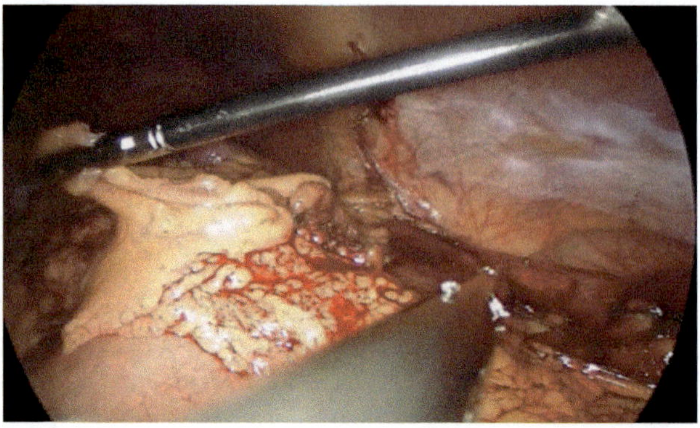

Fig. 25.12 Full splenic flexure and lateral colon mobilization is achieved with reduced-port laparoscopic assistance, allowing transanal extraction of the specimen and section of the proximal colon outside

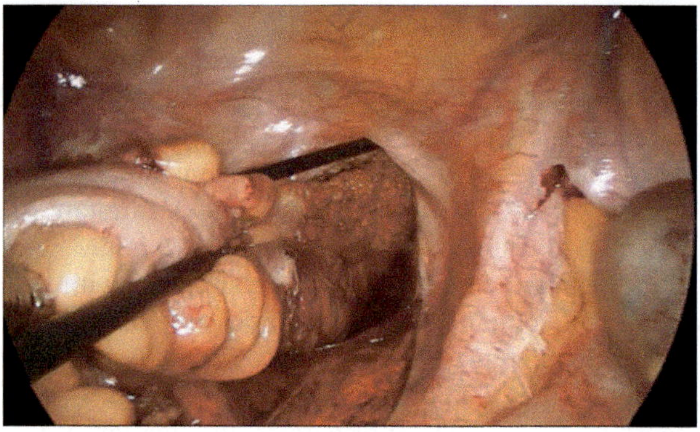

Fig. 25.13 Progression of the dissection into the pelvis to reach the simultaneous transanal dissection

(Covidien-Medtronic), an ultrasonic device (Ultracision®, Ethicon Endo-Surgery), or a mixed-energy device (Thunderbeat, Olympus Europa, Hamburg, Germany). The avascular plane is reached, and the left ureter is localized. After division of inferior mesenteric artery and vein, the complete left and left transverse colon including the splenic flexure is fully mobilized (Fig. 25.12). Entering the oncologic mesorectal plane from posterior and anterior allows the communication of both surgical sites, and then further dissection is facilitated (Fig. 25.13). The abdominal dissection is discontinued to permit only transanal insufflation. If the length of mobilization permits, the specimen is preferentially extracted transanally, and the proximal colon prepared outside for the anastomosis. In obese patients with fatty mesocolon and limited work room, preference is made to perform extraction through an umbilical single port (Fig. 25.14). Extraction of a bulky specimen through the future ileostomy site must be strongly avoided, as extension of this incision (and closure) is often associated with local complications as infection and parastomal hernia. With the proximal colon correctly placed presacrally without tension or rotations, the ileal loop is grasped and exteriorized at the level of the right lower trocar. A drainage can be placed through the right 5 mm trocar.

Fig. 25.14 If abdominal single port is used, specimen extraction, pouch construction, and anvil introduction can be performed by the transabdominal team

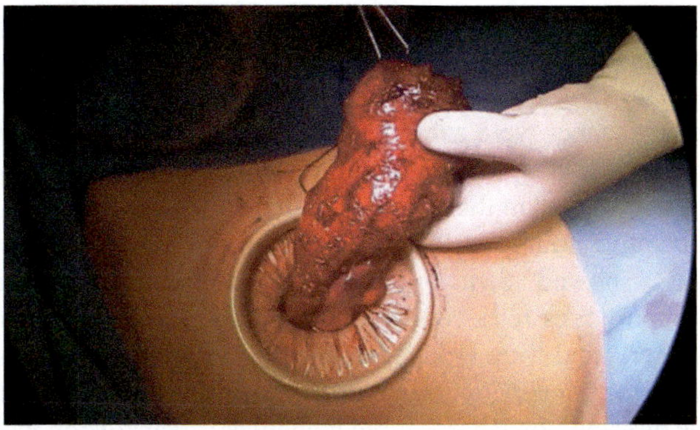

Fig. 25.15 Hand-sewn coloanal anastomosis after intersphincteric TAMIS-TME dissection in a lower rectal tumor

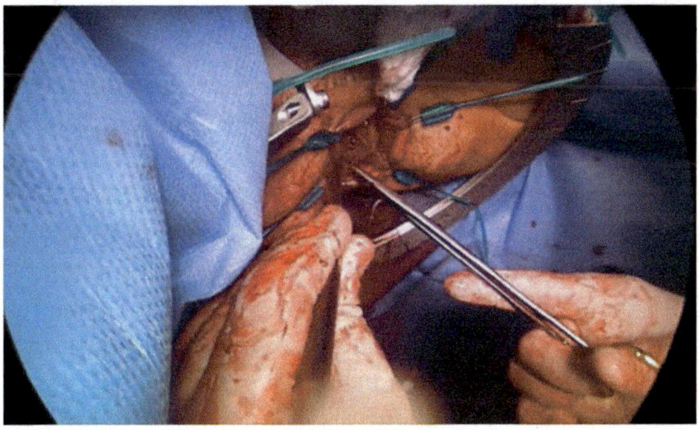

25.4.3 Anastomosis Phase

In most of the cases, it is possible to construct a colonic J-pouch of 5–6 cm. In obese patients and/or narrow pelvis, we indicate the creation of a small coloplasty or a stapled or sutured side-to-end anastomosis. The anastomotic technique is also different regarding the height of the tumor. For lower tumors, in which the transsphincteric dissection was made, a formal coloanal anastomosis using separate Vicryl sutures is indicated (Fig. 25.15). In patients in which the purse-string suture was created 3–4 cm from the dentate line, the rectal stump was closed by a second purse-string suture, and a stapled anastomosis is performed.

25.5 Clinical Results

Many clinical studies showed the feasibility of transanal TME. However, current data resumes to single-center studies with retrospective pilot series with smaller casuistic and with a short follow-up. Overall there are over 400 patients currently published in the literature, including two case-matched studies. Larger multicenter prospective registries are ongoing, but no randomized studies yet.

Our series of patients with elective surgical indication for oncologic resection for rectal cancer were submitted to down-to-up transanal NOTES TME with reduced-port assistance. The interventional team usually is composed by an abdominal and a transanal team that works simultaneously. Preliminary results showed good postoperative course of the patients with few complications recorded. Surgical specimens showed adequate circumferential and distal margins, with regular amount of lymph nodes retrieved. Operative times were long, especially in cases of flexible surgery, and were reduced using two simultaneous teams to around 180 min. There was one conversion to open surgery, in a patient with a bulky tumor that could not be dissected by laparoscopic maneuvers. Transfusion was not required, and complications were recorded in two patients. One patient claimed of transitory paresthesia of both feet due to intraoperative positioning that disappeared after 10 days. Two patients have a postoperative leak due to necrosis of the proximal anastomosis and required reoperation, one with colostomy and drainage and the second with a successful laparoscopic new coloanal anastomosis. Both were discharged without further complications.

Our group reported our early experience of down-to-up TME performed in 2009; some of these were two cases using a colonoscope to perform the mesorectal dissection and thereafter using a transanal inserted single port [7]. Sylla et al. described in 2010 the transanal dissection for rectal cancer in one female patient performing the access with a regular transanal endoscopic microsurgery (TEM) device [18]. The technique was performed using the principles of "down-to-up" dissection and produced adequate oncologic resection without complications. Lacy et al. recently reported transanal TME for rectal cancer in a series of 20 patients [19]. Evolving to a transanal single port and working with simultaneous transanal and transabdominal teams, the group obtained a mean operating time of 234 min and a mean circumferential margin of 1.8 cm. Contraindications at this point were stated for patients with preoperative T4, obese patients (BMI over 35 kg/m^2), and tumor recurrence.

Using the adaptation of new single-port platforms for rectal surgery, larger series are expected. The group of Larach in Orlando denominated the technique TAMIS (transanal minimally invasive surgery), performed over 50 cases including benign indications but also transanal TME [20, 21]. The technique currently seems to replace the earlier indications for transanally endoscopic microsurgery (TEM and TEO). Two recurrences were recorded (4%), at 4 and 18 months. He recognized advantages for the TAMIS technique are the short learning curve and the possibility to use a normal set of laparoscopic instruments.

With experience of over 80 cases, Veltcamp-Helbach et al. originally described down-to-up dissection using two SILS™ devices (Covidien, New Haven, CT, USA): one transanally inserted without fixation to the skin and a second transabdominal in the point chosen for the protective ileostoma [22]. In the casuistic, adequate mesorectal envelope integrity was achieved, with adequate margins and number of lymph nodes; other reports found similar results regarding safety and oncologic adequacy [23–26].

There are two comparative studies published suggesting the equivalence of transanal TME to laparoscopic TME. Fernandez-Hevia, with the researchers of Clínic Barcelona (Spain), compared a group of 37 patients with transanal TME to retrospective, non-matched laparoscopic cases with middle and low rectal cancer [27]. They showed oncologic equivalence regarding all parameters including mesorectal quality score. Flexure mobilization was more frequently needed in the transanal group (37% vs. 13.5%), along with the wider indication for coloanal anastomosis in this group. Besides, operative time was longer in the laparoscopic group (252 vs. 215 min), and readmissions were more frequent for the laparoscopic (22%) than for the transanal TME group (6%). Velthuis et al. compared 25 patients submitted to transanal TME with a laparoscopic TME group [28]. Although there was equivalence regarding circumferential resection margins and number of lymph nodes, there was a superiority for the mesorectal specimen for the transanal TME group. For this group, they found a complete TME specimen in 94%, and for the laparoscopic TME group, 72% of the specimens were classified as complete, 8% as nearly complete, and 20% as incomplete ($p < 0.05$).

The current standard of care of the treatment of rectal cancer implies in high ligation of the inferior mesenteric artery and total mesorectal resection with en bloc lymphadenectomy. The TME precise plane of dissection, described by Heald in early 1980s, resulted in a better oncologic anatomical specimen without cell spillage, improving results and reducing the indication of abdominoperineal resections [10, 11]. Clinical experience with transanal TME, an adequate dissection with preservation of the mesorectal envelope, can be achieved by the flexible or rigid technique. The dissection is performed in the same anatomical plane, performed in opposite direction (from anal to rectosigmoid junction), beginning the dissection by gaining access to the presacral plane between the presacral fascia and the mesorectal fascia. The progression of the cephalad dissection is improved by the retropneumoperitoneum inside this avascular plane.

These encouraging initial series and our institutional experience suggest that the down-to-up principle is feasible with low complication rates and good short-term oncologic results. Whether the oncologic and postoperative results are comparable facing current standard techniques is not clear yet, and this equivalence has still to be proven in further studies. Additionally, functional studies are needed to understand the potential prejudice of a prolonged intraoperative anal dilation to the sphincteric function in patients submitted to the technique.

25.6 Future Perspectives

Colorectal surgery is evolving, and minimizing the access trauma has shown significant progress in the last years. Recent advances in the therapy of rectal surgery, coming from laparoscopy, neoadjuvant therapy, and transanal resections, pointed that much can still be done to offer better options to our patients. Full transanal surgery without laparoscopic assistance is a goal for current transanal techniques and was achieved in 2013 in a pioneer study by Leroy et al. [29]. The authors performed TME for a low rectal using transanal endoscopic microsurgery (TEO) with two different lengths to achieve first, the local dissection of the rectum and TME, and second, the intraabdominal colonic mobilization and high ligation of the vessels. The authors recognized also the need for more dedicated platforms, with longer and steerable instruments to perform safely this procedure in a standard fashion. Currently, totally transanal TME without laparoscopic assistance can only be offered in selected cases.

The key to successful dissection in TME is visualization of the delicate areolar tissue surrounding the yellow mesorectal edge. In laparoscopic cases, the difficulty in maintaining this plane of dissection can occur in the distal 5 cm of the rectum, where the anatomy of the sacrum can lead to sharp angulation to the anal canal from the abdominal point of view. Moreover, the difficulty accentuates in obese male patients with a narrow pelvis. Increased risk of local cancer recurrence has been reported for patients after potentially curative resection, but had an incomplete or damaged specimen [13]. Transanal TME is particularly useful to avoid the risk of "coning in," a known limitation of open and laparoscopic techniques.

The indications for the transanal approach for TME are evolving. With the current growing experience in many centers and published casuistic with consistent oncologic results, dedicated teams incorporated the technique as a surgical alternative for difficult lower tumors. Other centers incorporated transanal TME as the standard therapy for middle and low rectal cancers. In the future, with the availability of long-term oncologic and functional results, it will be possible to evaluate the tendency of using the technique as the primary indication for almost all rectal cancers with surgical indication.

References

1. Kalloo AN, Singh VK, Jagannath BS, Niiyama H, Hill SL, Vaughn CA, Magee CA, Kantsevoy SV. Flexible transgastric peritoneoscopy: a novel approach to diagnostic and therapeutic interventions in the peritoneal cavity. Gastrointest Endosc. 2004;60(1):287–92.
2. Zorron R, Palanivelu C, Galvão Neto MP, Ramos A, Salinas G, Burghardt J, Decarli L, Henrique Sousa L, Forgione A, Pugliese R, Branco AJ, Balashanmugan TS, Boza C, Corcione F, D'Avila Avila F, Arturo Gómez N, Galvão Ribeiro PA, Martins S, Filgueiras M, Gellert K, Wood Branco A, Kondo W, Inacio Sanseverino J, de Sousa JA, Saavedra L, Ramírez E, Campos J, Sivakumar K, Rajan PS, Jategaonkar PA, Ranagrajan M, Parthasarathi R, Senthilnathan P, Prasad M, Cuccurullo D, Müller V. International multicenter trial on clinical natural orifice surgery-NOTES IMTN study: preliminary results of 362 patients. Surg Innov. 2010;17(2):142–58.
3. Whiteford M, Denk EM, Swanstrom L. Feasibility of radical sigmoid colectomy performed as natural orifice translumenal endoscopic surgery (NOTES) using transanal endoscopic microsurgery. Surg Endosc. 2007;21:1870–4.
4. Sylla P, Willingham FF, Sohn DK, Gee D, Brugge WR, Rattner DW. NOTES rectosigmoid resection using transanal endoscopic microsurgery (TEM) with transgastric endoscopic assistance: a pilot study in swine. J Gastrointest Surg. 2008;12(10):1717–23.
5. Leroy J, Cahill RA, Perretta S, Forgione A, Dallemagne B, Marescaux J. Natural orifice translumenal endoscopic surgery (NOTES) applied totally to sigmoidectomy: an original technique with survival in a porcine model. Surg Endosc. 2009;23:24–30.

6. Marks J, Mizrahi B, Dalane S, Nweze I, Marks G. Laparoscopic transanal abdominal transanal resection with sphincter preservation for rectal cancer in the distal 3 cm of the rectum after neoadjuvant therapy. Surg Endosc. 2010;24:2700–7.
7. Zorron R. Transcolonic NOTES-preliminary human experience: NOTES transrectal rectosigmoid resection and TME. Twelveth world congress of endoscopic surgery, Landover, Washington, DC, 17 Apr 2010.
8. Zorron R. Natural orifice surgery and single port access applied to colorectal surgery: the new era of intrarectal surgery? G Chir. 2010;31(6):205–9.
9. Zorron R. NOTES applied to colorectal surgery. World J Gastrointest Surg. 2010;27(2):35–8.
10. Heald RJ, Husband EM, Ryall RD. The mesorectum in rectal cancer surgery: the clue to pelvic recurrence? Br J Surg. 1982;69:613–6.
11. Heald RJ, Ryall RD. Recurrence and survival after total mesorectal excision for rectal cancer. Lancet. 1986;1(8496):1479–82.
12. Bonjer HJ, Deijen CL, Abis GA, Cuesta MA, van der Pas MH, de Lange-de Klerk ES, Lacy AM, Bemelman WA, Andersson J, Angenete E, Rosenberg J, Fuerst A, Haglind E, COLOR II Study Group. A randomized trial of laparoscopic versus open surgery for rectal cancer. N Engl J Med. 2015;372(14):1324–32.
13. Nagtegaal ID, van der Velde CJ, van der Worp E, Kapiteijn E, Quirke P, van Krieken JH. Macroscopic evaluation of rectal cancer resection specimen: clinical significance of the pathologist in quality control. J Clin Oncol. 2002;20:1729–34.
14. Bondeven P, Hegemann-Madsen RH, Laurberg S, Pedersen BG. Extent and completeness of mesorectal excision evaluated by postoperative magnetic resonance imaging. Br J Surg. 2013;100(10):1357–67.
15. Buess G, Kipfmüller K, Ibald R, Heintz A, Hack D, Brausntein S, Gabbert H, Junginger T. Clinical results of transanal endoscopic microsurgery. Surg Endosc. 1988;2:245–50.
16. Zorron R, Coelho D, Flach L, Lemos FB, Moreira MS, Oliveira PS, Barbosa AM. Perirectal NOTES access (PNA): down-to-up total mesorectal excision for rectal cancer. Surg Innov. 2012;19(1):11–9.
17. Zorron R, Phillips HN, Wynn G, Neto MP, Coelho D, Vassallo R. Down-to-up transanal total mesorectal excision for rectal cancer: preliminary series of 9 patients. J Minim Access Surg. 2014;10:144–50.
18. Sylla P, Rattner D, Delgado S, Lacy A. NOTES transanal rectal cancer resection using transanal endoscopic microsurgery and laparoscopic assistance. Surg Endosc. 2010;24(5):1205–10.
19. Lacy AM, Rattner DW, Adelsdorfer C, Tasende MM, Fernández M, Delgado S, Sylla P, Martínez-Palli G. Transanal natural orifice transluminal endoscopic surgery (NOTES) rectal resection: "down-to-up" total mesorectal excision (TME)-short term outcomes in the first 20 cases. Surg Endosc. 2013;27(9):3165–72.
20. Larach SW. Transanal endoscopic microsurgery (TEM) and transanal minimally invasive surgery (TAMIS). Cir Esp. 2012;90(7):418–20.
21. Albert MR, Atallah SB, de Beche-Adams TC, Izfar S, Larach SW. Transanal minimally invasive surgery (TAMIS) for local excision of benign neoplasms and early stage rectal cancer: efficacy and outcomes in the first 50 patients. Dis Colon Rectum. 2013;56(3):301–7.
22. Veltcamp Helbach M, Deijen CL, Velthuis S, Bonjer HJ, Tuynman JB, Sietses C. Transanal total mesorectal excision for rectal carcinoma: short-term outcomes and experience after 80 cases. Surg Endosc. 2016;30(2):464–70.
23. Serra-Aracil X, Mora-Lopez L, Casalots A, Pericay C, Guerrero R, Navarro-Soto S. Hybrid NOTES: TEO for transanal mesorectal excision: intracorporal resection and anastomosis. Surg Endosc. 2016;30(1):346–54.
24. Wang HS, Lin JK, Yang SH, Jiang JK, Chen WS, Lin TC. Prospective study of the functional results of transanal endoscopic microsurgery. Hepato-Gastroenterology. 2003;50(53):1376–80.
25. Tuech JJ, Bridoux V, Kianifard B, Schwarz L, Tsilividis B, Micholt F. Natural orifice total mesorectal excision using transanal port and laparoscopic assistance. Eur J Surg Oncol. 2011;37:334–5.

26. Velthuis S, van den Boezem PB, van der Peet DL, Cuesta MA, Sietses C. Feasibility study of transanal total mesorectal excision. Br J Surg. 2013;100(6):828–31.
27. Fernandez-Hevia M, Delgado S, Castells A, Tasende M, Momblan D, del Gobbo DD, DeLacy B, Balust J, Lacy AM. Transanal total mesorectal excision for rectal cancer: short-term outcomes in comparison with laparoscopic surgery. Ann Surg. 2015;261(2):221–7.
28. Velthuis S, Niewenhuis DH, Ruijter TE, Cuesta MA, Bonjer HJ, Sietses C. Transanal versus traditional laparoscopic total mesorectal excision for rectal carcinoma. Surg Endosc. 2014;28:3494–9.
29. Leroy J, Barry BD, Melani A, Mutter D, Marescaux J. No-scar transanal total mesorectal excision: the last step to pure NOTES for colorectal surgery. JAMA. 2013;148(3):226–30.

26 Transanal Laparoscopic TME with Single-Port Abdominal Laparoscopy

Giovanni Dapri

Abstract

In the last decade, single-port laparoscopy (SPL) gained interest as well as the application of transanal laparoscopy for rectal diseases. Different transanal procedures have been described. One of the most attractive transanal laparoscopic surgeries remains the realization of the total mesorectal excision (TME). In this chapter, the transanal TME assisted by SPL, with both colorectal and coloanal anastomoses, is described. The single-access site will be finally used for the temporary ileostomy placement.

Keywords

Transanal laparoscopy • Total mesorectal excision • Single-port laparoscopy

26.1 Introduction

In the last decade, thanks to the natural orifice transluminal endoscopic surgery (NOTES) [1], the application of laparoscopy through the anus took interest from both research and clinical point of views. This approach was already introduced in 1985 by Buess et al. [2] with the transanal endoscopic microsurgery (TEM), and recently it underwent to an evolution with the application of laparoscopy to the surgery of the rectum and rectal diseases. Hence, different transanal procedures

G. Dapri, M.D., Ph.D.
Department of Gastrointestinal Surgery, European School of Laparoscopic Surgery, Saint-Pierre University Hospital, 322, Rue Haute, 1000 Brussels, Belgium
e-mail: giovanni@dapri.net

G. Dapri, J.H. Marks (eds.), *Surgical Techniques in Rectal Cancer*,
https://doi.org/10.1007/978-4-431-55579-7_26

have been described like the resection of large rectal polyps, the colorectal resection, the total mesorectal excision (TME), and finally the control of perioperative problems like bleeding, leak, and stenosis. One of the most attractive procedures remains the realization of the TME transanally.

Besides NOTES, in the last decade, single-port laparoscopy (SPL) gained interest as well [3]. The union between SPL and transanal TME makes sense because the vascular dissection and the colic mobilization can be performed through the abdominal SPL and the abdominal access site can be used for the placement of the temporary ileostomy at the end of the procedure.

In this chapter, the transanal TME assisted by SPL, with both colorectal and coloanal anastomoses, is described.

26.2 Preoperative Preparation and General Anesthesia

Patient is asked not to eat for at least 8 h prior to the procedure. A bowel preparation is usually prescribed in the days before.

General anesthesia is induced intravenously (i.v.) with 0.2 mg/kg sufentanil, 2 mg/kg propofol, and 0.6 mg/kg rocuronium or 0.15 mg/kg cisatracurium. After tracheal intubation, anesthesia is maintained with 5–6% desflurane or 2% sevoflurane. In case of rapid sequence induction, 2 mg/kg etomidate or 2 mg/kg propofol and 1 mg/kg succinylcholine are used i.v., and a 0.2 mg/kg sufentanil and 0.1 mg/kg rocuronium are administered after the intubation.

Antibiotic and TVP prophylaxis are applied as well.

An arterial catheter, a central line, and a urinary catheter are placed.

26.3 Tools

26.3.1 Abdominal Table

- One scalpel, two tissue forceps, one monopolar electrode, two Farabeuf retractors, two Kocher-Ochsner curved forceps, one Mayo scissors, two Mayo-Hegar needle holders, two Pean-Rochester curved forceps, one purse-string suture device (DAPRI purse-string suture device, Karl Storz—Endoskope, Tuttlingen, Germany), and one monopolar electrode
- Sutures: one polydioxanon 1 (PDS 1, round tip, 1/2c, 36 mm), two polyglactin 1 (Vicryl 1, round tip, 1/2c, 27 mm), one polyamide 2/0 (Ethilon 2/0, straight needle, 60 mm), three polyglactin 2/0 (Vicryl 2/0, round tip, 1/2c, 36 mm), four polyglactin rapide 3/0 (Vicryl Rapide 3/0, triangular tip, 1/2c, 22 mm)
- One reusable 11-mm rigid trocar
- Two reusable 6-mm flexible trocars and rigid mandrils (DAPRI flex trocars, Karl Storz—Endoskope)
- One straight 10-mm, 30°, and regular length scope (Karl Storz—Endoskope)
- One reusable bicurved grasping forceps (DAPRI grasping forceps I, Karl Storz—Endoskope) (Fig. 26.1a)

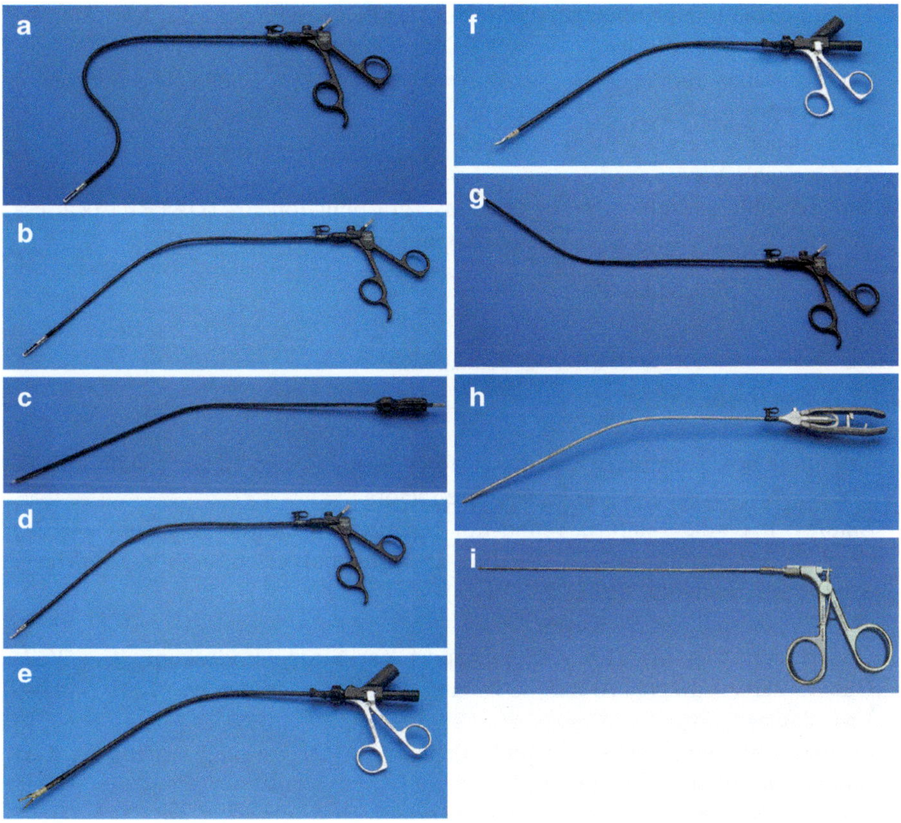

Fig. 26.1 (**a**–**i**) Reusable instruments according to DAPRI (Karl Storz—Endoskope, Tuttlingen, Germany): bicurved grasping forceps I (**a**), monocurved grasping forceps IV (**b**), monocurved coagulating hook (**c**), monocurved dissecting forceps (**d**), monocurved RoBi® bipolar grasping forceps (**e**), monocurved RoBi® bipolar scissors (**f**), monocurved scissors (**g**), monocurved needle holder I (**h**), straight 1.8-mm trocarless grasping forceps (**i**)

- One reusable monocurved grasping forceps (DAPRI grasping forceps IV, Karl Storz—Endoskope) (Fig. 26.1b)
- One reusable monocurved coagulating hook (DAPRI coagulating hook, Karl Storz—Endoskope) (Fig. 26.1c)
- One reusable monocurved dissecting forceps (DAPRI dissecting forceps, Karl Storz—Endoskope) (Fig. 26.1d)
- One reusable monocurved RoBi® bipolar grasping forceps (DAPRI bipolar grasping forceps, Karl Storz—Endoskope) (Fig. 26.1e)
- One reusable monocurved RoBi® bipolar scissors (DAPRI bipolar scissors, Karl Storz—Endoskope) (Fig. 26.1f)
- One reusable straight 5-mm clip applier
- One reusable monocurved scissors (DAPRI scissors, Karl Storz—Endoskope) (Fig. 26.1g)

- One reusable monocurved needle holder (DAPRI needle holder I, Karl Storz—Endoskope) (Fig. 26.1h)
- One reusable monocurved suction and irrigation cannula (Karl Storz—Endoskope)
- One reusable straight grasping forceps
- One reusable Veress needle
- One reusable straight 1.8-mm trocarless grasping forceps (DAPRI trocarless grasping forceps, Karl Storz—Endoskope) (Fig. 26.1i)
- One drain
- Ileostomy set

26.3.2 Perineal Table

- One monopolar electrode, two tissue forceps, one Mayo-Hegar needle holder, one Mayo scissors, and two Farabeuf retractors
- Sutures: five silk 0 (silk 0, round tip, 1/2c, 26 mm), three polypropylene 2/0 (Prolene 2/0, round tip, 1/2c, 26 mm), and three polyglactin rapide 3/0 (Vicryl Rapide 3/0, triangular tip, 1/2c, 22 mm)
- One non-reusable anal retractor
- One reusable transanal D-port (DAPRI port, Karl Storz—Endoskope) (Fig. 26.2)
- One reusable straight 10-mm, 30°, and regular length scope (Karl Storz—Endoskope)
- One reusable monocurved grasping forceps (DAPRI grasping forceps IV, Karl Storz—Endoskope) (Fig. 26.1b)
- One reusable straight grasping forceps
- One reusable monocurved needle holder (DAPRI needle holder I, Karl Storz—Endoskope) (Fig. 26.1h)
- One reusable monocurved scissors (DAPRI scissors, Karl Storz—Endoskope) (Fig. 26.1g)
- One reusable monocurved coagulating hook (DAPRI coagulating hook, Karl Storz—Endoskope) (Fig. 26.1c)
- One reusable monocurved RoBi® bipolar grasping forceps (DAPRI bipolar grasping forceps, Karl Storz—Endoskope) (Fig. 26.1e)
- One reusable monocurved RoBi® bipolar scissors (DAPRI bipolar scissors, Karl Storz—Endoskope) (Fig. 26.1f)
- One reusable monocurved suction and irrigation cannula (Karl Storz—Endoskope)
- One reusable monocurved anvil grasping forceps (DAPRI anvil grasping forceps, Karl Storz—Endoskope)
- One non-reusable plastic protector
- One non-reusable circular stapler
- Lidocaine 1% solution and syringe
- One rectal tube and syringe

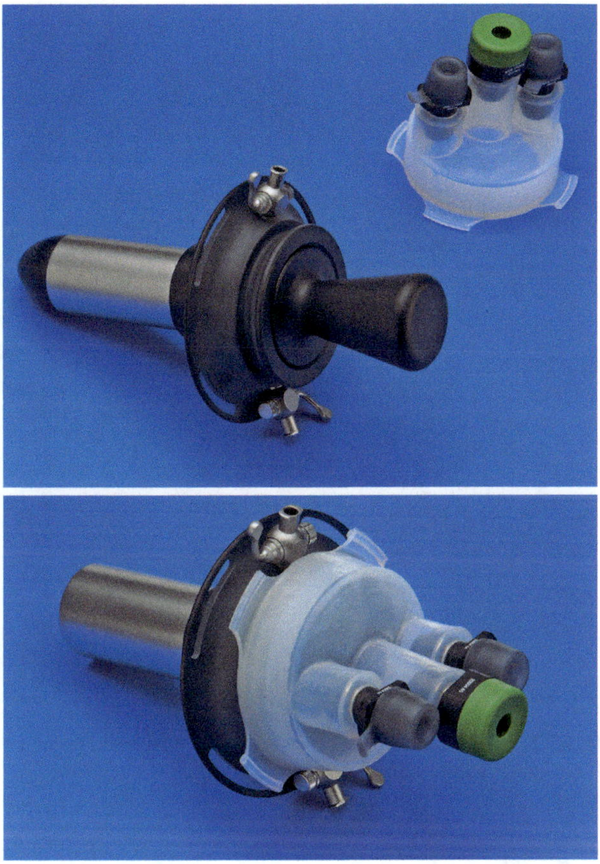

Fig. 26.2 Reusable transanal D-port according to DAPRI (Karl Storz—Endoskope)

26.4 Patient and Team Positioning

The patient is placed in a supine position, with the arms alongside the body and the legs apart. The arms, ankles, and legs are secured and protected. These latter are well secured to the operative table, and the left leg is positioned further up.

For the first part of the procedure, the surgeon stands to the patient's right and the camera assistant to the surgeon's right. The scrub nurse stands between the patient's legs. The video monitor is placed in front of the surgeon and camera assistant (Fig. 26.3).

After the mesocolic mobilization is made, the camera assistant moves to the surgeon's left and the scrub nurse to the surgeon's right.

During the perineal resection, the surgeon stands between the patient's legs, the camera assistant to the surgeon's right, and the scrub nurse to the surgeon's left. The video monitor is placed in front of the surgeon and camera assistant (Fig. 26.4).

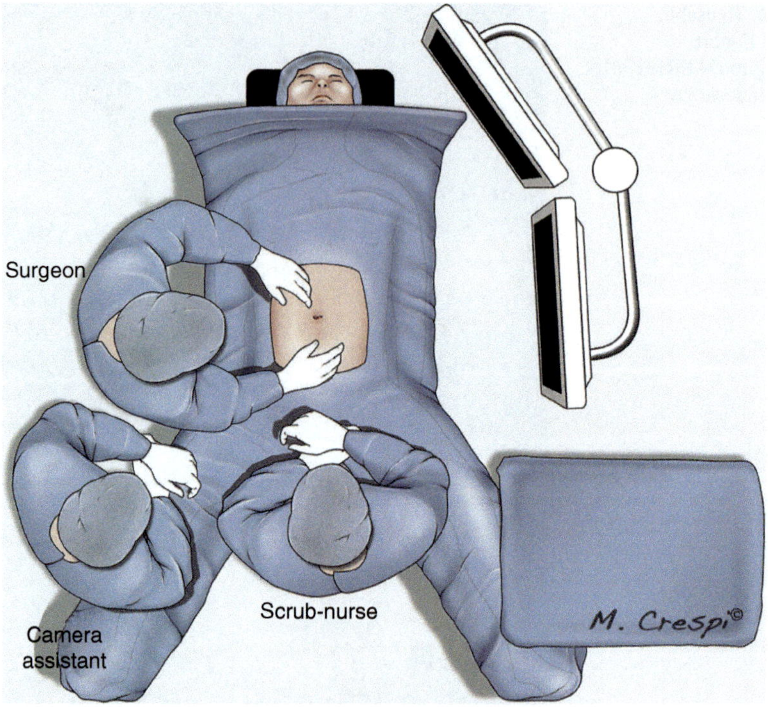

Fig. 26.3 Single-port abdominal laparoscopy: patient and team positioning.

26.5 Technique

26.5.1 Single-Port Abdominal Laparoscopy

A 3.5-cm vertical skin incision is made in the right flank, adjacent to the right rectus abdominis muscle and between the umbilicus and the superior right iliac spine (Fig. 26.5). The underlying fascia is divided in a pararectal fashion for 1.5 cm, which exposes the rectus abdominis muscle. The muscle is medially retracted, and a purse-string suture using PDS 1 is placed in the fascia, going inside and outside, respectively, at the 5, 7, 9, 11, 1, and 3 o'clock positions. The peritoneal sheet is entered through a 1-cm vertical incision, and a new purse-string suture using Vicryl 1 is placed, going inside and outside, respectively, at the 5, 7, 9, 11, 1, and 3 o'clock positions. Both sutures are kept externally with Pean-Rochester curved graspers.

An 11-mm rigid trocar is introduced into the peritoneal cavity inside the purse-string sutures, in order to create the pneumoperitoneum and to accommodate the 10-mm 30° scope.

A 6-mm flexible trocar is inserted at the 12 o'clock position with respect to the patient's head, outside the purse-string sutures and on the same vertical line

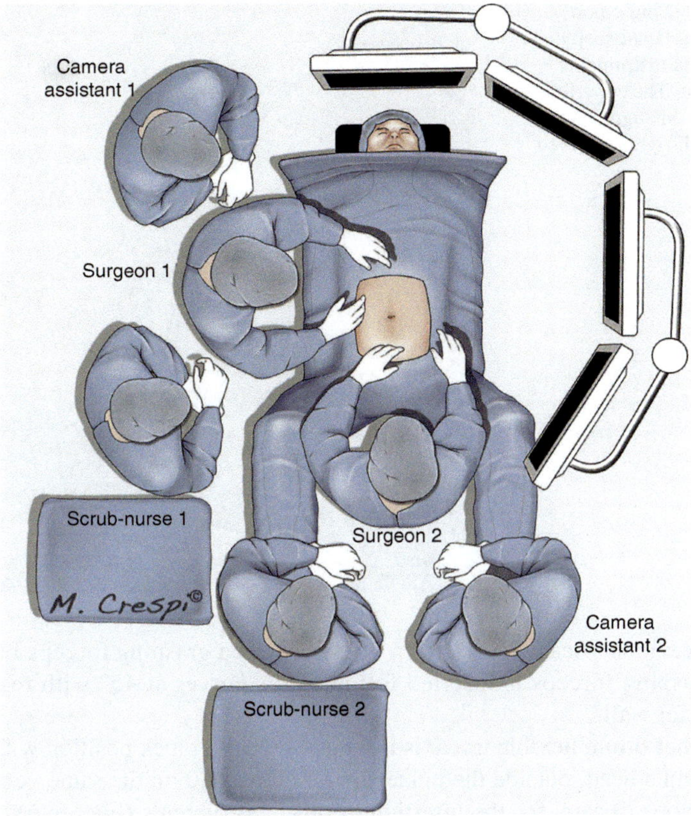

Fig. 26.4 Single-port abdominal laparoscopy: team positioning. The copyright holder of this figure is the author.

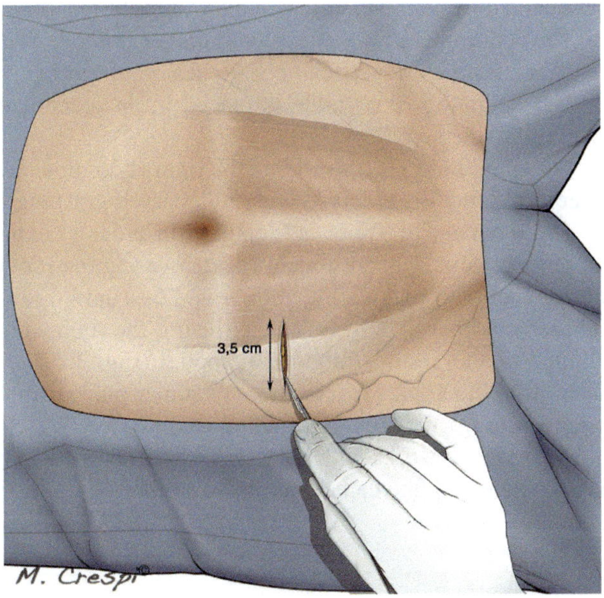

Fig. 26.5 Single-port abdominal laparoscopy: access site in the right flank. The copyright holder of this figure is the author.

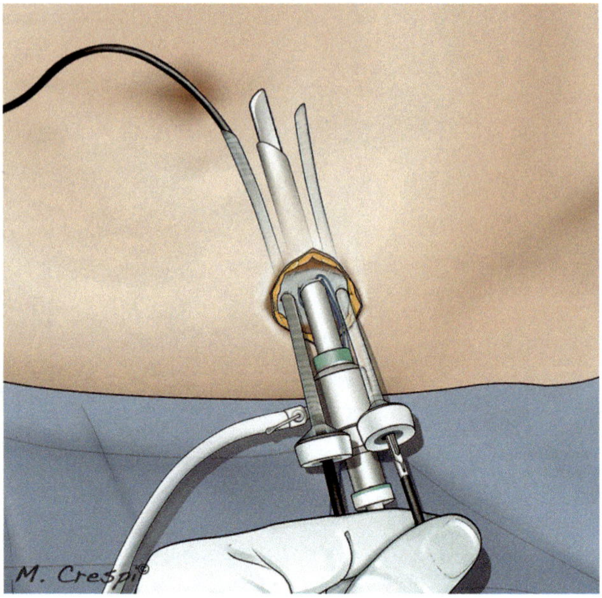

Fig. 26.6 Single-port abdominal laparoscopy: trocars and instruments placement. The copyright holder of this figure is the author. All rights reserved

as the previous trocar, for insertion of the bicurved grasping forceps I (Fig. 26.6). This grasping forceps is inserted following its curves at 45° with respect to the abdominal wall.

Another 6-mm flexible trocar is inserted at the 6 o'clock position with respect to the patient's head, outside the purse-string sutures and on the same vertical line as the previous trocars, for the insertion of other instruments (Fig. 26.6), such as the monocurved grasping forceps IV, the monocurved coagulating hook, the monocurved dissecting forceps, the monocurved bipolar forceps and scissors, the straight 5-mm clip applier, the monocurved scissors, the monocurved needle holder I, the suction and irrigation cannula, and the straight grasping forceps.

The abdominal cavity is explored and examined to rule out the presence of peritoneal metastases, superficial hepatic lesions, and free ascites.

The operating room table is placed in an accentuated Trendelenburg position with right-sided tilt.

The small bowel is moved into the right abdominal quadrants and above the right liver lobe using the bicurved and monocurved grasping forceps (Fig. 26.7).

The ligament of Treitz is identified in order to expose the root of the inferior mesenteric vein. The peritoneal sheet covering the root of this vein is incised with the monocurved coagulating hook (Fig. 26.8) until the Toldt's fascia is reached. The inferior mesenteric vein is isolated using the monocurved dissecting forceps and clipped by the 5-mm straight clip applier (Fig. 26.9). The left mesocolon is separated from the Toldt's fascia in an avascular plane using the monocurved coagulating hook or the monocurved suction cannula.

The surgeon works with curved instruments without crossing hands and without interference with the camera assistant's hand (Fig. 26.10).

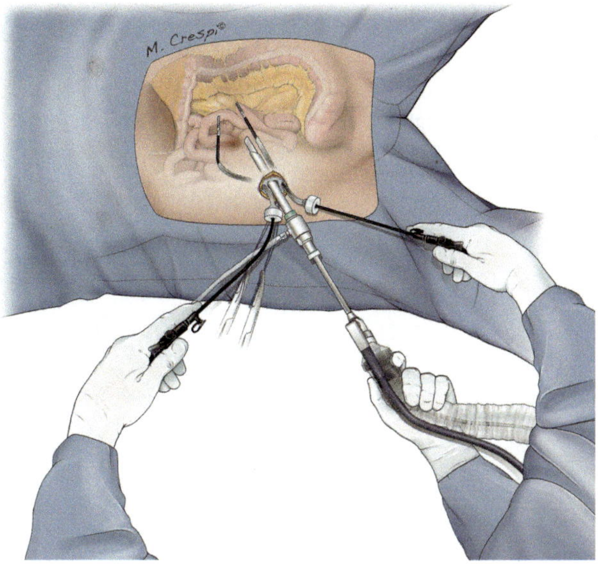

Fig. 26.7 Single-port abdominal laparoscopy: placement of the small bowel on the right liver. The copyright holder of this figure is the author. All rights reserved

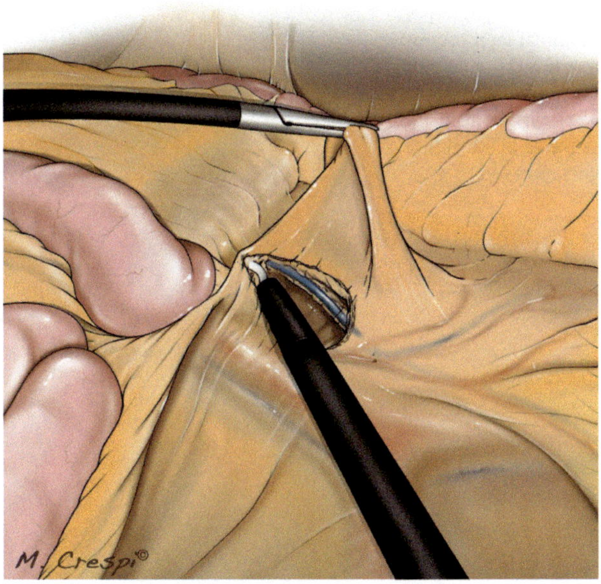

Fig. 26.8 Single-port abdominal laparoscopy: inferior mesenteric vein dissection. The copyright holder of this figure is the author. All rights reserved

The peritoneal sheet is incised along the abdominal aorta using the monocurved coagulating hook, until the origin of the inferior mesenteric artery is reached. The root of the artery is freed using the monocurved coagulating hook and the monocurved dissecting forceps, clipped by the 5-mm straight clip applier, and divided using the monocurved scissors (Fig. 26.11).

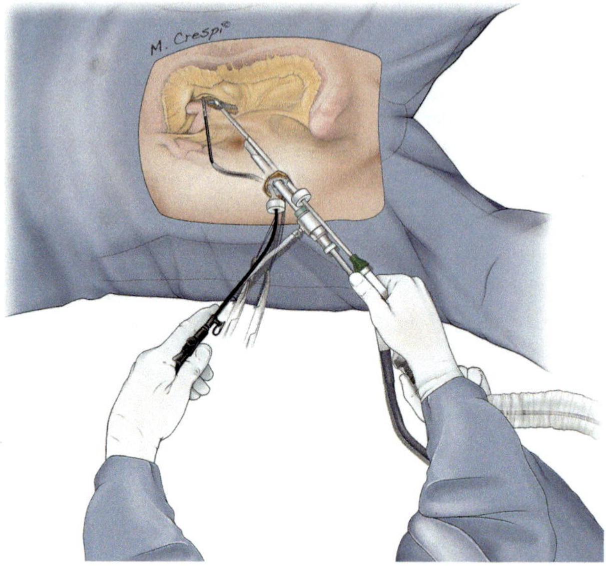

Fig. 26.9 Single-port abdominal laparoscopy: external view of the inferior mesenteric vein clipping. The copyright holder of this figure is the author. All rights reserved

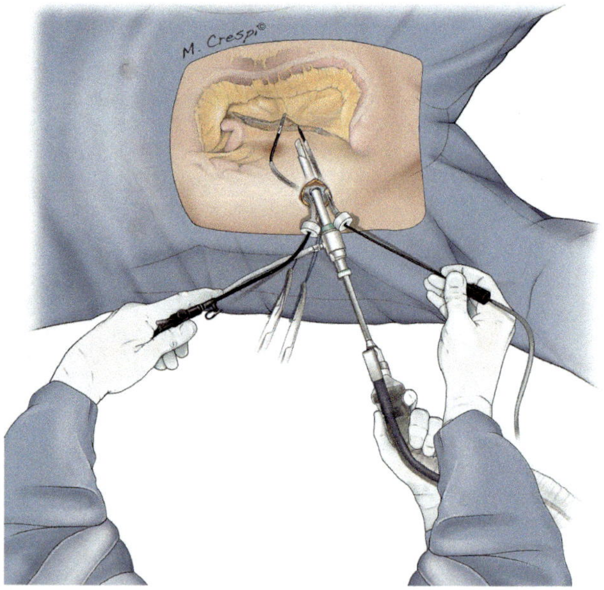

Fig. 26.10 Single-port abdominal laparoscopy: surgeon's ergonomy during left mesocolic dissection. The copyright holder of this figure is the author. All rights reserved

If necessary to improve the operative field's exposure, a straight 1.8-mm trocar-less grasping forceps can be inserted percutaneously via a skin puncture (created by a Veress needle) in the left suprapubic area. At the end of the procedure, this hole can be used for drain placement.

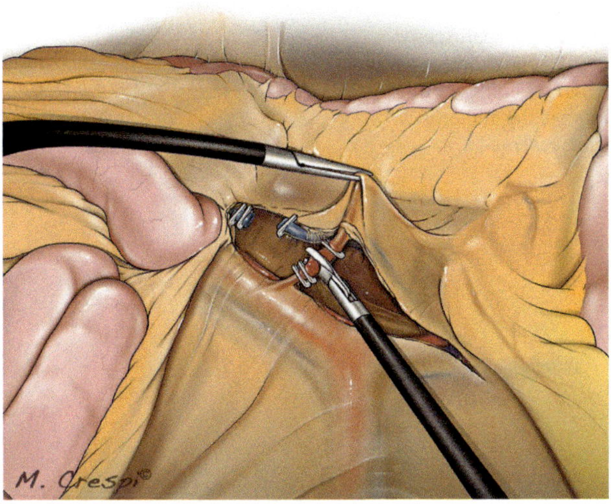

Fig. 26.11 Single-port abdominal laparoscopy: inferior mesenteric artery section. The copyright holder of this figure is the author. All rights reserved

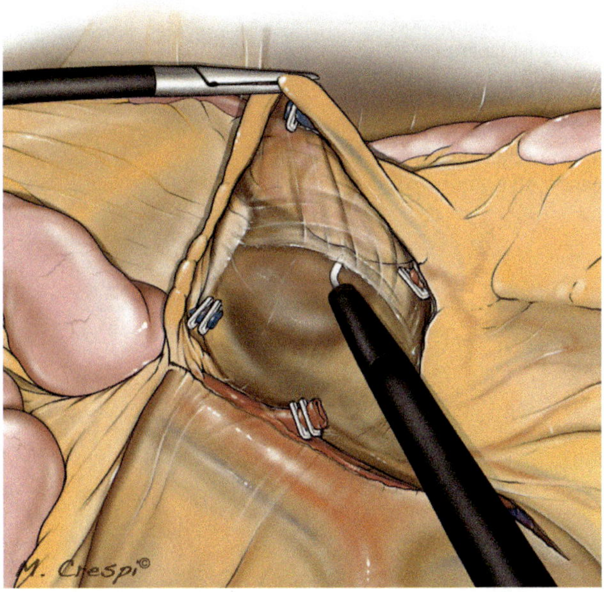

Fig. 26.12 Single-port abdominal laparoscopy: mesocolic dissection respecting the Toldt's fascia. The copyright holder of this figure is the author. All rights reserved

The left mesocolon is freed from the Toldt's fascia (Fig. 26.12), respecting the left Gerota's fascia and going in the direction of the pancreatic tail.

The sigmoid and left colons are moved away from the peritoneal attachments using the monocurved coagulating hook or scissors (Fig. 26.13) until reaching the splenic flexure, which is downloaded using a medial-to-lateral approach (Fig. 26.14).

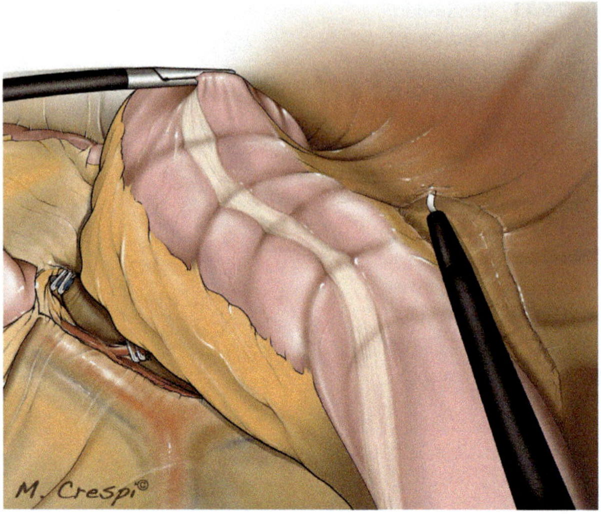

Fig. 26.13 Single-port abdominal laparoscopy: left paracolic section.

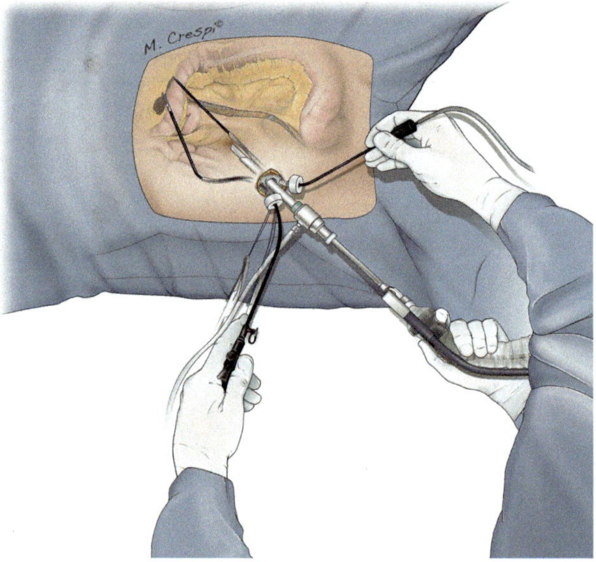

Fig. 26.14 Single-port abdominal laparoscopy: splenic flexure mobilization and surgeon's ergonomy.

The procedure is continued by moving the left mesocolon until the promontory is reached. The upper mesorectum is incised and dissected from the presacral fascia in an avascular plane using the monocurved coagulating hook and the monocurved bipolar grasping forceps and scissors (Fig. 26.15). The level of the left colon transection is chosen, and the mesocolon is dissected from this level going in the direction of the inferior mesenteric vein root, using the monocurved coagulating hook and bipolar tools.

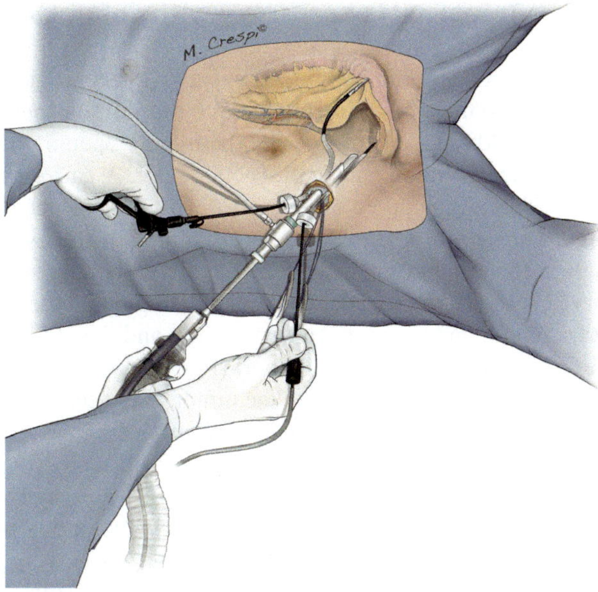

Fig. 26.15 Single-port abdominal laparoscopy: upper mesorectum mobilization and surgeon's ergonomy. The copyright holder of this figure is the author. All rights reserved

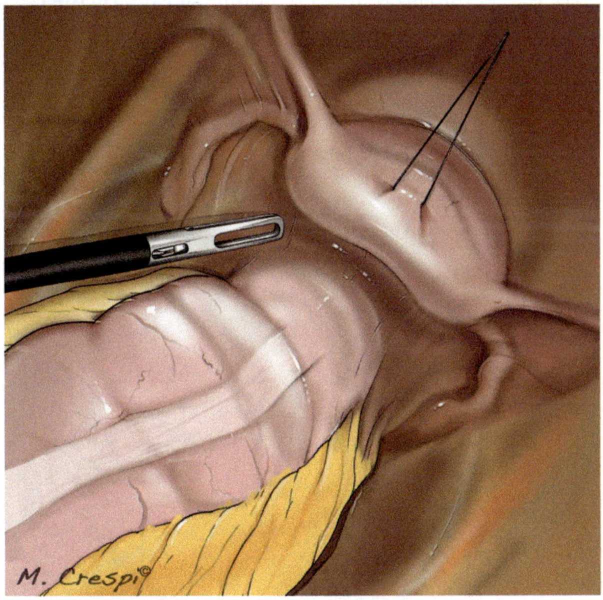

Fig. 26.16 Single-port abdominal laparoscopy: uterine fundus retraction (in female patients). The copyright holder of this figure is the author. All rights reserved

In female patients, a temporary percutaneous suture, using a straight Ethilon 2/0 needle, is placed in the uterine fundus to improve the operative field's exposure (Fig. 26.16).

The procedure continues with the TME performed from down-to-up. The operating room table is placed in a reduced Trendelenburg position and reduced right-sided tilt.

26.5.2 Transanal Laparoscopy with Colorectal Anastomosis

Both patient's legs are positioned upward (gynecologic positioning). The D-port is inserted into the anal canal and fixed to the skin by four silk 0 sutures (Fig. 26.17). A 10-mm 30° scope is inserted in the middle opening of the D-port, and the rectal lumen is checked to identify the rectal tumor. A gauze pad is pushed over the rectal tumor. The monocurved grasping forceps IV and the monocurved anvil grasping forceps are inserted at the 9 o'clock opening of the D-port. The other instruments, such as the straight grasping forceps, the monocurved needle holder I, the monocurved scissors, the monocurved coagulating hook, the monocurved bipolar forceps and scissors, and the monocurved suction and the irrigation cannula, are inserted at the 3 o'clock opening of the D-port (Fig. 26.17).

A safe margin, distally from the tumor, is chosen, and a purse-string suture using Prolene 2/0 is placed into the rectal mucosa, using the monocurved grasping forceps and the monocurved needle holder (Figs. 26.18 and 26.19). The suture is tied extracorporeally; the knot is pushed intraluminally and cut by the monocurved scissors. Then, the mucosa just under the purse-string suture is incised until past the entire rectal wall and reaching the perirectal fatty tissue (Fig. 26.20). The TME is performed from bottom to top, going first posteriorly (Fig. 26.21). Then, the mobilization of the rectum is completed, going laterally on the left (of the patient) (Fig. 26.22) and right side (of the patient) (Fig. 26.23). The dissection is finally performed anteriorly, taking care to dissect the correct plane between the rectum and the prostate

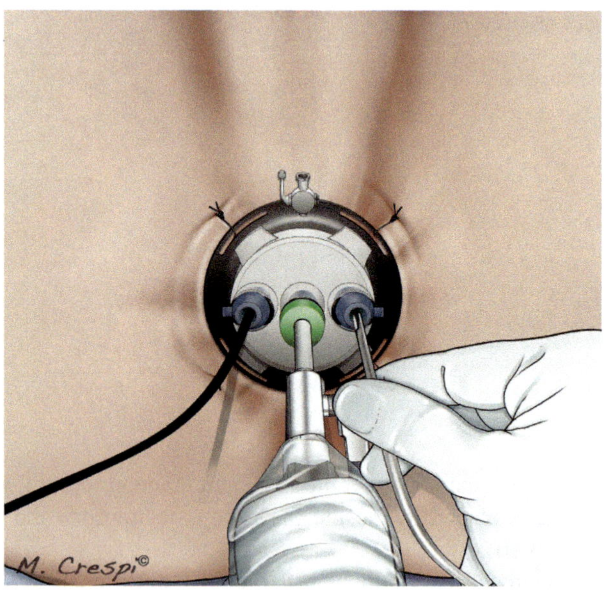

Fig. 26.17 Transanal laparoscopy with colorectal anastomosis: placement of the D-port and instruments into the anus. The copyright holder of this figure is the author. All rights reserved

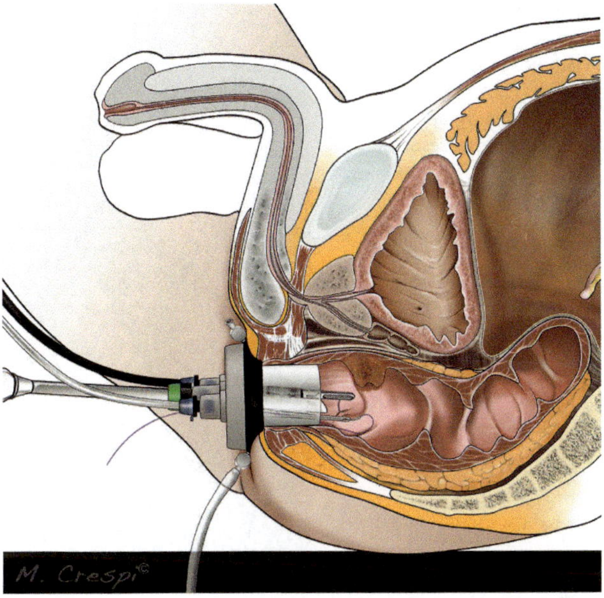

Fig. 26.18 Transanal laparoscopy with colorectal anastomosis: lateral view of the endoluminal rectum closure.

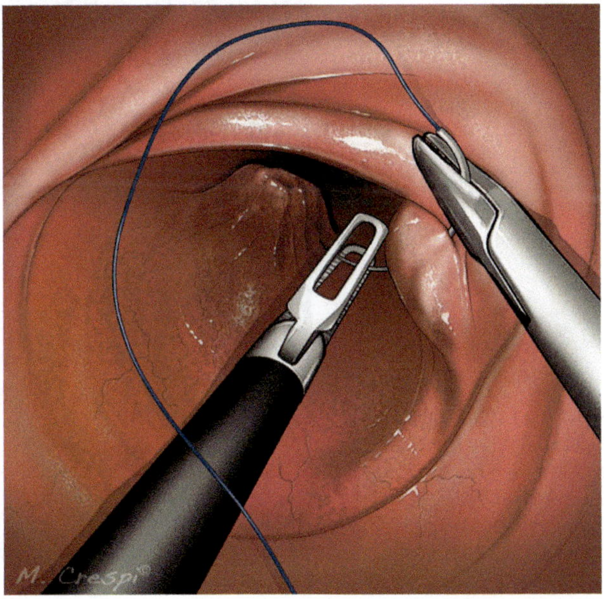

Fig. 26.19 Transanal laparoscopy with colorectal anastomosis: internal view of the endoluminal rectum closure.

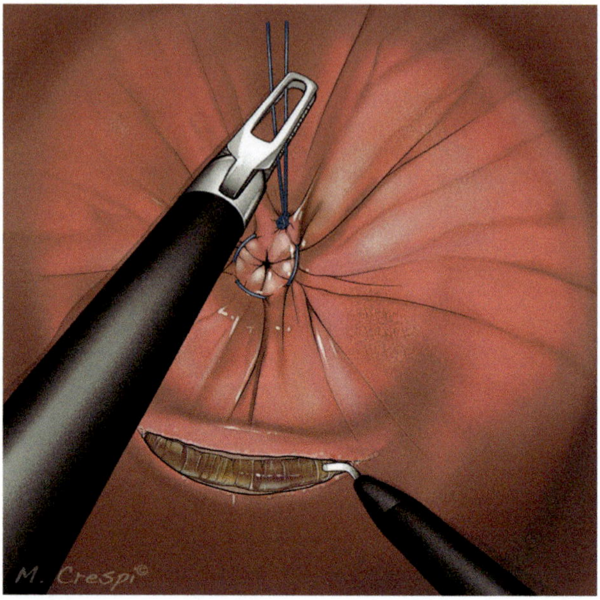

Fig. 26.20 Transanal laparoscopy with colorectal anastomosis: transrectal incision. The copyright holder of this figure is the author. All rights reserved

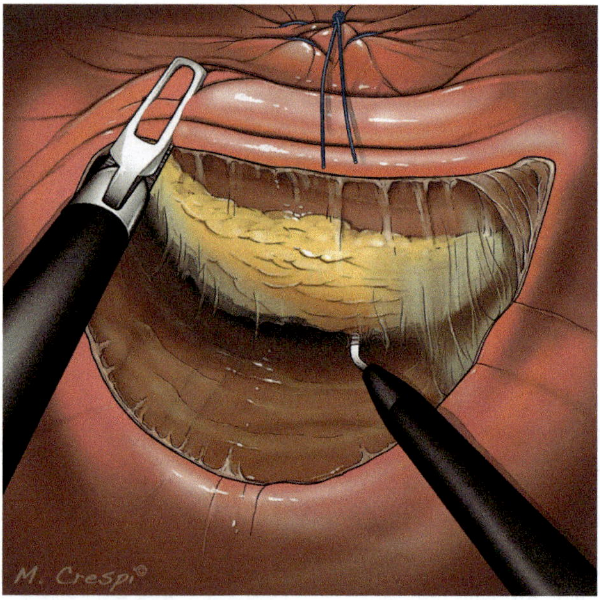

Fig. 26.21 Transanal laparoscopy with colorectal anastomosis: beginning of the posterior TME. The copyright holder of this figure is the author. All rights reserved

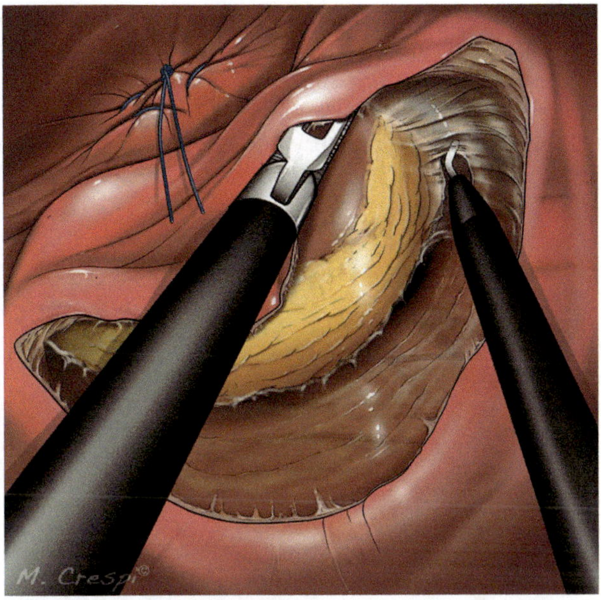

Fig. 26.22 Transanal laparoscopy with colorectal anastomosis: left (of the patient) lateral TME. The copyright holder of this figure is the author. All rights reserved

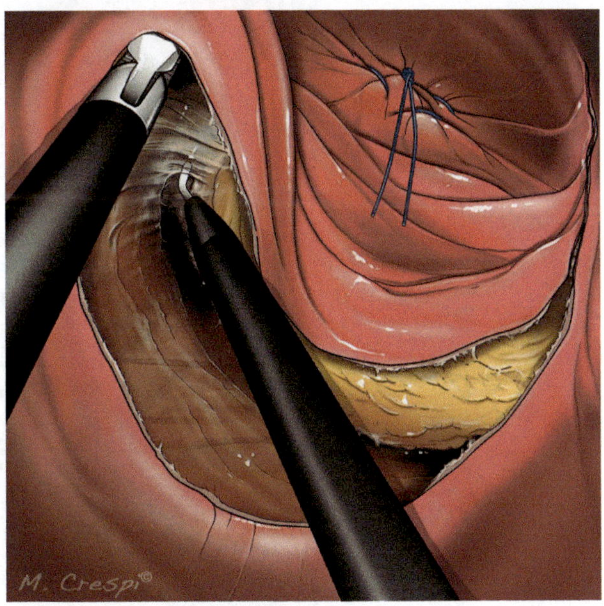

Fig. 26.23 Transanal laparoscopy with colorectal anastomosis: right (of the patient) lateral TME. The copyright holder of this figure is the author. All rights reserved

(male) or the vagina (female). The dissection is continued up, respecting the presacral fascia posteriorly (Fig. 26.24), until reaching the seminal vesicles (male) or the uterine cervix (female), using both monocurved coagulating hook and monocurved bipolar scissors. Finally, the transanal dissection joins the previous dissection started at the level of the promontory through the laparoscopic abdominal access, opening the Douglas' pouch (Fig. 26.25).

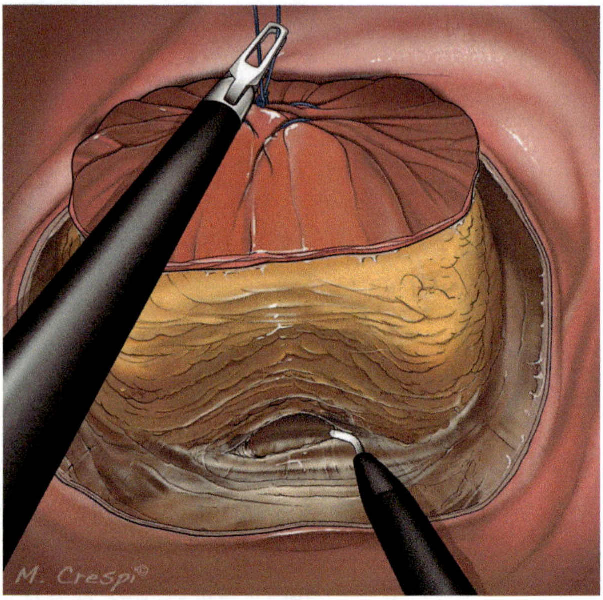

Fig. 26.24 Transanal laparoscopy with colorectal anastomosis: posterior TME. The copyright holder of this figure is the author. All rights reserved

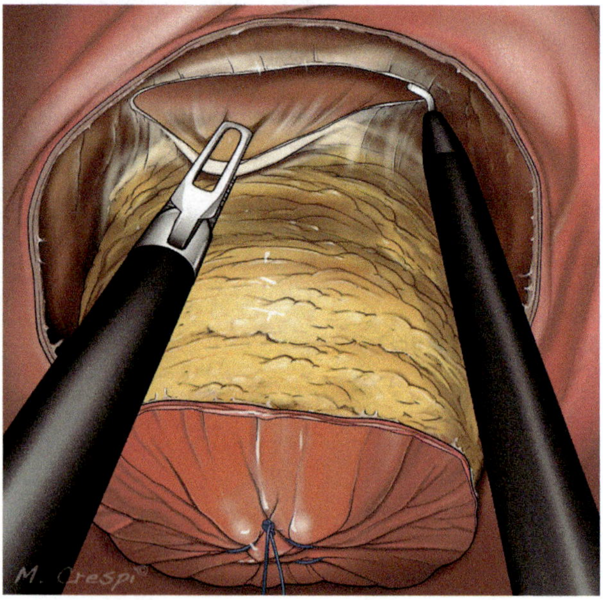

Fig. 26.25 Transanal laparoscopy with colorectal anastomosis: anterior TME and Douglas' pouch opening. The copyright holder of this figure is the author. All rights reserved

The rectal-sigmoid colon is encircled by a plastic protector and removed transanally, after having removed the D-port (Fig. 26.26). The level of the colic transection is found, and the left colon is sectioned and the specimen removed. The anvil of the circular stapler is introduced into the colic lumen, closing the latter with a Prolene 2/0 purse-string suture (Fig. 26.27). The colon and anvil are pushed inside the pelvis, and the D-port is repositioned. The rectal stump is closed transanally

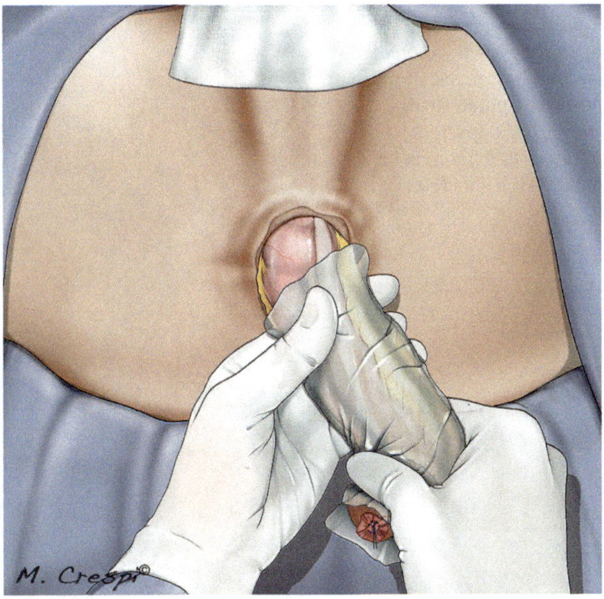

Fig. 26.26 Transanal laparoscopy with colorectal anastomosis: specimen's extraction. The copyright holder of this figure is the author. All rights reserved

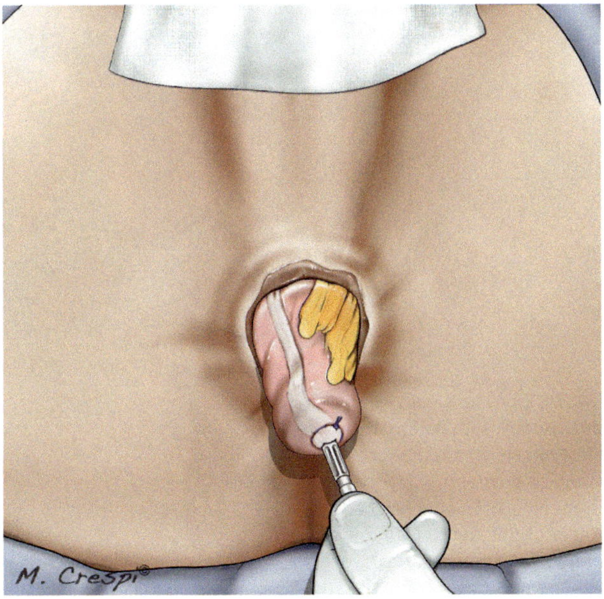

Fig. 26.27 Transanal laparoscopy with colorectal anastomosis: introduction of the circular anvil into the colon. The copyright holder of this figure is the author. All rights reserved

with a Prolene 2/0 purse-string suture, using the monocurved grasping forceps and the monocurved needle holder (Fig. 26.28). Then, the monocurved anvil grasping forceps keeps the anvil, while the suture is tightened by extracorporeal knot, pushed intraluminally and cut by the monocurved scissors. The D-port is removed again, and the circular stapler is introduced transanally (Fig. 26.29). The anvil is attached

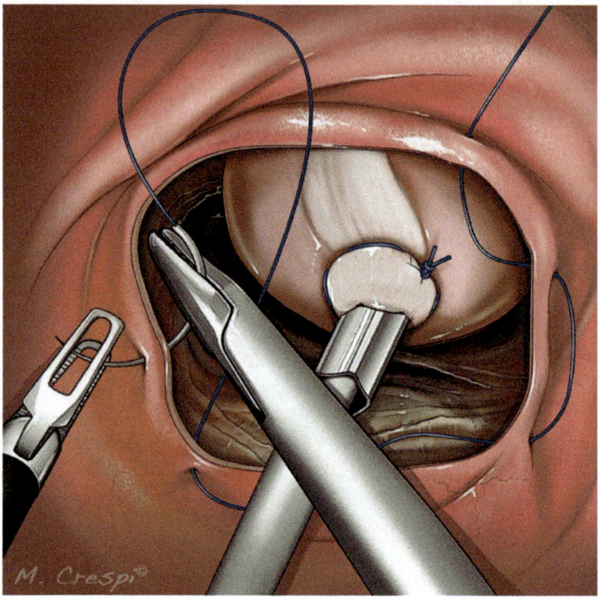

Fig. 26.28 Transanal laparoscopy with colorectal anastomosis: rectal stump closure by purse-string suture.

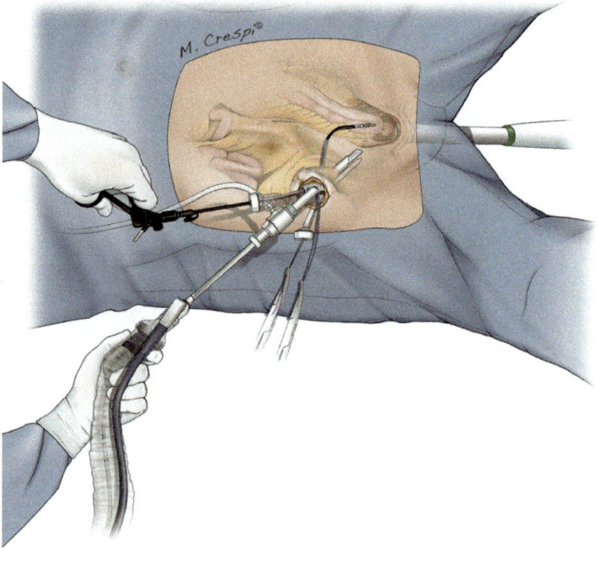

Fig. 26.29 Transanal laparoscopy with colorectal anastomosis: external view of the colorectal anastomosis.

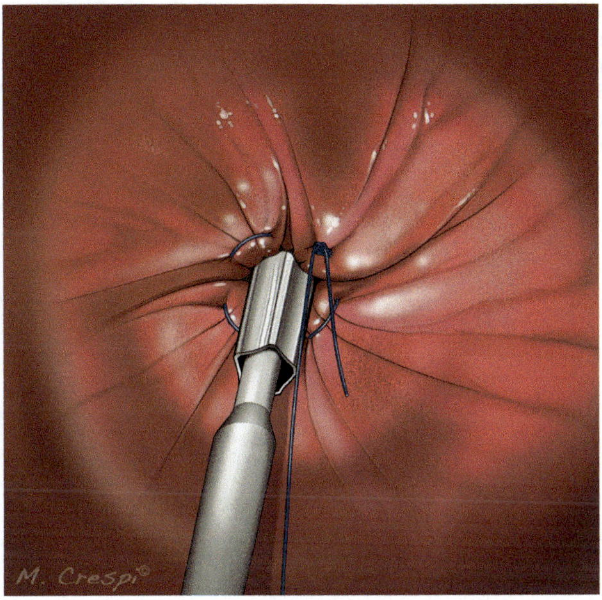

Fig. 26.30 Transanal laparoscopy with colorectal anastomosis: internal view of the colorectal anastomosis. The copyright holder of this figure is the author. All rights reserved

to the circular stapler by the monocurved anvil grasping forceps (Fig. 26.30), under abdominal laparoscopic control (Fig. 26.29). The stapler is closed and fired.

Through the abdomen, the monocurved suction and irrigation cannula is introduced, and the pelvis is immersed under physiologic solution. A leak test of the anastomosis, using insufflated air through the anus, is performed.

26.5.3 Transanal Laparoscopy with Coloanal Anastomosis

Both patient's legs are positioned upward (gynecologic positioning). A gauze pad is inserted in the anal canal to avoid potential fecal contamination. The anal retractor is positioned, and the anal mucosa is injected with lidocaine 1%. The pectineal line is incised using the monopolar electrode (Fig. 26.31). Once freed circumferentially, the anal mucosa is closed by a silk 0 purse-string suture (Fig. 26.32) and pushed into the pelvis.

The D-port is inserted and fixed to the skin by four silk 0 sutures (Fig. 26.33). A 10-mm 30° scope is inserted in the middle opening of the D-port. The monocurved grasping forceps IV is inserted at the 9 o'clock opening of the D-port. The other instruments, such as the monocurved coagulating hook, the monocurved bipolar forceps and scissors, and the monocurved suction and irrigation cannula, are inserted at the 3 o'clock opening of the D-port (Fig. 26.33).

The anal canal is mobilized circumferentially from down-to-up, going first posteriorly (Figs. 26.34 and 26.35), to the left side (of the patient) (Fig. 26.36), to the

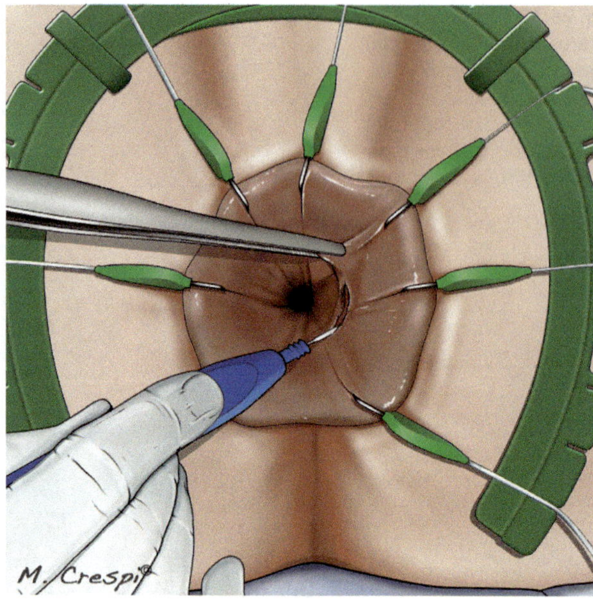

Fig. 26.31 Transanal laparoscopy with coloanal anastomosis: anal mucosa dissection.

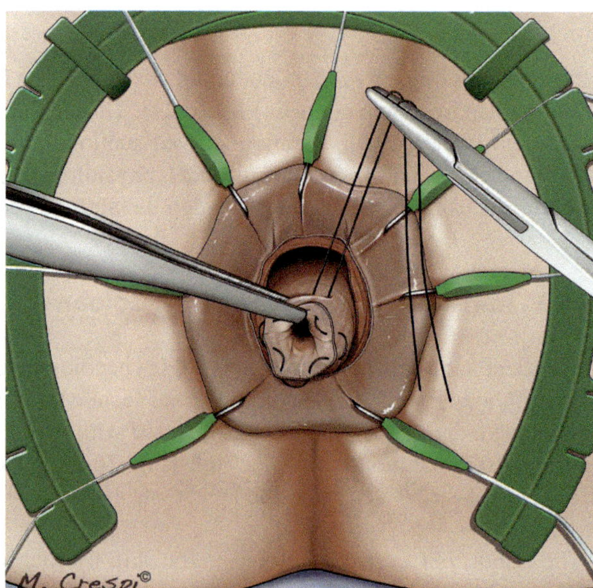

Fig. 26.32 Transanal laparoscopy with coloanal anastomosis: closure of the anal mucosa.

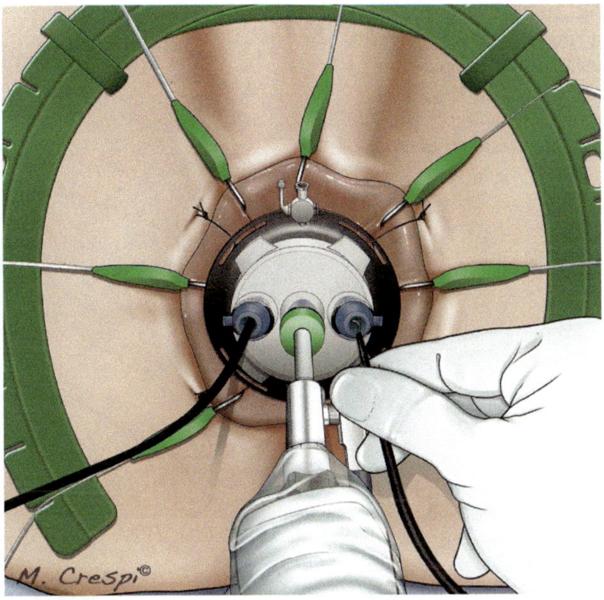

Fig. 26.33 Transanal laparoscopy with coloanal anastomosis: placement of the D-port and curved instruments. The copyright holder of this figure is the author. All rights reserved

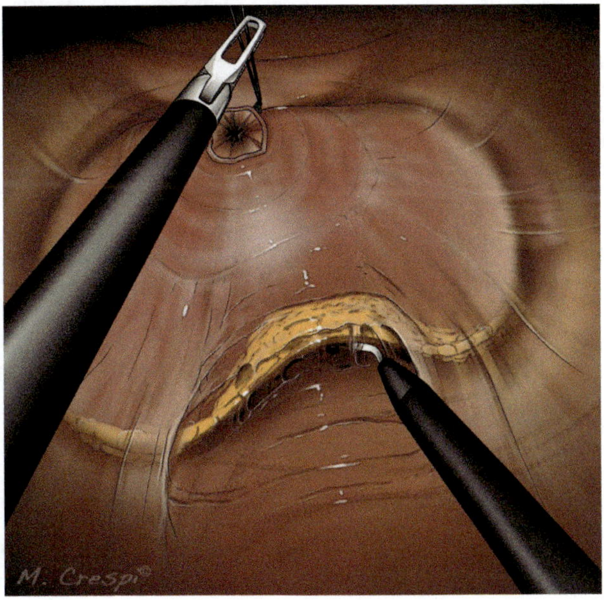

Fig. 26.34 Transanal laparoscopy with coloanal anastomosis: internal view of the beginning of TME. The copyright holder of this figure is the author. All rights reserved

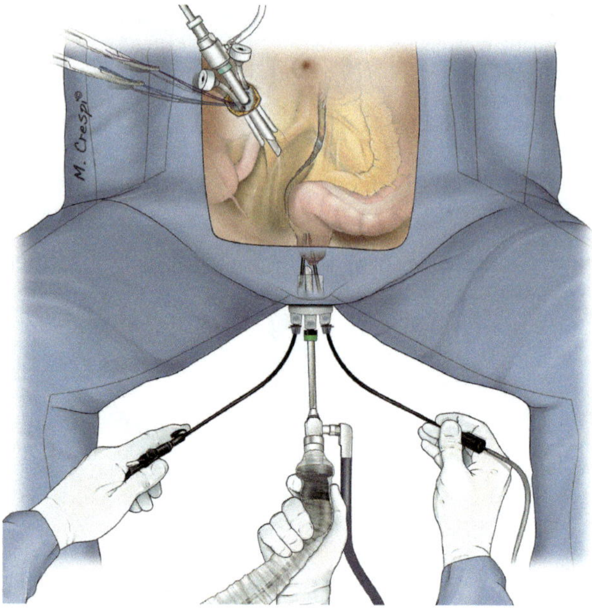

Fig. 26.35 Transanal laparoscopy with coloanal anastomosis: surgeon's ergonomy. The copyright holder of this figure is the author. All rights reserved

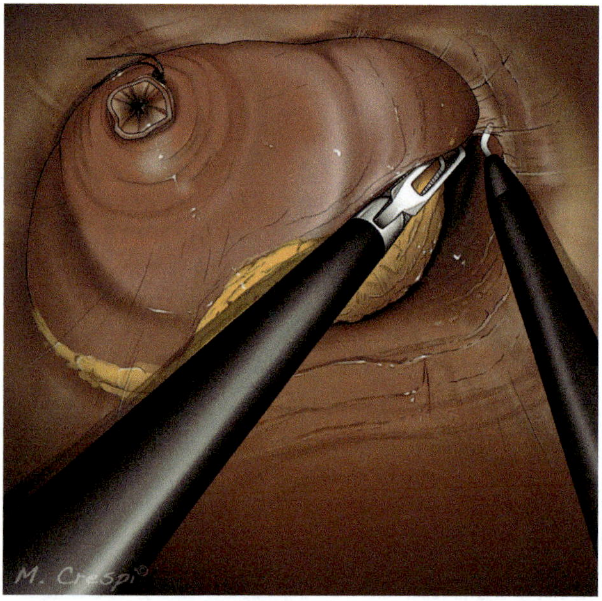

Fig. 26.36 Transanal laparoscopy with coloanal anastomosis: left (of the patient) lateral TME. The copyright holder of this figure is the author. All rights reserved

right side (of the patient) (Fig. 26.37), and, finally, anteriorly. Similarly, the lower rectum is mobilized circumferentially from down-to-up, going posteriorly (Fig. 26.38), to the left side, to the right side, and anteriorly, using the monocurved coagulating hook and the monocurved grasping forceps. The dissection is performed posteriorly and anteriorly finding the correct plane between the rectum and the prostate (male) or the vagina (female).

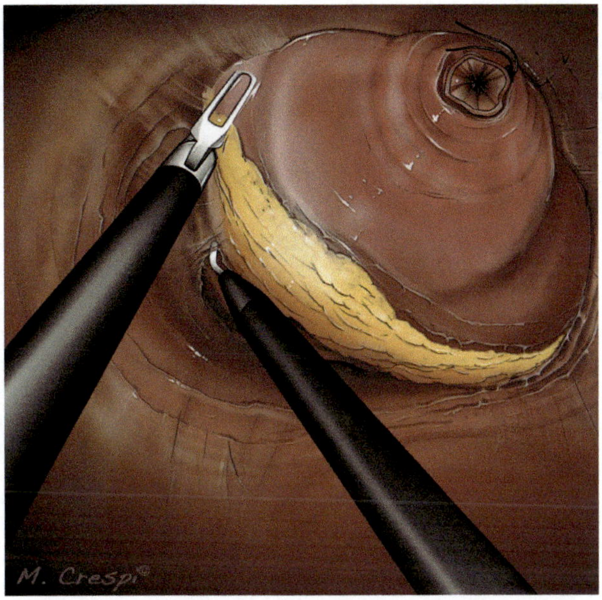

Fig. 26.37 Transanal laparoscopy with coloanal anastomosis: right (of the patient) lateral TME.

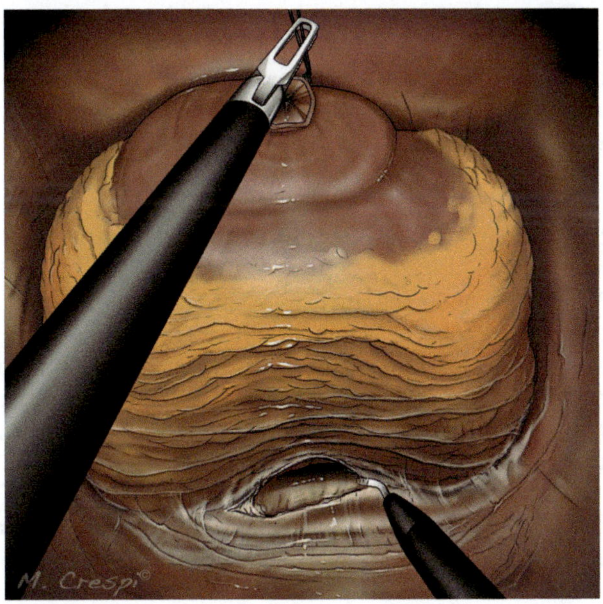

Fig. 26.38 Transanal laparoscopy with coloanal anastomosis: posterior TME.

The middle rectum is freed, taking care to respect the presacral fascia posteriorly and to find the correct plane between the rectum and the seminal vesicles (male) or uterine cervix (female) anteriorly. Both the monocurved coagulating hook and the monocurved bipolar scissors are used. Finally, the transanal dissection joins the previous dissection started at the level of the promontory through the laparoscopic abdominal access, opening the Douglas' pouch (Fig. 26.39).

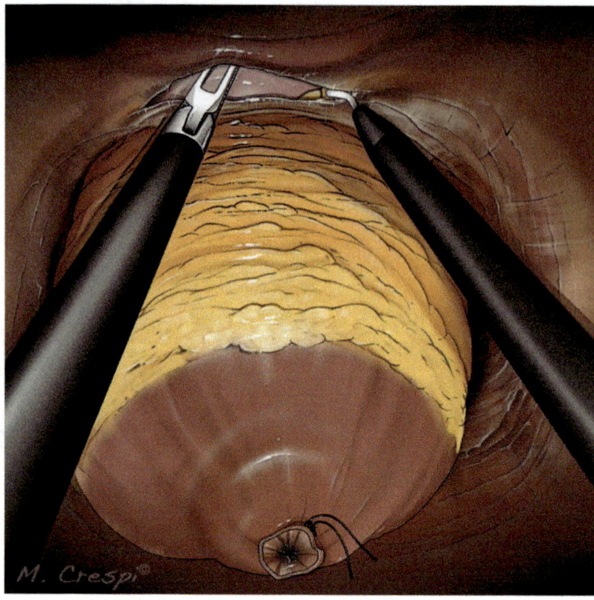

Fig. 26.39 Transanal laparoscopy with coloanal anastomosis: anterior TME and Douglas' pouch opening. The copyright holder of this figure is the author. All rights reserved

The rectal-sigmoid colon is encircled by a plastic protector and removed transanally, after having removed the D-port (Fig. 26.40). The level of the colic transection is found, and the left colon is sectioned, removing the specimen. A coloanal anastomosis is created using Vicryl Rapide 3/0 sutures (Fig. 26.41). The anal retractor is taken out.

26.5.4 End of Both Procedures and Temporary Ileostomy

Through the abdomen, the pelvic parietal peritoneum is closed and attached to the left colon by Vicryl 2/0 running sutures (a preformed knot at its extremity is useful to gain operative time), using the monocurved needle holder and the bicurved grasping forceps (Fig. 26.42). Then, the temporary percutaneous Ethilon 2/0 suture (female) is removed. The left mesocolic window is closed as well by a Vicryl 2/0 running suture. If necessary, a suprapubic drain is placed into the pelvis.

The operating room table is positioned without any Trendelenburg and tilt, and the small bowel is gently moved out of the right abdominal quadrants and over the left colon.

The distal bowel loop together with the ileocecal valve is searched. A loop, roughly 20 cm before the ileocecal valve, is grasped and extracted at the level of the abdominal single access, together with the trocars' removal and purse-string sutures. A temporary ileostomy is performed, placing the ileum outside the access (Fig. 26.43) and closing the fascia and the peritoneal sheet by Vicryl 1 sutures. The ileum is open, and mucocutaneous sutures using Vicryl Rapide 3/0 are positioned. An ileostomy set is finally placed.

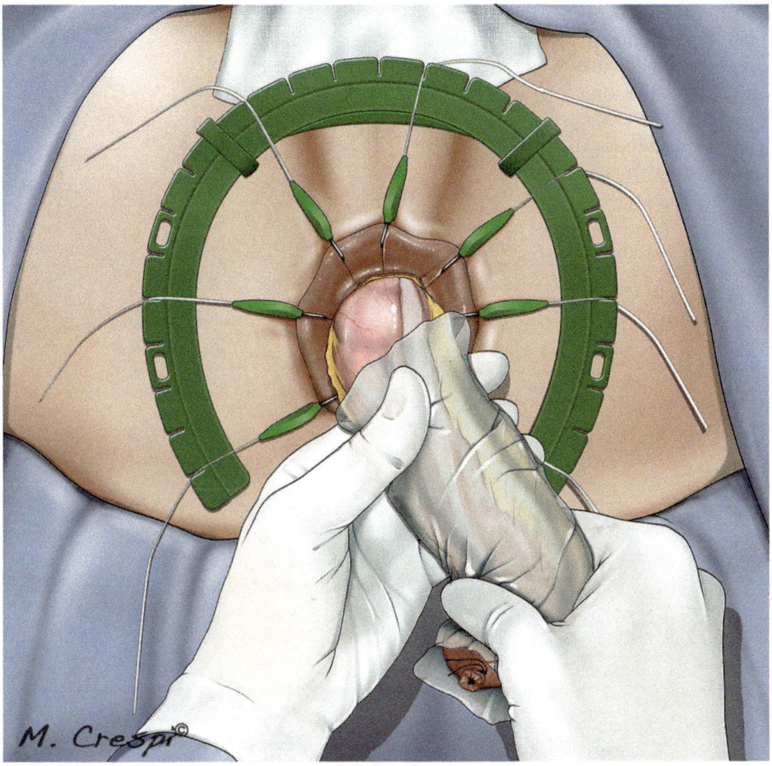

Fig. 26.40 Transanal laparoscopy with coloanal anastomosis: specimen's extraction.

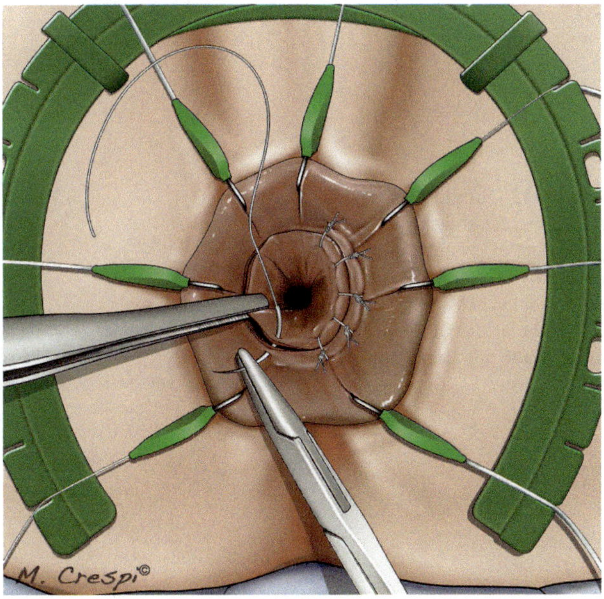

Fig. 26.41 Transanal laparoscopy with coloanal anastomosis: coloanal anastomosis.

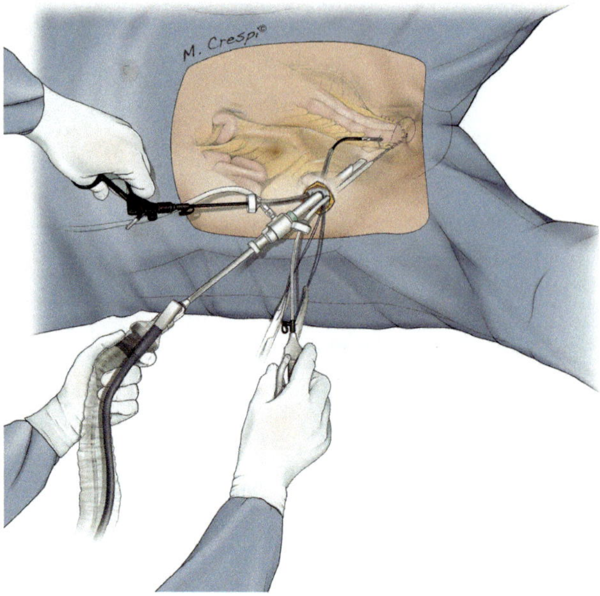

Fig. 26.42 Single-port abdominal laparoscopy: pelvic peritoneum closure under surgeon's ergonomy. The copyright holder of this figure is the author. All rights reserved

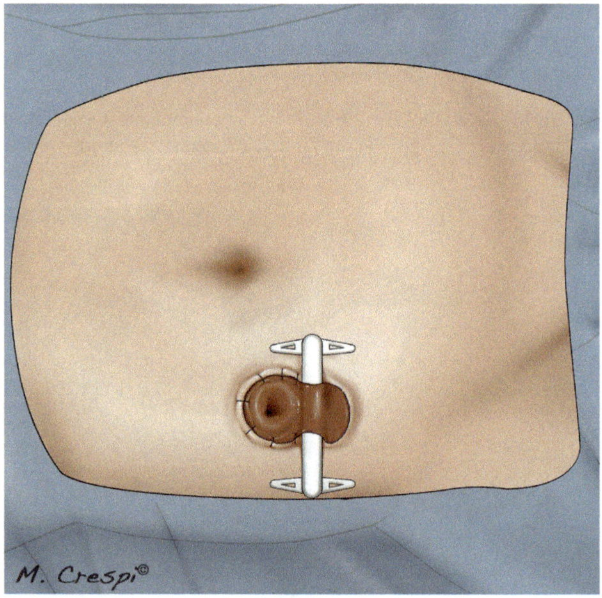

Fig. 26.43 Single-port abdominal laparoscopy: placement of the temporary ileostomy at the single abdominal access site. The copyright holder of this figure is the author. All rights reserved

26.6 Postoperative Care

One gram paracetamol is given i.v. at the end of the surgical procedure. Postoperative analgesia is given following the WHO visual analog pain scale (VAS). In the recovery room, the following scheme is followed: for VAS between 1 and 3, 1 g paracetamol i.v. is pushed; for VAS between 4 and 8, 100 mg tramadol i.v. is used; and for VAS greater than 8, 1 mg piritramide i.v. is incremented.

The arterial catheter is removed in the recovery room.

Once the patient leaves the recovery room, pain is assessed every 6 h, with 1 g paracetamol administered i.v. if VAS is between 1 and 3 and 100 mg tramadol administered i.v. if VAS is between 4 and 8.

Antibiotic prophylaxis is prescribed if necessary and TVP prophylaxis until the discharge of the patient from the hospital. The urinary catheter is removed after 5 days. The patient is allowed to drink water after 24 h and to tolerate a light diet from the third postoperative day. The management of the ileostomy is started after 48 h. If there are no complications, the patient is discharged on the 6th postoperative day, after having removed the abdominal drain (if used) and the central line.

Upon discharge, 1 g paracetamol perorally or 50 mg tramadol perorally is prescribed only if needed.

Office visits are scheduled at 10 days and 1 and 2 months. Usually the patient is scheduled for closure of temporary ileostomy after 2 months. Then, the patient is followed up by the surgeon and gastroenterologist/oncologist.

References

1. Rattner D. Introduction to NOTES white paper. Surg Endosc. 2006;20(2):185.
2. Buess G, Theiss R, Gunther M, Hutterer F, Pichlmaier H. Transanal endoscopic microsurgery. Leber Magen Darm. 1985;15(6):271–9.
3. Dapri G. Single-incision laparoscopy: a review of the indications, techniques and results after more than 700 procedures. Asian J Endosc Surg. 2014;7(2):102–16.

Transanal Laparoscopic TME with Robot-Assisted Abdominal Laparoscopy

27

Jean Salem and John H Marks

Abstract

Transanal total mesorectal excision (taTME) exists as an excellent new technique for sphincter-preserving surgery in the distal rectum. Convergence of this with a minimally invasive approach from above, albeit laparoscopically or robotically, allows for an extension of sphincter preservation and represents the ultimate application of a minimally invasive approach. In this chapter, we will describe a taTME approach using laparoscopy from below. The abdominal portion of the procedure including release of splenic flexure, high ligation of the inferior mesenteric artery and inferior mesenteric vein (IMV), mobilization of the colon, and completion of the TME dissection from above will be described using a robotic technique. Anatomic and technical approaches will be highlighted demonstrating the evolving field of rectal cancer surgery.

Keywords

Rectal cancer • Transanal abdominal transanal proctosigmoidectomy • TATA • taTME • Robotic surgery • Sphincter-preserving surgery

J. Salem
Division of Colorectal Surgery, Lankenau Medical Center, Wynnewood, PA 19096, USA

J.H. Marks (✉)
Department of Colorectal Surgery, Lankenau Medical Center, Main Line Healthcare, 100 Lancaster Avenue, Wynnewood, PA 19096, USA
e-mail: MarksJ@mlhs.org

G. Dapri, J.H. Marks (eds.), *Surgical Techniques in Rectal Cancer*, https://doi.org/10.1007/978-4-431-55579-7_27

27.1 Indication for Surgery

Transanal total mesorectal excision (taTME) surgery is employed in our practice for cancer in the distal third to half of the rectum that would otherwise require an abdominoperineal resection. This is utilized as an extension of the transanal abdominal transanal (TATA) procedure, which we have described extensively [1, 2]. The taTME approach is utilized after neoadjuvant therapy has downstaged the tumor and extends the possibility for sphincter preservation. Only those patients who are incontinent to begin with or whose cancer remains fixed 12 weeks after completion of their chemoradiotherapy undergo abdominoperineal resection. The other patients, who in our practice represent over 90% of the cases, are treated using the TATA technique [3]. This allows for a known distal margin from the tumor and includes incising and resecting the upper half of the internal sphincter. By extending this dissection transanally with the use of a port from below, the TME dissection can be carried out into the abdominal cavity. Using a minimally invasive approach from above, laparoscopically or robotically, allows for completion of the TME surgery. The specimen can then be delivered transanally and a temporary diverting stoma is created.

This evolving approach of rectal cancer surgery is highlighted throughout the book, and so indications and neoadjuvant treatment have been described elsewhere and will not be reiterated here.

27.2 Transanal Portion of TME Surgery: taTME (Table 27.1)

The operation is started with the patient in the extended lithotomy position in Skytron leg holders. The legs are positioned so as to have the anus hang 4 cm off the operative table. The yellowfin retractors are placed in maximal lithotomy to allow the best visualization of the area. The operation begins with infiltrating the perianal skin and levator musculature with a Xylocaine-epinephrine solution 1:200,000 concentration to minimize bleeding. Four Allis-Adair clamps are applied at the 12, 3, 6, and 9 o'clock position (Fig. 27.1). Often times a small Richardson retractor is utilized in the posterior (or 6 o'clock) position to better visualize the dentate line. A key aspect to the operation is to incise the mucosa circumferentially at the level of the dentate line using electrocautery (Fig. 27.2). It is essential that no mucosal bridges are left during this dissection. If the mucosa is not fully incised, a radial tear will result with the possibility of the extension tearing into the inferior margin of the tumor. The Metzenbaum scissors are then used to spread just off of the posterior midline to enter through the full thickness of the internal sphincter and into the intersphincteric plane.

Table 27.1 Initial steps of taTME

1	Incise mucosa circumferentially
2	Spread scissors to visualize glistening white of puborectalis
3	Transect rectal wall perpendicular to the axis of the rectum circumferentially

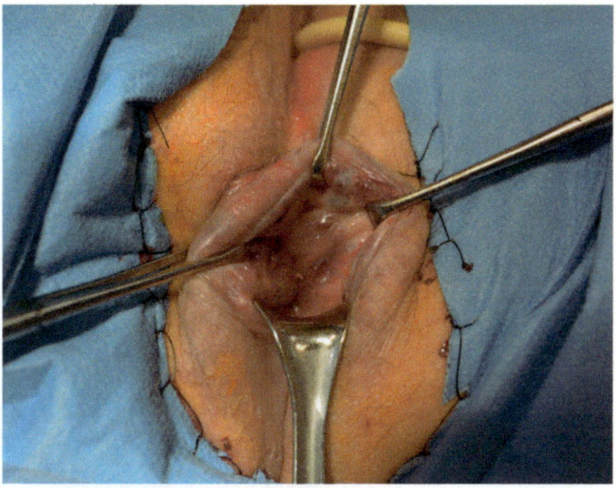

Fig. 27.1 Exposure of the dentate line

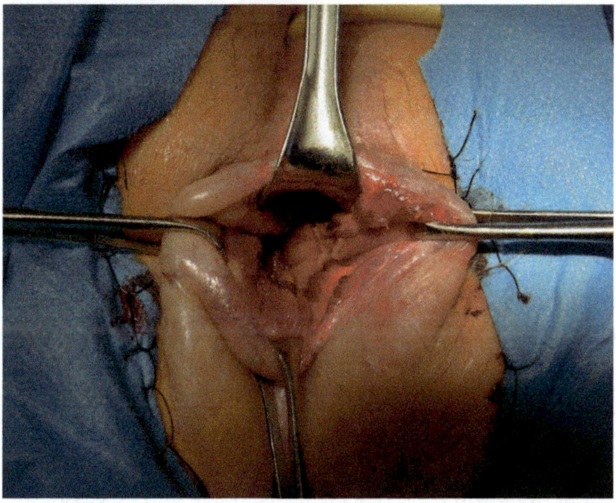

Fig. 27.2 Circumferential incision of the mucosa at the dentate line

The typical level for this is at the dentate line, but this can be modified distally or cephalad for 5 mm or so depending on the level of the cancer. The key anatomic area to see at this point of the operation is the glistening white aspect of the puborectalis (Fig. 27.3). This allows one to be certain that they have entered into the proper plane of dissection. This is the most critical aspect of the operation from an oncologic and functional standpoint. If the dissection is carried out too superficially, the rectal wall musculature will be sheared, and a positive margin will result, or a perforation of the rectum can occur. If the dissection is taken too deeply, the levator musculature will be injured and significant bleeding encountered, or the patient will have resultant fecal incontinence. An Allis-Adair clamp is then placed on the transected distal margin of the rectum, and a baby Deaver retractor is put into the intersphincteric plane to allow the area for transection to be put on stretch (Fig. 27.4). The dissection is

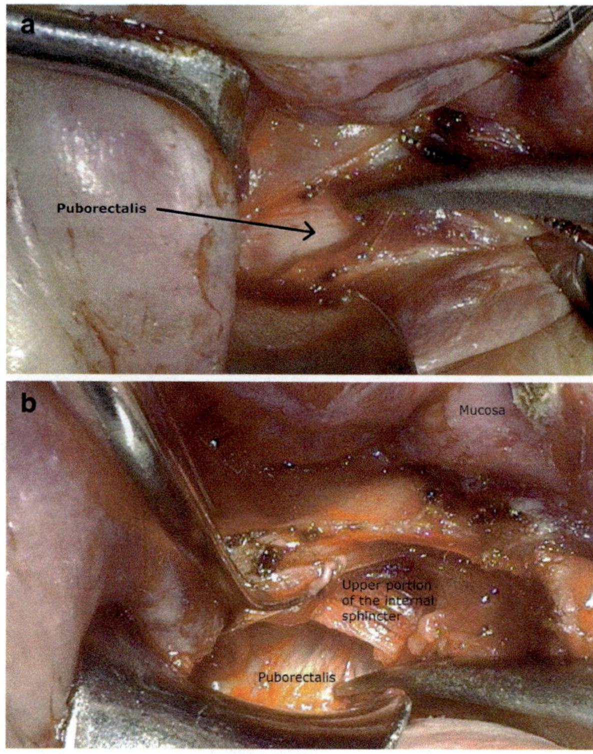

Fig. 27.3 (a, b) Intersphincteric plane with identification of the puborectalis muscle

taken circumferentially perpendicular to the axis of the anal canal. This is brought around to the right and the left side and then anteriorly. Typically in men, the anterior dissection is left to last as this is the most challenging aspect of the dissection. Except if there is a large bulky tumor in a different position, then that is generally the last position we dissect. In women, the anterior dissection is facilitated by a finger being placed into the vagina to better palpate the rectovaginal septum and fold. In a male patient, as a finger is placed transanally and is swept around in the intersphincteric space anteriorly, the puboprostatic sulcus is identified. Great care must be taken not to go anterior to the prostate. As surgeons have started to adopt this approach laparoscopically, reports of infraprostatic urethral injuries have surfaced, a potentially catastrophic morbidity that must be avoided at all costs and one we have never encountered to date with this described approach. The plane between the rectum and prostate or vagina should be a relatively avascular plane. Increased bleeding should alert the surgeon to the fact that they have taken the dissection too deeply into either the prostatic capsule or the posterior wall of the vagina. Once the dissection is completed circumferentially, one encounters, in the posterior midline, poorly described fibers of the puborectalis inserting into the rectum that need to be transected to mobilize the rectum fully (Fig. 27.5). The dissection is taken up as high as possible, generally to the level of the cervix in women and the level of the seminal vesicles in men. Once this is completed, a 0-Vicryl stitch is placed circumferentially in a

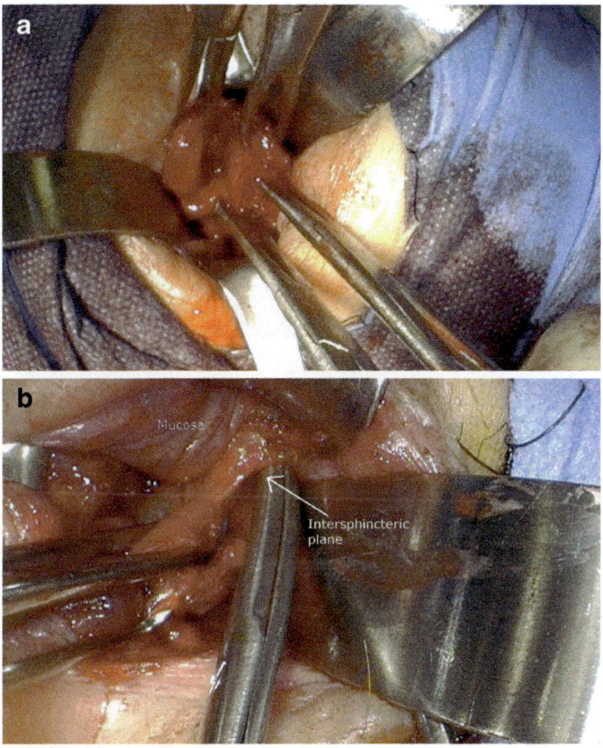

Fig. 27.4 Intersphincteric dissection. (**a**) Setup for exposure of the intersphincteric plane. (**b**) Mucosa and intersphincteric plane dissection with the transected end put on stretch

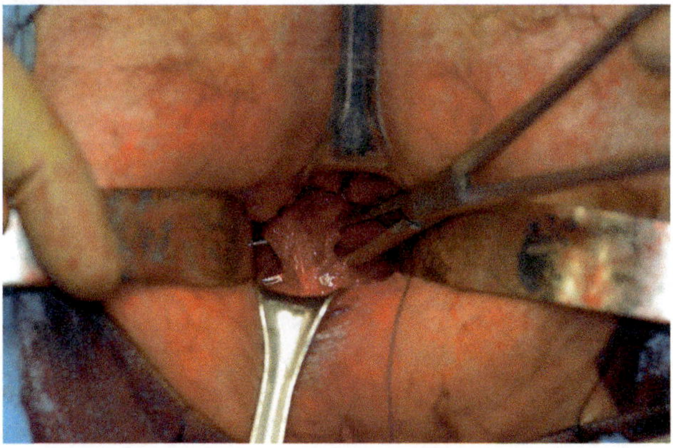

Fig. 27.5 Transection of poorly described fibers of the puborectalis muscle that insert into the rectum

seromuscular fashion on the mesorectum to turn in the transected end of the anus. The edges are turned inward in a horizontal mattress-running fashion, tightened after each stitch in order to avoid potential contamination with fecal matter or malignant cells (Fig. 27.6).

Finally when this is completed, a transanal laparoscopic port is placed from below. Different single-port platforms are available and have been described in

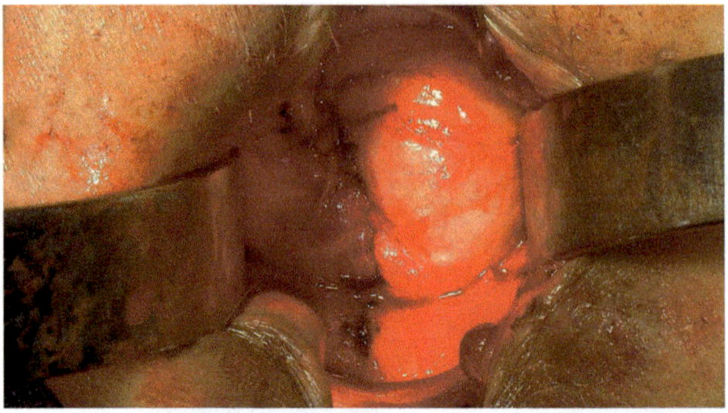

Fig. 27.6 Closure of the transected end of the rectum

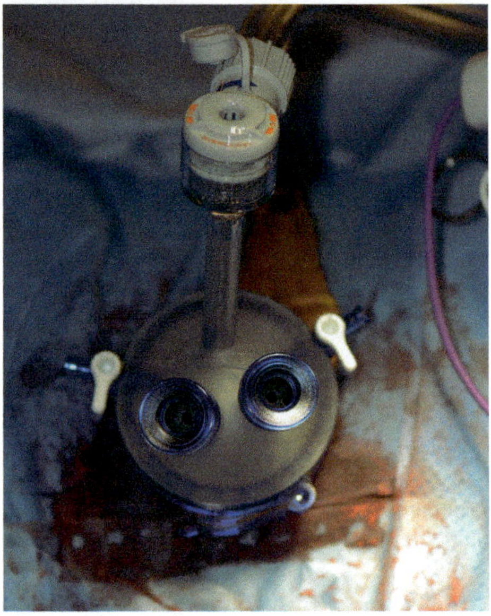

Fig. 27.7 Transanal port

different portions of this book. In our hands, generally, a SILS port (Covidien, New Haven, CT, USA) or a GelPOINT Path (Applied Medical, Rancho Santa Margarita, CA, USA) is used in order to assist with the dissection. CO_2 insufflation is carried out into the confines of the bony pelvis and the plane outside of the mesorectum. While not absolutely mandatory, we prefer the use of a high-insufflation AirSeal Port (AirSeal System Insufflator, SurgiQuest Inc, Mildford, CT, USA), which minimizes the billowing effect that occurs in a small space, such as the confines of the bony pelvis, when utilizing a typical insufflator [4]. A three-port configuration is used with the ports themselves in tight approximation (Fig. 27.7). Through this, preferably a 30° flexible tip 5 mm Olympus Videoendoscope (USA) is utilized at the top part of the triangle with a bariatric length fenestrated grasper in the left hand and a bariatric length scissors from below. The scissors are traded out with a vessel-sealing device, which in our hands is typically a LigaSure (Covidien) for bigger vessels. A key point to note is that smoke and blood in small amounts in this limited area can cause a great loss of visualization. For these reasons, preferably we utilize the scissors without electrocautery and maintain very precise hemostasis for the dissection.

Once the instrumentation is in place, the dissection can be brought around in a circumferential fashion. By performing the dissection in a circumferential, almost corkscrew, fashion, the areolar tissue plane is entered and directs the dissection in the proper plane (Fig. 27.8). Constant reorientation needs to be maintained during the dissection to avoid straying laterally into the obturator fossa on the right and the left side. There is potential for injury to the sacral nerve roots and/or hypogastric nerves and ureters on the lateral sidewall during this dissection. The easiest areas of dissection are in the posterior midline and the anterior midline. That being said, we prefer to maintain the dissection in a circular, almost corkscrew fashion to avoid tunneling too far in any one direction, which can potentially be

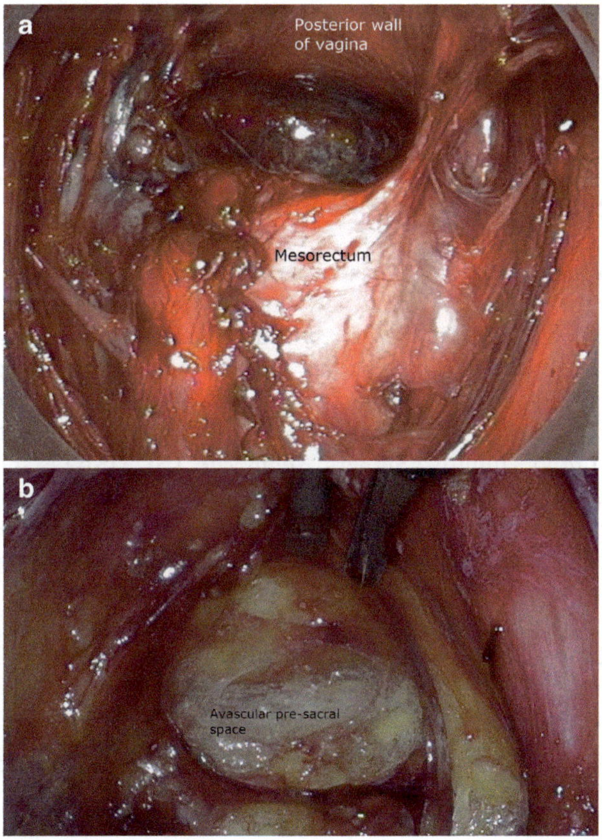

Fig. 27.8 (**a**, **b**) Transanal TME dissection

disorienting anatomically. In the posterior midline, the surgeon must remind himself that the presacral hollow curves superiorly, and if the dissection is taken straight back, the surgeon will enter into the presacral veins. While always a potentially disastrous problem, it is even more difficult to deal with if this occurs within the narrow confines of the pelvis with a laparoscope from below. While having no personal experience with bleeding in this fashion from this approach, the area would require control with pressure and likely packing the area and then approaching it from above.

The anterior dissection is carried out, the pouch of Douglas is incised, and the peritoneum is entered. Often times at this point, there is a loss of some visualization from above as pneumoperitoneum is established and pushes down onto the pelvis. That said, if time is given to allow this to equilibrate, one can usually continue from below. However, it is for this reason that we attempt to incise the peritoneum only as a later step in the dissection. If the dissection has gone smoothly from below, it is often times beneficial to rotate the rectum dissected from below through the opening in the pouch of Douglas into the peritoneal cavity and continue with dissection up to the sacral promontory. While we and others have experience with continued abdominal dissection from below, that is outside of the purvey of this chapter [5]. Once this is completed, gloves and gowns are changed, and we leave the insufflation from below, which is equilibrated from above, and then start the dissection transabdominally.

27.3 Abdominal Portion

After gowns, gloves, and instruments are changed, the patient's legs are moved from high lithotomy to low lithotomy position so that the thighs are flat to the abdomen. Pneumoperitoneum can be instituted via a Veress needle or in a thinner patient or someone who has had previous abdominal operations with a cutdown, depending on the surgeon's preference. Often times, there is already a pneumoperitoneum established from the dissection from below. Port placement for the XI and SI robot (Intuitive Surgery, Sunnyvale, CA, USA) is shown in Fig. 27.9. The first step always is a thorough exploration of the abdominal cavity laparoscopically to rule out any evidence of metastatic disease, particularly in the area of the liver. The table is then put in Trendelenburg position, airplaned right side down so the small bowel can be positioned out of the pelvis and to the right side of the abdomen, giving visualization of the inferior mesenteric artery (IMA), inferior mesenteric vein (IMV), and pelvis. Once the small bowel is positioned out of the field, the robot is brought in and docked. The two arms are placed to the left of the midline, the camera's port is placed at the midline above the umbilicus, and a 12 mm port is placed where the ileostomy site will ultimately go in the right lower quadrant. A target width of 8 cm is left between ports to minimize robotic arm clashing. The assistant

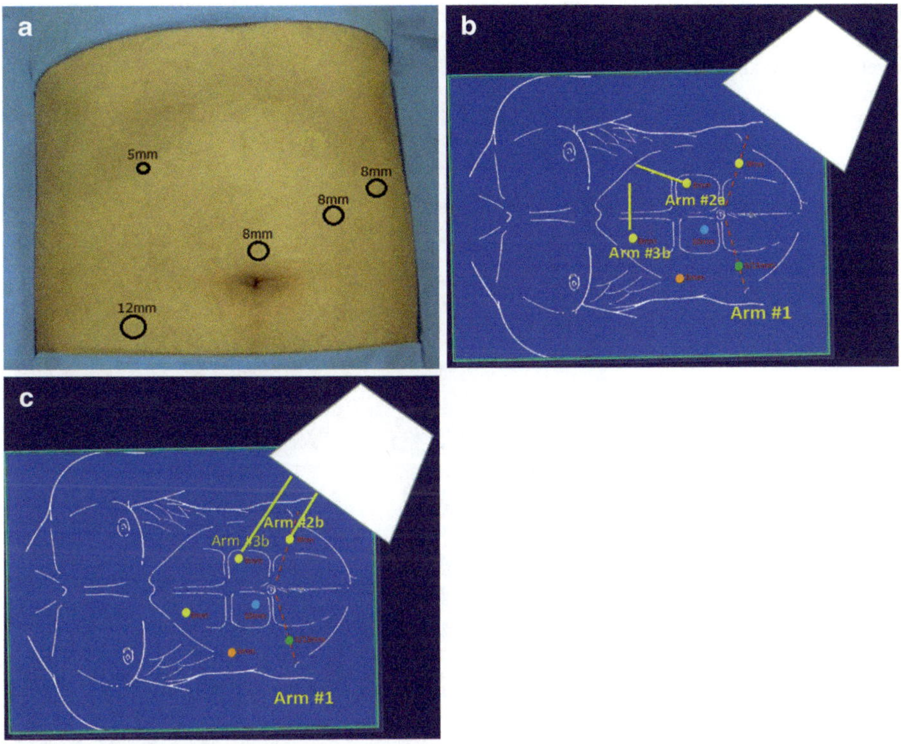

Fig. 27.9 Ports placement. (**a**) Ports placement for the da Vinci Xi robot. (**b**) Ports placement for the da Vinci Si robot. (**c**) Adjustment of the arms of the da Vinci Si robot for the pelvic dissection

port is in the right upper quadrant, and it is generally a 5 mm port. The assistant uses a bariatric length grasper or suction in order to reach down into the pelvis later at the case. We prefer to utilize a single-dock technique with inframesocolic release of the splenic flexure.

The operation commences by incising the peritoneum with the scissors and monopolar cautery from the sacral promontory up to the duodenojejunal junction (Fig. 27.10). The assistant is generally not very active in this portion of the operation. The mesentery of the sigmoid colon is retracted anteriorly using a bipolar grasper with the number 2 arm. If there is a redundant sigmoid colon, the number 1 arm with a wide mouth grasper is used to retract the sigmoid colon up and toward the left hip to get this out of the surgeon's field. If the sigmoid colon is not very large, oftentimes just two working hands are utilized for this portion of the operation. Either way, the hypogastric nerves are identified and swept posteriorly so that the left ureter can be identified and protected

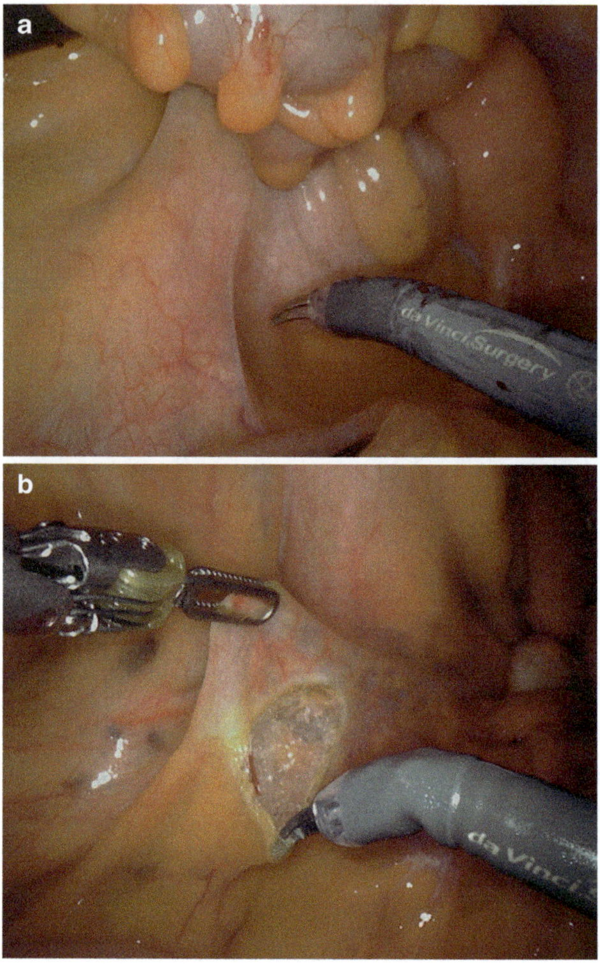

Fig. 27.10 (**a**, **b**) Incision of the peritoneum at the level of the sacral promontory

(Fig. 27.11). The dissection cephalad to the IMA is carried out posteriorly to the inferior mesenteric vein. This enters into the plane dissected from below and allows the IMA to be safely dissected free circumferentially (Fig. 27.12). If there is difficulty establishing a proper plane of orientation inferior to the IMA due to previous diverticulitis, radiation, or other factors, the plane superior to the IMA and posterior to the IMV is a very reliable one. By starting here and dissecting in the plane above the retroperitoneum, one enters into the proper plane inferior to the IMA from above. That said, it is our preference to identify the hypogastric nerves and sweep them posteriorly, as that serves the dual function of protecting the nerves while establishing a proper plane of orientation and will always bring you upon the ureter first and then the gonadal vessels lateral to them. Once the IMA is dissected circumferentially with the left ureter

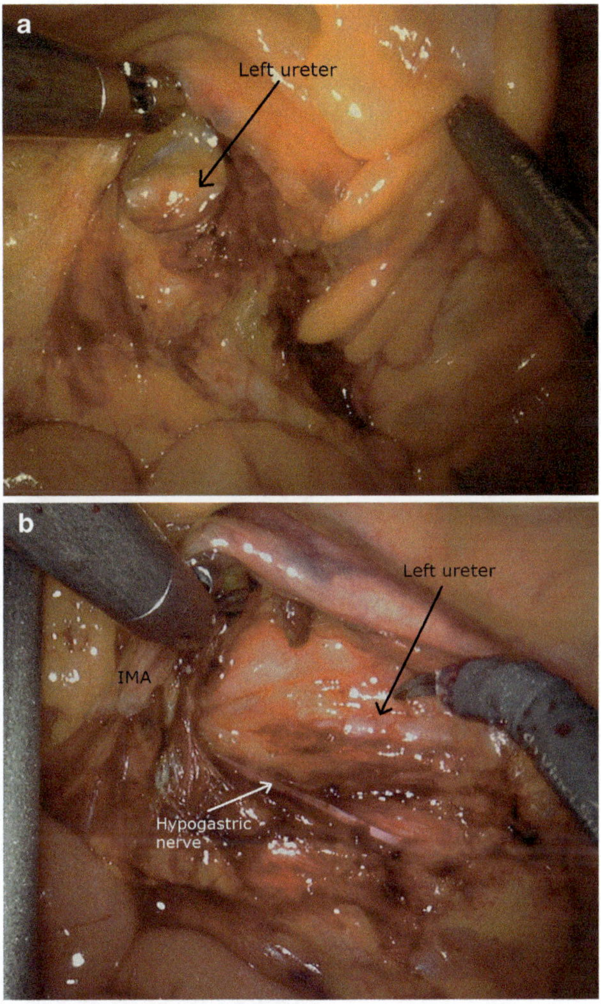

Fig. 27.11 (a, b) Mesenteric dissection with identification of the left ureter and hypogastric nerves

identified, the IMA is transected. This is generally done, in our hands, with a vessel-sealer device; however, this could be done with a vascular stapler or clips as well. The vessel is taken high, as this is a cancer operation, central to the takeoff of the left colic. We advocate leaving a 1 cm length of IMA off of the aorta so that if any problem with the vascular control and bleeding ensues, the IMA can be grasped and an endo-tie placed. When an endo-tie is necessary, it is placed by the assistant through the assistant port. In general, up until this part of the operation, the assistant is doing nothing more than aspirating smoke from cautery. An endo-tie is always placed in any instance where the patient has a history of coronary or peripheral vascular disease or hypertension because of the higher incidence of calcification of the IMA and vessel sealer failure.

At this point, the IMV is dissected free (Fig. 27.13). It is common at this time with the Xi system for the number 1 port to be used to hold up the mesentery of the distal transverse colon and descending colon. If using the Si system, an additional port has been placed subcostally in the right upper quadrant, and this is shown in the diagram. The number 2 arm is used there with number 1 arm retracting. That said, once exposure is established, the IMV is dissected free and transected centrally with the vessel-sealing device. Again, there is 1 cm length left on the IMV in case of problems with vessel sealing, which would allow an area of vessel to be grasped and endo-tie or clip placed on it if need be. Once this is done, dissection is carried out with scissors and electric cautery in the avascular plane extending out toward the

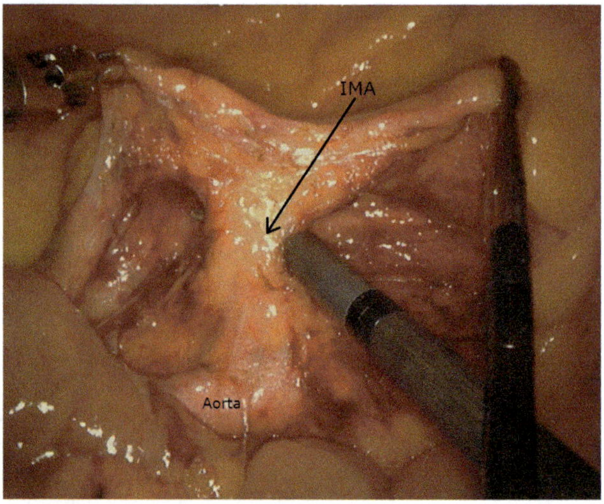

Fig. 27.12 IMA dissection

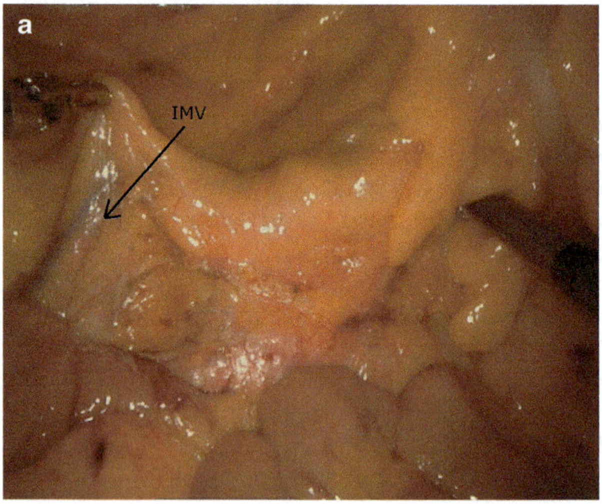

Fig. 27.13 (**a**, **b**) IMV dissection

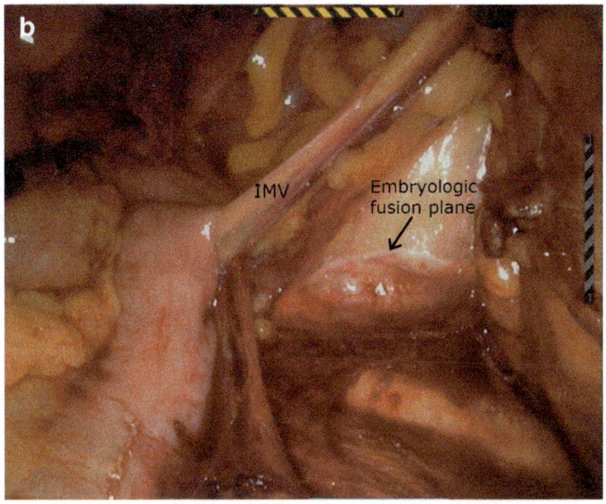

Fig. 27.13 (continued)

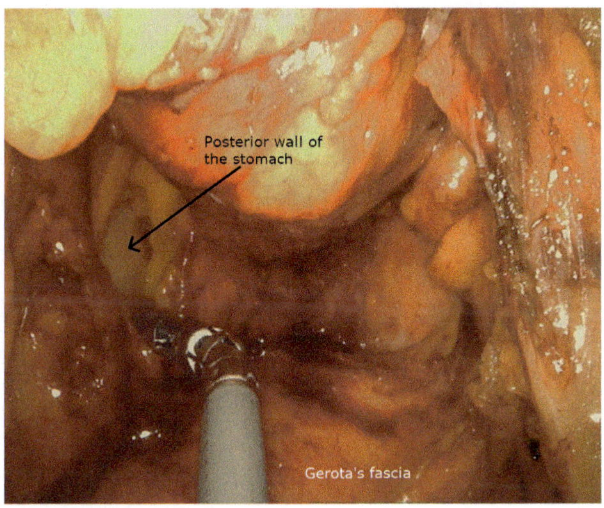

Fig. 27.14 Inframesocolic dissection

splenic flexure. The mesentery is dissected off of the retroperitoneum, and the plane is identified anteriorly to the pancreas (Fig. 27.14). This is often the most challenging aspect of the splenic flexure release, as one can go posterior to the pancreas and come upon the splenic vein. By going 1 cm anterior to the IMV, the proper plane is identified, and you can enter in the lesser sac anterior to the pancreas and posterior to the mesentery. If having challenges identifying this, the upper portion of the line of Toldt can be taken from above the mesentery and the dissection brought around medially (Fig. 27.15). Lastly if this remains confusing, the camera can be brought up above the mesentery, and using the assistant to retract up the greater omentum and the number 1 port to retract the colon medially, the scissors can be used to mobilize the upper portion of the line of Toldt and bring the dissection around medially.

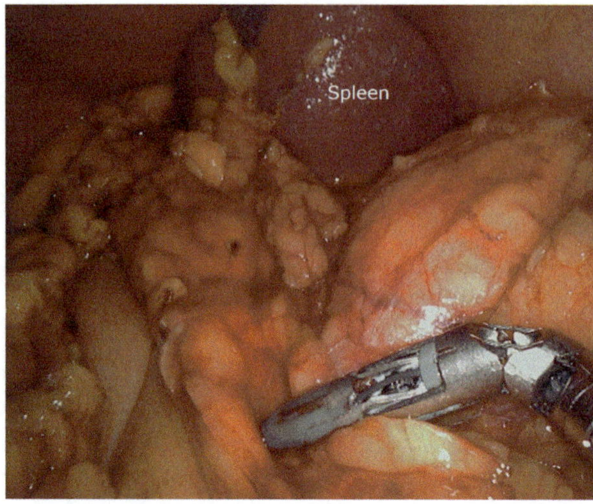

Fig. 27.15 Splenic flexure release

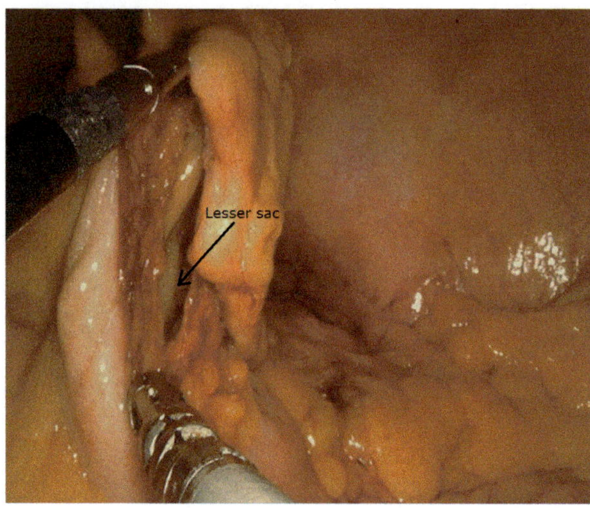

Fig. 27.16 Incision of the gastrocolic ligament

Once this is done, the vessel sealer is used to incise the gastrocolic ligament up to the middle portion of the transverse colon (Fig. 27.16). In this fashion, the splenic flexure is entirely mobilized. It is essential that there is a full release of the splenic flexure for these procedures, as a colo-anal anastomosis will be performed. For this anastomosis, there needs to be full mobility of the splenic flexure in order to have a tension-free, well-vascularized anastomosis.

Having completed the previous steps, the line of Toldt is freely mobilized. This is generally a very straightforward aspect of the operation, done with the electrocautery. The dissection has already been carried out in a mediolateral fashion, so just a band of peritoneum is holding the lateral attachment along the line of Toldt

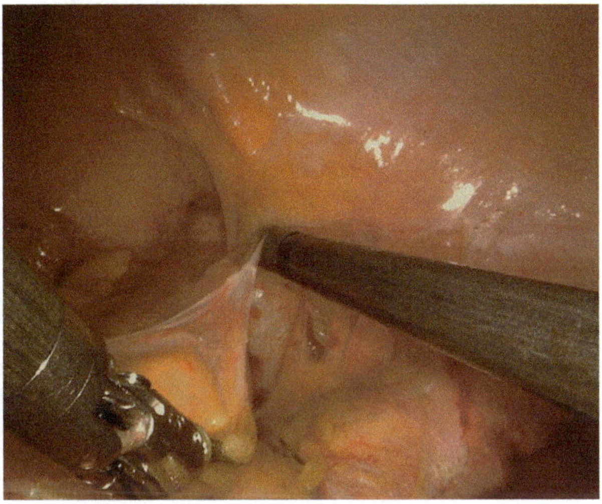

Fig. 27.17 Dissection of the line of Toldt

(Fig. 27.17). This is left in place until this portion of the operation, as it serves as a retractor for the descending and sigmoid colon with the patient airplaned to the right side for the previous aspects of the dissection. This is an ideal first step for the training surgeon to perform with the robot as he or she is learning. At this point, the attention is turned to the pelvis. The sigmoid colon is retracted medially, and the scissors are used to incise the lateral attachments. Almost immediately, the dissection should connect to the previous medial to lateral dissection. Once done, the dissection is continued cephalad, and the colon is entirely mobilized from the mid-transverse colon to the rectum.

27.4 Pelvic TME Dissection

Now, the joints of the arms of the Xi robot are shifted so that we are able to dissect into the pelvis. For the Si system, the arms are reconfigured so that 3 is placed in the left lateral position in a 3B position (which was the previous 2A position), from the 3A position, and the number 2 arm is switched to the left lateral position from 2A to 2B, as shown in the diagram (Fig. 27.9). At this time, the assistant's port is used to grasp the sigmoid colon and hold this in a cephalad fashion. It is essential to have good teamwork with the bedside assistant in order to have adequate mobility and retraction. One of the major benefits of the bottoms-up transanal TME approach is that the pelvic dissection is greatly facilitated. With the colon and rectum being retracted cephalad and to the left side, the right perirectal sulcus is incised, and then the left perirectal sulcus is incised (or what is left of this dissection) (Fig. 27.18). The hypogastric nerves are swept posteriorly, and the dissection begins in the posterior midline, in the avascular plane anterior to the hypogastric nerves (Fig. 27.19). Dissection is taken down toward the levators and usually by midway through the

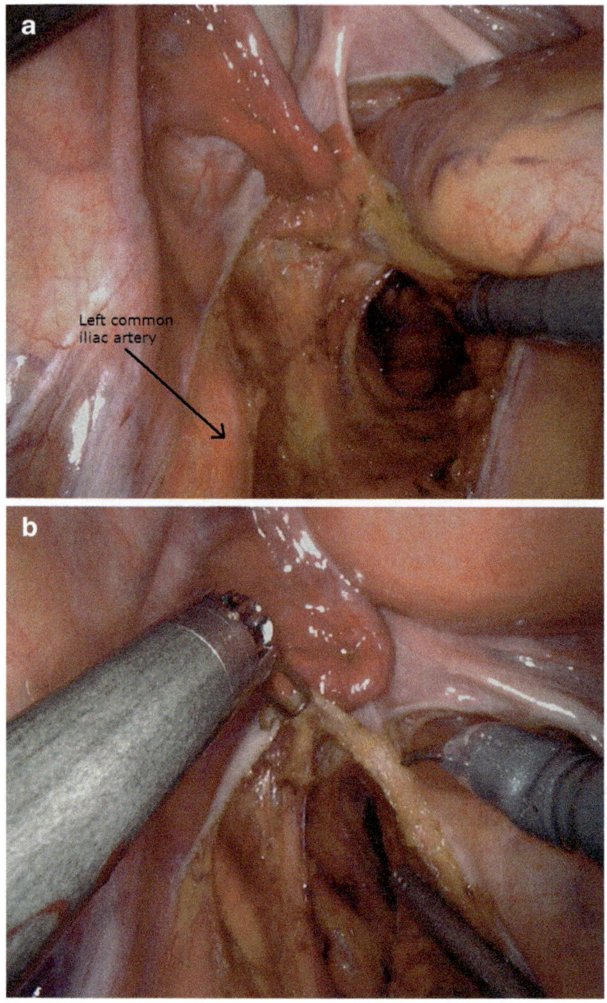

Fig. 27.18 (**a**, **b**) Incision of the right and left perirectal sulcus

dissection posteriorly, or earlier, the dissection is connected to the dissection from below (Fig. 27.20). The surgeon must remain mindful that there is an avascular plane behind the hypogastric nerves as well, and this constitutes the wrong plane, which will lead to nerve injury as well as bleeding. By utilizing the number 2 arm, the mesorectum is retracted cephalad and to the left shoulder, and hypogastric nerves and nervi erigentes are used as a landmark to carry the dissection down toward the pelvis and finish the dissection on the right side. Depending on the location of the tumor, the rectovesicular fold is incised at this point, taking the Denonvilliers' fascia 1 cm above the rectovesicular fold for an anteriorly based tumor or right at the fold for a posteriorly or laterally based tumor. Again, this aspect of the dissection is tremendously facilitated by the dissection from below and has often already been started as the peritoneal cavity has often been entered through

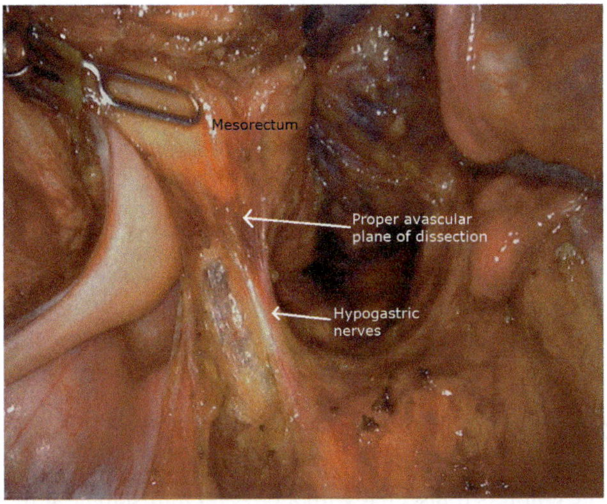

Fig. 27.19 Proper avascular plane of TME dissection with identification of the hypogastric nerves

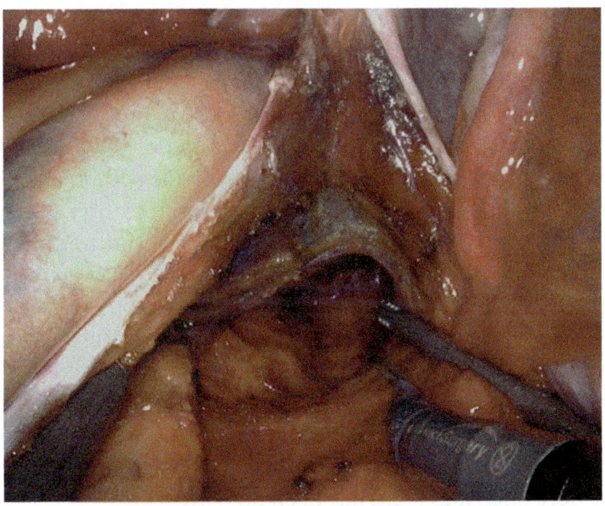

Fig. 27.20 TME dissection

the pouch of Douglas from below. Following this, the left lateral rectal sulcus is incised, the hypogastric nerves are protected and swept posteriorly, and the dissection is brought around circumferentially to connect with the dissection from below. With this completed, the mesorectum is brought out of the pelvis and the pelvis inspected to assure hemostasis and completeness of resection. Once this is completed, the mesentery of the left colon is transected up to the sigmoidocolic junction just cephalad to the left colic takeoff, coming through the IMA and IMV up to the area of distal descending colon. A Babcock is placed on the rectum from the assistant port. The robot is undocked, the patient is put in extended lithotomy position, and then using laparoscopic visualization from above, the surgeon goes below, a Babcock is placed through the anus, and the specimen is delivered from above and removed transanally. Once this is done, the decision is made regarding the type of anastomosis to be performed. There are three options for pelvic anastomosis: straight end-to-end colo-anal anastomosis, a side-to-end colo-anal anastomosis, or a colonic J-pouch. It is generally our preference presently to do a side-to-end anastomosis to gain a little bit of additional capacitance for functional benefit. If the patient has a wide pelvis and adequate length of the colon, a colonic J-pouch is fashioned. If there are challenges in terms of length or a very narrow pelvis, direct end-to-end colo-anal anastomosis is carried out. It should be noted that prior to performing the anastomosis, the team from above must determine that the bowel is properly oriented with no twisting of the mesentery, the mesentery lies without tension, and there is no small bowel herniating underneath the mesentery of the colon.

27.4.1 Side-to-End Anastomosis

The colon is transected with a GIA 60 mm stapler at the previously selected site of the sigmoidocolic junction. The staple line is then oversewn with a 3-0 Vicryl stitch. An incision is made approximately 4 cm proximal to this with the electrocautery on the antimesenteric portion of the colon. The staple line is brought in and pushed posteriorly in the midline, and then four cardinal sutures are placed. The first suture is placed anteriorly with a full-thickness bite of the colonic wall and then a full thickness bite through the transected end of the internal sphincter and the mucosa. A Kelly clamp is placed as a marker on the suture, and it is left untied. A stitch then is placed in the right lateral and left lateral position and then at the posterior midline. Care should be noted on placing the posterior midline stitch not to grab the back wall of the colon, as this can protrude in and inadvertently be included which would end up closing off the patient's lumen. Once these four cardinal stitches are placed and Kelly clamps are applied, the remaining sutures are placed using 0 Vicryl suture and full-thickness bites through the colonic wall and then through the transected end of internal sphincter and mucosa, and these are tied as we go. In general, each quadrant takes an additional one to two stitches to complete the anastomosis. That concludes the anastomosis, and digital examination is carried out to assure the lumen is widely open and there has been no narrowing.

27.4.2 Colonic J-Pouch Anastomosis

The colon is brought out from below. The area of the sigmoidocolic junction is transected with a GIA 60 mm stapler, and then the colon is folded back upon itself, and a J-pouch is created by incising the colonic wall approximately 4–6 cm distal to the staple line. It should be noted the staple line is oversewn with 3-0 Vicryl before this is done. The bowel is folded on itself, and with a single firing of a GIA 60 mm stapler, the colonic J-pouch is created. The pouch is created in an antimesenteric to antimesenteric fashion. The lumen is inspected to make sure there is no bleeding along the staple line. Once this is done, the pouch and anastomosis are carried out by taking full-thickness bites through the colonic wall, and then through the transected end of the internal sphincter and the mucosa at the 12, 6, 3, and 9 o'clock position, Kelly clamps are placed, and then the resultant quadrants are anastomosed, with usually between one and three stitches. These are tied as they are placed, unlike the cardinal sutures. Once this is done, the cardinal sutures are tied, the area is inspected to make sure that there are no gaps in the closure, and digital examination is carried out.

27.4.3 Direct Hand-Sewn End-to-End Colo-anal Anastomosis

While this anastomosis is often characterized in a negative fashion in the literature, it is our feeling that it is far better to have a well-vascularized direct colo-anal anastomosis without tension, as opposed to straining, to create a side-to-end anastomosis or colonic J-pouch and putting the mesentery on stretch. For the first two decades of performing the TATA, a direct colo-anal anastomosis was the only anastomosis performed. This is a particularly beneficial approach for male patients with a very narrow pelvis. Once the bowel is delivered below, the mesentery is stepped up to the colonic wall (if this wasn't already performed from above). The anterior antimesenteric portion of the colon is transected with the electrocautery, and then a full-thickness bite using a 0 Vicryl stitch is taken through the full-thickness of the colonic wall and through the anterior wall of the internal sphincter and mucosa. A Kelly clamp is placed, and then additional stitches are placed at the 3 and 9 o'clock position. Once these are completed, the resection of the bowel is completed with the electrocautery, and then a stitch is placed in the 6 o'clock position. The bowel wall is transected in a segmental fashion to avoid the possibility of coming through it all at once and having the colon retract into the pelvis. As in the other types of anastomoses, once these are done, these stitches are not tied, and then the intervening quadrants are closed with one to three sutures, taking full-thickness bites through the colonic wall and through the transected portion of the anus involving both the internal sphincter and the mucosa, and tied as we go. Once these are completed, the cardinal stitches are tied, and digital examination is carried out to make sure there is no stenosis. The anastomosis is inspected and probed to make sure there are no gaps that exist.

Once this is completed, all instruments are changed, and we go back above for the last time, irrigate out the pelvis, and inspect the IMA and IMV, as well as the left upper quadrant to make sure there is no bleeding, as well as no bleeding anywhere else. A loop of ileum is identified approximately 30 cm proximal to the ileocecal valve, brought out, making sure it is properly oriented, through the right lower quadrant port, and then matured over a red rubber catheter in a standard Brooke fashion.

27.5 Postoperative Care

Generally the patients are ambulated the day of surgery or the following day. They are started on a clear liquid diet the day of surgery or the following day once they have recovered from anesthesia. After 24 h, the diet is advanced to gastrointestinal soft diet, assuming there is no gross distention of the abdomen with concomitant nausea and/or vomiting. Perioperative antibiotics are generally maintained for 7–10 days' time using doxycycline intravenously. This has been our standard of practice for three decades, stemming from the difficulty of eradicating infection in radiated tissue. While extended antibiotic use has currently gone out of favor, we have been very pleased with our low infection rates in the pelvis and therefore continue this practice. The Foley catheter is left in place for 5 days' time, unless the patient is felt to be able to go home before that. In that case, the night prior to planned discharge, the Foley catheter is removed at midnight. Patients are seen at the 2-week mark, and gentle digital examination is carried out [6]. It is important that this is done at the 2-week and 4–6-week period to avoid any apposition of the anastomosis. Sometimes synechiae form, which are gently dilated without problem. If left unmolested, the synechiae progress to a fixed stenosis that will require a formal repair. The stoma is left in place for 3 months' time or until they have completed and recovered from postoperative chemotherapy, depending on their course [6]. We recently published our long-term outcomes of patients who underwent TATA and showed low local recurrence rates and excellent overall survival [6]. We also showed that satisfaction with quality of life and functional outcomes is high after TATA [7]. Patients clearly preferred this approach over having a permanent stoma [7].

References

1. Marks G, Mohiuddin M, Goldstein SD. Sphincter preservation for cancer of the distal rectum using high dose preoperative radiation. Int J Radiat Oncol Biol Phys. 1988;15:1065–8.
2. Marks G, Bannon J, Marks J. Transanal-abdominal transanal radical proctosigmoidectomy with coloanal anastomosis for distal rectal cancer. In: Baker R, Fisher J, Nyhus L, editors. Mastery of surgery. 3rd ed. Boston, MA: Little, Brown and Company Inc.; 1996. p. 1524–34.
3. Marks JH, Frenkel JL, D'Andrea AP, Greenleaf CE. Maximizing rectal cancer results: TEM and TATA techniques to expand sphincter preservation. Surg Oncol Clin N Am. 2011;20(3):501–20.
4. Nicholson G, Knol J, Houben B, et al. Optimal dissection for transanal total mesorectal excision using modified CO_2 insufflation and smoke extraction. Colorectal Dis. 2015;17(11):265–7.
5. Marks JH, Lopez-Acevedo N, Krishnan B, Johnson MN, Montenegro GA, Marks G. True NOTES TME resection with splenic flexure release, high ligation of IMA, and side-to-end hand-sewn coloanal anastomosis. Surg Endosc. 2016;30(10):4626–31.
6. Marks JH, Myers EA, Zeger EL, Denittis AS, Gummadi M, Marks GJ. Long-term outcomes by a transanal approach to total mesorectal excision for rectal cancer. Surg Endosc. 2017; https://doi.org/10.1007/s00464-017-5597-7.
7. Marks JH, Salem JF, Valsdottir EB, Yarandi SS, Marks GJ. Quality of life and functional outcome after transanal abdominal transanal proctectomy for low rectal cancer. Dis Colon Rectum. 2017;60(3):258–65.

Pure Transanal Laparoscopic TME without Abdominal Laparoscopy

28

Joel Leroy, Usmaan Hameed, Ntourakis Dimitrios, and Frédéric Bretagnol

Abstract

Transanal rectal dissection was put forward by Toupet 60 years ago in 1950. The objective was to preserve the anal sphincter in low rectal tumors in patients with a narrow pelvis.

At present, there is a renewed interest due to the use of video endoscopes which allow for an excellent visualization of anatomical structures by transanal way. Following the studies of John Marks who described the laparoscopic transanal transabdominal (TATA) surgical procedure, hybrid techniques combining the transanal approach with laparoscopic assistance have increased.

Here, the authors propose a full resection technique of the rectum and of its meso using a purely transanal approach. The different steps of this technique and the required armamentarium have been perfectly described and illustrated.

J. Leroy (✉)
Hanoi High Tech & Digestive Center, Saint Paul Hospital,
12 Chu Văn An, Dien Bien Phu, Ba Dinh, Hanoi, Vietnam

IRCAD/EITS (Research Institute Against Digestive Cancer/European Institute of TeleSurgery), Strasbourg 67075, France

48 Route de la Colline, 62172 Bouvigny-Boyeffles, France
e-mail: joelleroy002@me.com

U. Hameed
Department of Surgical Oncology, M3-130, Princess Margaret Cancer Centre, University of Toronto, 610 University Avenue, Toronto M5G 2M9, Canada

N. Dimitrios
IRCAD/EITS (Research Institute Against Digestive Cancer/European Institute of TeleSurgery), Strasbourg 67075, France

F. Bretagnol, M.D., Ph.D.
Department of Digestive Surgery, Louis Mourier Hospital, Paris, France

G. Dapri, J.H. Marks (eds.), *Surgical Techniques in Rectal Cancer*,
https://doi.org/10.1007/978-4-431-55579-7_28

Keywords
Pure transanal TME • Rectal cancer • PROGRESS • TATA • NOTES

28.1 Introduction

Heald et al. introduced the concept of total mesorectal excision (TME) for the treatment of rectal cancer in 1982 [1]. It is the "gold standard" worldwide in the surgical treatment of advanced rectal cancer. Maintaining the integrity of the mesorectum while achieving a negative distal margin can be particularly difficult due to limited exposure and reach, particularly in obese male patients with a deep, narrow pelvis. While laparoscopic resection has been shown to be oncologically equivalent as compared to open resection, resection of low rectal neoplasms in these patients has its challenges. In order to address some of these technical challenges, transanal TME has had a recent resurgence in popularity. However, the concept is not a new one. Marks et al. described transanal abdominal transanal (TATA) proctosigmoidectomy with coloanal anastomosis [2, 3]. While hybrid laparoscopic endoscopic TME using various platforms has risen in popularity [4–16], purely natural orifice transluminal endoscopic surgery (NOTES) in colorectal surgery has remained elusive.

Pure NOTES TME has been described in experimental settings both in porcine [17–22] and cadaveric models [22–25]. As of now, there have been *three* case reports [26–28] and one series [26] published on no-scar transanal NOTES TME. Marks et al. reported on four operations of true NOTES TME with splenic flexure relesease, high ligation of the IMA/IMV, and side-to-end anastomosis [29]. Zhang et al. have described an alternate approach, where the anterior rectovaginal or rectoprostatic dissection and entry into the peritoneal cavity through the anterior peritoneal reflection are performed early [27]. In this approach, a significant portion of the mesorectal and mesocolic dissection is performed within the abdominal cavity.

Our technique described below relies on a mesorectal and mesocolic dissection performed through a retroperitoneal endoscopic approach known as perirectal oncologic gateway to retroperitoneal endoscopic surgery (PROGRESS). All of this has been described in both experimental and clinical settings [18, 26–28].

In this chapter, our aim is to outline the rationale and the steps of this approach.

28.2 Pure Transanal Retroperitoneal Endoscopic TME

28.2.1 Rationale

Today, the gold standard for an oncological resection of the rectum is to use either laparoscopy or laparotomy. The transanal approach has been used for some time now. First, Toupet in the 1950s and more recently Gerald Marks in the 1980s put forward the transanal route for low rectal tumors after radiochemotherapy (RCT) and in fragile patients or patients with a difficult pelvic access. In the 1990s, his son

John Marks updated this approach by combining it with laparoscopy. All these techniques are hybrid techniques that combine two approaches.

Using our own experience in minimally invasive and transanal surgery, as we have the chance to use the latest endorectal surgical equipment, we progressively reconsidered our transanal approach.

The idea of PROGRESS was inspired by the Japanese experience which described right and left colectomy techniques using an oncological minimally invasive laparoscopic retroperitoneal approach [30]. The authors concluded that it represented a huge advantage in obese patients in which the retraction of digestive loops can sometimes be difficult. Following their work, I imagined the possibility to dissect the retroperitoneal space by going through or around the rectum in order to allow the lowering of the left colon and perform a colorectal or coloanal anastomosis, after a resection of the sigmoid colon and/or the rectum. The first step was experimental in order to check feasibility in an animal model and in a cadaver.

In human patients, the experiment was performed in a stepwise fashion. We were actually performing NOTES without even knowing it. Our experience in transanal surgery dates back to the 2000s and stemmed from the work of Gerhard Buess on transanal endoscopic microsurgery (TEM) in the early 1980s. Our first complete oncological resection of the rectum and its meso using a purely transanal approach was performed in June 2010. Since then, we have refined and standardized the steps of the procedure in a better way. Consequently, indications are still limited to our experience in small-sized tumors.

28.2.2 Patient Selection

We stress that this approach is experimental and not a standard of care.

As such, surgeons attempting this technique should have significant technical experience with transanal endoscopic microsurgery or transanal minimally invasive surgery and should follow their patients within the context of a prospective clinical trial.

Patient selection is paramount when considering a NOTES TME approach. After a thorough discussion concerning risks, benefits, and alternative approaches, consenting patients are included in our prospective trial for NOTES transanal TME. We select patients with mid-to-low, early rectal cancers. Currently, we exclude patients with locally advanced (T3, T4) disease.

28.3 Surgical Technique

28.3.1 Armamentarium (Fig. 28.1a, b)

Instrumentation is essential to the success of this approach.

The TEO® device platform (Karl Storz, Tuttlingen, Germany) was used. The platform includes 4 cm-diameter tubes at the oblique distal extremity (the superior

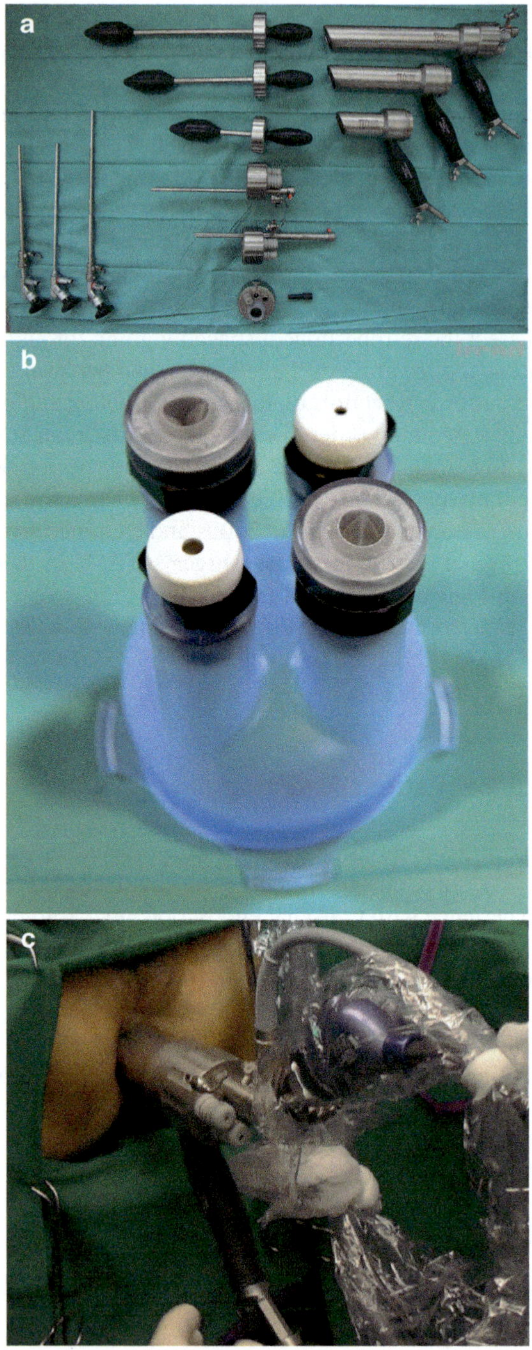

Fig. 28.1 (**a**) Transanal endoscopic operation (TEO) platform (Karl Storz, Tuttlingen, Germany). (**b**) TEO flexible cap (Karl Storz, Tuttlingen, Germany). (**c**) TEO platform fixed on articulated arm (Karl Storz, Tuttlingen, Germany)

border is the longest) and at the proximal orifice, which allows the connection of cups of different shapes and functions. There are three tube lengths (the "short" one which is 7.5 cm long, the "medium" one which is 15 cm long, and the "long" one which is 20 cm long). Once introduced into the rectum, the tube is maintained by a support fixed to the operating table. The TEO® can be mobilized during the intervention. This is important, as the working space is limited by the size and by the length of the tube and of the instruments.

Instrumentation is the same as that of conventional laparoscopic surgery, specific to the TEO® and the S-Portal® system (Karl Storz), especially long instruments and double-curved instruments with a rotating tip according to Leroy. Monopolar electrosurgery can be connected to any type of adapted instruments. We are also fond of the LigaSure™ Advance™ (Covidien, New Haven, CT, USA). This relies on two types of energy, known as "intelligent" monopolar and bipolar, which limits smoke production. The surgeon works in a seated position between the patient's legs with an assistant who will manipulate the TEO® in order to change its position during the surgical maneuver. Insufflation is performed by means of carbon dioxide. Light comes from a cold light source connected to the TEO®'s handle by a cable. The tip of the scope is angulated over 30° downward. It is a scope with a diameter of 5 mm. One of the advantages of the TEO® is the possibility to introduce a flexible operating endoscope (up to 2 cm in diameter) into the appropriate cup (e.g., a double-channel colonoscope or even the ISIS-SCOPE® (Karl Storz)), specifically designed for this kind of intervention. The camera used is a high-definition one (Image 1 Full HD, Karl Storz). It is connected to the scope itself and introduced into its support situated at the upper part of the cup fixed to the TEO®. There are two lengths (21 and 27 cm) of scope available. The 21 cm scope is used with the 7.5 and 15 cm TEO® and the 27 cm scope for the 20 cm TEO®. Any type of conventional laparoscope which can be introduced into one of the holes of the cup fixed to the TEO® can be used. Considering such options, choosing the soft cup of the silicone S-Port is better. Obtaining a clear visual field is one of the issues in such a confined operating space. It can be achieved by soft exsufflation controlled by means of a cannula introduced into one of the cup's holes.

28.3.2 Setup

All patients were administered our standard preoperative bowel preparation: 3–8 days of low-residue diet and admission one day prior to the operation with enemas given as inpatients. The step-by-step procedure has been previously published and described in detail [28]. Once the patient has been put under general anesthesia, he/she is placed supine in a lithotomy position, well strapped onto the electrically controlled operating table to allow for remote control changes in positioning. The patient's buttocks should extend slightly beyond the inferior edge of the table (Fig. 28.1c).

The final control monitoring screen is placed above the pubis in the visual axis of the operator.

For safety reasons, the different control panel elements (carbon dioxide pressure, carbon dioxide output, insufflated volume, power of used energies) should be visually and rapidly accessible to the operator.

The laparoscopic equipment should be prepared in the operating room in case of conversion or should a hybrid technique be required.

28.3.3 Dissection

Step 1 (Fig. 28.2a, b)—placing the purse-string suture

A purse-string suture is placed just distal to the tumor in order to prevent fecal and cancer cell contamination and to avoid colonic insufflation. The distal rectum is irrigated copiously with Betadine in an attempt to sterilize the distal anorectum.

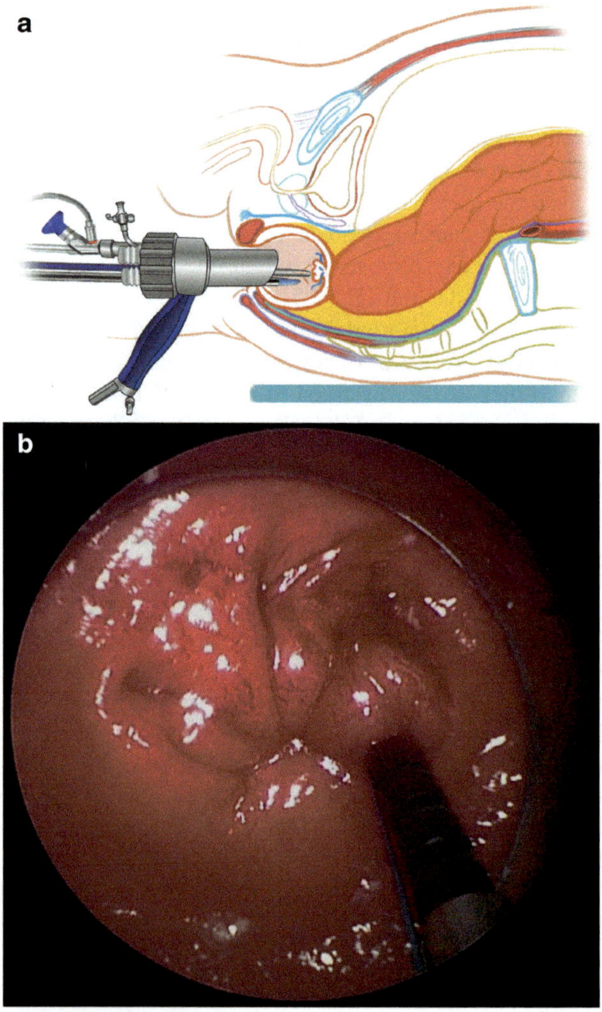

Fig. 28.2 (**a**) Placing the purse-string suture. (**b**) Placing the purse-string photo

Step 2 (Fig. 28.3a, b)—posterior rectal transection

The rectal mucosa is initially scored and then transected posteriorly from a 2 o'clock to a 10 o'clock position. The plane of dissection begins just posteriorly to the presacral fascia and is developed at a 6 o'clock position in the posterior midline. The pneumodissection performed using insufflation facilitates the identification of this space.

Step 3 (Fig. 28.4a, b)—extending rectal transection covering an area that spans from the 2 o'clock to 10 o'clock position posteriorly

It should be noted that the plane initially entered is not the "holy plane" described by Heald but rather the presacral space just posterior to the presacral fascia. Care must be taken to avoid going too posteriorly into the presacral veins. While entering the presacral space is initially quite straightforward, it becomes more challenging as progress is made more cranially and laterally.

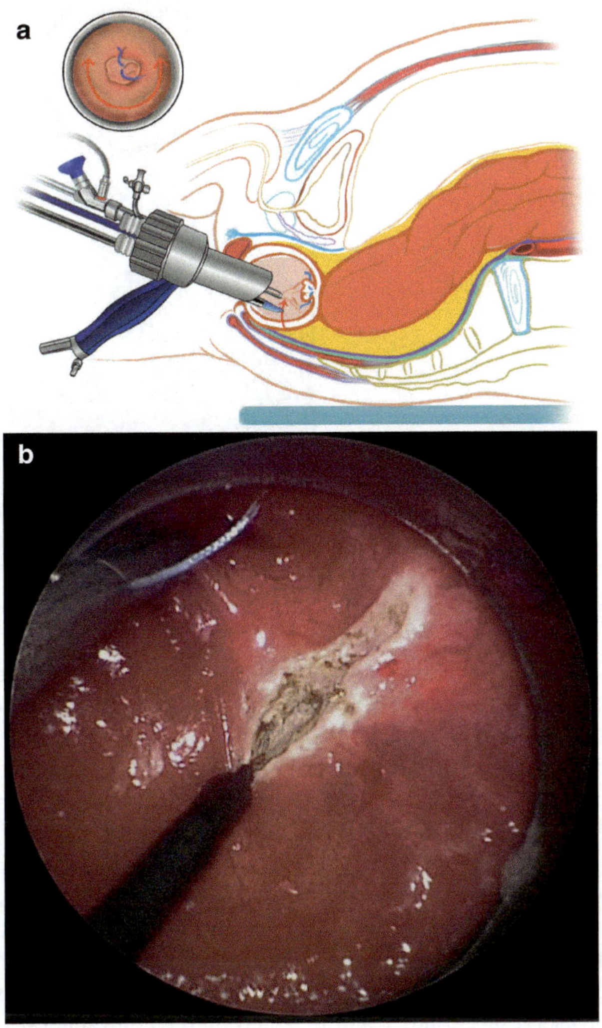

Fig. 28.3 (**a**) Posterior rectal transection. (**b**) Endoscopic view of posterior opening of the rectal wall

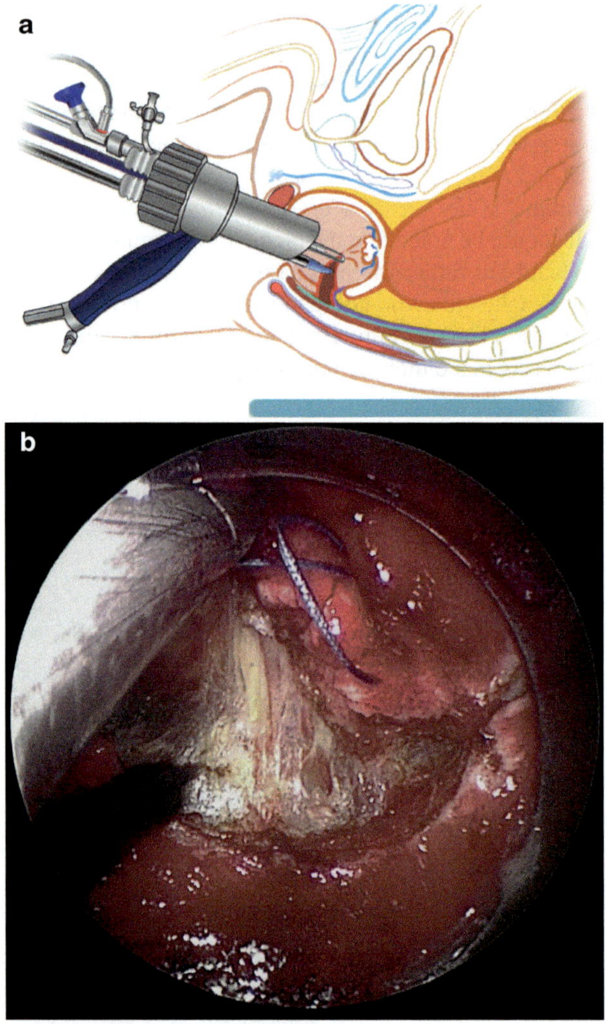

Fig. 28.4 (**a**) Extending rectal transection to the 2 o'clock–10 o'clock position posteriorly. (**b**) Extending rectal transection to the 2 o'clock–10 o'clock position posteriorly

Step 4 (Fig. 28.5)—entering the "holy plane"

Posteriorly, at the root of Waldeyer's fascia, the presacral fascia should be incised to open the space between the fascia propria of the mesorectum and the presacral fascia to enter the true "holy plane." The posterior dissection is continued proximally to the level of the sacral promontory. The TEO® device facilitates navigation in the presacral space by retracting the mesorectum anteriorly.

Step 5 (Fig. 28.6a–c)—extending the rectal dissection laterally

The presacral fascia is then incised laterally, and the surface of the lateral endopelvic fascia is followed as it curves medially. The nerves, lymphatics, and vascular branches crossing from the pelvic sidewall fascia to the fascia propria of the rectum are identified and divided. The middle rectal vessels are divided with the LigaSure™ (Covidien) vessel-sealing system. The lateral dissection is performed to the level of the sacral promontory and repeated on the contralateral side.

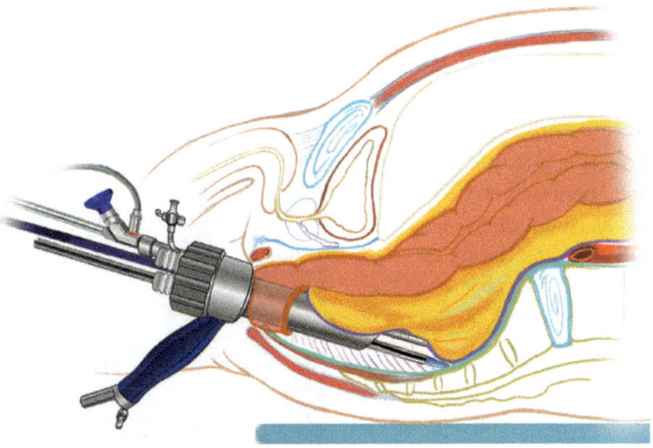

Fig. 28.5 Entering the "holy plane"

Step 6 (Fig. 28.7)—extending the rectal dissection anteriorly

Once the posterior and lateral dissection of the mesorectum has been completed, the remainder of the distal rectal transection is performed anteriorly from a 2 o'clock to a 10'clock position. The rectovaginal plane in women and the rectoprostatic plane in men are developed until the level of the peritoneal reflection.

Step 7 (Fig. 28.8)—developing the anterior plane and dividing the anterior peritoneal reflection

This maneuver reveals the rectouterine pouch (Douglas' pouch) in women and the rectovesicular pouch in men. As in transabdominal resections, this step is more difficult in men. In men with anterior lesions, Denonvilliers' fascia is kept on the mesorectum, and care is taken to prevent injury to the prostate, seminal vesicles, and urethra.

Step 8 (Figs. 28.9 and 28.10)—retracting the rectum toward the abdominal cavity

Once the anterior peritoneal reflection has been transected, the rectum is gently pushed cephalad into the peritoneal cavity. This results in tenting of the sigmoid mesentery and lateral peritoneal attachments.

Step 9 (Fig. 28.11)—extending the "holy plane" dissection toward the root of the mesosigmoid

The TEO® device is advanced through the viscerotomy toward the promontory by dissecting planes posteriorly. Care is taken to prevent injury to presacral veins posteriorly, to the mesorectal envelope medially, and to pelvic nerves, ureters, and distal branches of iliac vessels running laterally.

Step 10 (Fig. 28.12a–c)—identifying the origin of the inferior mesenteric artery

The "short" TEO® device is switched to a "long" 20 cm device. The retroperitoneal dissection of the mesorectum of the retroperitoneum is continued to reveal the origin of the inferior mesenteric artery (IMA). If desired for oncological purposes, a high ligation of the IMA is performed. Otherwise for benign lesions, a distal transection of the superior rectal artery is performed with the LigaSure™ (Covidien) vessel-sealing system.

Step 11 (Fig. 28.13a, b)—ligating the inferior mesenteric vessels

Distal or high divisions of the inferior mesenteric vessels are performed using the LigaSure™ (Covidien) system or clips.

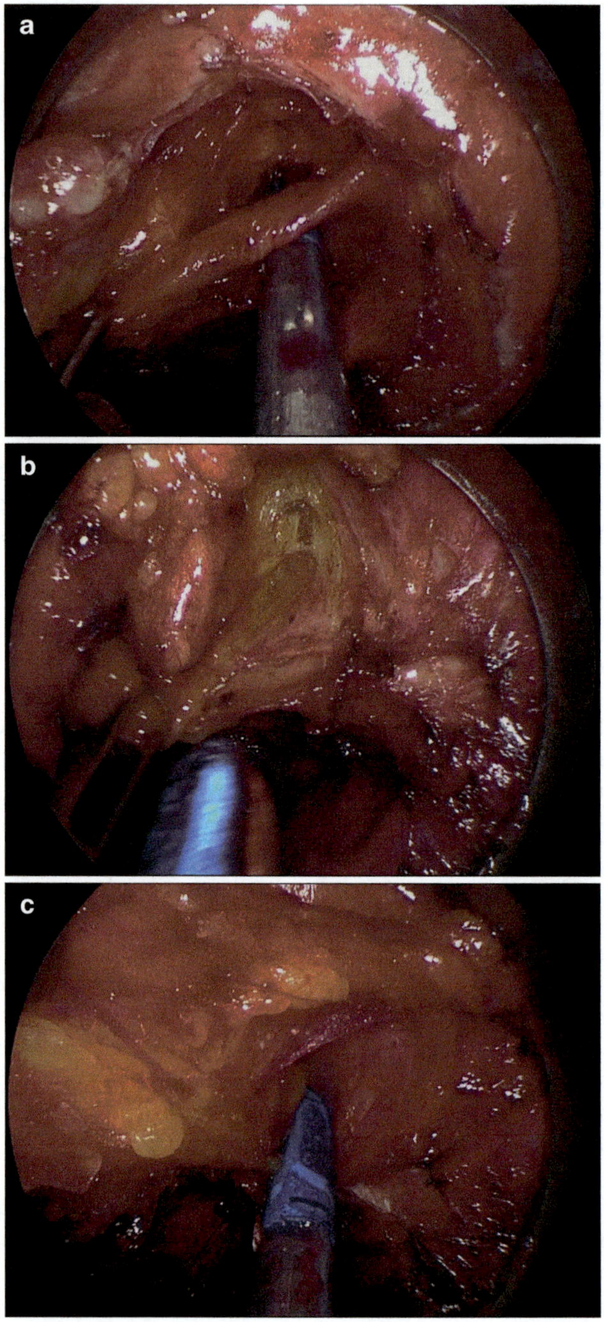

Fig. 28.6 (**a**) Extending the rectal dissection laterally: left mid-rectal artery isolated. (**b**) Extending the rectal dissection laterally: left rectal neurovegetative nerves isolated. (**c**) Extending the rectal dissection laterally: left rectal neurovegetative nerves division

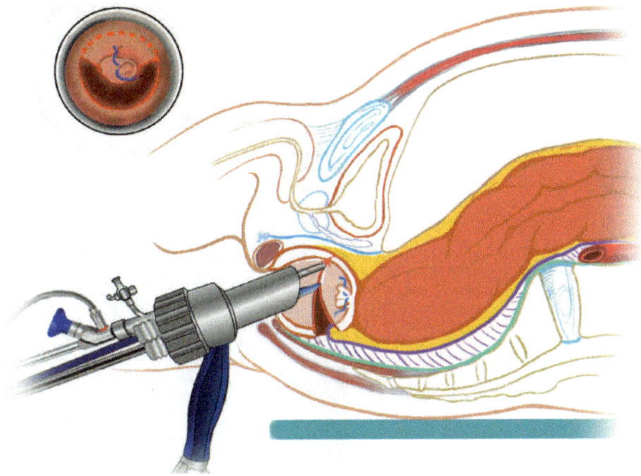

Fig. 28.7 Extending the rectal transection anteriorly

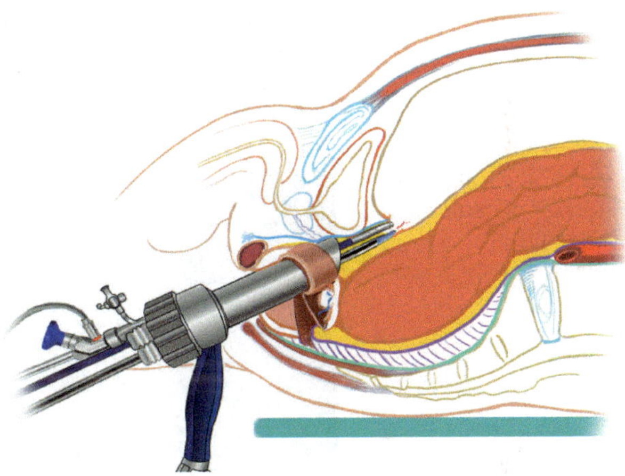

Fig. 28.8 Developing the anterior plane and dividing the anterior peritoneal reflection

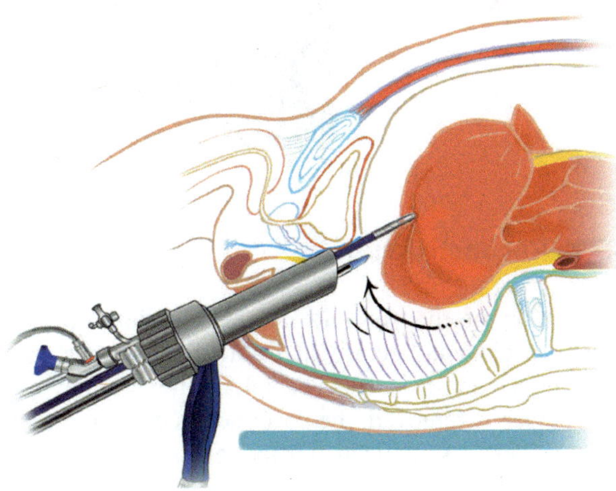

Fig. 28.9 Returning the rectum to the abdomen

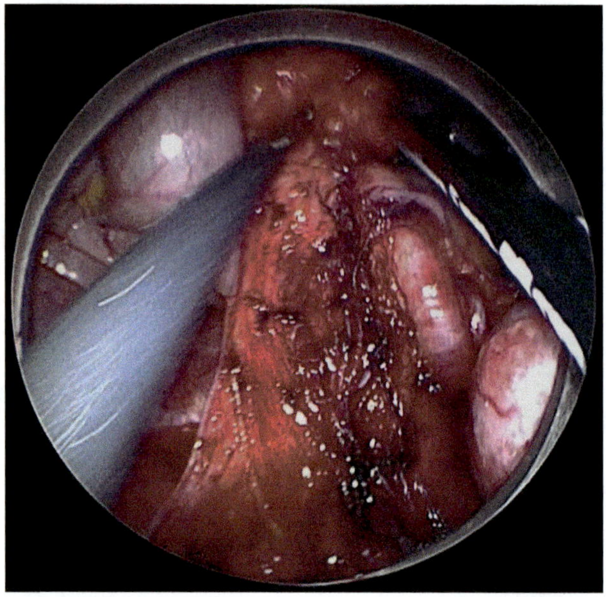

Fig. 28.10 Retracting the rectum toward the abdominal cavity

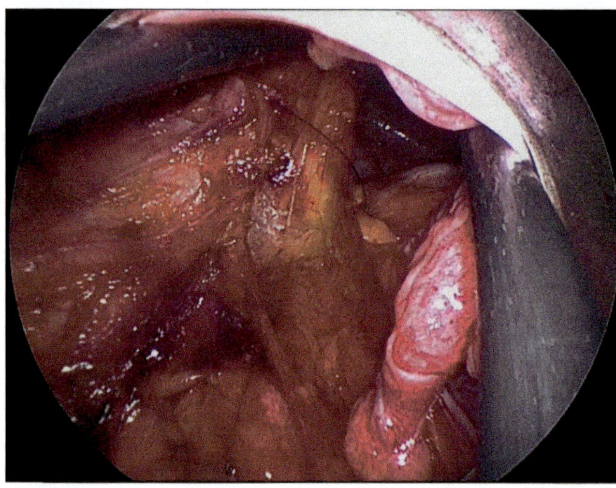

Fig. 28.11 Extending the "holy plane" dissection to the root of the mesosigmoid

28.3.4 Reconstruction

Mobilization of the sigmoid colon posteriorly off of the retroperitoneum and Gerota's fascia, and laterally at Toldt's fascia is performed as high as necessary for a tension-free anastomosis. The splenic flexure may be mobilized if required. The TEO® device is removed, the specimen is delivered transanally, and an appropriate proximal well-vascularized transection is chosen. The specimen is inspected for margins and to ensure the quality of the TME (Fig. 28.14).

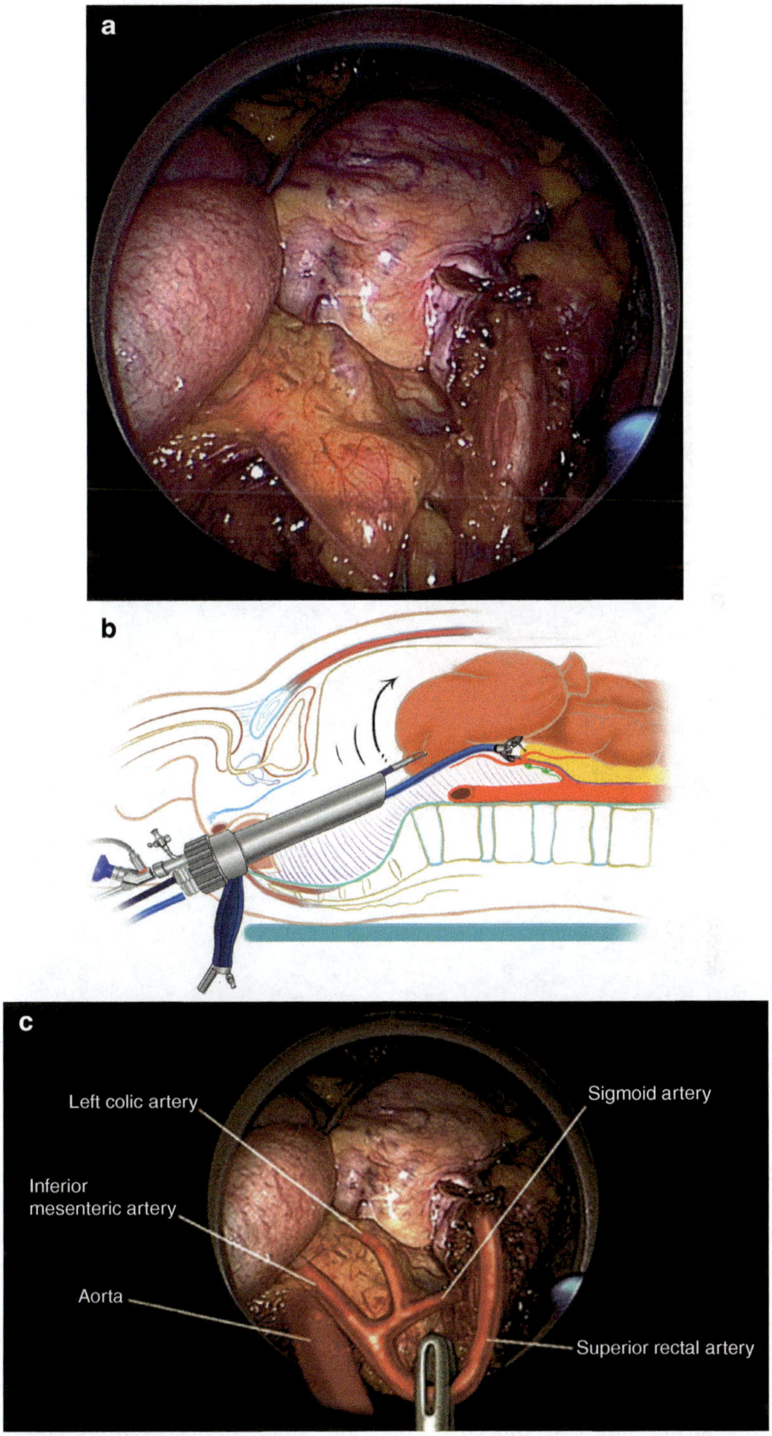

Fig. 28.12 (**a**) Intra abdominal identification of IMA trunk. (**b**) Retro-peritoneal identification of IMA. (**c**) Origin of IMA and branches

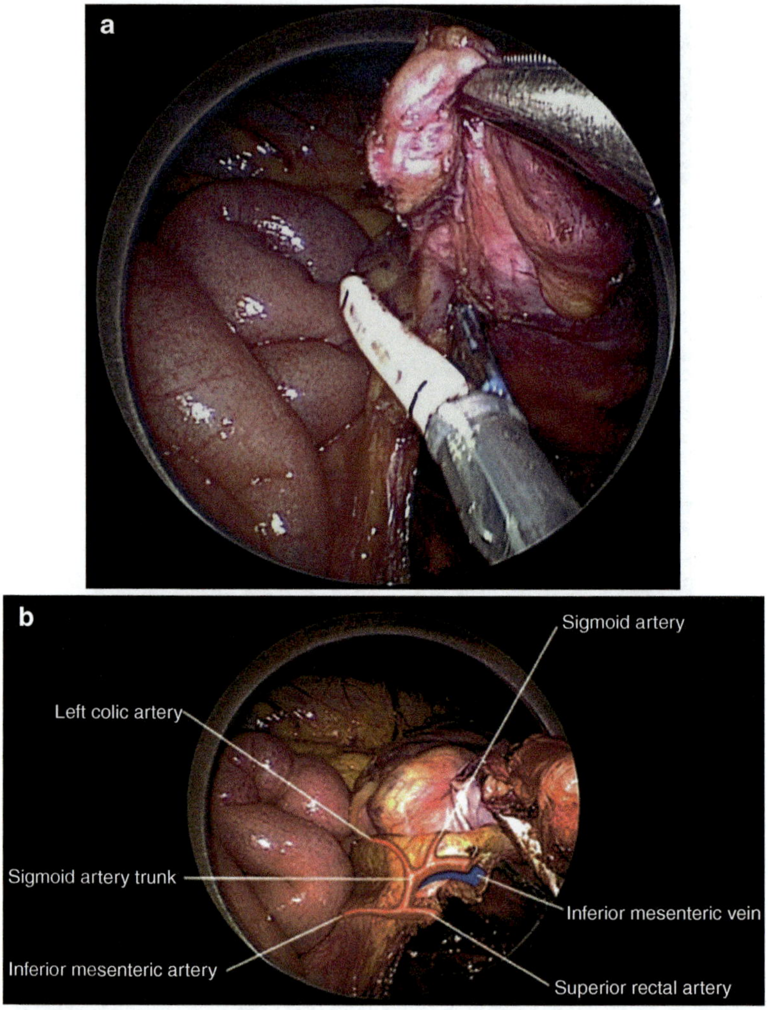

Fig. 28.13 (**a**) Distal division of IMV with LigasureTM. (**b**) Distal division IMA and Sigmoid artery trunk

The anastomosis may be an end-to-end or a side-to-end colorectal or colo-anal anastomosis. It can be stapled or hand-sewn depending on the clinical scenario.

In a side-to-end anastomosis, a colotomy is made just distal to the well-vascularized area of colon desired for the anastomosis. The spike of the anvil is pushed through the colotomy and brought out through the antimesenteric side of the proximal colon. The colon is then transected with a single firing of a linear stapling device, just distal to the anvil and proximal to the colotomy (Fig. 28.15).

A purse-string suture is placed around the spike of the anvil. A catheter is attached over the spike of the anvil to be used as a handle to prevent excessive retraction of the anvil cranially into the abdomen. The anvil is pushed back into the

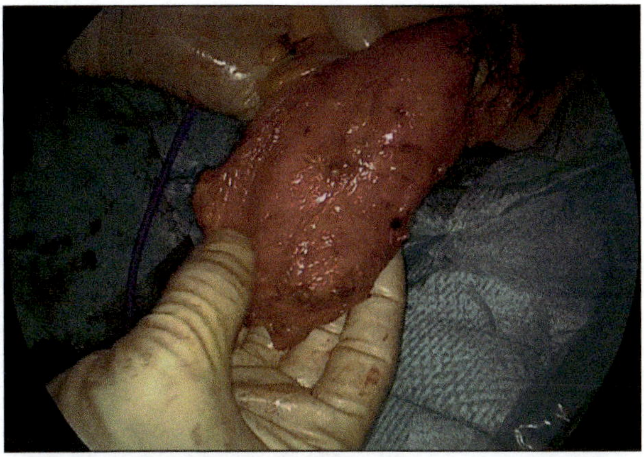

Fig. 28.14 Transanal specimen extraction

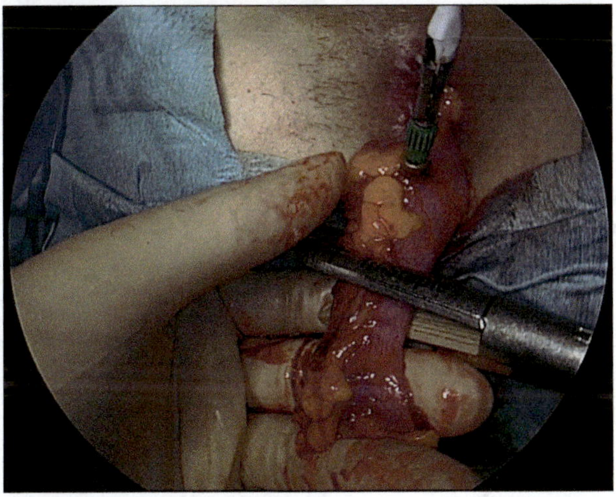

Fig. 28.15 Proximal preparation of mechanical anastomosis

pelvis and the short TEO® is reinserted. The pelvis is inspected for hemostasis, and orientation of the proximal bowel is controlled to ensure that it is not twisted. A purse-string suture is placed to close the orifice around the spike of the anvil. Prior to synching the purse-string suture, a drain is briefly advanced into the pelvis to evacuate any residual pneumoperitoneum. The catheter on the spike is removed, and the spike is maintained with a Kelly forceps. The circular stapler is inserted, connecting the spike to the anvil before performing the anastomosis and controlling it with endoscopy (Figs. 28.16, 28.17, and 28.18).

28.3.5 Postoperative care

Each patient followed our enhanced recovery after surgery (ERAS) protocol, and standard analgesia is offered (paracetamol and oral opiates). Sips of fluid are given on the evening of surgery and diet started the next day. Early patient mobilization is encouraged.

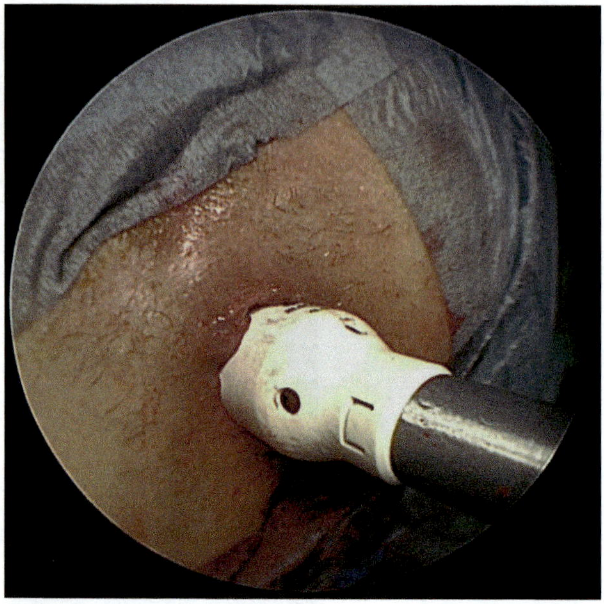

Fig. 28.16 Transanal circular mechanical anastomosis

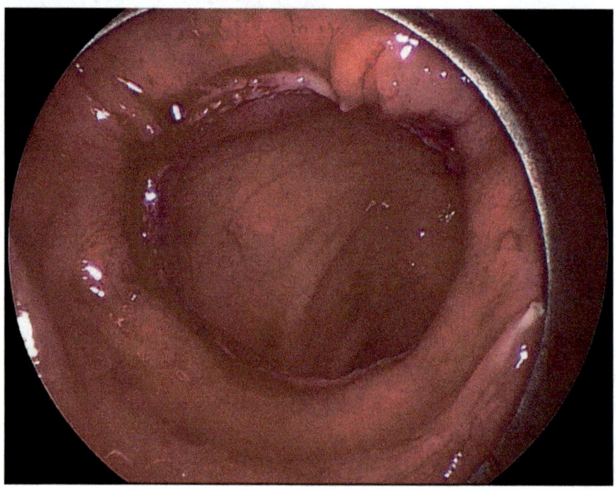

Fig. 28.17 End-to-end mechanical anastomosis

Conclusion

Performing a pure oncologic transanal NOTES TME with a retroperitoneal dissection is feasible. In our primary experience, a diverting stoma may be avoided in patients in whom there is no neoadjuvant radiochemotherapy.

Patient selection is highly important. The best indications for this approach are currently for early rectal cancers of the mid-rectum with or without neoadjuvant therapy and voluminous benign rectal tumors for which a complete endoscopic excision is impossible. Its current limitations seem to be locally advanced rectal and sigmoid cancer and obesity.

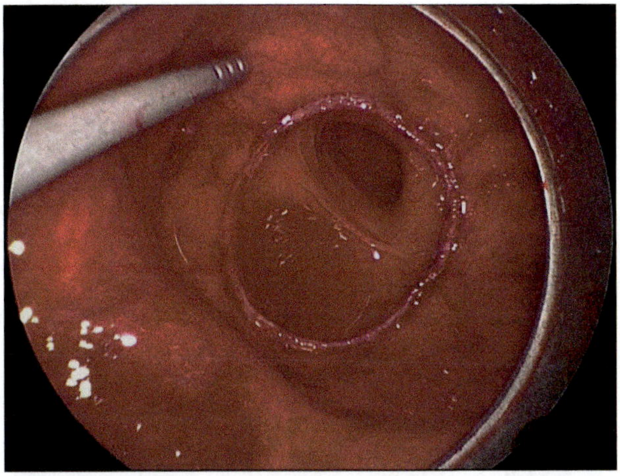

Fig. 28.18 Side-to-end mechanical anastomosis

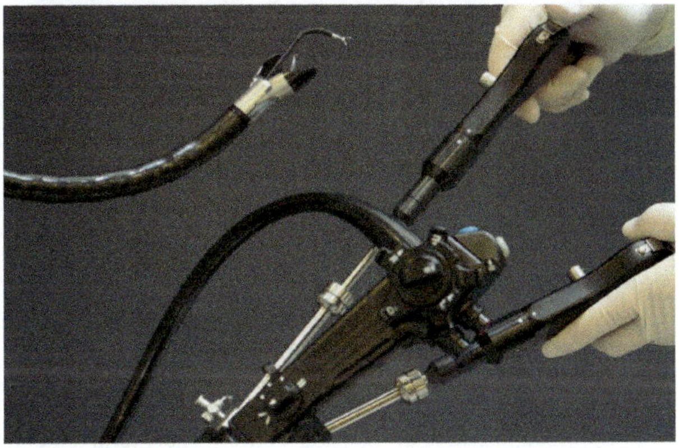

Fig. 28.19 Operative fibroscope solution by STORZ™: ISIS-Scope™

We recommend that it should be applied in specialized colorectal departments with highly skilled surgeons in laparoscopic colorectal and transanal dissection techniques.

Our team is currently working to enhance this procedure and to develop tools that may render it more accessible. In the near future, we hope to combine the PROGRESS procedure with augmented reality, in order to create an image-guided technique using flexible operative devices such as the ISIS-SCOPE® (Karl Storz) to reach the retrosplenic area more easily (Fig. 28.19).

References

1. Heald RJ, Husband EM, Ryall RD. The mesorectum in rectal cancer surgery--the clue to pelvic recurrence? Br J Surg. 1982;69(10):613–6.
2. Marks G, Mohiuddin M, Goldstein SD. Sphincter preservation for cancer of the distal rectum using high dose preoperative radiation. Int J Radiat Oncol Biol Phys. 1988;15(5):1065–8.

3. Marks J, Mizrahi B, Dalane S, Nweze I, Marks G. Laparoscopic transanal abdominal transanal resection with sphincter preservation for rectal cancer in the distal 3 cm of the rectum after neoadjuvant therapy. Surg Endosc. 2010;24(11):2700–7.
4. Tuech JJ, Karoui M, Lelong B, De Chaisemartin C, Bridoux V, Manceau G, et al. A step toward NOTES total mesorectal excision for rectal cancer: endoscopic transanal proctectomy. Ann Surg. 2015;261(2):228–33.
5. Zorron R, Phillips HN, Wynn G, Neto MP, Coelho D, Vassallo RC. "Down-to-Up" transanal NOTES Total mesorectal excision for rectal cancer: preliminary series of 9 patients. J Minim Access Surg. 2014;10(3):144–50.
6. Wolthuis AM. de Buck van Overstraeten A, D'Hoore A. Dynamic article: transanal rectal excision: a pilot study. Dis Colon Rectum. 2014;57(1):105–9.
7. Velthuis S, Nieuwenhuis DH, Ruijter TE, Cuesta MA, Bonjer HJ, Sietses C. Transanal versus traditional laparoscopic total mesorectal excision for rectal carcinoma. Surg Endosc. 2014;28(12):3494–9.
8. Delgado S, Fernandez M, Lacy AM. Laparoscopic-assisted total mesorectal resection through the transanal route. Cir Esp. 2014;92(Suppl 1):21–9.
9. Atallah S, Martin-Perez B, Albert M, deBeche-Adams T, Nassif G, Hunter L, et al. Transanal minimally invasive surgery for total mesorectal excision (TAMIS-TME): results and experience with the first 20 patients undergoing curative-intent rectal cancer surgery at a single institution. Tech Coloproctol. 2014;18(5):473–80.
10. Velthuis S, van den Boezem PB, van der Peet DL, Cuesta MA, Sietses C. Feasibility study of transanal total mesorectal excision. Br J Surg. 2013;100(6):828–31, discussion 31.
11. Sylla P, Bordeianou LG, Berger D, Han KS, Lauwers GY, Sahani DV, et al. A pilot study of natural orifice transanal endoscopic total mesorectal excision with laparoscopic assistance for rectal cancer. Surg Endosc. 2013;27(9):3396–405.
12. Rouanet P, Mourregot A, Azar CC, Carrere S, Gutowski M, Quenet F, et al. Transanal endoscopic proctectomy: an innovative procedure for difficult resection of rectal tumors in men with narrow pelvis. Dis Colon Rectum. 2013;56(4):408–15.
13. Han Y, He YG, Zhang HB, Lv KZ, Zhang YJ, Lin MB, et al. Total laparoscopic sigmoid and rectal surgery in combination with transanal endoscopic microsurgery: a preliminary evaluation in China. Surg Endosc. 2013;27(2):518–24.
14. de Lacy AM, Rattner DW, Adelsdorfer C, Tasende MM, Fernandez M, Delgado S, et al. Transanal natural orifice transluminal endoscopic surgery (NOTES) rectal resection: "down-to-up" total mesorectal excision (TME)--short-term outcomes in the first 20 cases. Surg Endosc. 2013;27(9):3165–72.
15. Zorron R, Phillips HN, Coelho D, Flach L, Lemos FB, Vassallo RC. Perirectal NOTES access: "down-to-up" total mesorectal excision for rectal cancer. Surg Innov. 2012;19(1):11–9.
16. Tuech JJ, Bridoux V, Kianifard B, Schwarz L, Tsilividis B, Huet E, et al. Natural orifice total mesorectal excision using transanal port and laparoscopic assistance. Eur J Surg Oncol. 2011;37(4):334–5.
17. Araujo SE, Seid VE, Horcel Lde A. Transanal endoscopic proctectomy: a case in swine. Hepatogastroenterology. 2014;61(130):333–5.
18. Leroy J, Diana M, Barry B, Mutter D, Melani AG, HS W, et al. Perirectal oncologic gateway to retroperitoneal endoscopic single-site surgery (PROGRESSS): a feasibility study for a new NOTES approach in a swine model. Surg Innov. 2012;19(4):345–52.
19. Trunzo JA, Delaney CP. Natural orifice proctectomy using a transanal endoscopic microsurgical technique in a porcine model. Surg Innov. 2010;17(1):48–52.
20. Sylla P, Sohn DK, Cizginer S, Konuk Y, Turner BG, Gee DW, et al. Survival study of natural orifice translumenal endoscopic surgery for rectosigmoid resection using transanal endoscopic microsurgery with or without transgastric endoscopic assistance in a swine model. Surg Endosc. 2010;24(8):2022–30.
21. Leroy J, Cahill RA, Perretta S, Forgione A, Dallemagne B, Marescaux J. Natural orifice translumenal endoscopic surgery (NOTES) applied totally to sigmoidectomy: an original technique with survival in a porcine model. Surg Endosc. 2009;23(1):24–30.

22. Sylla P, Willingham FF, Sohn DK, Gee D, Brugge WR, Rattner DW. NOTES rectosigmoid resection using transanal endoscopic microsurgery (TEM) with transgastric endoscopic assistance: a pilot study in swine. J Gastrointest Surg. 2008;12(10):1717–23.
23. Telem DA, Han KS, Kim MC, Ajari I, Sohn DK, Woods K, et al. Transanal rectosigmoid resection via natural orifice translumenal endoscopic surgery (NOTES) with total mesorectal excision in a large human cadaver series. Surg Endosc. 2013;27(1):74–80.
24. Rieder E, Spaun GO, Khajanchee YS, Martinec DV, Arnold BN, Smith Sehdev AE, et al. A natural orifice transrectal approach for oncologic resection of the rectosigmoid: an experimental study and comparison with conventional laparoscopy. Surg Endosc. 2011;25(10):3357–63.
25. Whiteford MH, Denk PM, Swanstrom LL. Feasibility of radical sigmoid colectomy performed as natural orifice translumenal endoscopic surgery (NOTES) using transanal endoscopic microsurgery. Surg Endosc. 2007;21(10):1870–4.
26. Chouillard E, Chahine E, Khoury G, Vinson-Bonnet B, Gumbs A, Azoulay D, et al. NOTES total mesorectal excision (TME) for patients with rectal neoplasia: a preliminary experience. Surg Endosc. 2014;28(11):3150–7.
27. Zhang H, Zhang YS, Jin XW, Li MZ, Fan JS, Yang ZH. Transanal single-port laparoscopic total mesorectal excision in the treatment of rectal cancer. Tech Coloproctol. 2013;17(1):117–23.
28. Leroy J, Barry BD, Melani A, Mutter D, Marescaux J. No-scar transanal total mesorectal excision: the last step to pure NOTES for colorectal surgery. JAMA Surg. 2013;148(3):226–30, discussion 31.
29. Marks JH, Lopez-Acevedo N, Krishnan B, Johnson MN, Montenegro GA, Marks GJ. True NOTES TME resection with splenic flexure release, high ligation of IMA, and side-to-end hand-sewn colonal anastomosis. Surg Endsoc. 2016;30:4626–31.
30. Hideo Y. Laparoscopic colectomy using retroperitoneal approach method. Gastroenterologic Surg. 2004;27(6):861–9.

Transanal Robot-Assisted TME with Multiport Abdominal Laparoscopy

29

Vikram Attaluri and Elisabeth C. McLemore

Abstract

Transanal total mesorectal excision (taTME) is a "bottom-up" rather than "top-down" approach to radical proctectomy for rectal cancer. The surgical tools utilized to perform taTME continue to evolve. This chapter will review the robotic technical approach to performing taTME and summarize the published experience to date. Lastly, the perceived benefits and drawbacks associated with robotic taTME will be discussed.

Keywords

Rectal cancer • Total mesorectal excision • Transanal TME • taTME • Robotic

29.1 Introduction

Transanal total mesorectal excision (taTME) is the latest advancement in the minimally invasive surgical approach to restorative proctectomy with TME for rectal cancer [1–3]. The taTME technique builds upon the foundation of the transabdominal-transanal (TATA) approach developed by Gerald and John Marks [1] and was pioneered by leaders in natural orifice surgery (NOS), Patricia Sylla and Antonio Lacy [3]. The taTME technique has many potential advantages, including improved precision of the distal rectal transection, accuracy in determining the distal margin length, and improved visibility during the total mesorectal excision (TME) dissection, especially in the distal third of the rectum [4].

V. Attaluri, M.D., F.A.C.S. • E.C. McLemore, M.D., F.A.C.S., F.A.S.C.R.S. (✉)
Colon and Rectal Surgery, Department of Surgery, Kaiser Permanente Los Angeles Medical Center, 4760 Sunset Blvd, 3rd Floor, Los Angeles, CA 90027, USA
e-mail: Elisabeth.C.McLemore@kp.org

G. Dapri, J.H. Marks (eds.), *Surgical Techniques in Rectal Cancer*,
https://doi.org/10.1007/978-4-431-55579-7_29

From a transabdominal approach, the distal third of the TME dissection can be the most challenging portion of the operation. Robotic-assisted surgery in the deep pelvis has significantly improved the surgeon's subjective impression of dexterity and visibility. However, the working space in the deep pelvis can be on the order of millimeters in size, even when using a robotic platform. The technical difficulty and challenges can be high, especially in a narrow, male pelvis as well as in patients with morbid obesity.

Multiple transanal access devices are being utilized and evaluated for taTME dissection and are similar to the currently available platforms used when performing transanal endoscopic surgery (TES) [5]. The three most widely utilized transanal access platforms include rigid platforms (transanal endoscopic microsurgery, TEM, Richard Wolf Medical Instruments Corporation, Vernon Hills, IL 60061; transanal endoscopic operation, TEO, KARL STORZ GmbH & Co., Tuttlingen, Germany) and disposable platforms (GelPOINT Path, Applied Medical, Rancho Santa Margarita, CA; SILS™ port, Covidien, Mansfield, MA). The rigid platforms and disposable platforms all have their advantages and disadvantages. In addition, the robotic single-port surgery platform and the second-, third-, and fourth-generation robotic platforms (Da Vinci® robot, Intuitive Surgical, Inc., Sunnyvale, CA, USA) have been employed to perform robotic-assisted taTME [6]. To date, there is not a transanal access platform or device that has been specifically designed to perform taTME. Instead, transanal access devices utilized for TES as well as robotic instrumentation are being utilized to perform the taTME dissection.

The potential benefits of a robotic taTME approach include improved operator control of the visualized fields and instrumentation through the use of stereotactic cameras and robotic arm controls at the surgeon operator console. In addition, there is a greater degree of instrument rotation with the second–fourth-generation robotic instrumentation that may afford improved ease of access and dissection in the limited working space in the deep pelvis. Another potential benefit is the improved ergonomics and working space for the surgeon within the confines of the robotic surgeon console rather than the confines of the lithotomy position. However, it is difficult to perform a simultaneous transabdominal and transanal TME with the current robotic patient carts. This is the main limitation of a robotic approach compared to the other platforms currently being utilized for taTME at this time. However, robotic- and computer-assisted surgical technology continues to rapidly evolve, and transanal robotic platforms specifically designed for TES and taTME are expectant in the near future which may allow for simultaneous robotic transabdominal and transanal dissection to be performed [7].

The robotic-assisted taTME technique is currently being evaluated in select tertiary referral centers, and various approaches are under investigation. The robotic platform has been utilized to perform both the abdominal and pelvic dissection in the same patient, abdominal dissection only, and pelvic dissection only. Atallah from the USA, Ruiz from Spain, and Verheijen from the Netherlands have published their preliminary experience [7–9]. While only a limited number of cases have been reported in the literature to date, the technical approach has been described by these authors and is summarized in the following section.

29.2 Patient Selection and Surgical Technique

29.2.1 Spain Experience

Ruiz et al. described their approach with five patients during 2013 and 2014. Eligible patients were those patients with T2 or T3 rectal cancer including N0 or N1 disease. Stage 3 patients underwent standard neoadjuvant chemoradiation with 50.4 Gy and capecitabine followed by surgery 8 weeks later. Only tumors within 10 cm from the anal verge on rigid proctoscopy and 1 cm from the anorectal ring were considered eligible. Patients older than 70 years and those with extensive prior abdominal or pelvic surgery were excluded.

The procedure begins with the robotic patient cart docked over the left side of the patient for the transabdominal dissection. After transection of the inferior mesenteric vein and artery and complete mobilization of the left colon from the splenic flexure down to the sacral promontory, the robotic patient cart is undocked. The patient is placed in Trendelenburg position and right side down for the transanal portion. The robotic patient cart is then docked (Fig. 29.1). Distal rectal transection is initiated at least 1 cm below the tumor, with partial intersphincteric resection for tumors at 3 cm from the anal verge (Fig. 29.2). After extending the dissection for 1–2 cm, the lumen is occluded with a purse-string suture. Ruiz et al. utilize the "transanal access port" proctoscope (PAT, Developia-HUMV, Santander, Spain) and a GelPOINT Path (Applied Medical, Rancho Santa Margarita, CA) system (Fig. 29.3). Through the GelPOINT Path, a four-port approach is used: robotic camera, two robotic ports, and a 12 mm assistant port. Monopolar scissors are used to perform the TME dissection. The assistant port is primarily used for suction and retraction. Simultaneous laparoscopic assistance is utilized during the robotic taTME dissection. Once dissection is complete, the specimen is extracted through an Alexis wound retractor (Applied Medical, Rancho Santo Margarita, CA). Depending on the distance from the anal verge, a hand-sewn or double-purse-string stapled anastomosis is performed. A pelvic drain and diverting loop ileostomy are utilized [8].

29.2.2 US Experience

Atallah et al. published their experience of three patients in 2013. Selected patients had rectal cancer in the lower third of the rectum (5 cm of anal verge). The abdominal portion including splenic flexure mobilization and high ligation of the inferior mesenteric vein and artery is performed and completed first using a laparoscopic

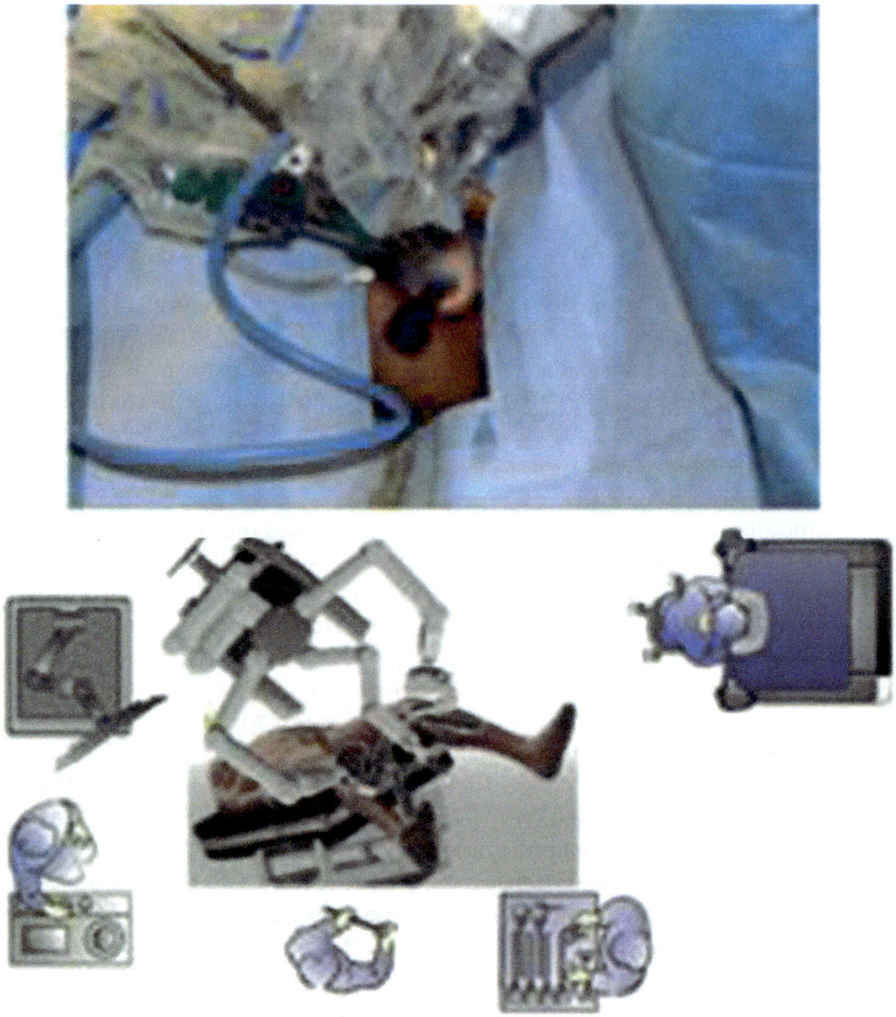

Fig. 29.1 Robotic patient cart: left-side docking

approach. Distal rectal transection is initiated, and the distal rectum is closed with a purse-string suture. taTME dissection is carried out using manual cautery for circumferential distal rectal transection followed by placement of the transanal access platform. The robotic patient cart is then docked via the GelPOINT Path transanal access platform (Fig. 29.4). The preferred taTME dissection approach is to start with the posterior and lateral dissection first before completing the anterior dissection and entering the peritoneum through the anterior side. Lastly, the specimen is extracted through a Pfannenstiel incision prior to performing a hand-sewn colorectal anastomosis [7, 10].

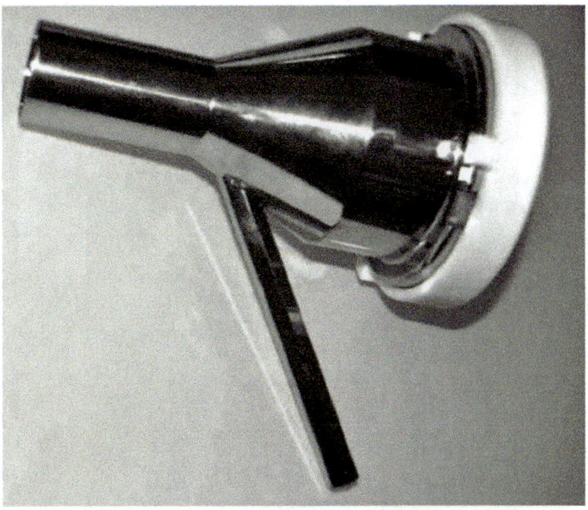

Fig. 29.2 Transanal Port/Access [8]

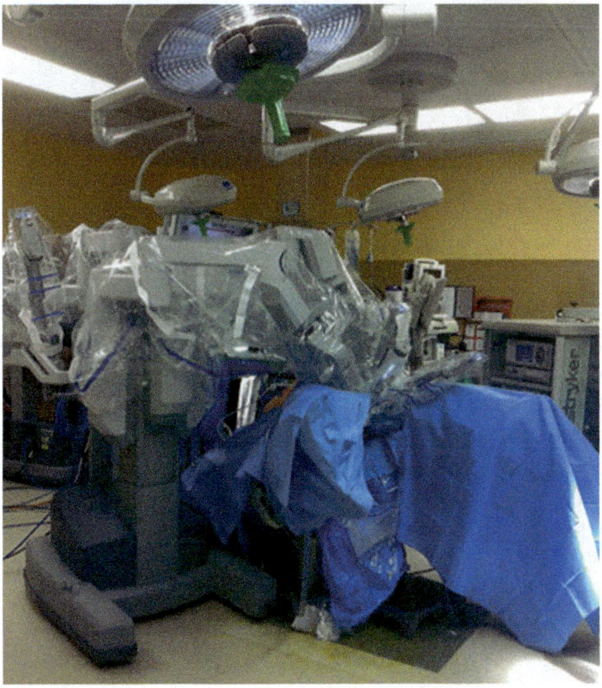

Fig. 29.3 Robotic patient cart: right side docking [8]

29.2.3 Netherlands Experience

Verheijen et al. published their experience with their initial robotic taTME in 2014. The patient was a 48-year-old woman with a circumferential T3N2 rectal located 8 cm from the anal verge. The patient underwent preoperative chemoradiotherapy with 50.4 Gy and capecitabine for 6 weeks. The abdominal portion was performed

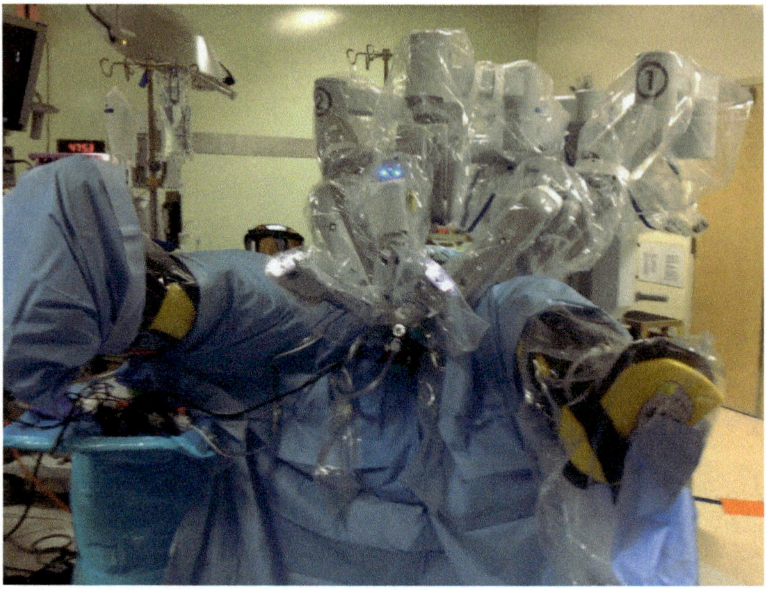

Fig. 29.4 Specialized transanal port [10]

first, similar to prior reports, and included laparoscopic splenic flexure mobilization, and high ligation of the inferior mesenteric vein and artery is performed and completed first using four 5 mm trocars. The GelPOINT Path was placed transanally. The robotic patient cart was docked on the left side of the patient. Three 8.5 mm robotic ports were utilized and one 5 mm assistant port. An 8.5 mm camera was utilized. Pneumorectum was created and the tumor was identified. A purse-string suture was placed 2 cm distal to the rectal cancer. The rectal wall was then transected circumferentially with monopolar diathermy followed by robotic taTME dissection. The specimen was extracted through the anus. A double-purse-string end-to-end circular stapler was utilized to create the anastomosis. A diverting loop ileostomy was created as well [9].

29.2.4 Demographic and Perioperative Data

The age of the patients in the groups ranged from 26 to 67 years old. Whereas all of the patients from Ruiz were cT2N1 or cT2N0, Atallah's series included two patients with cT4N1 disease. Operative time ranged from 270 to 440 min, with transanal time ranging from 39 to 190 min. Blood loss ranged from 25 to 300 cm^3 (Table 29.1). There were no conversions to open operation. All surgical margins were negative, but two out of three patients with TME grade available had a grade of 2. Postoperative complications include high-output ileostomy, pulmonary embolus, and one anastomotic leak. Mean length of stay was 5.4 days. Not all patients had undergone ileostomy reversal at time of publication (Table 29.2).

Table 29.1 Patient characteristics and operative data

Patient	Age	Sex	BMI	Clinical stage	Distance from AV (cm)	Operative time (min)	Abdominal time	taTME time	EBL	Intraoperative complications	Anastomosis
MR1	55	M	26	cT2N1	4	370	120	130	120	None	Handsewn
MR2	57	M	31	cT2N1	6	440	110	100	100	None	Stapled
MR3	38	F	25	cT2N1	4	270	82	39	35	None	Handsewn
MR4	67	M	26	cT2N1	6	343	150	130	25	None	Stapled
MR5	46	M	22	Dysplasia T2N0	5	450	80	190	100	None	Stapled
SA1	51	F	36	cT4N1	3	380	*	*	200	*	*
SA2	59	M	38.5	cT4N2	5	409	*	*	300	*	*
SA3	26	M	21	pT1Nx	4	339	*	*	100	*	*
SA4	41	M	21	cT3N2	2	140	*	*	50	*	*
PV1	48	F	23.6	cT3N1	8	205	*	65		*	*

MR = Ruiz et al.
SA = Atallah et al.
PV = Verheigen
* = data not available

Table 29.2 Postoperative and pathologic data

Patient	LOS	Pathology	Distal margin (mm)	CRM	TME grade	Lymph nodes	Complication
MR1	7	Complete response	10	Negative	*	7	None
MR2	6	ypT2N0	15	Negative	*	29	Anastomotic leak
MR3	5	ypT3N1b	10	Negative	*	17	None
MR4	7	ypTisN0	30	Negative	*	5	None
MR5	5	dysplasia	25	Negative	*	12	None
SA1	4	ypT2N0	*	Negative	2	35	Pulmonary embolus
SA2	5	ypT2N1	10	Negative	2	18	Dehydration from ileostomy
SA3	4	pT1N0	*	Negative	1	39	None
SA4	5	ypT3N2		Negative	2	15	None
PV1	3	Complete response	20	Negative	*	*	None

MR = Ruiz et al.
SA = Atallah et al.
PV = Verheigen
* = data not available

Conclusion

Hompes has described robotic taTME as the possible "sweet spot for robotics in colorectal surgery" [11]. Compared to other transanal access platforms currently utilized to perform taTME, the robotic taTME approach requires a major capital investment and annual service maintenance fee in the robotic patient cart, surgeon console, and robotic equipment. This has remained one of the major impediments to universal acceptance of this platform for a wider variety of surgical procedures. In addition, the robotic platform adds to the cost of the disposable transanal access platform, as the currently available robotic platform requires a transanal access port in order to perform the robotic taTME dissection.

The bulky nature of the current robotic patient carts also makes it difficult to perform surgery from the transabdominal top-down and transanal bottom-up approach simultaneously, thereby eliminating one of the potential benefits of reduced operative time associated with the taTME approach. This would result in potentially longer operative times as well as increased overall operative costs. Other potential drawbacks to a robotic approach relate to the nature of transanal endoscopic surgery, which is similar to single-port surgery. Limited maneuverability may result in the robotic patient cart arms interfering and colliding with each other. Similarly for the camera, as the robotic camera cannot rotate 360°, one may need to remove and reposition the camera to move the dissection from the posterior aspect to the anterior aspect. However, despite these potential drawbacks and limitations of the robotic platform, the ergonomics, motion scaling, and instrumentation with multiple degrees of freedom remain attractive features

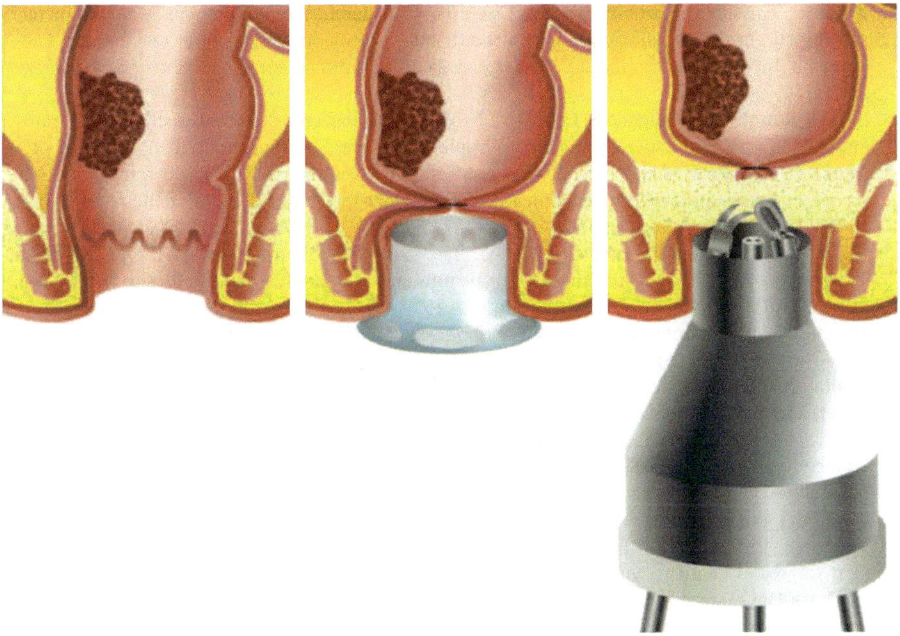

Fig. 29.5 Specialized transanal port [8]

unique to the robotic platform and are ideal features when working in a confined space such as the pelvis.

At this time, the published robotic taTME results include only small series or case reports. Vital information is lacking in some of these reported cases, namely, the quality of the TME specimen. Currently, taTME is an investigational minimally invasive technique for performing restorative radical proctectomy for rectal cancer. The current technique of complete abdominal splenic flexure mobilization and high ligation of the inferior mesenteric vein and artery first followed by taTME pelvic dissection alone or in combination with an abdominal approach appears to be the most widely accepted practice in published reports. Robotic- and computer-assisted surgical technology continues to rapidly evolve, and a transanal robotic platform specifically designed for TES and taTME is expected in the near future which may allow for simultaneous robotic transabdominal and transanal TME dissection. The key operative finding, regardless of the technique, is the quality of the TME dissection and specimen TME grade in addition to margin status and lymph node harvest, which should be reported in any new technical approach to radical proctectomy with TME for rectal cancer (Fig. 29.5).

References

1. Marks JH, Frenkel JL, D'Andrea AP, Greenleaf CE. Maximizing rectal cancer results: TEM and TATA techniques to expand sphincter preservation. Surg Oncol Clin N Am. 2011;20(3):501–20. viii–ix

2. Marks J, Nassif G, Schoonyoung H, DeNittis A, Zeger E, Mohiuddin M, et al. Sphincter-sparing surgery for adenocarcinoma of the distal 3 cm of the true rectum: results after neoadjuvant therapy and minimally invasive radical surgery or local excision. Surg Endosc. 2013;27(12):4469–77.
3. Sylla P, Rattner DW, Delgado S, Lacy AM. NOTES transanal rectal cancer resection using transanal endoscopic microsurgery and laparoscopic assistance. Surg Endosc. 2010;24(5):1205–10.
4. Marks J, Mizrahi B, Dalane S, Nweze I, Marks G. Laparoscopic transanal transabdominal resection with sphincter preservation for rectal cancer in the distal 3 cm of the rectum after neoadjuvant therapy. Surg Endosc. 2010;24(11):2700–7.
5. McLemore EC, Weston LA, Coker AM, Jacobsen GR, Talamini MA, Horgan S, et al. Transanal minimally invasive surgery for benign and malignant rectal neoplasia. Am J Surg. 2014;208(3):372–81.
6. Huscher CGS, Bretagnol F, Ponzano C. Robotic-assisted Transanal Total Mesorectal Excision. Ann Surg. 2015;261(5):e120–1.
7. Atallah S, Nassif G, Polavarapu H, deBeche-Adams T, Ouyang J, Albert M, et al. Robotic-assisted transanal surgery for total mesorectal excision (RATS-TME): a description of a novel surgical approach with video demonstration. Tech Coloproctol. 2013;17(4):441–7.
8. Gómez Ruiz M, Parra IM, Palazuelos CM, Martín JA, Fernández CC, Diego JC, et al. Robotic-assisted laparoscopic transanal total mesorectal excision for rectal cancer. Dis Colon Rectum. 2015;58(1):145–53.
9. Verheijen PM, Consten ECJ, Broeders IAMJ. Robotic transanal total mesorectal excision for rectal cancer: experience with a first case. Int J Med Robot Comput Assist Surg. 2014;10(4):423–6.
10. Atallah S, Martin-Perez B, Parra-Davila E, deBeche-Adams T, Nassif G, Albert M, et al. Robotic transanal surgery for local excision of rectal neoplasia, transanal total mesorectal excision, and repair of complex fistulae: clinical experience with the first 18 cases at a single institution. Tech Coloproctol. 2015;19(7):401–10.
11. Hompes R. Robotics and transanal minimal invasive surgery (TAMIS): the "'sweet spot'" for robotics in colorectal surgery? Tech Coloproctol. 2015;19(7):377–8.

Transanal Robot-Assisted TME with Reduced Port Abdominal Laparoscopy

30

Teresa deBeche-Adams, Matthew Albert, and John Burke

Abstract

Total mesorectal excision (TME) remains the gold standard in the curative surgical treatment of rectal cancer. The principle of performing a TME, obtaining a complete and intact mesorectal envelope with a negative circumferential resection margin (CRM), is the greatest predictor of locoregional control. Technical challenges to minimally invasive techniques for proctectomy leading to high conversion rates, increased operative times, and inferior pathological outcomes have prompted the development of alternative approaches. Transanal TME (TaTME) has recently evolved in the last decade as a technique in which TME is performed utilizing a perineal approach. Precise definition of the distal resection margin, clarity of lower third and anterior rectal mobilization, and ease in obese and male patients are the proposed advantages. Following the description of transanal minimally invasive surgery (TAMIS), robotic TAMIS was soon reported. Synthesis of these techniques led to the performance of robotic TaTME. Robotic TaTME with single-port abdominal colonic mobilization via the required temporary ostomy site represents an innovative, minimally invasive technique for performing curative proctectomy for rectal cancer. This technique represents advancement in the evolution of natural orifice transluminal endoscopic surgery (NOTES) for the treatment of rectal cancer, which adheres to the principle tenants of oncologic surgery.

T. deBeche-Adams, M.D. (✉) • M. Albert, M.D. (✉)
Department of Colorectal Surgery, Florida Hospital, Orlando, FL, USA

Center for Colon and Rectal Surgery, Florida Hospital,
2415 N. Orange Ave, Suite 300, Orlando, FL 32804-5505, USA
e-mail: debeche.adams@gmail.com; matthew.albert.md@flhosp.org

J. Burke, M.D., Ph.D.
Department of Colorectal Surgery, Florida Hospital, Orlando, FL, USA

General and Colorectal Surgery, Beaumont Hospital, Dublin, Ireland

G. Dapri, J.H. Marks (eds.), *Surgical Techniques in Rectal Cancer*,
https://doi.org/10.1007/978-4-431-55579-7_30

Keywords
Transanal TME • Robotic transanal surgery • Robotic transanal TME Single-port laparoscopy

Key Points

- Transanal total mesorectal excision (TaTME) is an approach developed for the treatment of benign and malignant conditions of the rectum, where TME is performed from a transanal approach in a "down-to-up" fashion.
- Although TaTME has been performed and reported completely utilizing a pure "NOTES" approach with transanal left colon and splenic flexure mobilization, traditionally it is performed with abdominal assistance using multiport laparoscopy since fecal diversion is usually required.
- Single-incision laparoscopy for left colon and splenic flexure mobilization is an ideal approach for TaTME where abdominal single-port access can be positioned at the future stoma site in the right lower quadrant.
- Robotic transanal surgery was initially described in 2009 for the endoluminal resection of benign and malignant rectal tumors.
- Robotic TaTME has been demonstrated in small case series to be an effective modality for performing proctectomy with improved access to the pelvis, the goal being achieving a completely intact mesorectal specimen.
- Currently, experience in robotic transanal surgery remains somewhat limited due to incompatible transanal ports combined with ongoing technical challenges including instrument conflict, exterior arm collisions, as well as the need for additional transanal assistance for a third working port.
- Single-port robots will likely provide an improved platform for multi-instrument dissection under three-dimensional visualization to deliver optimal transanal access for complex rectal surgery.

30.1 Introduction to Robotic Transanal Total Mesorectal Excision

Total mesorectal excision (TME) is the criterion standard treatment for the management of rectal cancer [1], and surgical quality has a direct impact on local control and survival [2, 3]. In the pathological assessment of rectal cancer specimens, the circumferential resection margin (CRM) and the plane of surgery achieved have been demonstrated to be independent predictors of local recurrence [4, 5]. Despite the advances in operative approach and neoadjuvant treatment, contemporary CRM positivity rates have reached a nadir of approximately 10% [2, 6]. Risk factors for a positive CRM include advanced T stage [7], male sex, and large tumor size [8]. In the setting of laparoscopic proctectomy for rectal cancer, male gender, high body mass index (BMI), visceral obesity, and a narrow pelvis predict intraoperative difficulty [9], which in turn is associated with local recurrence [10]. But even in experienced hands, TME can be challenging in a male patient with visceral obesity, increasing the risk of incomplete mesorectal excision. Since the introduction of laparoscopic resection techniques, the adoption rate of this approach has remained low with high rates of conversion to open laparotomy because of the unique challenges of laparoscopic pelvic dissection [11]. While randomized multicenter trials comparing laparoscopic with open approaches for rectal cancer treatment have shown short-term advantages to laparoscopic surgery [6, 12], recent data has demonstrated that from the perspective of specimen quality, laparoscopic surgery is not non-inferior to open surgery [13, 14]. These anatomic and technical challenges have led to the investigation of performing TME not only from an abdominal approach but also utilizing transanal mobilization, termed transanal TME or TaTME.

TaTME is not a novel concept as approaching rectal mobilization transanally for cancer was first reported 30 years ago by Gerald Marks [15]. However, recent data suggests it may be an oncologically superior approach [16]. Following an initial cadaveric description using a transanal endoscopic microsurgery (TEM) platform to mobilize the rectum [17], several case reports emerged using this technique to perform proctectomy for rectal cancer [18, 19]. As transanal access platforms became more accessible and interest in the perceived benefits of this approach grew, several centers began assessing the safety of this technique for the resection of low rectal cancer [20–24]. This approach has been suggested to enhance distal rectal access and visualization [25, 26] and improve resection quality by allowing optimal radial and distal margins with an adequate lymph node dissection, especially in male subjects who are obese and have a narrow pelvis [20].

Our center has previously developed the technique of transanal minimally invasive surgery (TAMIS) [27] and demonstrated its ability to perform high-quality local excision of rectal neoplasia [28]. The technique of TAMIS evolved and was utilized to perform TaTME [29, 30]. As robotic surgery and laparoscopy are analogous to one another, the natural progression from TAMIS was robotic transanal surgery [31]. A number of case series have demonstrated the feasibility of robotic TaTME with excellent specimen quality and short-term perioperative outcomes [31–34]. The present chapter describes our technique for robotic TaTME and details the benefits and outcomes.

30.1.1 Indications for Robotic Transanal TME

In broad terms, robotic TaTME may be applied in any case where a complete proctectomy is required. In practice, the published literature on robotic TaTME is limited to adenocarcinoma of the rectum within 10 cm from the anal verge where sphincter preservation is possible. Following clinical evaluation, patients are staged locally with magnetic resonance imaging (MRI) of the rectum and distantly with a computerized tomography (CT) of the thorax, abdomen, and pelvis. After multidisciplinary team discussion, patients with locally advanced tumors undergo long-course preoperative chemoradiotherapy with surgery scheduled 8–12 weeks following the completion of treatment. Relative contraindications to performing robotic TaTME include a T4 tumor, extensive previous abdominal or pelvic surgery, or contraindications to restoring intestinal continuity (e.g., invasion of tumor into sphincter complex and poor sphincter function).

30.2 Procedure for Robotic Transanal TME with Reduced Port Abdominal Laparoscopic Mobilization

30.2.1 Room Setup

Surgical technique and specifically robotic setup are somewhat more challenging and less standardized given the youthfulness of the procedure. In addition to standard laparoscopic equipment, the operating room should be fitted with the da Vinci® Robotic System (Intuitive Surgical, Sunnyvale, CA, USA) as well as with a second CO_2 insufflator. We strongly recommend using a device that will provide stable, continuous pneumorectum for better visualization (e.g., AirSeal, SurgiQuest, Milford, CT, USA).

30.2.2 Patient Positioning

The patient is situated in lithotomy position using Allen stirrups at the start of the laparoscopic segment. After the abdominal portion of the operation has been completed, the abdominal field is kept sterile, and the legs are elevated to high dorsal lithotomy for placement of the transanal port. The operating table is tilted in a moderate Trendelenburg position. The patient's legs can then be lowered to a modified lithotomy position to allow docking of the robotic cart without encroachment. This is done parallel to the patient along the right, so that the robotic arms are able to swing over the abdomen and be directed transanally. If a simultaneous team will be working transabdominally, the robotic cart can alternatively be docked on the left side to allow the abdominal team room to operate.

30.2.3 Initial Approach: Above or Below?

As with any oncologic abdominal surgery, an inspection of the abdomen and viscera is critical to evaluate for unexpected peritoneal or hepatic disease. The primary tumor should also be evaluated for local extension if applicable. For the purposes of maintaining reduced port surgery, the port used for initial exploration should be used in the expected location of a pelvic drain suprapubically, hidden in the umbilicus, or in the right lower quadrant through the stoma site. Intuitively, performing the abdominal mobilization initially might seem superior, as it would facilitate the surgeon working in the normal existing planes, with identification of key pelvic structures such as the ureters and sympathetic trunks early in the pelvic dissection. Dissection would continue above until retraction and exposure becomes difficult, with subsequent transition to the transanal approach to complete the dissection of extraperitoneal rectum and perform the anastomosis. Additionally, an initial abdominal approach prevents the possibility of colonic distention, which may occur with an incomplete purse string, or severe pneumoretroperitoneum, which has transpired on several occasions and is nonhazardous yet causes significant distortion of the anatomic planes from the "bottom-first" approach. Finally, performing the abdominal approach first can minimize the time during which the anal canal remains continuously dilated by the transanal port.

On the other hand, initial precise division of the rectal wall, with immediate "holy plane" dissection of the distal extraperitoneal rectum, is perhaps the single greatest advantage of initiating the surgery from a transanal approach. Tumor visualization, location, and assessment are performed simultaneously, and early assessment of sphincter preservation can be determined at the onset of the operation. Early division and mobilization of the rectum transanally can also minimize the forceful traction and manipulation of the rectum often required when performing both open and laparoscopic proctectomy, hypothetically decreasing the risk of tumor fracture and implantation. Finally, an initial transanal approach avoids blood or fluid rundown after peritoneal entry when the upper rectum has already been dissected abdominally.

A simultaneous transanal and transabdominal approach has the obvious value of minimizing the operating time. Two skilled operative teams working synchronously above and below can simplify retraction and deep pelvic exposure. The lower extremities have to be positioned in such a way as to permit both surgeons to operate comfortably and freely without collisions, which is possible but challenging with the current robotic platforms.

30.2.4 Laparoscopic Reduced Port Abdominal Mobilization

A tension-free anastomosis with adequate blood supply to the distal colon is essential for all safe intestinal anastomoses. A surgeon must also adhere to traditional oncologic principles of rectal cancer surgery while dealing with body habitus, disease states, and varying comorbidities. One must also consider functional outcomes of patients undergoing low anterior resection. The sigmoid colon is commonly a poor conduit, especially when narrowed and thickened with diverticular disease. Furthermore, adequate colonic mobilization to permit reconstruction with a colonic J pouch should be strongly considered. Even more colonic mobilization may be required when one is considering reconstruction with colonic J pouch. Lastly one must reflect on the need for temporary fecal diversion with loop ileostomy in high-risk patients with a low pelvic anastomosis, especially in the setting of neoadjuvant chemoradiation.

To accomplish the above, complete splenic flexure mobilization to the middle colic trunk, with high ligation of the inferior mesenteric artery (IMA) below the takeoff of the left colic artery, and division of the inferior mesenteric vein (IMV) provide the maximal colonic length and appear mandatory. However, critics often cite routine splenic flexure mobilization as timely, usually unnecessary, and having the potential of decreasing distal colonic perfusion [35]. At our institution, routine splenic flexure mobilization is performed on all patients in a medial-to-lateral approach beginning at the mesoduodenal ligament. Although colonic mobilization can be achieved in a multiport fashion, this can be also performed with reduced port surgery safely and efficiently, while more challenging dissection deeper in the pelvis is unnecessary due to the transanal dissection.

Single-port colonic surgery has been well described in large numbers with varying non-standardized techniques and port location. For left colonic surgery, single-port devices have been utilized in the umbilicus, suprapubic position (Pfannenstiel incision) in addition to the right lower quadrant [36]. Given the potential need for fecal diversion in the majority of patients, access through the right lower quadrant at the site of the future ileostomy is the obvious best choice. Single-port deployment in this area should provide sufficient access to the splenic flexure superiorly and to the upper rectum in the pelvis inferiorly while offering a potential extraction site for the colon and rectum. Synchronous transanal and transabdominal surgery is possible with this orientation as well, with the abdominal operating team adequately away from the robotic cart and arms docked on the opposite side of the patient. Extraction through the ileostomy site can prove to be challenging in patients with a bulky tumor or mesorectum, and/or a thick abdominal wall, but can be facilitated by a wound protector included in many commercially available ports. In our experience, enlarging the fascial opening to facilitate extraction is superior to specimen fracture or mesenteric injury and can be performed in a temporary fashion without undue risk of hernia. In addition, although transanal extraction and transperineal construction of a J pouch is feasible, it requires a significant colonic segment and can more easily be constructed from above and transferred below.

The initial setup for splenic flexure mobilization includes a traditional stoma incision created in the right lower quadrant at the pre-marked ileostomy site. A single-port device can then be deployed through this incision. An additional 5 mm port can be placed suprapubically for either a camera or retraction and can be the site of a pelvic drain. Complete abdominal exploration is performed to evaluate for unexpected liver, peritoneal, or other sites of extrarectal disease. The patient is placed in moderate Trendelenburg position and in steep, right-sided tilt to allow the small bowel contents to be completely displaced to the right side of the abdomen. The omentum is reflected superiorly and pushed over the transverse colon (Fig. 30.1). The ligament of Treitz and bordering IMV are identified. Frequently, the mesoduodenal ligament running from the left lateral border of the duodenum to the left colon mesentery is present and divided to adequately expose the IMV and root of the mesentery (Fig. 30.2).

With the inferior mesenteric vein grasped and placed on tension toward the abdominal wall, a transverse incision is created at the base of the mesentery from just below the IMV following the contour of the left colic artery as it joins the IMA (Fig. 30.3a, b). The correct plane between the mesocolon and retroperitoneum is easily identified, and medial-to-lateral dissection is performed on top of Gerota's and Toldt's fasciae up to the inferior edge of the pancreas, laterally under the colon to the abdominal sidewall and underneath the splenic flexure (Fig. 30.4a–c). The inferior mesenteric vein is isolated and divided at the base of the pancreas, below the left colic vein, between clips or with an energy device.

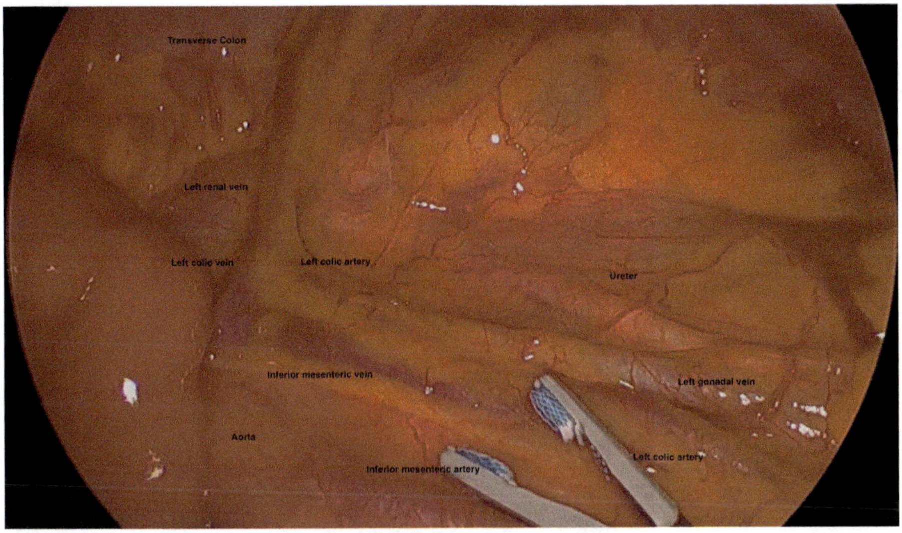

Fig. 30.1 The anatomy of the left mesocolon is critical to complete mobilization of the splenic flexure and prepare an adequate conduit for low pelvic and coloanal anastomosis without urologic or major vascular injury

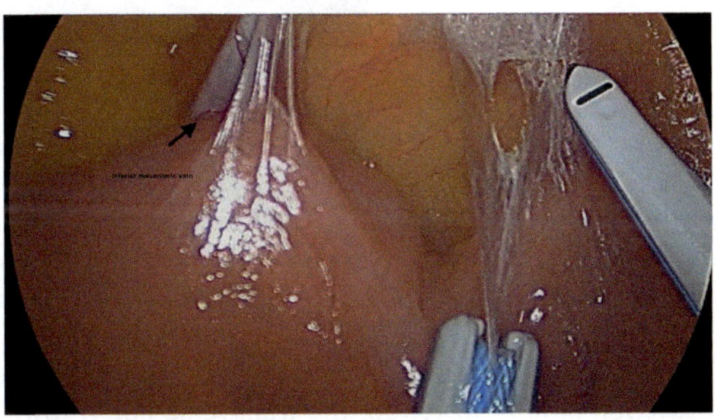

Fig. 30.2 The patient is placed in full right lateral tilt in order to displace all of the small bowel contents to the right of the abdomen and identify the ligament of Treitz where the mesoduodenal ligament is divided

Of note, a meandering mesenteric artery, when present, can be seen and/or injured at this location (Fig. 30.5).

The initial peritoneal incision is continued inferiorly to the origin of the inferior mesenteric artery, along the origin of the mesosigmoid and mesorectum toward the pelvic inlet (Fig. 30.6). From a medial-to-lateral approach, the mesocolon is mobilized off of the retroperitoneum identifying the hypogastric nerves, left ureter, and gonadal vessels while working toward the lateral sidewall. At this point, the instrument in the right hand can be placed below and behind the superior rectal artery, exposing the origin of the IMA proximal to the left colic branch for division with an energy device and clips (Fig. 30.7). The left colic branch is also divided at this time to prevent avulsion and facilitate extraction.

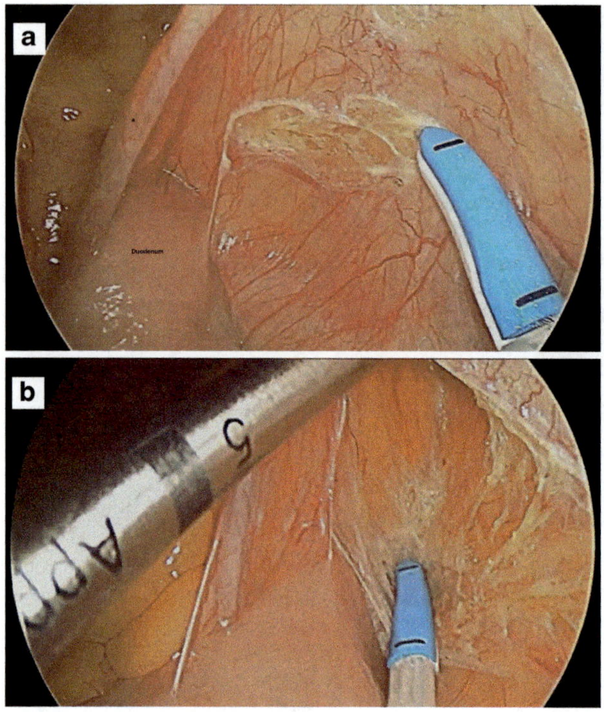

Fig. 30.3 (**a**, **b**) An incision is made at the root of the mesocolon just below the inferior mesenteric vein (*asterisk*) and left colic artery. The plane between the mesocolon and retroperitoneum is identified

With the sigmoid colon pulled medially using an atraumatic bowel grasper in the right hand, the peritoneal attachments in the mesosigmoid fossa can be incised over the "bruise" created from the previous retroperitoneal dissection, and the two planes are joined (Fig. 30.8a, b). With an instrument under the mesocolon to provide traction, the white line of Toldt can be incised to the splenic flexure along the lateral edge of the descending colon.

A third instrument to improve triangulation is beneficial during the omental dissection simply to retract the transverse colon toward the pelvis. This can be accomplished with an accessory port or through a single-port platform, which will accommodate an additional trocar. With the operating surgeon facing cephalad, the greater omentum is retracted over the transverse mesocolon and grasped near the attachments of epiploic fat and transverse mesocolon. With an energy device in the right hand, the omentum is divided and the lesser sac entered. Once lesser sac entry is established, the left hand instrument can be placed inside the lesser sac underneath the omentum to more easily retract. Following division of the omentum to communicate with the lateral plane previously dissected, the mesocolic plane at the inferior edge of the pancreas is identified and incised, again communicating with the previously established retroperitoneal plane (Fig. 30.9a, b. The final splenocolic ligaments are divided, completely releasing the splenic

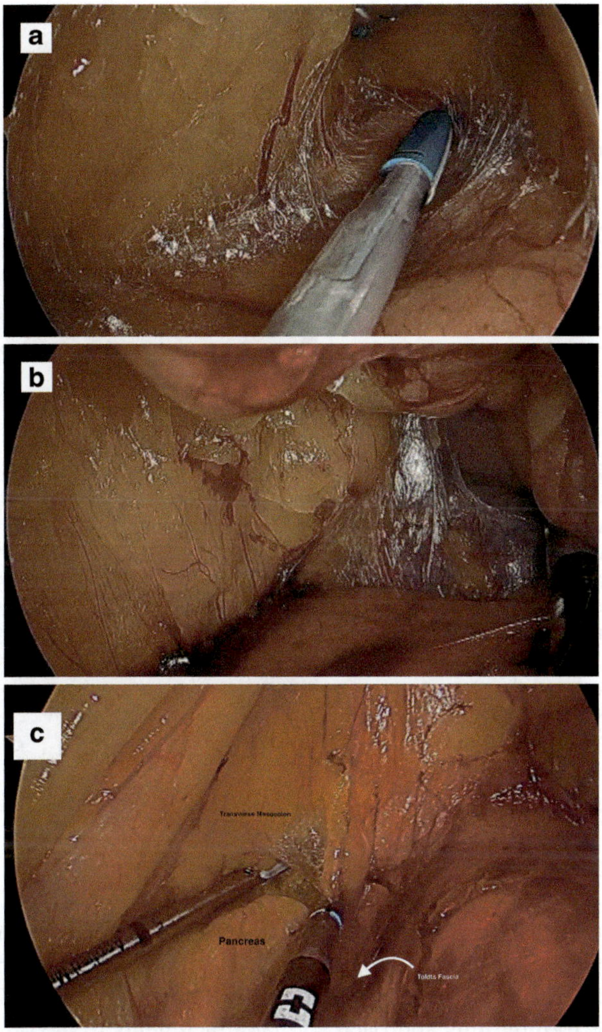

Fig. 30.4 (**a**–**c**) Medial-to-lateral dissection is performed maintaining the integrity of Toldt's and Gerota's fasciae. This is continued to the abdominal side wall beneath the colon and to the spleen. At the level of the pancreas, continued dissection along Toldt's fascia will be posterior to the pancreas and splenic vein. It is critical to stop the dissection posteriorly and instead incise the base of the transverse mesocolon at the inferior edge of the pancreas

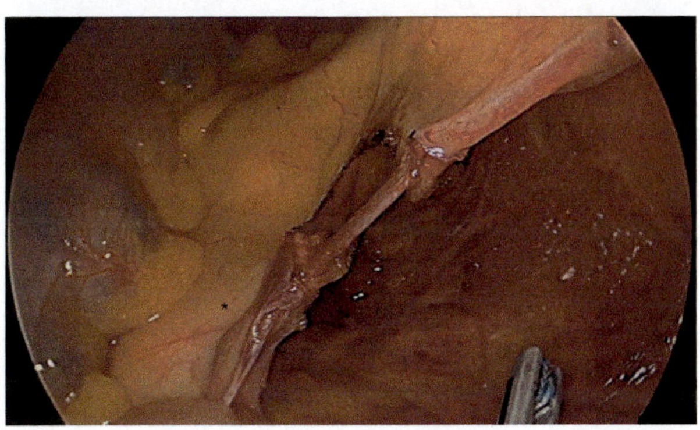

Fig. 30.5 The inferior mesenteric vein is skeletonized and divided with an energy device at the base of the pancreas (*asterisk*) to achieve maximal mesenteric length

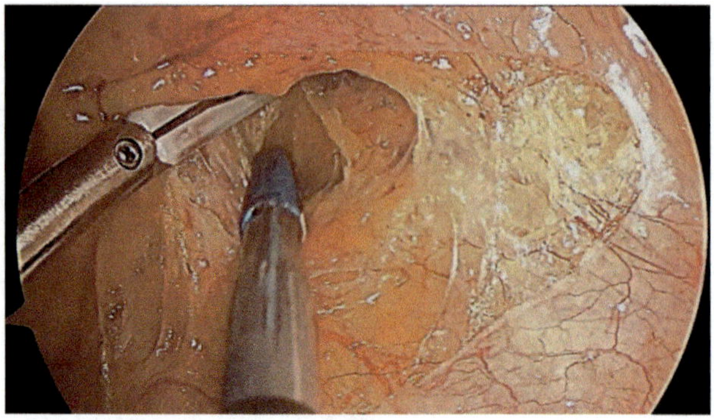

Fig. 30.6 The initial mesenteric incision is extended inferiorly over the inferior mesenteric artery. The appropriate plane is again identified below the superior hemorrhoidal vessel and hypogastric nerve trunks

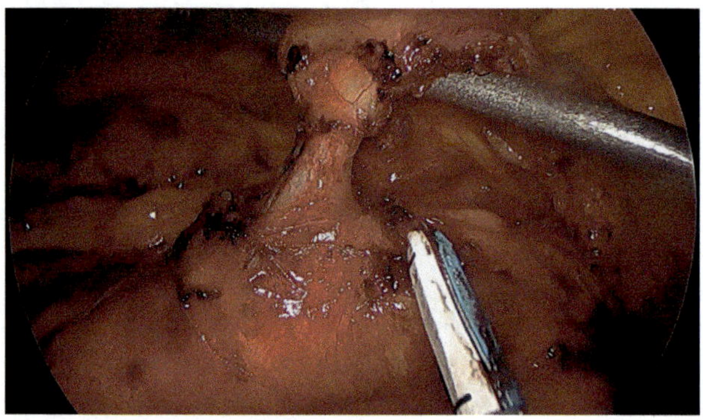

Fig. 30.7 The inferior mesenteric artery is skeletonized and divided between clips and an energy device. Exposure is facilitated by passing an instrument through the accessory suprapubic port to elevate the mesocolon away from the retroperitoneum

flexure up to the middle colic pedicle. Alternatively, the lesser sac can be more quickly entered adjacent to the gastroepiploic arcade, which will detach the omentum and transverse colon together from the stomach. Care must be taken when performing this approach so that attachments to the omentum at the angle of the splenic flexure are not tethering the descending colon and hindering its mobilization into the pelvis.

Upper rectal mobilization may now proceed with the patient returned to the steep Trendelenburg position. The presacral plane is entered in the midline and dissection continued until the previously performed transanal dissection is met (Fig. 30.10).

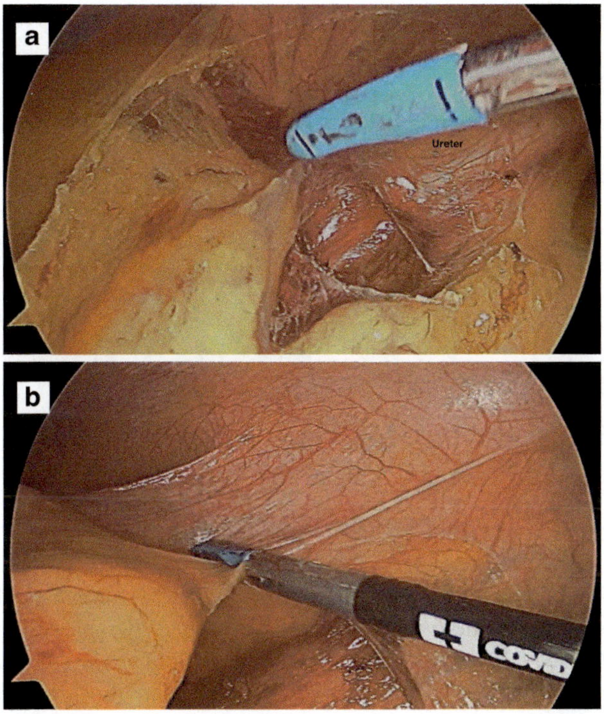

Fig. 30.8 (**a**, **b**) The sigmoid and descending colons are then mobilized, incising the lateral attachments and joining the previous medial-to-lateral dissection to the splenic flexure

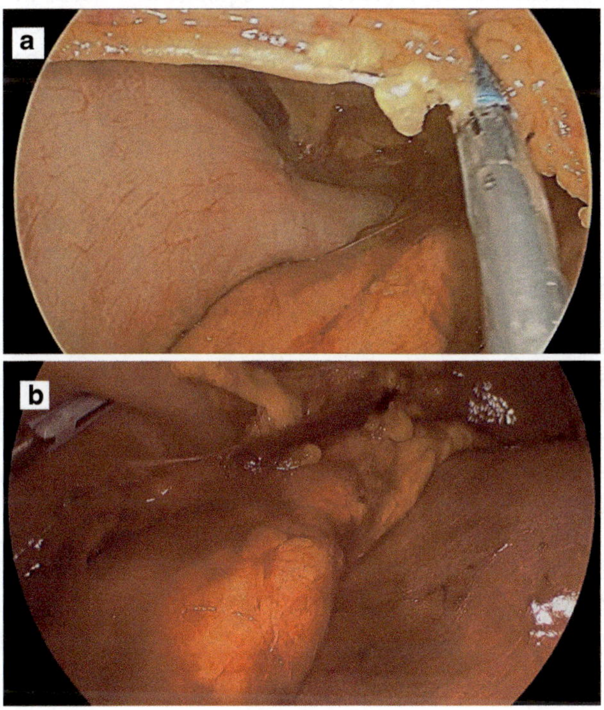

Fig. 30.9 (**a**, **b**) The gastrocolic ligament is divided along the gastroepiploic arcade, leaving the omentum on the colon. The lesser sac is entered. After dividing the omentum to join the lateral dissection, the entire left mesocolon is completely mobilized to the level of the middle colic pedicle for maximal length

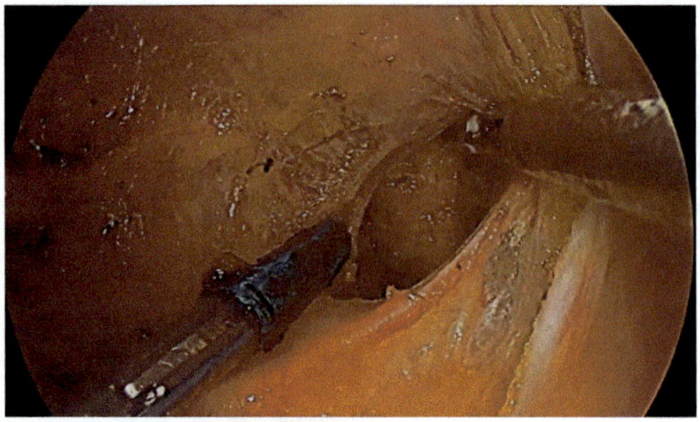

Fig. 30.10 Mesorectal dissection begins in the posterior midline. The transanal dissection plane is quickly met facilitating retraction and division of the final peritoneal reflection attachments

30.2.5 Robotic Docking and Port Placement

While the robotic setup might seem cumbersome and time-consuming, the docking time significantly reduces with experience. For robotic transanal surgery, several ports have been described. The GelPOINT Path transanal access platform (Applied Medical, Rancho Santa Margarita, CA, USA) consists of a rigid cylindrical sleeve, which may help protect against injury to the sphincter mechanism. The sleeve is lubricated with petroleum jelly and introduced into the anal canal using an obturator provided by the manufacturer. Once seated above the anorectal ring, the sleeve is secured to the skin with 2-0 silk sutures. Next, three GelPOINT Path cannulas are introduced through the cap at an equilateral distance in the shape of a triangle. The da Vinci® robotic 5-mm trocars (Intuitive Surgical, Inc.) are passed through the cannulas. A variation on this technique has been described using a "transanal access port" proctoscope (PAT, Developia-HUMV, Santander, Spain) inserted transanally, followed by insertion of a GelPOINT device to occlude the proctoscope and for trocar placement [33].

Alternatively, a glove port technique can be employed as described for robotic TAMIS [37]. This involves using a circular anal dilator (CAD), wound protector, and standard surgical glove. Instruments are introduced through the fingers of the glove with the thumb of the glove facing superiorly, in the so-called "thumbs-up" position. The transanal glove port may simplify the robotic setup, allowing increased flexibility and enabling docking of the cannulas farther away from the limited workspace when the patient is in lithotomy position. The glove port also allows for better mobility of instruments inside the rectum, enabling improved triangulation, rotation, and the ability to cross instruments. In addition, inherent to this setup is the maximal separation of the robotic arms externally, which reduces collision between the robotic arms and camera.

TaTME has been described using the da Vinci® Robotic Surgical System with both the Si and Xi models (Intuitive Surgical) [31–34, 38]. Docking is best accomplished parallel to the base of the operating table along the patient's right side. Again, this can be modified to the patient's left side if the abdominal team will be working simultaneously (Fig. 30.11). The robotic arms are then brought over the

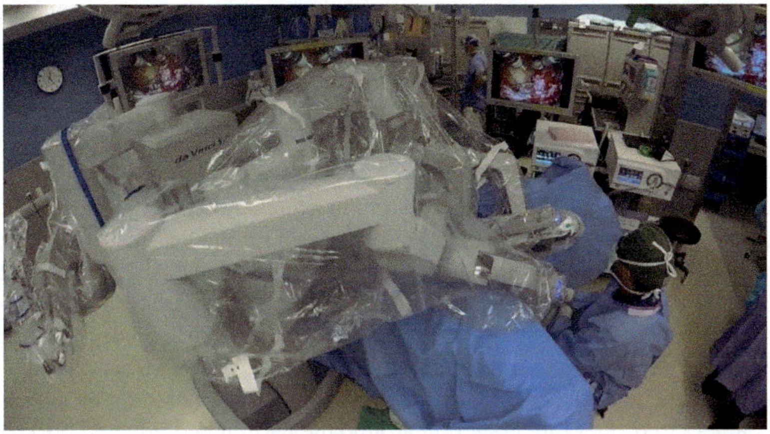

Fig. 30.11 The robot is shown docked to the patient's right hip with arms directed toward the perineum

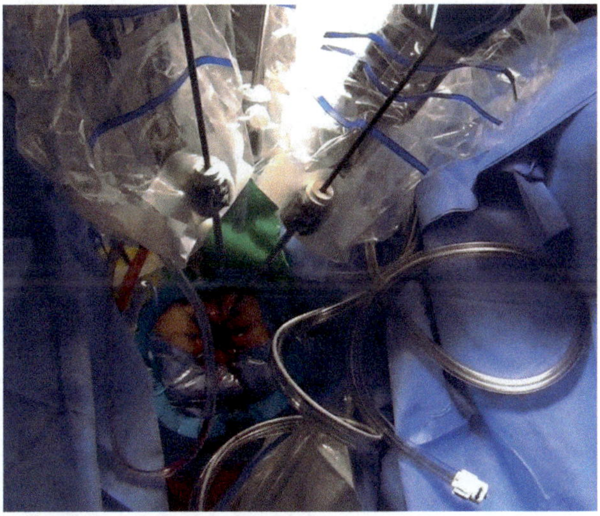

Fig. 30.12 Robotic arms are positioned over the abdomen and directed toward the perineum, positioned to interface with a transanal port for transanal access

abdomen and directed toward the perineum where they interface with the transanal platform (Fig. 30.12). The port device is connected to insufflation set to 15–18 mmHg using CO_2. Two 5-mm working arms and an 8-mm downward-looking 30° lens are delivered through the cannulas. A 5-mm monopolar cautery and 5-mm grasper of the surgeon's choice are utilized [34]. We prefer hook cautery and Maryland graspers. Scissors and bipolar fenestrated graspers have also been described [33]. An additional 5-mm laparoscopic trocar can be inserted and utilized by a bedside assistant for suction of fluid and smoke, as well as with retraction when required. For low-lying lesions, an intersphincteric dissection can be performed prior to robotic docking. The dissection is begun with a handheld Hill-Ferguson retractor and monopolar cautery dissection. A Lone Star Retractor System® (Cooper Surgical, Trumbull, CT, USA) or a PPH anoscope (Ethicon Endo-Surgery, Cincinnati, OH, USA) may also be introduced to complete the circumlinear division distal to the tumor. The lumen is then closed with 0-Prolene purse-string suture to avoid any fecal contamination. The retractors are removed and the transanal port is introduced into the anal canal and seated.

After the purse-string suture and port are placed, electrocautery is used to mark a circular incision distal to the purse string. The rectum is then incised through all layers of the wall (Fig. 30.13). Initially, it was thought that beginning the dissection posteriorly and leaving the anterior portion for later in the dissection was simpler. We have since noted that developing the anterior plane first and continuing along Denonvilliers' fascia provides a safer initial dissection to prevent injury to the membranous urethra. The dissection can be started using a 0° camera and then switched to a 30° camera to further the dissection around the rectum laterally and posteriorly. Dissection can be accomplished with cautery and small amounts of blunt dissection or "bumps" which allows the pneumo-dissection to advance.

In the first portion of the dissection (distal 5 cm of rectum), working space is limited, and movement of the robotic arms is constrained much more than when performing TaTME with standard laparoscopic instruments. As the dissection progresses, there is usually an increase in working space within the pelvis. With the aid of pneumo-dissection, TaTME is significantly easier, particularly in the mid-rectum (Fig. 30.14a, b). The upper rectum is more challenging to dissect using robotic-assisted TaTME, as the working angles necessary to complete the dissection are difficult to obtain. Important anatomic landmarks are well visualized with robotic-assisted TaTME. In particular, the ureters and nerve bundles, including the nervi erigentes, and the closely associated middle rectal arteries are appreciated with an enhanced view. The hypogastric plexus and nerves are clearly visible with the robotic approach from below, allowing for preservation of the nerves. Once the

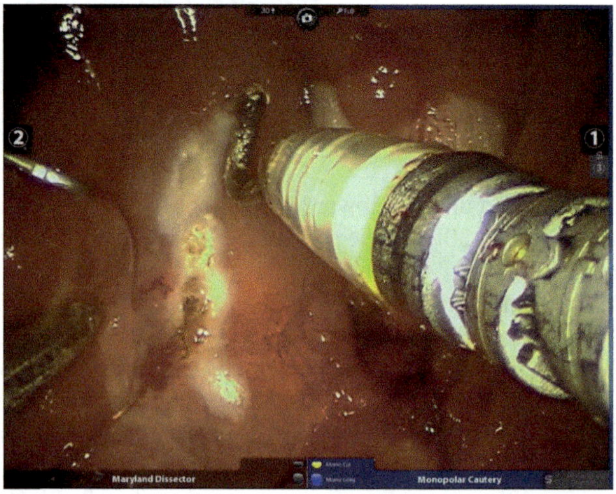

Fig. 30.13 Cautery marks are placed circumferentially distal to the tumor and purse-string suture. This dissection is then continued through all the layers of the rectal wall

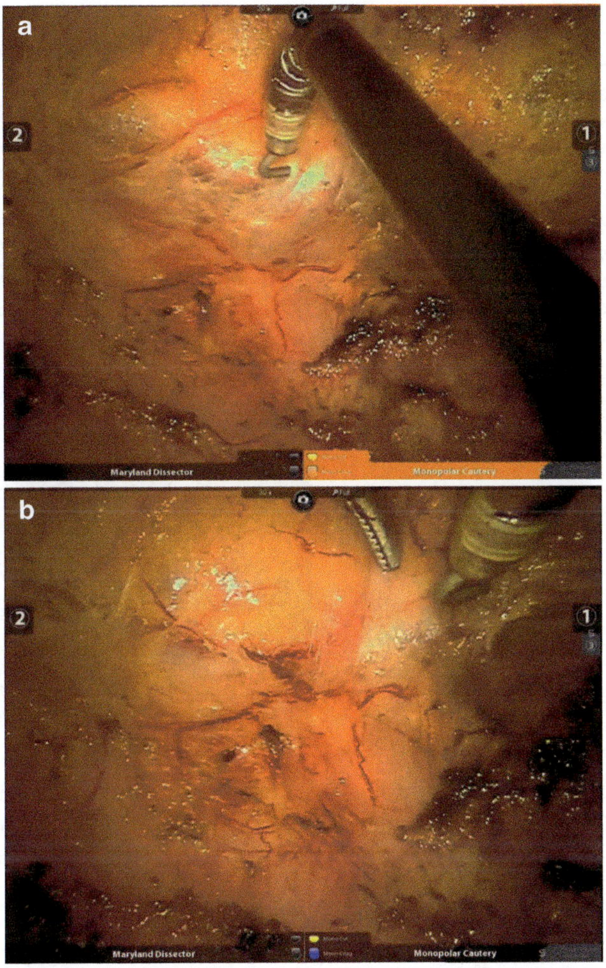

Fig. 30.14 (a, b) Posterior dissection showing the embryologic plane for TaTME, which is made more evident with the aid of pneumodissection from the insufflation

dissection progresses cephalad to the level of the peritoneum, the planes of dissection can be communicated with the abdominal team.

Following the posterior "rendezvous," dissection is continued from the midline out laterally to either side, displacing the hypogastrics to their lateral location and better defining the lateral plane. The cut peritoneal edge on either side of the upper rectum is identified, grasped, and retracted, and an incision is made along the lateral rectal sulcus on either side to join the anterior peritoneotomy created by the transanal dissection (Fig. 30.15a, b). It is at this portion of the procedure that a synchronous approach can show the most benefit creating traction from multiple approaches to provide an excellent mesorectal dissection and avoiding the inferior hypogastric plexus laterally.

Either a transanal or transabdominal extraction can be used to extract the surgical specimen. If transanal extraction is planned, the mesentery of the colonic conduit

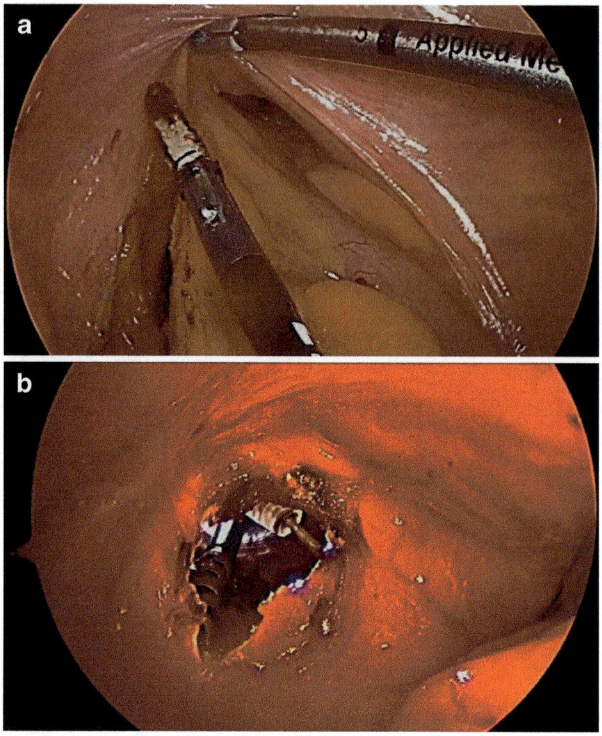

Fig. 30.15 (**a**) The incision along the lateral rectal sulcus and the anterior peritoneotomy are shown just before the two working groups have communicated anteriorly. (**b**) Intra-abdominal view of robotic instruments working transanally to connect the planes of dissection anteriorly

can be divided prior to extraction as described above. This will prevent avulsion of the marginal artery and devascularization of the conduit during the pull-through. The colon can then be delivered through the transanal access channel by the perineal team, bringing the specimen out transanally under direct vision to avoid twisting or injuring the mesentery. It is then divided and prepared for the anastomosis. With visceral obesity and a bulky tumor and/or mesentery, particularly in a narrow male pelvis, specimens can be extracted transabdominally through the stoma site. This may prevent tearing of the specimen or injury to the blood supply of the conduit.

30.2.6 Coloanal Anastomosis

The two most common techniques for an anastomosis are a hand-sewn coloanal anastomosis and a stapled double purse-string technique. The option of a hand-sewn coloanal anastomosis is favored when the rectum is divided extremely distally and there is little room for a staple fire. This technique is generally accomplished with interrupted 2-0 Vicryl sutures. The channel of the transanal port can be left in place and used as a retractor during the hand-sewn anastomosis. If it has been removed, standard transanal retractors can be used to accomplish the anastomosis.

If enough of a rectal cuff is remaining to perform a stapled anastomosis, the descending colon conduit is prepared in standard fashion with the anvil of a circular stapler and a purse-string suture. A second purse-string suture is performed at the rectal cuff using a 0-Prolene stitch. The pin of the circular stapler is then inserted through the rectal stump purse string for firing of the stapler. A conventional stapled side-to-end coloanal anastomosis has also been described [34], and the option for colonic J pouch construction is available if there is adequate length to the colon conduit. A pelvic drain should be placed, and temporary loop ileostomy should be performed on all patients routinely, especially in the setting of preoperative chemoradiotherapy.

30.2.7 Ileostomy

After extraction and anastomosis, the pelvis should be inspected, and a pelvic drain can be placed through the suprapubic port. The ileum is grasped and retracted through the single port in the right lower quadrant. The ileostomy is then oriented appropriately and matured in a loop fashion.

30.3 The Evidence for Robotic TaTME

At the time of writing this chapter, the published experience of robotic TaTME is limited to 17 highly select cases (Table 30.1). The range of tumor distance from the anal verge was 2–8 cm, and the operative time ranged from 166 to 398 min. No case of an incomplete mesorectal specimen or positive CRM has yet been reported, and lymph node yields have been adequate. Abdominal colonic mobilization was achieved laparoscopically in three series [31, 32, 34] and robotically in one [33].

30.4 Discussion and Conclusions

Technological advances have made minimally invasive surgery possible for rectal cancer treatment with an improved postoperative recovery. However, the technical and patient-specific challenges associated with these procedures have resulted in limited adoption, high conversion rates, and sometimes inadequate pathological outcomes.

Table 30.1 Published experience of robotic TaTME

	Huscher [34]	Gómez Ruiz [33]	Atallah [31]	Verheijen [32]
n	7	5	4	1
Body mass index (kg/m^2)	29.9	25.8	29	23.6
Distance from the anal verge (cm)	2	5	3	8
Operative time (min)	165.7	398	317	250
Incomplete mesorectum	0%	0%	0%	0%
Lymph nodes retrieved	14	14.9	26.8	NR
CRM positive	0%	0%	0%	0%

CRM circumferential resection margin, *NR* not reported

TaTME represents a synthesis of a number of significant developments in rectal cancer surgery [24] including TME, the transanal-abdominal-transanal (TATA) procedure, advanced laparoscopy, and minimally invasive approaches to the rectum such as the lap TATA, TEM, and TAMIS. The principle advantage of TaTME is improved access, particularly to the distal one-third of the rectum—especially for male patients with a narrow, deep pelvis and visceral obesity. Theoretically, improved access can result in improved visualization, which then directly translates into an ability to more completely excise the rectum and mesorectum. As a result, it has been suggested that TaTME could represent a solution to the "Achilles' heel" of rectal cancer surgery [34, 39]. In the largest published TaTME series to date, the CRM positivity rates range from 2.5 to 6.4% [21, 22].

Data on TaTME remains limited to that obtained from nonrandomized published series of early adopters, often retrospective in nature. Notwithstanding, the preliminary data has been encouraging, particularly when compared to laparoscopic TME. It has been shown that when compared to conventional laparoscopic mobilization, TaTME results in a significantly longer distal resection margin [40], a lower rate of CRM positivity [16], and improved TME quality [41]. The suggested advantages of robotic TaTME include low conversion rates [34], low blood loss, and successful transanal specimen extraction [33]. The advantage of transanal extraction is that it spares the patient an abdominal incision and its inherent morbidity—including the potential for infection, postoperative pain, and hernia formation. However, a bulky rectal mesentery can be difficult to deliver through the anal canal and may result in shearing of the surgical specimen, and if this is the case, oncological principals should not be sacrificed to save an extraction incision. Other advantages include the stable camera view, three-dimensional high-definition vision, and 7° of freedom with endowristed instruments and better ergonomics, offering the surgeon the ability to develop surgical planes that are optimal and precise in a relatively fixed anatomic space. The superior visualization and magnification are harder to quantify, but are suggested to confer an improved view of Denonvilliers' fascia, the presacral fascia, and the neurovascular bundles running behind the presacral fascia on the right and left sides [34]. The prolonged operative times observed are expected, as is seen in the early development of any new application for robotic surgery. In the future, a combined abdominal and transanal team approach and the development of single-port robotics will likely improve operative times.

It must be noted that results for TaTME and particularly robotic TaTME are limited by a paucity of functional and long-term oncological outcome data, which is essential in fully understanding the utility of TaTME. The ongoing European and North American registries along with the proposed COLOR III study, which will compare TaTME to laparoscopic TME for rectal cancer in a randomized trial, will be of great value in validating the utility and safety of TaTME in the future. It can be concluded however that the technique of robotic TaTME is feasible and can result in a high-quality rectal cancer resection specimen, but further data is needed before generalized adoption can be advised. Appropriate training is critical for the safe introduction of this technique to ensure the best outcomes for patients with rectal cancer.

References

1. Heald RJ, Husband EM, Ryall RD. The mesorectum in rectal cancer surgery—the clue to pelvic recurrence? Br J Surg. 1982;69:613–6.
2. Quirke P, Steele R, Monson J, Grieve R, Khanna S, Couture J, O'Callaghan C, Myint AS, Bessell E, Thompson LC, Parmar M, Stephens RJ, Sebag-Montefiore D, MRC CR07/NCIC-CTG CO16 Trial Investigators; NCRI Colorectal Cancer Study Group. Effect of the plane of surgery achieved on local recurrence in patients with operable rectal cancer: a prospective study using data from the MRC CR07 and NCIC-CTG CO16 randomised clinical trial. Lancet. 2009;373:821–8.
3. Martling A, Singnomklao T, Holm T, Rutqvist LE, Cedermark B. Prognostic significance of both surgical and pathological assessment of curative resection for rectal cancer. Br J Surg. 2004;91:1040–5.
4. Birbeck KF, Macklin CP, Tiffin NJ, Parsons W, Dixon MF, Mapstone NP, Abbott CR, Scott N, Finan PJ, Johnston D, Quirke P. Rates of circumferential resection margin involvement vary between surgeons and predict outcomes in rectal cancer surgery. Ann Surg. 2002;235:449–57.
5. Nikberg M, Kindler C, Chabok A, Letocha H, Shetye J, Smedh K. Circumferential resection margin as a prognostic marker in the modern multidisciplinary management of rectal cancer. Dis Colon Rectum. 2015;58:275–82.
6. van der Pas MH, Haglind E, Cuesta MA, Furst A, Lacy AM, Hop WC, Bonjer HJ, COlorectal cancer Laparoscopic or Open Resection II (COLOR II) Study Group. Laparoscopic versus open surgery for rectal cancer (COLOR II): short-term outcomes of a randomised, phase 3 trial. Lancet Oncol. 2013;14:210–8.
7. den Dulk M, Marijnen CA, Putter H, Rutten HJ, Beets GL, Wiggers T, Nagtegaal ID, van de Velde CJ. Risk factors for adverse outcome in patients with rectal cancer treated with an abdominoperineal resection in the total mesorectal excision trial. Ann Surg. 2007;246:83–90.
8. Oh SJ, Shin JY. Risk factors of circumferential resection margin involvement in the patients with extraperitoneal rectal cancer. J Korean Surg Soc. 2012;82:165–71.
9. Targarona EM, Balague C, Pernas JC, Martinez C, Berindoague R, Gich I, Trias M. Can we predict immediate outcome after laparoscopic rectal surgery? Multivariate analysis of clinical, anatomic, and pathologic features after 3-dimensional reconstruction of the pelvic anatomy. Ann Surg. 2008;247:642–9.
10. Kang SB, Park JS, Kim DW, Lee TG. Intraoperative technical difficulty during laparoscopy-assisted surgery as a prognostic factor for colorectal cancer. Dis Colon Rectum. 2010;53:1400–8.
11. Guillou PJ, Quirke P, Thorpe H, Walker J, Jayne DG, Smith AM, Heath RM, Brown JM, MRC CLASICC trial group. Short-term endpoints of conventional versus laparoscopic-assisted surgery in patients with colorectal cancer (MRC CLASICC trial): multicentre, randomised controlled trial. Lancet. 2005;365:1718–26.
12. Kang SB, Park JW, Jeong SY, Nam BH, Choi HS, Kim DW, Lim SB, Lee TG, Kim DY, Kim JS, Chang HJ, Lee HS, Kim SY, Jung KH, Hong YS, Kim JH, Sohn DK, Kim DH, Oh JH. Open versus laparoscopic surgery for mid or low rectal cancer after neoadjuvant chemoradiotherapy (COREAN trial): short-term outcomes of an open-label randomised controlled trial. Lancet Oncol. 2010;11:637–45.
13. Stevenson AR, Solomon MJ, Lumley JW, Hewett P, Clouston AD, Gebski VJ, Davies L, Wilson K, Hague W, Simes J, ALaCaRT Investigators. Effect of laparoscopic-assisted resection vs. open resection on pathological outcomes in rectal cancer: the ALaCaRT randomized clinical trial. JAMA. 2015;314:1356–63.
14. Fleshman J, Branda M, Sargent DJ, Boller AM, George V, Abbas M, Peters WR Jr, Maun D, Chang G, Herline A, Fichera A, Mutch M, Wexner S, Whiteford M, Marks J, Birnbaum E, Margolin D, Larson D, Marcello P, Posner M, Read T, Monson J, Wren SM, Pisters PW, Nelson H. Effect of laparoscopic-assisted resection vs. open resection of stage II or III rectal cancer on pathologic outcomes: the ACOSOG Z6051 randomized clinical trial. JAMA. 2015;314:1346–55.

15. Marks G, Mohiuddin M, Borenstein BD. Preoperative radiation therapy and sphincter preservation by the combined abdominotranssacral technique for selected rectal cancers. Dis Colon Rectum. 1985;28:565–71.
16. Denost Q, Adam JP, Rullier A, Buscail E, Laurent C, Rullier E. Perineal transanal approach: a new standard for laparoscopic sphincter-saving resection in low rectal cancer, a randomized trial. Ann Surg. 2014;260:993–9.
17. Whiteford MH, Denk PM, Swanstrom LL. Feasibility of radical sigmoid colectomy performed as natural orifice translumenal endoscopic surgery (NOTES) using transanal endoscopic microsurgery. Surg Endosc. 2007;21:1870–4.
18. Sylla P, Rattner DW, Delgado S, Lacy AM. NOTES transanal rectal cancer resection using transanal endoscopic microsurgery and laparoscopic assistance. Surg Endosc. 2010;24:1205–10.
19. Leroy J, Barry BD, Melani A, Mutter D, Marescaux J. No-scar transanal total mesorectal excision: the last step to pure NOTES for colorectal surgery. JAMA Surg. 2013;148:226–30. discussion 31
20. Rouanet P, Mourregot A, Azar CC, Carrere S, Gutowski M, Quenet F, Saint-Aubert B, Colombo PE. Transanal endoscopic proctectomy: an innovative procedure for difficult resection of rectal tumors in men with narrow pelvis. Dis Colon Rectum. 2013;56:408–15.
21. Lacy AM, Tasende MM, Delgado S, Fernandez-Hevia M, Jimenez M, De Lacy B, Castells A, Bravo R, Wexner SD, Heald RJ. Transanal total mesorectal excision for rectal cancer: outcomes after 140 patients. J Am Coll Surg. 2015;221:415–23.
22. Veltcamp Helbach M, Deijen CL, Velthuis S, Bonjer HJ, Tuynman JB, Sietses C. Transanal total mesorectal excision for rectal carcinoma: short-term outcomes and experience after 80 cases. Surg Endosc. 2016;30(2):464–70.
23. Tuech JJ, Karoui M, Lelong B, De Chaisemartin C, Bridoux V, Manceau G, Delpero JR, Hanoun L, Michot F. A step toward NOTES total mesorectal excision for rectal cancer: endoscopic transanal proctectomy. Ann Surg. 2015;261:228–33.
24. Atallah S. Transanal minimally invasive surgery for total mesorectal excision. Minim Invasive Ther Allied Technol. 2014;23:10–6.
25. Atallah S. Transanal total mesorectal excision: full steam ahead. Tech Coloproctol. 2015;19:57–61.
26. Heald RJ. A new solution to some old problems: transanal TME. Tech Coloproctol. 2013;17:257–8.
27. Atallah S, Albert M, Larach S. Transanal minimally invasive surgery: a giant leap forward. Surg Endosc. 2010;24:2200–5.
28. Albert MR, Atallah SB, deBeche-Adams TC, Izfar S, Larach SW. Transanal minimally invasive surgery (TAMIS) for local excision of benign neoplasms and early-stage rectal cancer: efficacy and outcomes in the first 50 patients. Dis Colon Rectum. 2013;56:301–7.
29. Atallah S, Albert M, DeBeche-Adams T, Nassif G, Polavarapu H, Larach S. Transanal minimally invasive surgery for total mesorectal excision (TAMIS-TME): a stepwise description of the surgical technique with video demonstration. Tech Coloproctol. 2013;17:321–5.
30. Atallah S, Martin-Perez B, Albert M, deBeche-Adams T, Nassif G, Hunter L, Larach S. Transanal minimally invasive surgery for total mesorectal excision (TAMIS-TME): results and experience with the first 20 patients undergoing curative-intent rectal cancer surgery at a single institution. Tech Coloproctol. 2014;18:473–80.
31. Atallah S, Martin-Perez B, Parra-Davila E, deBeche-Adams T, Nassif G, Albert M, Larach S. Robotic transanal surgery for local excision of rectal neoplasia, transanal total mesorectal excision, and repair of complex fistulae: clinical experience with the first 18 cases at a single institution. Tech Coloproctol. 2015;19:401–10.
32. Verheijen PM, Consten EC, Broeders IA. Robotic transanal total mesorectal excision for rectal cancer: experience with a first case. Int J Med Robot. 2014;10:423–6.
33. Gomez Ruiz M, Parra IM, Palazuelos CM, Martin JA, Fernandez CC, Diego JC, Fleitas MG. Robotic-assisted laparoscopic transanal total mesorectal excision for rectal cancer: a prospective pilot study. Dis Colon Rectum. 2015;58:145–53.
34. Huscher CG, Bretagnol F, Ponzano C. Robotic-assisted transanal total mesorectal excision: the key against the Achilles' heel of rectal cancer? Ann Surg. 2015;261:e120–1.

35. Chand M, Miskovic D, Parvaiz A. Is splenic flexure mobilization necessary in laparoscopic anterior resection? Dis Colon Rectum. 2012;55(11):1195–7.
36. Fung AK, Aly EH. Systematic review of single-incision laparoscopic colonic surgery. Br J Surg. 2012;99(10):1353–64.
37. Hompes R, Rauh SM, Ris F, Tuynman JB, Mortensen NJ. Robotic transanal minimally invasive surgery for local excision of rectal neoplasms. Br J Surg. 2014;101(5):578–81.
38. Atallah S, Martin-Perez B, Pinan J, Quinteros F, Schoonyoung H, Albert M, Larach S. Robotic transanal total mesorectal excision: a pilot study. Tech Coloproctol. 2014;18(11):1047–53.
39. Atallah SB, Larach S, deBeche-Adams TC, Albert MR. Transanal minimally invasive surgery (TAMIS): a technique that can be used for retrograde proctectomy. Dis Colon Rectum. 2013;56:931.
40. Fernandez-Hevia M, Delgado S, Castells A, Tasende M, Momblan D, Diaz del Gobbo G, DeLacy B, Balust J, Lacy AM. Transanal total mesorectal excision in rectal cancer: short-term outcomes in comparison with laparoscopic surgery. Ann Surg. 2015;261:221–7.
41. Velthuis S, Nieuwenhuis DH, Ruijter TE, Cuesta MA, Bonjer HJ, Sietses C. Transanal versus traditional laparoscopic total mesorectal excision for rectal carcinoma. Surg Endosc. 2014;28:3494–9.

Transanal Robot-Assisted TME with Single-Port Abdominal Laparoscopy

31

Cristiano Germano Sigismondo Hüscher, Cecilia Ponzano, and Gilda Marzullo

Abstract

Transanal total mesorectal excision (taTME) is a new approach to perform minimally invasive rectal resection. It has special applications in case of low tumors, narrow pelvis, obese patients, and anteriorly located cancers. It was developed to overcome some drawbacks of laparoscopic TME, basically the difficulty of a low division of the rectum with intracorporeal stapling with a known negative distal margin.

Different platforms have been used to perform this approach, and we herein present the technique and the preliminary results of a small series of robotic transanal TME. More data is necessary to determine whether the robotic approach gives a true advantage compared with other platforms, but the robotic technique certainly gives the advantage of an extremely precise dissection under perfect tridimensional vision in a very narrow space. If this precision will reflect in better oncological and functional outcomes for patients will be the matter for further investigations.

Keywords

Rectal cancer • Transanal total mesorectal excision • Robotic TME • TaTME

31.1 Introduction

Since 1982 when Bill Heald [1] revolutionized the history of rectal cancer introducing the concept of total mesorectal excision (TME), the amount of knowledge about natural history, prognostic factors, diagnosis, adjuvant and neo-adjuvant therapies, and surgical technique has continued to grow.

C.G.S. Hüscher, M.D., F.A.C.S., F.R.C.S (✉) • C. Ponzano, M.D. • G. Marzullo, M.D.
General and Oncologic Surgery Department, Rummo Hospital,
Via dell'Angelo 1, Benevento, Italy
e-mail: cristiano.huscher@gmail.com

G. Dapri, J.H. Marks (eds.), *Surgical Techniques in Rectal Cancer*,
https://doi.org/10.1007/978-4-431-55579-7_31

There is probably no other field in general surgery where the interest and work of clinical investigators has been so active. There are many reasons for this. First, surgical technique by itself is able to heavily change the course of an otherwise aggressive disease. Less local recurrence actually means more long-term survival [2]. This certainly pushed surgeons toward better knowledge of the TME technique and trying to achieve the "perfect specimen." A natural progression was also achieved in terms of functional results. Preserving the integrity of the mesorectum turned gradually in a more and more precise respect of the delicate neural and visceral structures around it. Minimal disturbance to these structures may bring profound functional effects that lead to a severe impairment in the quality of life of the patients. Sexual and urological dysfunction are certainly reduced by precise surgical dissection, but studies on this specific topic are still very few in the medical literature.

When laparoscopy appeared as a new surgical option, many concerns were raised about its oncological adequacy. Current evidence suggests that "primary markers" of a good-quality oncologic resection (number of nodes harvested; proximal, distal, and radial margins; length of the specimens; all surrogate indicators of local and distant recurrence rate and ultimately of survival) are not compromised by the laparoscopic approach to rectal cancer and may be equivalent to those of open surgery [3].

As time has gone on, some of the benefits of the laparoscopic approach to TME have started to be appreciated even by the "old guard" of open surgeons. Additionally, laparoscopy has the advantage to show to everybody the whole procedure and thus the ability to teach surgery in a way not previously possible. This explained the widespread use of live demonstrations with expert surgeons showing a well-standardized and reproducible technique which potentially has resulted in a better oncological outcome for all [4]. Laparoscopic magnification and visualization are advances of critical import in the constant drive toward greater precision in cancer surgery [5].

As the technique was adopted around the world, some unique drawbacks to the laparoscopic approach started to become evident. Division of the rectum using intracorporeal stapling devices is technically difficult due to their width and limited roticulation. More than one cartridge is often required to transect the rectum, and this is a well-known factor affecting the leak rate [6, 7].

Even more problematic in low rectal cancers is stapling across or just below the tumor with inadequate margin, a risk which is higher than in open surgery where, in fact, the triple-stapling technique was developed in order to minimize this redoubtable mistake [8]. Although distal tumor margins are a justifiable concern, the focus over recent years has rightly shifted toward obtaining clean lateral (or radial) margins as well [9–11]. The lower tumors are not only surgically more difficult to excise, but because of the closer association with the distal mesorectum than the higher cancers [12], tearing the mesorectum carries a higher risk of leaving cancer cells in the pelvis.

Big, low, tumors in a narrow pelvis, especially anteriorly located, are mostly unsuitable for a laparoscopic approach. As in open surgery, these cancers are the most difficult cases to deal with [5].

Meanwhile, many companies developed new instruments and tools with the aim of further reducing the access trauma to the abdominal wall. Single-port surgery and natural orifice transluminal endoscopic surgery (NOTES) were investigated by many authors almost in the same time frame. After initial enthusiastic reports on feasibility and potential benefits, technical drawbacks and limited indications emerged for both techniques, and nowadays we can affirm that NOTES and single-port surgery are elegant techniques whose clinical applications are still limited to few centers with high laparoscopic and endoscopic expertise and to selected cases.

One of the major obstacles to NOTES diffusion concerned the opening of an otherwise healthy organ and the technical difficulties in closing the opened organ with the existing instruments.

The endoscopic platform, developed by Gerard Buess in 1983 in Tubingen, for transanal endoscopic microsurgery (TEM), seemed to be the right answer to the question of a reliable access platform and visceral closure, for NOTES. This seemed especially appealing after the fear of short-term complications arising by fecal contamination of the abdominal cavity was overcome [13–16]. Moreover, in colorectal resections this risk also applies to laparoscopic and open resections where microscopic fecal contaminations routinely occur. As a result of this, rectosigmoid resection becomes the most attractive target for NOTES. In 2010 Sylla et al. published the first case of NOTES transanal resection of a rectal cancer with TME (taTME) under laparoscopic assistance [17]. In 2013 Sylla and Lacy published the results of the first cases of down-to-up TME where total mesorectal excision was performed transanally with laparoscopic assistance for vascular ligation and colonic mobilization. The major finding from those papers was that dissection from below, in low cancer, narrow pelvis, and anteriorly located tumors, was much easier than either minimally invasive or open surgery from above [18, 19].

In an editorial published in 2013 by Heald, he predicted that 2013 would have been the year of endoscopic transanal approach to radical low rectal resection and anastomosis [20]. Successively many authors published case reports and case series of transanal endoscopic TME [21–26], and a potential further step forward was the introduction of transanal robot-assisted TME, first proposed by Atallah as a real advantage in the use of the Da Vinci robotic system (Intuitive Surgical, Sunnyvale, CA, USA) [27–30].

Before entering in the technical aspects of the robotic procedure, which is the topic of this chapter, it is worthwhile to note that the transanal approach to low rectal cancers has been developed in 1984 by Gerald Marks, who coined the name transanal transabdominal (TATA) procedure with coloanal hand-sewn anastomosis, to avoid a permanent colostomy for low-lying cancers [31]. In 2010 John Marks et al. published the results of laparoscopic TATA for rectal cancer in the distal 3 cm of the rectum, with a very low recurrence rate (2.5%) and a high percentage of sphincter preservation (90%) despite very low tumor locations. In this technique the dissection begins transanally to ensure a maximal and known distance from the tumor, with a full-thickness incision through the anal canal. An intersphincteric dissection between the puborectalis and the internal sphincter is then performed, the rectum is mobilized transanally to the level of the cervix in the female and to the seminal vesicles in the male, and here is where the transanal procedure stops and laparoscopic procedure starts. In half of the patients in this series, the specimen was extracted transanally, and a hand-sewn anastomosis was performed in all cases. A diverting stoma was performed in all cases [32]. So the major difference between the TATA technique and the "new" transanal taTME approach basically lies in the use of dedicated platforms.

31.2 Platforms

Without entering in the details of the different platforms used to achieve pure or laparoscopically assisted transanal TME, which have been extensively described elsewhere in this book, we would like to briefly discuss what are, in our opinion, the major advantages and drawbacks of every system in order to clarify what technical aspects have led us to the use of the GelPOINT system (Applied Medical Inc., Rancho Santa Margarita, CA, USA) for the robot-assisted approach to the transanal TME.

The SILS system (Covidien, New Haven, CT, USA) has the advantage of being a small, soft system, easily introduced in the anal canal, but has three major disadvantages: first, both the operating surgeon and the camera assistant must find place between the patient's legs; second, it requires the use of a 5 mm camera; and third, this platform is not suitable for the robotic approach because it has predesigned ports that don't fit with the 8 mm port (for instruments) and 12 mm port (for camera) of the robot. If the robotic ports are inserted using and enlarging the existing holes, the system becomes very fragile and is easily displaced outside the anal canal by the movements of the robotic arms.

The transanal endoscopic operation (TEO) rigid platform (KARL STORZ Endoskope, Tuttlingen, Germany) is a very attractive system to work with. It is, in fact, a very stable platform connected to the operating room table that doesn't require the presence between the patient's legs of a second surgeon. The system allows the use of a 10 mm scope, doesn't require the use of specifically designed instruments, and acts itself as a retractor when properly orientated inside the rectum. It also has the great advantage of being produced in two different lengths (9 and 15 cm) that allows for a more precise dissection and visualization until the peritoneal cavity is reached (and even further). The major disadvantage of this system is the fixed position of the camera, which requires the surgeon to zoom in as the dissection advances, with a relative loss in the quality of visual definition. This platform also has the limitation of pre-shaped hole for the ports that does not allow the utilization of robotic ports.

The multiport rectal device GelPOINT has the advantage of being a large platform that allows the introduction of as many ports as needed and doesn't have a fixed location or dimension for the insertion of the cannulas. When used "traditionally," it has the same disadvantages of the SILS system, namely, the contemporary presence of two operating surgeons between the patient's legs. It allows the use of a 3-D flexible-tip endoscope (3-D EndoEye 5 mm flexible-tip video laparoscope (Olympus KeyMed, Europe)), which helps to overcome some of the difficulties of working with parallel instruments. With this device it is possible to place the robotic ports setting their position according to patient characteristics and tumor location.

31.3 Operating Theater

When working with the Da Vinci system (Intuitive Surgical), the operating room needs to be carefully set up in order to avoid collision between the laparoscopic and robotic towers, to leave enough space for the all equipment, and to maintain the sterility of the robotic arms during all the procedure. While all of these items may sound obvious, in fact, especially with a new technique being established, they are not at all. Any robotic procedure is performed by a team. In this team, the only person that seems to enjoy the robotic dissection is the operating surgeon (and probably later the patient), who sits comfortably at the console and benefits from 3-D vision, appreciating the great ergonomic advantage of the robotic system.

The rest of the team has many practical problems that one needs to know if considering adopting this new procedure.

The anesthesiologist, once the patient cart is positioned, has all his/her "sacred" space almost fully invaded by the patient cart. This means that it will be very difficult for anesthesia to check the position, for instance, of the endotracheal tube (there is almost always some cephalad movement of the endotracheal tube assuming the lithotomy from the supine position), to access intravascular lines and electrodes, and to control the position of the patient during the whole transanal dissection. By discussing these aspects with your anesthesiologist, beforehand you can be sure he/she will be happier and collaborative. The other aspect that must be discussed in advance is the patient's position. In fact, once the robotic arms are docked, the table cannot be moved, unless undocking the robot. For the entire transanal phase of the procedure, the patient must remain in a deep Trendelenburg position. Make this point clear before beginning the transanal dissection and fix properly the patient to the table, with shoulder supports with soft pads placed in between to reduce the risks of shoulder or nerve injury.

The scrub nurse is the second person that must be well trained in this new approach.

The role of the scrub nurse as usual starts before the procedure begins. He/she has to drape the robotic arms and to attach and calibrate the optic and is usually involved in positioning the patient cart into the sterile field. He/she has a working space that is unusual, because he/she must stay far enough from the robotic arms to avoid the risk of being inadvertently hit, but close enough to be ready to help the patient-side assistant surgeon in changing the instruments, cleaning the scope, inserting clip or stapling instruments, etc. The scrub nurse also has a role in controlling that there is not any clashing between the robotic arms and between the robotic arms and the patient.

The assistant surgeon also plays a key role in this team. He/she is the one that has to communicate with the lead surgeon sitting at the console and watching the 3-D monitor. This communication is not always simple as the surgeon console is placed outside the sterile field. Because the operating surgeon is watching his/her own monitor, and because the system lacks any tactile feedback, he/she cannot realize when an external arm clashing occurs or when a robotic arm is against the patient's abdominal wall or, as in the technique described below, against the patient's legs.

The assistant surgeon is also the person responsible for robot docking, instrument exchange, manipulation of laparoscopic instruments, application of hemostatic instruments, clips, lavage, and aspiration. His/her position on the sterile field is almost always an uncomfortable one between the robotic arms, with a high probability to clash against the robot (who invariably wins). Within the very narrow field of the transanal procedure, the ergonomics for the assistant surgeon are very poor and need to be improved.

With these points made clear to the entire team, the procedure can start.

For all rectal cancer surgery, our standard preparation of the patient includes a 7-day low-residue diet and a mechanical bowel preparation for 2 days preceding the operation. Preoperative workup includes endorectal ultrasonography, pelvic magnetic resonance according to the MERCURY Protocol [33], and a total body CT scan.

Antibiotics are administered as a single dose 30 min prior to skin incision, and a second dose is repeated if the procedure lasts more than 3 h.

31.4 Surgical Technique

Robot-assisted transanal TME is performed with a hybrid approach with the abdominal portion of the operation first completed either laparoscopically, with multiple- or single-access device or with an open approach. In this chapter we describe the transanal TME assisted by single-port abdominal laparoscopy.

The procedure starts laparoscopically with the patient positioned in modified lithotomy with the legs in Allen stirrups. As we always protect the colorectal/anal anastomosis with a loop ileostomy, the single-port device is positioned at the future ileostomy site.

The operation starts by ligating the inferior mesenteric vein and artery and achieving wide splenic flexure mobilization. Then the descending colon is mobilized from medial to lateral in the avascular plane between the Toldt and Gerota fascia and along the left parietocolic groove downward till the sacral promontory is reached. At this point the laparoscopic phase ends, and the pneumoperitoneum is deflated, the single-port left in place, and the abdominal field kept sterile.

The legs are brought up to the high dorsal lithotomy position, the more apart as possible. This will help in avoiding collisions between patient's thighs and the robotic arms. The perineum is prepared and draped appropriately after a lavage with betadine solution has been performed transanally.

The sleeve portion of the GelPOINT Path Transanal Access Platform (Applied Medical Inc.) is positioned and secured with sutures to the skin (Fig. 31.1). For a lower tumor, a circular dissection starts 1 cm above the dentate line to free 2 cm of the rectum using a Lone Star Retractor System (Cooper Surgical, Trumbull, CT, USA). A purse string is placed to tightly occlude the rectum with a measured, known distal free margin from the tumor (Fig. 31.2). Before attaching the GelPOINT to the sleeve, it is preferable to insert the trocars in the desired position to avoid a blind insertion through the gel part with the risk of making an injury to the rectal mucosa (Fig. 31.3).

The GelPOINT is then secured to the sleeve (Fig. 31.4) and the robotic cart is docked along the patient's right side to enable the robotic arms to swing over the abdomen and to be directed transanally (Figs. 31.5 and 31.6).

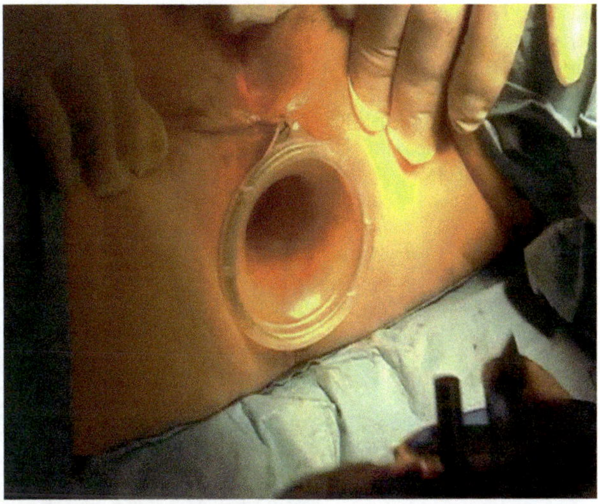

Fig. 31.1 The sleeve portion of the GelPOINT platform is inserted and secured to the perianal skin with sutures

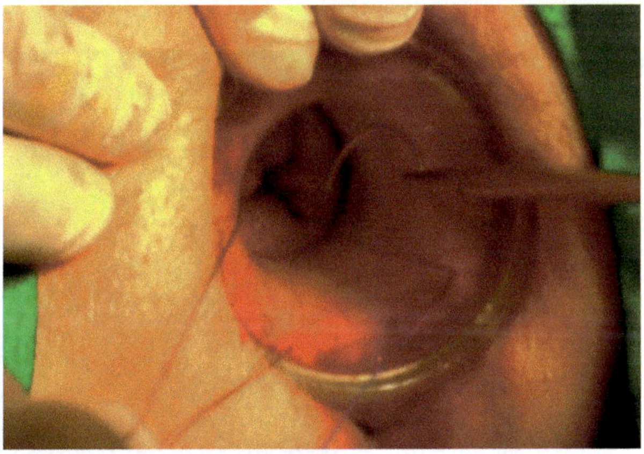

Fig. 31.2 A purse string is fashioned to tightly occlude the rectum at a measured, controlled, distal margin from the tumor

The scope is positioned in the 10–12 mm superior trocar, and once the camera is locked, we find useful to exercise on this trocar a little traction upward with the robotic arm to gain more space between the ports that can help to reduce the risk of collision between the robotic arms outside and between the instruments inside the rectum (Fig. 31.7). This traction is made possible thanks to the elastic consistency of the GelPOINT. The port device is connected to CO_2 insufflation with the setting of 20 mmHg.

A bipolar forceps is inserted in the left port and a monopolar hook in the right one.

The rectal mucosa is scored circumferentially with the monopolar hook starting distally to the purse string (Fig. 31.8), and the incision is deepened to obtain a full-thickness dissection which starts anteriorly. The rectum is separated from the posterior vagina or from prostate and seminal vesicles remaining in a plane posterior to the Denonvilliers' fascia (Figs. 31.9, 31.10, 31.11, and 31.12).

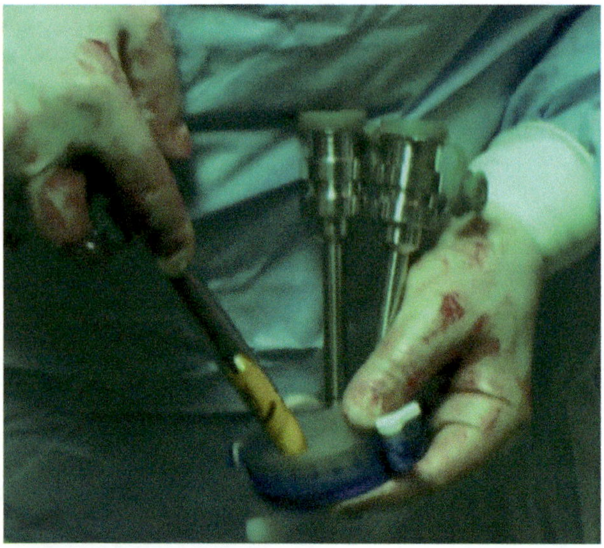

Fig. 31.3 Trocars are inserted in the gel portion of the GelPOINT in the desired position before securing it to the sleeve in order to minimize the risk of injury to the rectal mucosa

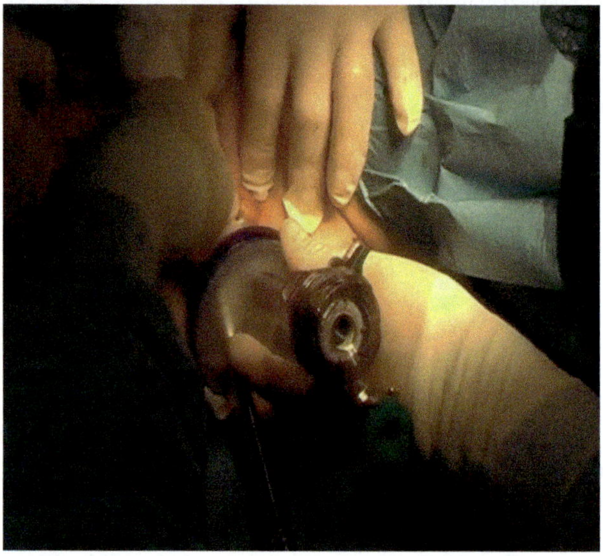

Fig. 31.4 The GelPOINT is then attached to the sleeve

Then the posterior dissection is achieved following the holy plane of Heald (Figs. 31.13 and 31.14). Care must be taken during this phase not to open the Waldeyer's fascia with the risk of bleeding from the presacral vessels which can make the dissection very tedious, as even small bleeding in the very limited posterior space reduces enormously the quality of the vision and thus the precision of the dissection.

Once the anterior and posterior planes have been dissected, the lateral stalks, containing connective tissue and sometimes branches of the middle rectal artery, can be divided. A gentle lateral traction rightward and leftward can be applied on

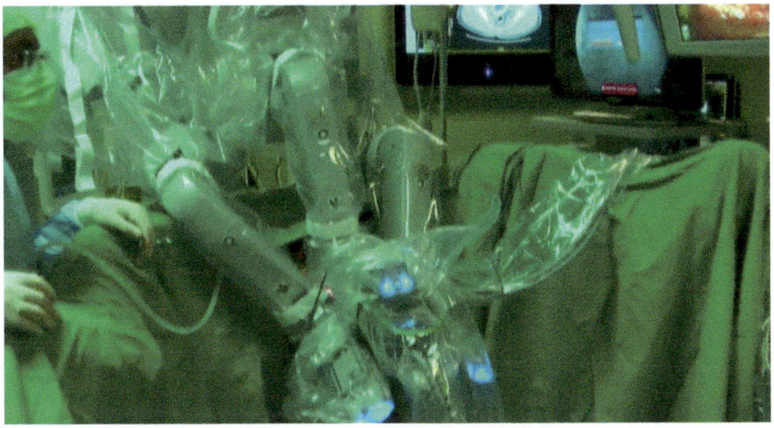

Fig. 31.5 The robotic cart is docked along the patient's right side

Fig. 31.6 Detail of the position of the robotic arms that swing over the abdomen and are directed transanally in the limited space between patient's legs

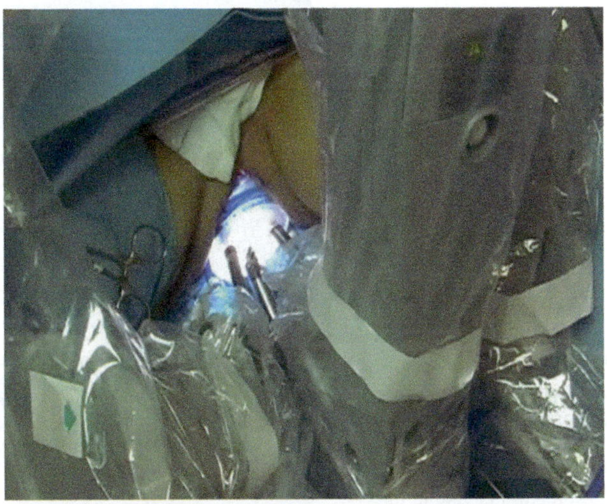

Fig. 31.7 The scope is positioned in the upper trocar, and once the camera is locked, a little traction upward can be applied on this trocar to gain more space between the trocars. This maneuver can reduce the risk of collision between robotic arms outside and between working instruments inside the rectum

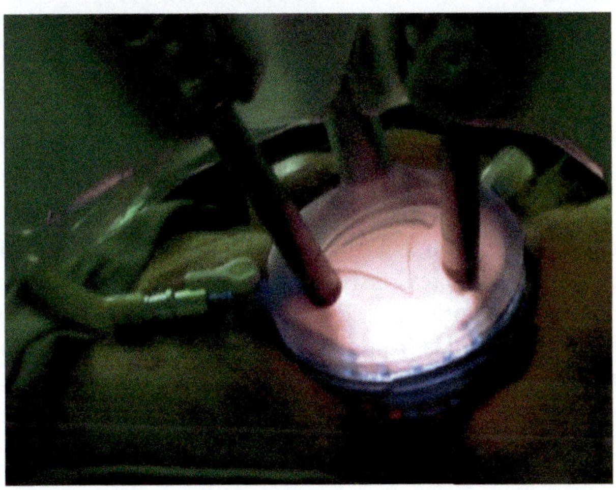

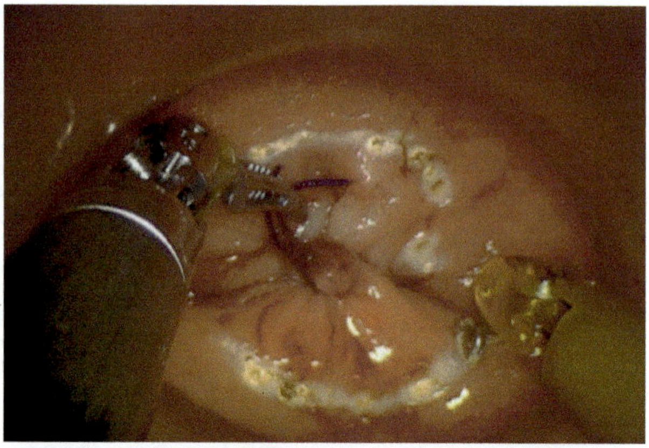

Fig. 31.8 Gently pulling on the purse string, rectal mucosa is scored circumferentially with monopolar hook

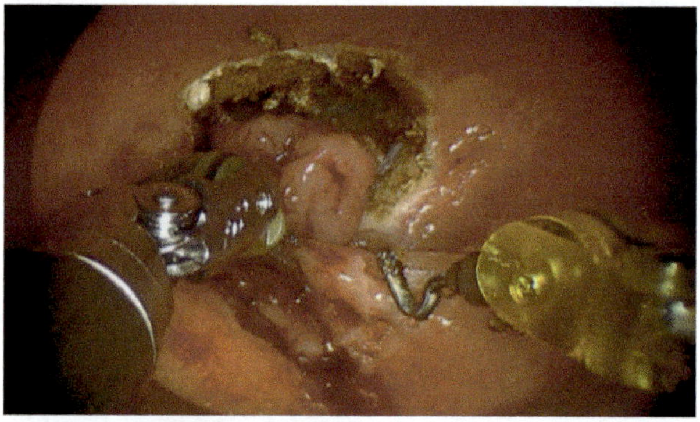

Fig. 31.9 The full-thickness dissection stars anteriorly

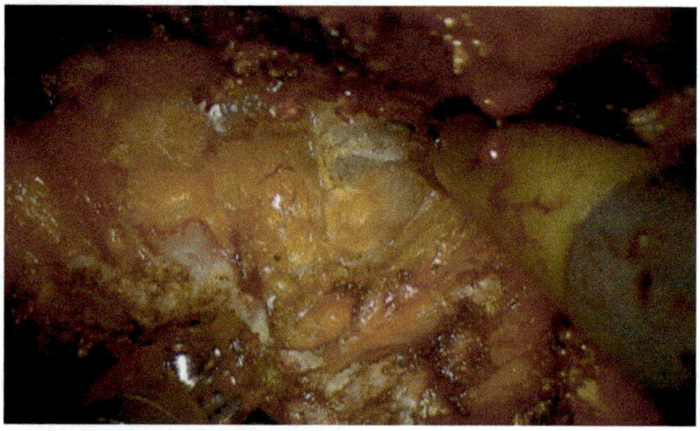

Fig. 31.10 The anterior dissection proceeds upward, and the boundary between the Denonvilliers' fascia and the thin anterior mesorectum is visible in the field

the tail of the purse string to facilitate this division and to expose the right plane connecting the previously dissected anterior and posterior planes.

Further anterior dissection is often necessary at this point to reach and open the pouch of Douglas from below. With all the rectal dissection completed, the specimen is pushed into the abdominal cavity and the robotic cart can be undocked.

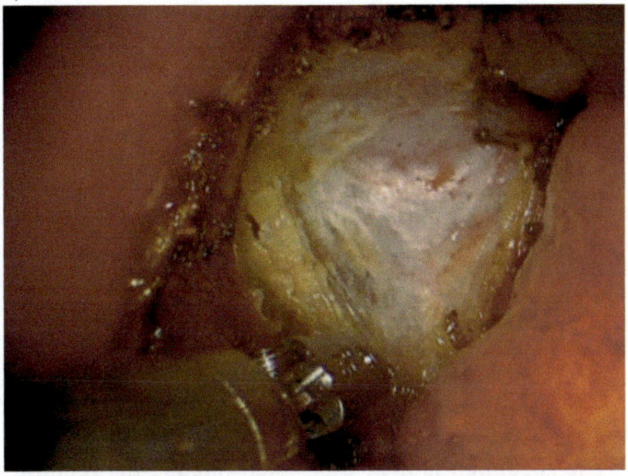

Fig. 31.11 Anteriorly, in male patients, the prostate is always very well visible even in a narrow pelvis, which represents one of the major advances of this approach

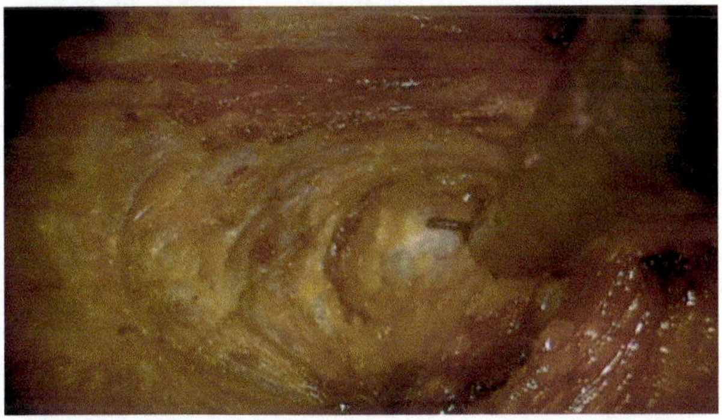

Fig. 31.12 The tiny neurovascular branches are evidenced anteriorly much more than through the abdominal approach

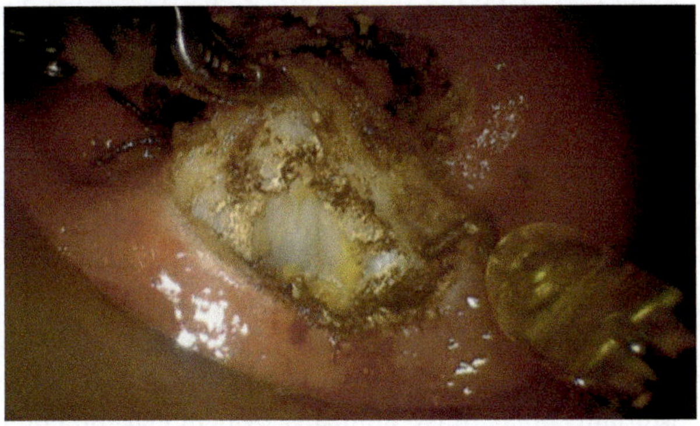

Fig. 31.13 The posterior dissection follows the holy plane

With the two dissections connected, the procedure goes back to the abdominal side, leaving in place the GelPOINT to maintain the pneumoperitoneum, and later the sleeve portion of the device is used for easier and protected transanal specimen extraction.

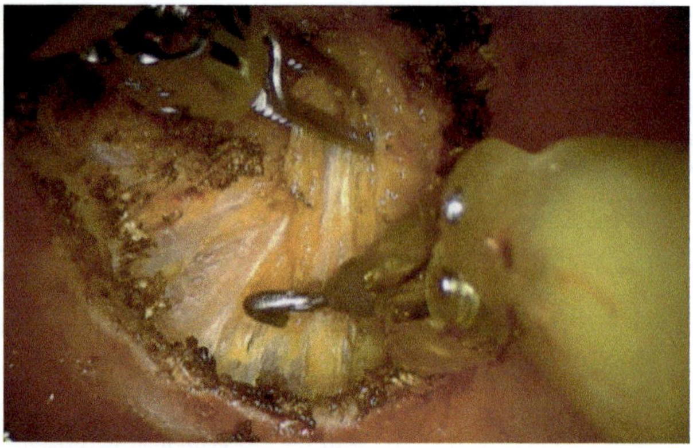

Fig. 31.14 In the posterior plane, great care must be taken not to go too posteriorly in the unsafe plane behind Waldeyer's fascia. This plane is still a safe plane for the oncologic dissection, but there is a high risk of bleeding from the presacral vessels and of damaging of the nerves

The specimen is then transected outside the rectum, and a purse string is fashioned to insert the anvil of a circular stapler.

A second purse string is fashioned on the distal rectal stump with the sleeve of the GelPOINT still in place, and a stapled end-to-end or side-to-end anastomosis is performed.

A pelvic drain is usually left in place and a temporary loop ileostomy at the site of the single access always fashioned.

31.5 Personal Experience

The preliminary results of our experience have been published recently [29].

Seven patients were submitted to the described technique. The mean age was 63.2 ± 9.7 years (range 48–74), the body mass index was 29.9 ± 6.1 kg/m^2 (range 21.5–37.5), and ASA grade was 1 in 4, 2 in 1, and 3 in 2 patients. The median tumor distance from the anal verge was 20 mm (range 10–65). Preoperative tumor stage included 5T2 and 3T3 tumors, all with negative nodes. Thus, in this set of patients, chemoradiotherapy was not used preoperatively.

The mean number of lymph node harvested was 14 ± 3 (range from 10 to 20). A R0 resection was achieved in all patients. The mean distal margin was 27 ± 20 mm (range from 10 to 65), and circumferential margin was 3.2 ± 1.8 (range from 1.4 to 5). Macroscopic assessment of the specimen showed complete mesorectum in six cases and nearly complete in one case.

Postoperative TNM stage was pT1N0 in two patients, pT2N0 in two, pT3N0 in three, and pT3N1 in one case.

Mortality was nil. No clinically evident anastomotic leak was recorded, and the only major complication occurred in this group was a rectal bleeding on postoperative day 2 treated conservatively with blood transfusion. The mean hospital stay was 4.8 ± 0.6 days (range from 4 to 6).

References

1. Heald RJ, Ryall RDH. The mesorectum in rectal cancer surgery—the clue to pelvic recurrence? Br J Surg. 1982;69:613–6.
2. Heald RJ. The "Holy Plane" of rectal surgery. J R Soc Med. 1988;81:503–8.
3. Anderson C, Uman G, Pigazzi A, et al. Oncologic outcomes of laparoscopic surgery for rectal cancer: a systematic review and meta-analysis of the literature. Eur J Oncol. 2008;34:1135–42.
4. Chand M, Heald RJ. Laparoscopic rectal cancer surgery. Br J Surg. 2011;98:166–7.
5. Heald RJ. Rectal cancer patients are often not suitable for laparoscopic surgery. Commentary. Color Dis. 2010;12:31–2.
6. Ito M, Sugito M, Kobayashi A, Nishizawa Y, Tsunoda Y, Saito N. Relationship between multiple numbers of stapler firings during rectal division and anastomotic leakage after laparoscopic rectal resection. Int J Color Dis. 2008;23:703–7.
7. Park JS, Choi GS, Kim SH, Kim HR, Kim NK, et al. Multicenter analysis of risk factors for anastomotic leakage after laparoscopic rectal cancer excision: the Korean laparoscopic colorectal surgery study group. Ann Surg. 2013;257:665–71.
8. O'Rourke N, Moran BJ, Heald RJ. A laparoscopic triple stapling technique that facilitates anterior resection for rectal cancer. J Laparoendosc Surg. 1994;4(4):261–3.
9. Quirke P, Durdey P, Dixon M. Local recurrence of rectal carcinoma due to inadequate surgical resection. Histopathological study of lateral tumour spread and surgical excision. Lancet. 1986;2:996.
10. Quirke P, Steele R, Monson J, Grieve R, Khanna S, et al. Effect of plane of surgery achieved on local recurrence in patients with operable rectal cancer: a prospective study using data from the MRC CR07 and NCIC-CTG C016 randomised clinical trial. Lancet. 2009;373:821–8.
11. Mark JH, Frenkel JL, D'Andrea AP, Greenleaf CE. Maximizing rectal cancer results: TEM and TATA techniques to expand sphincter preservation. Surg Oncol Clin N Am. 2011;20:501–20.
12. Heald RJ, Ryall RDH. Recurrence and survival after total mesorectal excision for rectal cancer. Lancet. 1986;1:1479–82.
13. Gagavan JV, Whiteford MH, Swanstrom LL. Full-thickness intraperitoneal excision by transanal endoscopic microsurgery does not increase short-term complications. Am J Surg. 2004;187:630–4.
14. Tsai BM, Finne CO, Nordestam JF, Christoforidis D, Madoff RD, Mellgren A. Transanal endoscopic microsurgery of rectal tumors: outcome and recommendations. Dis Colon Rectum. 2010;53(1):16–23.
15. Cataldo PA, O'Brien S, Osler T. Transanal endoscopic microsurgery: a prospective evaluation of functional results. Dis Colon Rectum. 2005;48:1366–71.
16. Whiteford MH, Denk PM, Swanstrom LL. Feasibility of radical sigmoid colectomy performed as natural orifice translumenal endoscopic surgery (NOTES) using transanal endoscopic microsurgery. Surg Endosc. 2007;21:1870–4.
17. Sylla P, Rattner DW, Delgado S, Lacy AM. NOTES transanal rectal cancer resection using transanal endoscopic microsurgery and laparoscopic assistance. Surg Endosc. 2010;24:1205–10.
18. Sylla P, Bordeianou LG, Berger D, Han KS, Lauwers GY, Sahani DV, Sbeih MA, Lacy A, Rattner DW. A pilot study of natural orifice transanal endoscopic total mesorectal excision with laparoscopic assistance for rectal cancer. Surg Endosc. 2013;27:3396–405.
19. Lacy AM, Rattner DW, Adelsdorfer C, Tasende MM, Fernandez M, Delgado S, Sylla P, Martinez-Palli G. Transanal natural orifice transluminal endoscopic surgery (NOTES) rectal resection: "down-to-up" total mesorectal excision (TME)- short term outcomes in the first 20 cases. Surg Endosc. 2013;27:3165–72.
20. Heald RJ. A new solution to some old problem: transanal TME. Tech Coloproctol. 2013;17:257–8.

21. Rouanet P, Mourregot A, Azar CC, Carrere S, Gutowski M, Quenet F, Saint-Aubert B, Colombo PE. Transanal endoscopic proctectomy: an innovative procedure for difficult resection of rectal tumors in men with narrow pelvis. Dis Colon Rectum. 2013;56:408–15.
22. Atallah S, Martin-Perez B, Albert M, deBeche-Adams T, Nassif G, Hunter L, Larach S. Transanal minimally invasive surgery for total mesorectal excision (TAMIS-TME): results and experience with the first 20 patients undergoing curative-intent rectal cancer surgery at a single institution. Tech Coloproctol. 2014;18(5):473–80.
23. Velthius S, van den Boezem PB, van der Peet DL, Cuesta MA, Sietses C. Feasibility study of transanal total mesorectal excision. Br J Surg. 2013;100:828–31.
24. Zhang H, Zhang YS, Jin XW, Li MZ, Fan JS, Yang ZH. Transanal single-port laparoscopic total mesorectal excision in the treatment of rectal cancer. Tech Coloproctol. 2013;17:117–23.
25. Choi BJ, Lee SC, Kang WK. Single port laparoscopic total mesorectal excision with transanal resection (transabdominal transanal resection) for low rectal cancer: initial experience with 22 cases. Int J Surg. 2013;11:858–63.
26. McLemore EC, Coker AM, Devaraj B, Chakedis J, Maawy A, Inui T, Talamini M, Horgan S, Peterson MR, Sylla P, Ramamoorthy S. TAMIS-assisted laparoscopic low anterior resection with total mesorectal excision in a cadaveric series. Surg Endosc. 2013;27:3478–84.
27. Cahill RA. Single port surgery for rectal cancer—going up or down? Dis Colon Rectum. 2013;56:1199–200.
28. Atallah S, Nassif G, Polavarapu H, deBeche-Adams T, Ouyang J, Albert M, Larach S. Robotic-assisted transanal surgery for total mesorectal excision (RATS-TME): a description of a novel surgical approach with video demonstration. Tech Coloproctol. 2013;17:441–7.
29. Huscher CGS, Bretagnol F, Ponzano C. Robotic-assisted transanal total mesorectal excision the key against the Achilles' heel of rectal cancer? Ann Surg. 2015;261(5):e120–1.
30. Sylla P. Robotically assisted transanal total mesorectal excision: an exciting new trend in rectal cancer surgery. Ann Surg. 2015;261(5):e122.
31. Marks G, Mohiuddin M, Goldstein SD. Sphincter preservation for cancer of the distal rectum using high dose preoperative radiation. Int J Radiat Oncol Biol Phys. 1988;15:1065–8.
32. Marks J, Mizrahi B, Dalane S, Nwezw I, Marks G. Laparoscopic transanal abdominal transanal resection with sphincter preservation for rectal cancer in the distal 3 cm of the rectum after neoadjuvant therapy. Surg Endosc. 2010;24:2700–7.
33. MERCURY Study Group. Extramural depth of tumor invasion at thin-section MR in patients with rectal cancer: results of the MERCURY study. Radiology. 2007;243(1):132–9.

Transanal Robot-Assisted TME with Robot-Assisted Abdominal Laparoscopy

32

Marcos Gómez Ruiz

Abstract

Open anterior resection with total mesorectal excision (TME) is the standard method of rectal cancer resection. However, this procedure remains technically difficult and has a high morbidity associated. Minimally invasive approaches may help to reduce these morbidities even though they still have some technical limitations. A robotic transanal approach could overcome some of these limitations and reduce the morbidities improving oncological and functional outcomes.

The feasibility of robotic transanal TME and set-up has been evaluated in different pilot studies.

Using the robotic technology and a specifically designed port for robotic transanal access, TME was shown to be feasible, and one specific preferred set-up was determined. Further clinical trials are still necessary to assess the safety and efficacy of this technique. In this chapter we describe a standardized technique after our initial clinical experience.

The standardization of this technique may help in this assessment and in the evolution to a natural orifice translumenal endoscopic surgery proctectomy with TME in the future.

Keywords

Rectal cancer • Robotic transanal surgery

M. Gómez Ruiz, MD, PhD, CBC (Hon.), EBSQ-Coloproctology
Unidad de Cirugía Colorrectal, Servicio de Cirugía General y Aparato Digestivo, Hospital Universitario Marqués de Valdecilla, Santander, Spain

Secretaría de Cirugía General y Aparato Digestivo, Pabellón 19 Bajo, Hospital Universitario Marqués de Valdecilla, Av. Valdecilla s/n, 39008 Santander, Spain
e-mail: marcgomez@humv.es

G. Dapri, J.H. Marks (eds.), *Surgical Techniques in Rectal Cancer*,
https://doi.org/10.1007/978-4-431-55579-7_32

32.1 Introduction

32.1.1 Minimally Invasive Surgery for Rectal Cancer

The anatomical location and its anatomical relations determine the difficulty of the surgical resection of the rectum. The rectum is placed in a narrow muscle-skeleton tunnel with an abdominal entrance and a perineal end. Inside this tunnel and with a huge relation to the rectum, we can also find the genital apparatus, the bladder, the urethra and a plexus of nerves with great importance in faecal, urinary and sexual function. This anatomical location makes the rectum a difficult structure to visualize and dissect. Conventional surgical techniques have a significant number of complications associated with this difficulty, making the surgeon factor a crucial element in the results of the surgical procedure. Overcoming these challenges is only possible with the application of the best knowledge of the disease, the best image techniques and over all the development of technologies that assist the surgeon to solve the barriers derived from the anatomical location [1].

In the last 30 years, the improvement in surgical results and the advances in surgical techniques and in the adjuvant therapies have changed the mentality of many surgeons. Bill Heald introduced in 1979 the total mesorectal excision (TME) concept [2]. In 1982, he performed the first description of non-nodal metastatic disease in the mesorectum distal to the tumour in the specimen of proctectomies [3], and in 1986, he published the results of the first 112 cases with large decrease of local recurrence (2.7% 5-year rate) and an increase of the survival rate (81.7% 5-year rate). These were the best results reported so far. The description of the "holy plane" by Heald [4] allowed the standardization of the TME technique.

On the other hand, there has been an evolution in the surgical mentality in order to achieve good oncological results at the same time that we obtain good functional results. In the last years, there has been a tendency to abandon the Miles procedure [5] as the "gold standard" for the treatment of lower third rectal tumours. Sphincter preservation techniques have been developed grounded in the knowledge about transmural extension of the disease [6]. Even the 5 cm of the distal margin rule was modified to 2 cm in the 1980s and more recently to 1 or even less [7]. Marks described the transanal-abdominal-transanal (TATA) resection in 1984 for cancers in the lower one third of the rectum, and Schiessel et al. developed intersphincteric resection with colo-anal anastomosis in 1994 [8, 9]. Nowadays, the European Association for Endoscopic Surgery has the following recommendation: a patient with a rectal cancer 3–4 cm from the anal verge, without infiltration of the pelvic floor or external sphincter, should undergo an intersphincteric dissection and a colo-anal anastomosis. If the patient suffers incontinence, an ultralow Hartmann's procedure should be considered (consensus 100%). Transanal intersphincteric resection should start at the dentate line (consensus 92.9%) [10].

Advances in optics and the application of optic fibre allowed the development of the flexible endoscopy. The technological complexity of the colonoscopes limited its use until the 1960s. Fifteen years later, they were as perfect as the gastroscopes, being possible to explore the complete colon and even the distal ileum in around 90% of the cases.

Even though the drawbacks that fiberscopes had were improved, the real revolution in the endoscopic field happened with the arrival of the video endoscope. Welch Allyn Incorporated presented their first video endoscope in 1983. The main feature of this endoscope was the use of a chip to generate images, being able to obtain a two-dimensional vision on a screen. Nowadays, the reduced diameter and perfect flexibility of the endoscopes allow their use without local or general anaesthesia. Their axial vision offers a perfect examination and the complete exploration of the colonic mucosa. They also make possible the accomplishment of biopsies and the treatment of some lesions [11].

This technology allowed better understanding and detection of the polypoid lesions of the colon and the sequence adenoma-adenocarcinoma. Most of these lesions can be removed endoscopically. Because of the size, location or histology, endoscopic excision may not be possible in some cases. In this situation, major surgical techniques have to be used (Park, Kraske, York-Mason or bowel resections).

In this context, the transanal endoscopic microsurgery (TEM) originally described by Gerhard Buess [12] in the 1980s has gained more and more relevance.

TEM is a minimally invasive technique that uses the transanal approach. Through a 3D vision system, access to the mid-superior third of the rectum is facilitated. Its use is widely accepted for resection of rectal adenomas and for T1 carcinomas.

Jacobs et al. described colorectal laparoscopic resection in 1991 [13]. Several prospective, randomized and multicentric clinical trials [14–16] have demonstrated the advantages in postoperative recovery, complications and oncological safety of the laparoscopic surgery in the treatment of colon cancer. However, there is still little clarity in the case of rectal cancer. Many retrospective studies show tendencies in favour of the laparoscopic approach, but there is a lack of evidence. Recently, 3-year follow-up results of COLOR II study were presented [17]. This trial concludes that the laparoscopic approach in the hands of expert surgeons in selected patients is as safe as the open surgery with similar resection margins and better postoperative recovery. Conversion rate in this trial was 17% even though expert surgeons performed the procedures in selected patients.

A new technological advance, the Da Vinci Robotic Surgical System (Intuitive Surgical, Inc., Sunnyvale, CA, USA), provides 3D endoscopic vision with an image magnification up to ×10, endowristed instruments and a tremor filter. These features may potentially decrease the technical difficulties that involve the anatomy of the rectum. After the initial use of this surgical system in other surgical fields, Delaney et al. reported their first experience in colorectal robotic surgery in 2003 [18]. Pigazzi et al. were the first to report a robotic low anterior resection with total mesorectal excision in 2006 [19].

In the last few years, the Da Vinci Robotic Surgical System (Intuitive Surgical, Inc.) has had different developments with new versions (S, Si, Xi®) that progressively included the fourth arm and more recently the possibility of having instrumentation for single-site procedures or fluorescence imaging (Firefly®). The number of centres that are performing robotic colorectal surgery is increasing in the world, but most of these centres are still in their learning curve phase. Very few centres in the world have performed a large number of cases.

The results of different single-institution studies, most of them retrospective, conclude that robotic colorectal surgery is feasible and safe, with very low conversion rates to open surgery and low blood loss. This technology may be specially indicated to perform very low anterior resections with sphincter preservation technique. Some studies show better functional outcomes in urinary and sexual function [20]. Cost-effectiveness results are an important issue due to the cost of the Da Vinci Robotic Surgical System (Intuitive Surgical, Inc.). A narrow view of the process, limited to the surgical procedure, may certainly conclude that robotic surgery is more expensive than open or conventional laparoscopic surgery. It is necessary to perform studies that include the input of the robotic system in a very complex process and that consider the entire benefits of using this technology. With this wider vision and analysis, maybe the use of the robotic instrumentation may have cost-effectiveness advantages as was demonstrated with the conventional laparoscopic approach [21].

The concept of a minimally invasive surgery through natural orifices (NOTES) started to be clinically applied in some surgical procedures like transvaginal cholecystectomy. In 2007, Whiteford et al. demonstrated the feasibility of a transanal sigmoidectomy in a cadaver model using the TEM platform and an endoscopic platform with no need of abdominal wounds [22]. Sylla et al. demonstrated in 2010 the feasibility of the transanal proctectomy using this technique in a swine model [23]. Trunzo and Delaney did demonstrate the feasibility of the transanal endoscopic proctectomy with endoscopic assistance [24]. Using the transanal endoscopic operation (TEO, KARL STORZ Endoskope, Tuttlingen, Germany) platform and a flexible endoscope, Leroy et al. demonstrated the feasibility of the transanal proctectomy in a swine model in 2009 [25]. They published a case report of this technique in 2013 [26]. Nonetheless, and mainly because of the technical difficulties due to the lack of technical development, researchers in the field of the transanal proctectomy have orientated their studies to hybrid procedures with laparoscopic assistance [27]. In 2010, Sylla et al. reported the first proctectomy with total mesorectal excision for the treatment of a mid-rectal cancer [28]. Although this technique is a bit far away from the NOTES concept, it adds some potential advantages, like approaching the "holy plane" from the abdominal approach and the transanal approach. In 2011, Tuech et al. published their first transanal proctectomy performed with the Endorec® trocar (Aspide Medical, La Talaudiere, France) and a single-site port at the ileostomy site. This access made possible the oncological excision of the rectum with a total mesorectal excision and the splenic flexure mobilization [29]. In the following years, different groups in the world have published short series of cases or case reports using different platforms [30, 31].

Lacy et al. published their initial 20 cases with this technique in 2013, concluding that this technique is safe in expert hands, allowing a better visualization and dissection of the pelvis with a good quality of the surgical specimen [32]. Tuech and the multicentre French group have recently reported their experience in a series of 56 cases treated with the transanal approach and with a follow-up between 3 and 5 years. No mortality or intraoperative complications were reported. Morbidity was 26%. TME was complete in 84% of the cases and nearly complete in 16%. The median number of lymph nodes retrieved was 12 (range 7–29) per patient. R0 resection was achieved in 94.6% of the patients with adequate circumferential and distal margins. Functional outcomes were assessed and median Wexner score was 4 (range 3–12) with stool fragmentation and difficult evacuation in 28% of the cases. This study shows that this technique is feasible, a possible alternative to the abdominal laparoscopic approach for rectal cancer and a step forward to NOTES rectal surgery [33].

Simultaneously, Lacy et al. published a retrospective comparative study of a cohort of 37 patients who underwent conventional laparoscopic surgery for rectal cancer compared with 37 patients who underwent a transanal procedure with laparoscopic assistance. In this study they observed that patients who underwent laparoscopic surgery have less colo-anal anastomosis with shorter distal margins and longer operative times. Readmissions were higher in the conventional laparoscopic group. They concluded that the evaluation of short-term outcomes demonstrated that transanal TME is a feasible and safe technique associated with a shorter surgical time and a lower early readmission rate [34].

32.1.2 Robotic Transanal Proctectomy with TME

Clinical experience of robotic transanal TME started in 2013 when Atallah et al. reported their first clinical case in a patient with familiar adenomatous polyposis and two synchronic tumours [35] for transanal access and 5 mm robotic instruments.

Our group published our robotic transanal TME experience in a cadaver model using the PAT platform (Developia-HUMV, Santander, Spain), a self-designed platform, and the GelPOINT (Applied Medical, Rancho Santa Margarita, CA, USA) [36]. In 2014 we reported our first clinical case [37].

Very few publications are available to date about robotic transanal resections with TME, and all are about early experiences [38] or reporting a short series of cases. Huscher et al. have recently published a short series of cases, concluding that this technique is feasible and safe [39].

Atallah et al. also published their initial experience [40]. We have reported the results of our pilot study with our first five cases concluding that this technique is feasible, with good pathological results and postoperative outcomes [41].

To date, the available clinical data make some surgeons think that the transanal approach is feasible and safe, with some potential benefits for the lower third dissection in distal rectal tumours reducing the conversion rate, making unnecessary the use of expensive technologies as robotic instrumentation [42].

Others think that the use of robotic instrumentation could add some potential benefits because of the endowristed instrumentation, excellent vision and future developments of this instrumentation [43].

32.2 Surgical Technique

Surgical technique is divided in two phases. One is the abdominal phase to explore the abdominal cavity and mobilize the left colon. Second is the transanal phase with abdominal assistance to perform the proctectomy and total mesorectal excision.

32.2.1 Abdominal Phase

After general anaesthesia, a urinary catheter is inserted, and patients are placed in supine position using stirrups (Lloyd-Davies position). Nasogastric tube is inserted during the procedure if necessary. Digital examination and rigid proctoscopy are performed to confirm tumour location. A Veress needle is inserted in the left upper quadrant, and the abdomen is insufflated with CO_2 to an average pressure of 10–12 mmHg. Trocars are inserted in the right upper quadrant (12–15 and 8 mm), right lower quadrant (two 8 mm trocars) and periumbilical region (12–15 mm). The patient is then positioned in a 20° right tilt, and the peritoneal cavity is first inspected through a standard laparoscope. After confirming the absence of significant intra-abdominal adhesions and no evidence of carcinomatosis or distal tumour extension, the Da Vinci Surgical System (Intuitive Surgical, Inc.) with instruments and accessories is docked perpendicular to the patient's left side a few centimetres above the level of the umbilicus (Figs. 32.1 and 32.2). Monopolar curved scissors are placed in arm #1, a fenestrated bipolar grasper is placed in arm #2, and a double fenestrated grasper is used in arm #3. A 30°-down 12 or 8.5 mm endoscope is used.

The splenic flexure is taken down with dissection and division of the inferior mesenteric vein (IMV) below the pancreas and inferior mesenteric artery (IMA) at its root. This is routinely performed as this technique is used at the moment for mid-low rectal tumours, and the left colon should be fully mobilized for a tension-free anastomosis. A medial to lateral approach over the pancreas is used for splenic flexure takedown. The descending and sigmoid colon are mobilized finishing the dissection at the sacral promontory. Left iliac vessels and left ureter are routinely identified before the transanal phase of the procedure begins. The hypogastric nerve dissection should also be started at this phase. The Da Vinci Surgical System (Intuitive Surgical, Inc.) is undocked and the patient repositioned in Trendelenburg with slight right tilt for the next phase of the operation.

32.2.2 Transanal Phase

32.2.2.1 Dissection

Low Rectal Tumours

Partial intersphincteric resection (pISR) is performed in these cases before the robotic transanal dissection begins. Special care has to be taken with the anterior plane as urethral injuries have been described during this part of the procedure. A Lone Star retractor (Lone Star Medical Products Inc., Houston, TX, USA) or a PPH anoscope (Ethicon Endo-Surgery, Cincinnati, OH, USA) is positioned, and the mucosa and internal sphincter muscle are dissected circumferentially beginning at least 1 cm below the distal margin of the tumour. Intersphincteric dissection is extended cephalad for a distance of 2–3 cm, and a 00 braided purse-string suture is placed to occlude the rectum below the tumour.

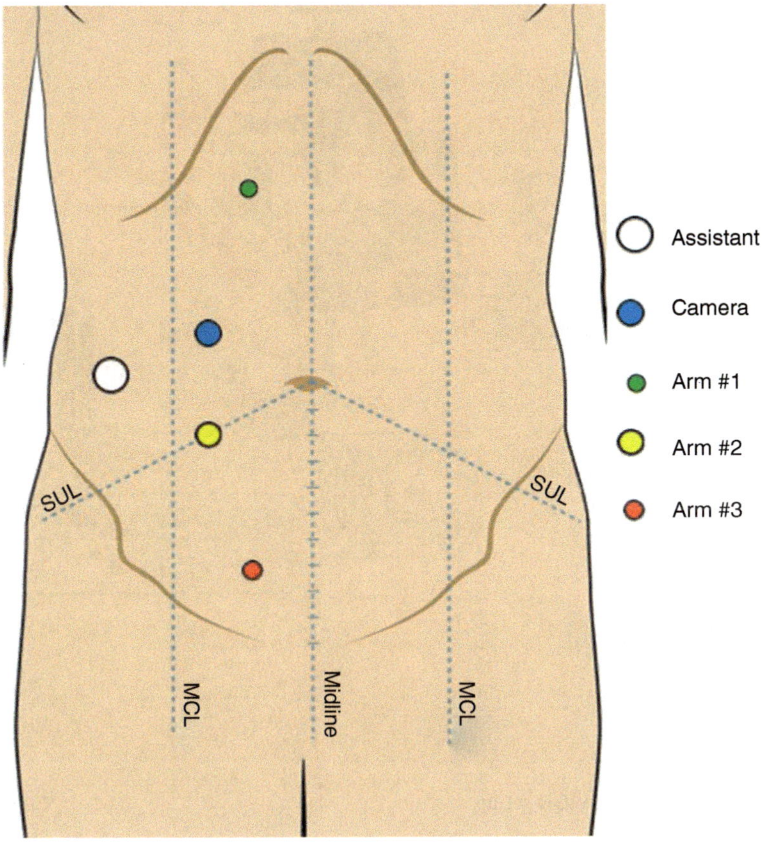

Fig. 32.1 Abdominal trocar set-up

Following rectal occlusion, a "transanal access port" proctoscope (PAT, Developia-HUMV) (Fig. 32.3) is inserted transanally, and a GelPOINT (Applied Medical) is used to occlude the proctoscope and for trocar placement. A 12 or 8.5 mm trocar is used for the optical port. Two 8 mm trocar ports are inserted with a distance of at least 4 cm for robotic instruments, and an accessory 12 mm trocar is inserted for the assistant port. The Da Vinci patient cart is then docked over the left hip of the patient (Figs. 32.4 and 32.5). The fenestrated bipolar grasper is placed in arm #1 and monopolar scissors in arm #2, and a 30°-up endoscope is placed through the 12 mm trocar (Fig. 32.6). The assistant trocar is used primarily to aid in tissue counter-traction or to apply suction or irrigation.

Mid-rectal Tumours

The PAT proctoscope (PAT, Developia-HUMV) is placed transanally after rectal lumen occlusion and fixed to the table. A GelPOINT (Applied Medical) is used to occlude the proctoscope and for trocar placement. Trocars and instruments are

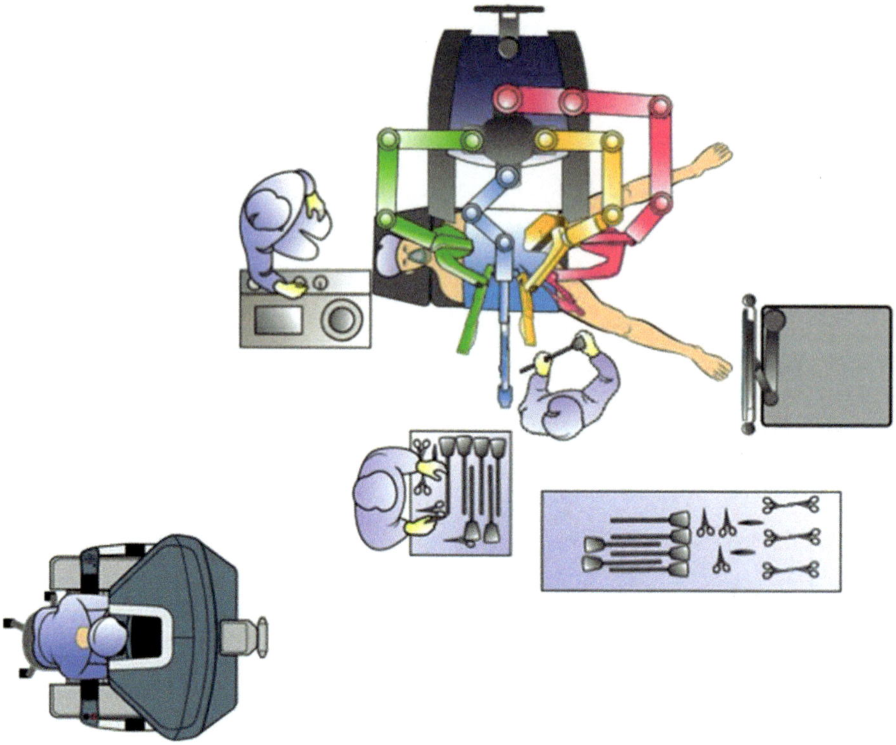

Fig. 32.2 Abdominal phase OR set-up

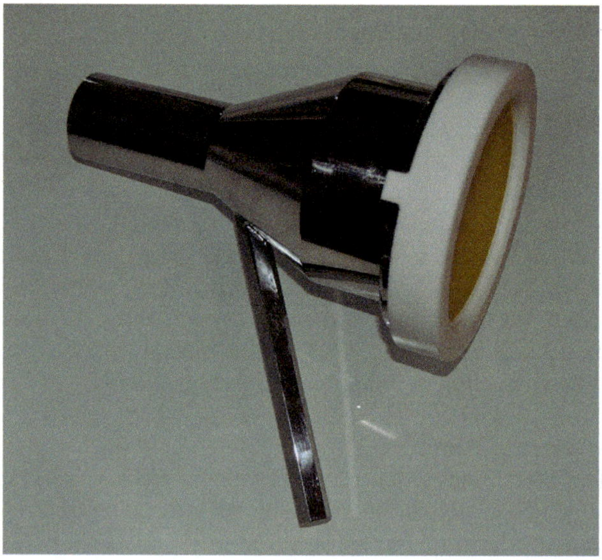

Fig. 32.3 PAT proctoscope

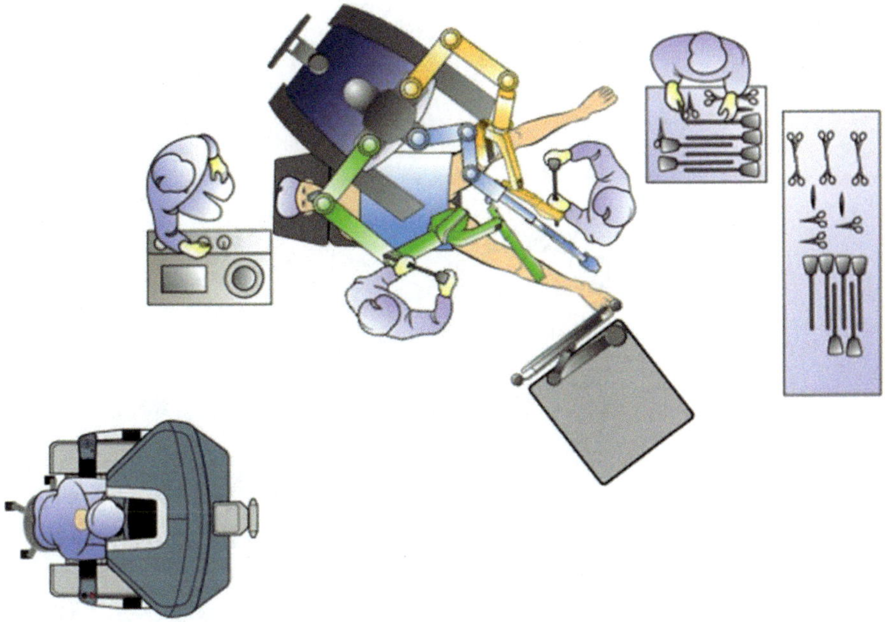

Fig. 32.4 Transanal phase OR set-up

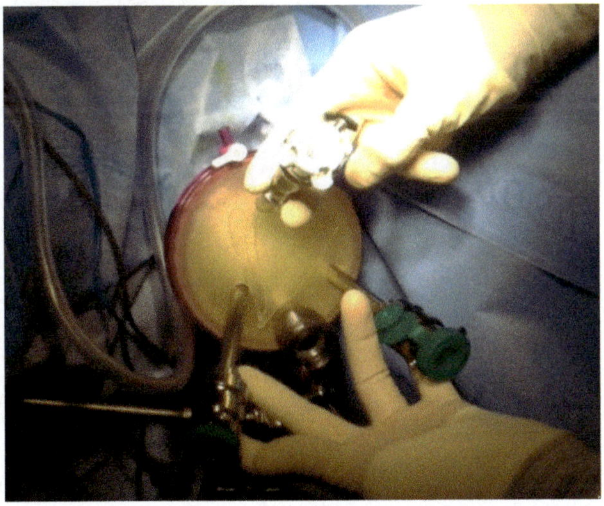

Fig. 32.5 Transanal trocar set-up

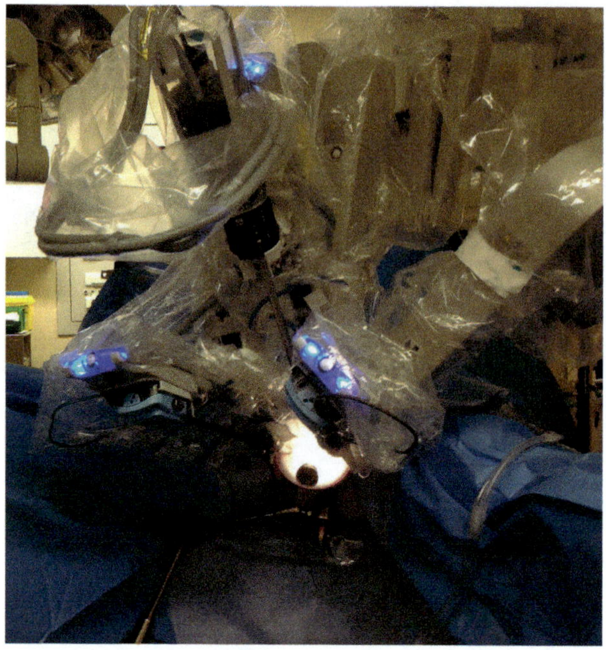

Fig. 32.6 Transanal docking

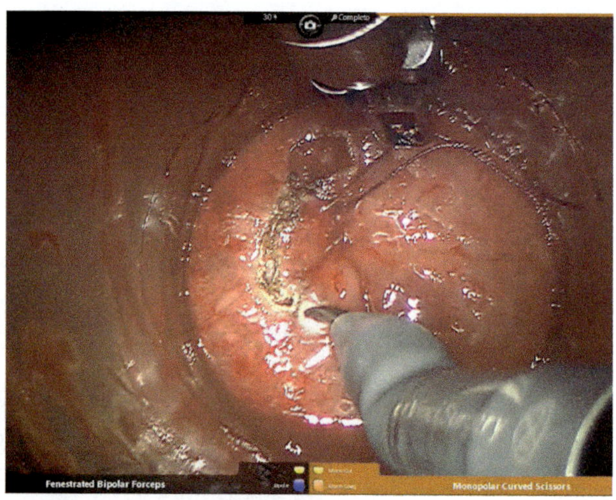

Fig. 32.7 Rectal purse string

placed as described for the low rectal tumours. The rectum is insufflated with CO_2 to a pressure of 8–10 mmHg. The rectal mucosa is then scored circumferentially with monopolar cautery beginning distal to the purse string and followed by full-thickness rectal dissection (Fig. 32.7). After rectal wall division, the pelvic space around the remnant anal canal is insufflated to facilitate pelvic dissection and TME. Anteriorly, the rectum is dissected from the posterior vagina or prostate following Denonvilliers' fascia until the peritoneal reflection/Douglas sack is reached and divided. In the cases in which the tumour is anterior, Denonvilliers' fascia is included in the specimen. Posterior and lateral mesorectal dissection is performed

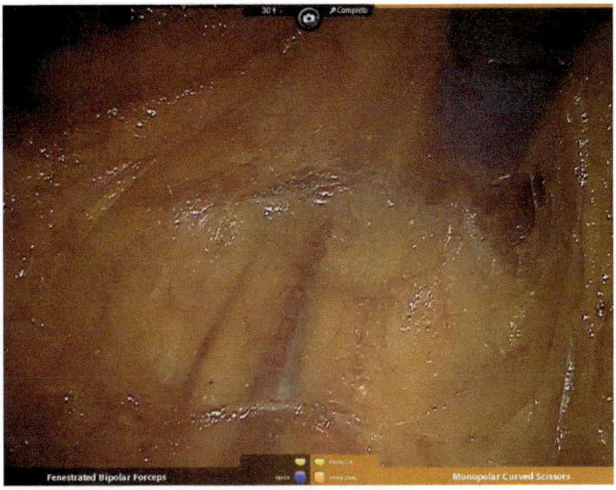

Fig. 32.8 Promontory and plexus

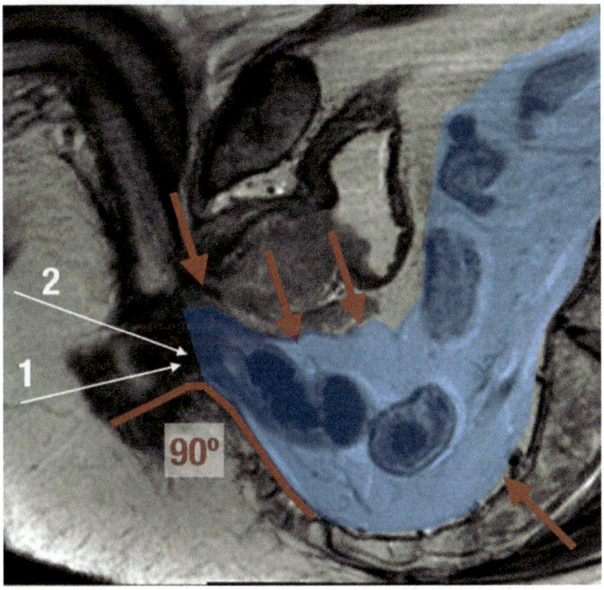

Fig. 32.9 Anatomical landmarks

using the transanal approach with laparoscopic assistance. Once the peritoneal reflection is opened, the abdominal assistant pulls from the 00 braided suture at the end of the rectum to facilitate posterior and lateral dissection.

Special care has to be taken in this approach to posterior dissection (Fig. 32.8). Common mistakes are to divide the mesorectum at the initial dissection in the lower third, as the initial access from below is nearly perpendicular to the mesorectum. It is not difficult to injure the sacral venous plexus at the mid-third of the dissection if your plane is too deep. The magnetic resonance image of each case may be of particular help to avoid these mistakes. To avoid this, we should dock our transanal port in position 1 initially (more parallel to our dissection plane) and then switch it to position 2 in order to continue towards the promontory (Fig. 32.9). Once we reach

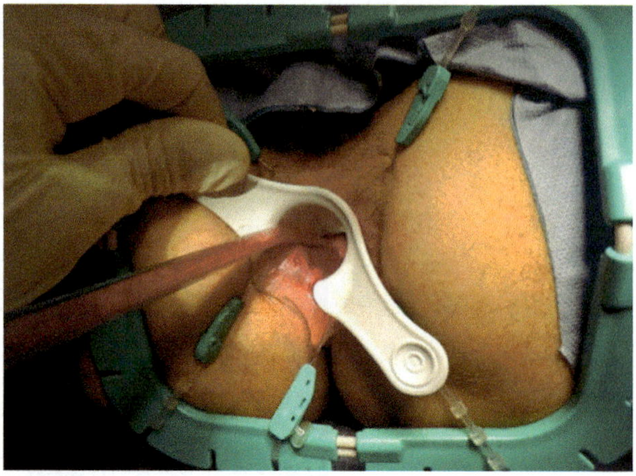

Fig. 32.10 Transanal exposure for second purse string

the upper third in the posterior dissection, we must keep an eye on the hypogastric nerves, as it may be easy to injure them during this step of the procedure.

Following adequate colonic mobilization and rectal dissection, the mesocolon is divided, and the rectum is grasped and exteriorized transanally under laparoscopic visualization through a small Alexis wound retractor (Applied Medical).

32.2.2.2 Anastomosis

Lower Third Tumours

Once the rectum is exteriorized, the colon is divided, and a handsewn end-to-end colo-anal anastomosis is performed with a 0000 monofilament suture. A diverting loop ileostomy was created and a pelvic drain was placed intra-abdominally.

Mid-third Tumours

Once the rectum is exteriorized, the colon is divided and a 00 monofilament purse-string suture is placed at the distal end of the colon. A 29/33 mm anvil is placed in the colon. A second 00 monofilament purse-string suture is performed transanally at the rectal cuff and closed over the anvil tip (Fig. 32.10). A mechanical end-to-end colorectal anastomosis is then performed. A diverting loop ileostomy is created and a pelvic drain is placed intra-abdominally.

References

1. Gomez Fleitas M. From Miles' procedure to robotic transanal proctectomy. Cir Esp. 2014;92(8):507–9. doi:10.1016/j.ciresp.2014.01.001.
2. Heald RJ. A new approach to rectal cancer. Br J Hosp Med. 1979;22(3):277–81.
3. Heald RJ, Husband EM, Ryall RD. The mesorectum in rectal cancer surgery—the clue to pelvic recurrence? Br J Surg. 1982;69(10):613–6.
4. Heald RJ. The 'Holy Plane' of rectal surgery. J R Soc Med. 1988;81(9):503–8.

5. WE M. A method of performing abdomino-perineal excision for carcinoma of the rectum and of the terminal portion of the pelvic colon. Lancet. 1908;2:1812–3.
6. Law WL, Chu KW. Anterior resection for rectal cancer with mesorectal excision: a prospective evaluation of 622 patients. Ann Surg. 2004;240(2):260–8.
7. Bujko K, Rutkowski A, Chang GJ, Michalski W, Chmielik E, Kusnierz J. Is the 1-cm rule of distal bowel resection margin in rectal cancer based on clinical evidence? A systematic review. Ann Surg Oncol. 2012;19(3):801–8. doi:10.1245/s10434-011-2035-2.
8. Schiessel R, Wunderlich M, Waneck R. Results of colo-anal anastomosis in deep-seated tumors of the rectum. Chirurg. 1986;57(12):792–6.
9. Marks G, Mohiuddin M, Borenstein B. Preoperative radiation therapy and sphincter preservation by the combined abdominotranssacral technique for selected rectal cancers. Dis Colon Rectum. 1985;28(8):565–71.
10. Siegel R, Cuesta MA, Targarona E, Bader FG, Morino M, Corcelles R, et al. Laparoscopic extraperitoneal rectal cancer surgery: the clinical practice guidelines of the European Association for Endoscopic Surgery (EAES). Surg Endosc. 2011;25(8):2423–40. doi:10.1007/s00464-011-1805-z.
11. DiMarino Benjamin AJ. Gastrointestinal disease an endoscopic approach. 2nd ed. Thorofare, NJ: Ed Snack Incorporated; 2002.
12. Buess G, Theiss R, Gunther M, Hutterer F, Pichlmaier H. Transanal endoscopic microsurgery. Leber Magen Darm. 1985;15(6):271–9.
13. Jacobs M, Verdeja JC, Goldstein HS. Minimally invasive colon resection (laparoscopic colectomy). Surg Laparosc Endosc. 1991;1(3):144–50.
14. Fleshman J, Sargent DJ, Green E, Anvari M, Stryker SJ, Beart RW Jr, et al. Laparoscopic colectomy for cancer is not inferior to open surgery based on 5-year data from the COST Study Group trial. Ann Surg. 2007;246(4):655–662.; discussion 62–4. doi:10.1097/SLA.0b013e318155a762.
15. Veldkamp R, Kuhry E, Hop WC, Jeekel J, Kazemier G, Bonjer HJ, et al. Laparoscopic surgery versus open surgery for colon cancer: short-term outcomes of a randomised trial. Lancet Oncol. 2005;6(7):477–84. doi:10.1016/S1470-2045(05)70221-7.
16. Jayne DG, Guillou PJ, Thorpe H, Quirke P, Copeland J, Smith AM, et al. Randomized trial of laparoscopic-assisted resection of colorectal carcinoma: 3-year results of the UK MRC CLASICC Trial Group. J Clin Oncol. 2007;25(21):3061–8. doi:10.1200/JCO.2006.09.7758.
17. van der Pas MH, Haglind E, Cuesta MA, Fürst A, Lacy AM, Hop WC, Bonjer HJ, COlorectal cancer Laparoscopic or Open Resection II (COLOR II) Study Group. Laparoscopic versus open surgery for rectal cancer (COLOR II): short-term outcomes of a randomised, phase 3 trial. Lancet Oncol. 2013;14(3):210–8.
18. Delaney CP, Lynch AC, Senagore AJ, Fazio VW. Comparison of robotically performed and traditional laparoscopic colorectal surgery. Dis Colon Rectum. 2003;46(12):1633–9. doi:10.1097/01.DCR.0000098941.42470.D9.
19. Pigazzi A, Ellenhorn JD, Ballantyne GH, Paz IB. Robotic-assisted laparoscopic low anterior resection with total mesorectal excision for rectal cancer. Surg Endosc. 2006;20(10):1521–5. doi:10.1007/s00464-005-0855-5.
20. Luca F, Valvo M, Ghezzi TL, Zuccaro M, Cenciarelli S, Trovato C, et al. Impact of robotic surgery on sexual and urinary functions after fully robotic nerve-sparing total mesorectal excision for rectal cancer. Ann Surg. 2013;257(4):672–8. doi:10.1097/SLA.0b013e318269d03b.
21. Jensen CC, Prasad LM, Abcarian H. Cost-effectiveness of laparoscopic vs. open resection for colon and rectal cancer. Dis Colon Rectum. 2012;55(10):1017–23. doi:10.1097/DCR.0b013e3182656898.
22. Whiteford MH, Denk PM, Swanstrom LL. Feasibility of radical sigmoid colectomy performed as natural orifice translumenal endoscopic surgery (NOTES) using transanal endoscopic microsurgery. Surg Endosc. 2007;21(10):1870–4. doi:10.1007/s00464-007-9552-x.
23. Sylla P, Sohn DK, Cizginer S, Konuk Y, Turner BG, Gee DW, et al. Survival study of natural orifice translumenal endoscopic surgery for rectosigmoid resection using transanal endo-

scopic microsurgery with or without transgastric endoscopic assistance in a swine model. Surg Endosc. 2010;24(8):2022–30. doi:10.1007/s00464-010-0898-0.

24. Trunzo JA, Delaney CP. Natural orifice proctectomy using a transanal endoscopic microsurgical technique in a porcine model. Surg Innov. 2010;17(1):48–52. doi:10.1177/1553350609359516.
25. Leroy J, Cahill RA, Perretta S, Forgione A, Dallemagne B, Marescaux J. Natural orifice translumenal endoscopic surgery (NOTES) applied totally to sigmoidectomy: an original technique with survival in a porcine model. Surg Endosc. 2009;23(1):24–30. doi:10.1007/s00464-008-0102-y.
26. Leroy J, Barry BD, Melani A, Mutter D, Marescaux J. No-scar transanal total mesorectal excision: the last step to pure NOTES for colorectal surgery. JAMA Surg. 2013;148(3):226–30. discussion 31
27. Telem DA, Han KS, Kim MC, Ajari I, Sohn DK, Woods K, et al. Transanal rectosigmoid resection via natural orifice translumenal endoscopic surgery (NOTES) with total mesorectal excision in a large human cadaver series. Surg Endosc. 2013;27(1):74–80. doi:10.1007/s00464-012-2409-y.
28. Sylla P, Rattner DW, Delgado S, Lacy AM. NOTES transanal rectal cancer resection using transanal endoscopic microsurgery and laparoscopic assistance. Surg Endosc. 2010;24(5):1205–10. doi:10.1007/s00464-010-0965-6.
29. Tuech JJ, Bridoux V, Kianifard B, Schwarz L, Tsilividis B, Huet E, et al. Natural orifice total mesorectal excision using transanal port and laparoscopic assistance. Eur J Surg Oncol. 2011;37(4):334–5. doi:10.1016/j.ejso.2010.12.016.
30. Zorron R, Phillips HN, Coelho D, Flach L, Lemos FB, Vassallo RC. Perirectal NOTES access: "down-to-up" total mesorectal excision for rectal cancer. Surg Innov. 2012;19(1):11–9. doi:10.1177/1553350611409956.
31. Dumont F, Goere D, Honore C, Elias D. Transanal endoscopic total mesorectal excision combined with single-port laparoscopy. Dis Colon Rectum. 2012;55(9):996–1001. doi:10.1097/DCR.0b013e318260d3a0.
32. de Lacy AM, Rattner DW, Adelsdorfer C, Tasende MM, Fernandez M, Delgado S, et al. Transanal natural orifice transluminal endoscopic surgery (NOTES) rectal resection: "down-to-up" total mesorectal excision (TME)—short-term outcomes in the first 20 cases. Surg Endosc. 2013;27(9):3165–72. doi:10.1007/s00464-013-2872-0.
33. Tuech JJ, Karoui M, Lelong B, De Chaisemartin C, Bridoux V, Manceau G, et al. A step toward NOTES total mesorectal excision for rectal cancer: endoscopic transanal proctectomy. Ann Surg. 2015;261(2):228–33. doi:10.1097/SLA.0000000000000994.
34. Fernandez-Hevia M, Delgado S, Castells A, Tasende M, Momblan D, Diaz del Gobbo G, et al. Transanal total mesorectal excision in rectal cancer: short-term outcomes in comparison with laparoscopic surgery. Ann Surg. 2015;261(2):221–7. doi:10.1097/SLA.0000000000000865.
35. Atallah S, Nassif G, Polavarapu H, deBeche-Adams T, Ouyang J, Albert M, et al. Robotic-assisted transanal surgery for total mesorectal excision (RATS-TME): a description of a novel surgical approach with video demonstration. Tech Coloproctol. 2013;17(4):441–7. doi:10.1007/s10151-013-1039-2.
36. Gomez Ruiz M, Martin Parra I, Calleja Iglesias A, Stein H, Sprinkle S, Manuel Palazuelos C, et al. Preclinical cadaveric study of transanal robotic proctectomy with total mesorectal excision combined with laparoscopic assistance. Int J Med Robot. 2015;11(2):188–93. doi:10.1002/rcs.1581.
37. Gomez Ruiz M, Palazuelos CM, Martin Parra JI, Alonso Martin J, Cagigas Fernandez C, del Castillo Diego J, et al. New technique of transanal proctectomy with completely robotic total mesorrectal excision for rectal cancer. Cir Esp. 2014;92(5):356–61. doi:10.1016/j.ciresp.2013.12.007.
38. Verheijen PM, Consten EC, Broeders IA. Robotic transanal total mesorectal excision for rectal cancer: experience with a first case. Int J Med Robot. 2014;10(4):423–6. doi:10.1002/rcs.1594.
39. Huscher CG, Bretagnol F, Ponzano C. Robotic-assisted transanal total mesorectal excision: the key against the Achilles' heel of rectal cancer? Ann Surg. 2015;261(5):e120–1. doi:10.1097/SLA.0000000000001089.

40. Atallah S, Martin-Perez B, Pinan J, Quinteros F, Schoonyoung H, Albert M, et al. Robotic transanal total mesorectal excision: a pilot study. Tech Coloproctol. 2014;18(11):1047–53. doi:10.1007/s10151-014-1181-5.
41. Gomez Ruiz M, Parra IM, Palazuelos CM, Martin JA, Fernandez CC, Diego JC, et al. Robotic-assisted laparoscopic transanal total mesorectal excision for rectal cancer: a prospective pilot study. Dis Colon Rectum. 2015;58(1):145–53. doi:10.1097/DCR.0000000000000265.
42. Wexner SD, Berho M. Transanal total mesorectal excision of rectal carcinoma: evidence to learn and adopt the technique. Ann Surg. 2015;261(2):234–6. doi:10.1097/SLA.0000000000000886.
43. Sylla P. Robotically assisted transanal total mesorectal excision: an exciting new trend in rectal cancer surgery. Ann Surg. 2015;261(5):e122. doi:10.1097/SLA.0000000000001090.

Printed in the United States of America